Neuroengineering

Neuroengineering

Edited by Evelyn Page

hayle
medical

New York

Hayle Medical,
750 Third Avenue, 9th Floor,
New York, NY 10017, USA

Visit us on the World Wide Web at:
www.haylemedical.com

ISBN: 978-1-63241-895-1

Cataloging-in-Publication Data

Neuroengineering / edited by Evelyn Page.
   p. cm.
Includes bibliographical references and index.
ISBN 978-1-63241-895-1
1. Biomedical engineering. 2. Neural networks (Neurobiology). 3. Neurology. I. Page, Evelyn.
R856 .N49 2020
610.28--dc23

Table of Contents

Preface

I am honored to present to you this unique book which encompasses the most up-to-date data in the field. I was extremely pleased to get this opportunity of editing the work of experts from across the globe. I have also written papers in this field and researched the various aspects revolving around the progress of the discipline. I have tried to unify my knowledge along with that of stalwarts from every corner of the world, to produce a text which not only benefits the readers but also facilitates the growth of the field.

Neuroengineering is a field of science which studies the properties and functions of neural systems, with the objective of enhancing, repairing or replacing neural function. This field builds on the foundations of experimental and computational neuroscience, electrical engineering, clinical neurology and signal processing of living neural tissue. It also integrates robotics, neural tissue engineering, nanotechnology, etc. By using the fundamentals of neural networks, neural relations and nervous system functions, devices that can control and interpret signals and produce meaningful responses can be designed. The research in neural engineering is driven by the use of techniques that study how the nervous system functions or malfunctions. Neuroimaging techniques such as MRI, fMRI, PET and CAT scans, neural networks that model neural systems, neural prostheses that replace or supplement impaired nervous functions, etc. are some of the applications of neuroengineering. Research in this domain is focused on the rehabilitation of brain malfunction or brain damage arising from spinal cord injury, peripheral nerve injury, etc. There has also been a concerted effort to develop scaffolds for the regrowth of the spinal cord for management of neurological problems. This book discusses the fundamentals as well as modern approaches of this field. It elucidates the concepts and innovative models of neuroengineering around prospective developments with respect to rehabilitation. This book, with its detailed analyses and data, will prove immensely beneficial to professionals and students involved in this area at various levels.

Finally, I would like to thank all the contributing authors for their valuable time and contributions. This book would not have been possible without their efforts. I would also like to thank my friends and family for their constant support.

Editor

Biomechanics and energetics of walking in powered ankle exoskeletons using myoelectric control versus mechanically intrinsic control

Jeffrey R. Koller[1]* (iD), C. David Remy[1] and Daniel P. Ferris[2,3]

Abstract

Background: Controllers for assistive robotic devices can be divided into two main categories: controllers using neural signals and controllers using mechanically intrinsic signals. Both approaches are prevalent in research devices, but a direct comparison between the two could provide insight into their relative advantages and disadvantages. We studied subjects walking with robotic ankle exoskeletons using two different control modes: dynamic gain proportional myoelectric control based on soleus muscle activity (neural signal), and timing-based mechanically intrinsic control based on gait events (mechanically intrinsic signal). We hypothesized that subjects would have different measures of metabolic work rate between the two controllers as we predicted subjects would use each controller in a unique manner due to one being dependent on muscle recruitment and the other not.

Methods: The two controllers had the same average actuation signal as we used the control signals from walking with the myoelectric controller to shape the mechanically intrinsic control signal. The difference being the myoelectric controller allowed step-to-step variation in the actuation signals controlled by the user's soleus muscle recruitment while the timing-based controller had the same actuation signal with each step regardless of muscle recruitment.

Results: We observed no statistically significant difference in metabolic work rate between the two controllers. Subjects walked with 11% less soleus activity during mid and late stance and significantly less peak soleus recruitment when using the timing-based controller than when using the myoelectric controller. While walking with the myoelectric controller, subjects walked with significantly higher average positive and negative total ankle power compared to walking with the timing-based controller.

Conclusions: We interpret the reduced ankle power and muscle activity with the timing-based controller relative to the myoelectric controller to result from greater slacking effects. Subjects were able to be less engaged on a muscle level when using a controller driven by mechanically intrinsic signals than when using a controller driven by neural signals, but this had no affect on their metabolic work rate. These results suggest that the type of controller (neural vs. mechanical) is likely to affect how individuals use robotic exoskeletons for therapeutic rehabilitation or human performance augmentation.

Keywords: Exoskeleton Control; Gait; Kinematics; Power; Electromyography

*Correspondence: jrkoller@umich.edu
[1]Department of Mechanical Engineering, University of Michigan, 2350 Hayward, 48109 Ann Arbor, MI, USA
Full list of author information is available at the end of the article

Background

When it comes to designing the control of lower extremity assistive robotic devices, such as exoskeletons or prostheses, there are a wide variety of control strategies to choose from. Ideally, with the correct control architecture and proper tuning, these devices can work in parallel with the user to aid in their locomotion [1–5]. There have been many different control strategies explored in research, but there is a lack of knowledge in knowing what type of control to use for certain applications and why.

Lower extremity robotic devices have traditionally been separated into two main approaches for device control. The device assistance can either be driven by *neural signals* or *mechanically intrinsic signals*. Control driven by neural signals relies on the already existing control architecture of the human body. By tapping into physiological electrical signals, such as brain activity or muscle activity, these controllers can decode human intention and actuate the device accordingly [6–8]. Control driven by mechanically intrinsic signals relies on measures that are intrinsic to the device itself, such as detected gait events, joint angles, or forces [9–12]. In doing so, these devices are trying to infer human intention from secondary information to drive actuation. For example, a joint angle may be used as a phasing variable for the onset of a predefined actuation signal [13].

Each of these control approaches has its own advantages and disadvantages. For example, control driven by neural signals is often argued to have better human-device synchronization over control driven by mechanically intrinsic signals [14]. Neural signals can be measured before force generation at the muscle has actually occurred due to the electromechanical delay of the body [15]. Therefore, there is a buffer of time between sensing of a neural signal and delivering actuation that is synchronous with the user's movement. In contrast, mechanically intrinsic signals can only be sensed after movement has already occurred. This creates an inherent lag behind the user when using control driven by mechanically intrinsic signals, yet if designed properly this lag may be indistinguishable by the user [16, 17]. Another advantage for control driven by neural signals is that it can allow for direct control by the user. With proportionality in the control scheme, users can directly control the timing and amplitude of actuation at any time instance using the same neurological control they would adjust their own muscle contraction timing and amplitude. This proportionality can lead to a more natural means of control and adaptation compared to a controller driven by mechanically intrinsic signals [18]. One big advantage of using mechanically intrinsic signals to drive control is the reduced complexity over neural signals. Sensors used to measure mechanically intrinsic signals can be self-contained in the device and produce consistent and repeatable measurements. With neural signals,

the electrodes used for electroencephalography (EEG) or electromyography (EMG) can have large variability depending upon placement and skin conditions. With relatively high noise content, neural signals require extensive decoding or filtering before they can be used in real time.

Despite the prevalence of these two types of controller designs, to date, there does not exist any systematic and fair comparison of how they differently affect the biomechanics and energetics of individual users. In the work presented here, we designed an experiment to make a close comparison between a controller driven by neural signals (a proportional myoelectric controller based on soleus muscle recruitment) and a controller driven by mechanically intrinsic signals (a timing-based mechanically intrinsic controller based on gait events). We tested both controllers with healthy subjects wearing bilateral ankle exoskeletons and aimed to better understand users' biomechanical and energetic responses to each during steady-state treadmill walking (Fig. 1). We designed these two controllers to have the *same average* actuation signal such that the main difference between them was the way in which the actuation was driven. To ensure the same average actuation signal, we created the actuation profile for the timing-based controller directly from the average of control signals seen during use with the proportional myoelectric controller. In previous work, we have mathematically derived the inherent relationship between muscle activation and device output when using a proportional myoelectric controller [19]. The timing-based controller we are showing here does not have such dependency so the actuation signal was consistently the same regardless of the user's soleus muscle recruitment. Our primary hypothesis was that the human nervous system would identify this key difference between controllers and therefore use each in a distinct way, thus resulting in a difference in metabolic work rate between the two controllers. We have investigated where some of these differences in use may be by analyzing subject's muscle recruitment, joint kinematics, and joint dynamics.

Methods

Subjects

In this study we tested eight healthy subjects with no prior experience walking in powered exoskeletons (male, 21 ± 1 years, 74.0 ± 2.7 kg, 180.0 ± 2.8 cm; mean $\pm$ standard error of the mean). We pre-screened all participants for exoskeleton hardware fit prior to testing. All subjects gave informed written consent to participate in the study in accordance to the University of Michigan Medical School's Institutional Review Board.

Exoskeleton hardware

The bilateral ankle exoskeletons that we used in this study were similar in design to our previous work [8, 20–22];

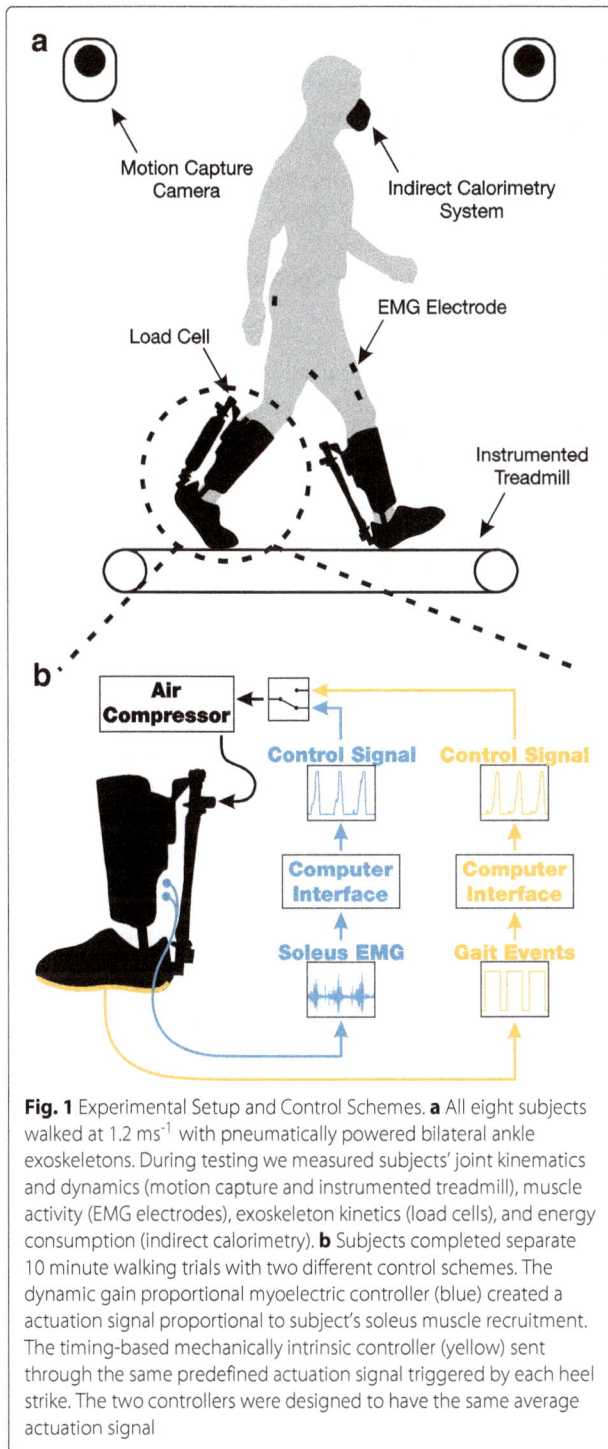

Fig. 1 Experimental Setup and Control Schemes. **a** All eight subjects walked at 1.2 ms⁻¹ with pneumatically powered bilateral ankle exoskeletons. During testing we measured subjects' joint kinematics and dynamics (motion capture and instrumented treadmill), muscle activity (EMG electrodes), exoskeleton kinetics (load cells), and energy consumption (indirect calorimetry). **b** Subjects completed separate 10 minute walking trials with two different control schemes. The dynamic gain proportional myoelectric controller (blue) created a actuation signal proportional to subject's soleus muscle recruitment. The timing-based mechanically intrinsic controller (yellow) sent through the same predefined actuation signal triggered by each heel strike. The two controllers were designed to have the same average actuation signal

the exoskeleton's motion to plantar flexion and dorsiflexion. The shank component was made from stainless steel rods and plastic cuffs. We used ratchet straps on the cuffs to fit the shank to different subject sizes. The shoe component was a standard orthotic shoe that we outfitted with metal attachments for actuation and joint coupling. The exoskeleton could accommodate subjects that wore between a 9 and 11 U.S. men's shoe size.

We actuated the exoskeletons using custom built artificial pneumatic muscles attached posteriorly. These actuation units only provided plantar flexion assistance to the user [20]. We attached a load cell in series (Omega Engineering, Stamford, Connecticut) with the actuator to measure actuation kinetics. The shoe, shank, actuator, and load cell combined to a total mass of 2.08 kg (approximately 0.81 kg at the foot and 1.27 kg at the shank).

Exoskeleton control

In this study we used two different controllers, a dynamic gain proportional myoelectric controller and a timing-based mechanically intrinsic controller, on the same exoskeleton hardware. We built both of these controllers in Simulink (The MathWorks, Inc., Natick, MA) and compiled them to run on a real-time control board (dSPACE, Inc., Northville, MI).

Dynamic gain proportional myoelectric control

The proportional myoelectric controller was driven by user's soleus EMG activity. We measured subjects' soleus activity in real time using EMG surface electrodes (sample rate: 1000 Hz; Biometrics, Ladysmith, VA). The designed controller then processed the recorded signal into its linear envelope by high-pass filtering (2nd order Butterworth, cutoff frequency 80 Hz), full-wave rectifying, and then low-pass filtering (2nd order Butterworth, cutoff frequency 4 Hz) the raw signal.

The controller multiplied the calculated linear envelope by a gain to linearly map the small voltage of the processed EMG signal into a larger control voltage that was sent to the pneumatic pressure control valves (MAC Valves, Wixom, MI). We applied a threshold to this control signal such that the commanded pneumatic pressure needed to be greater than 20 pounds per square inch (p.s.i) in order to actuate as the pneumatic muscles were pretensioned with this pressure to allow for a faster response time. The maximum output pressure of our pressure source was 90 p.s.i. and control signals were saturated beyond this point. The controller was designed to continuously tune the linear mapping gain on a subject-specific basis using a dynamically adaptive algorithm as described in [19]. This algorithm tuned the gain such that the average peak EMG signal over the previous 50 strides mapped to a desired maximum control signal voltage. We chose

however, we designed these exoskeletons to be more adjustable and versatile to fit a number of subject sizes. These were the same exoskeletons as presented in [19].

The exoskeletons consisted of an adjustable shank component attached to a shoe component by a single degree of freedom rotational joint. The rotational joint constrained a desired maximum control voltage that resulted in the peak of the average control signals to be the maximum output pressure of the valves (90 p.s.i.). This created a controller that, on average, supplied maximal peak actuation to the user at the same moment when they reached their maximal peak soleus activity for that given stride. In this control scheme, the user could adapt their own muscle activity to whatever level they felt comfortable with, while still receiving maximal peak power output from the device.

Timing-based mechanically intrinsic control

The timing-based mechanically intrinsic controller was driven by detected heel strikes as sensed by an instrumented treadmill (Bertec Corporation, Columbus, OH). We designed this controller to have the same average actuation signal as that of the proportional myoelectric controller (Fig. 2). To generate the actuation profile for this timing-based controller, we first normalized the actuation signals from the final 100 strides of a subject's walking bout using the proportional myoelectric controller by their percent gait cycle (heel strike to heel strike). We then averaged these 100 normalized actuation signals. We calculated the root mean squared error (RMSE) for each of the 100 individual stride's actuation signal compared to this average and then discarded the 20 strides with the largest RMSE values to safely remove any outliers. We then averaged the remaining 80 strides' actuation signals to generate the actuation profile for the timing-based mechanically intrinsic controller. This whole process was performed separately for each individual subject and leg.

During walking, the timing-based controller would assist with plantar flexion upon each detected heel strike. This process was equivalent to pressing a "play" button on the predefined actuation signal with each heel strike. If a stride was shorter than the averaged control signal, the signal would start over immediately. If a stride was longer than the averaged control signal, the actuators remained at a pressure that resulted in zero force generation until the next detected heel strike occurred.

Testing protocol

We trained all participating subjects in this study to walk with the powered ankle exoskeletons prior to the data collection presented here. All subjects had no experience with walking in a powered assistive device prior to this training. In recruiting a naive subject pool, we have ensured that all subjects were given the same amount of time to adapt and learn to walk in the exoskeletons. The training consisted of three separate days of walking with the exoskeletons using the dynamic gain proportional myoelectric controller. During these training sessions, subjects walked continuously on a treadmill at a fixed speed in the exoskeletons for 50 minutes, the middle 30 of which were powered. A more detailed description of these sessions and subjects' adaptations is described in [19].

After completing the three training sessions, we tested subjects on a separate fourth day to collect the data presented here. During this final testing session, subjects participated in four walking bouts that were each 10 minutes long. Subjects were given a seated rest period

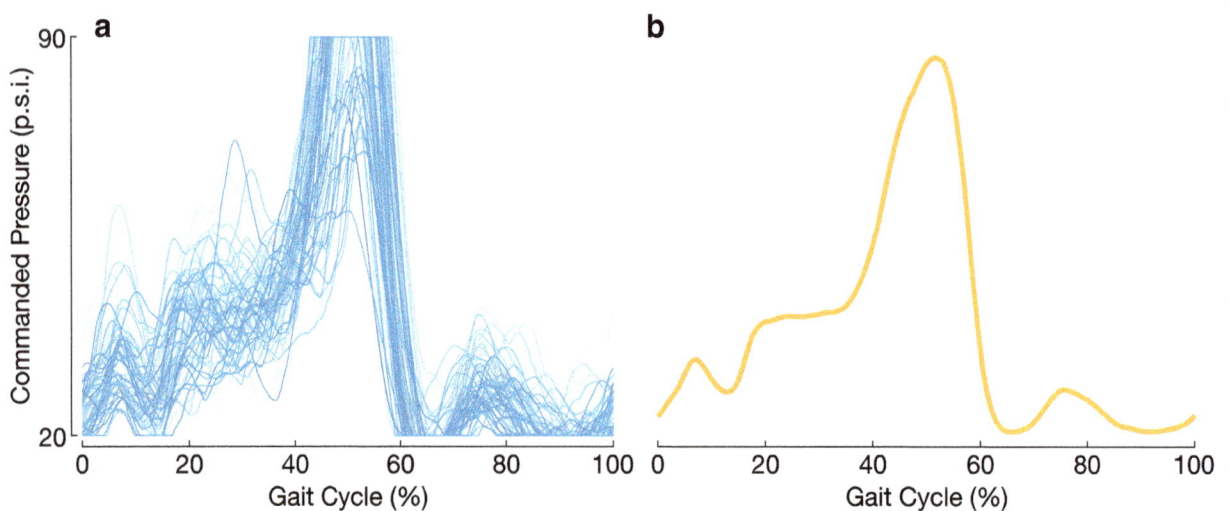

Fig. 2 Creating the Timing-Based Control Signal for a Representative Subject. **a** The actuation signals from 80 of the final 100 strides of a subject's walking bout with the dynamic gain proportional myoelectric controller were considered in creating the actuation signal for the timing-based controller. Those 80 strides are shown here for a single representative subject and from a single leg. The darker the color of the actuation signal, the later in the walking bout it occurred. **b** The actuation signal for the timing-based mechanically intrinsic controller was generated from the average of the 80 strides considered from the walking bout with the myoelectric controller

of 5-10 minutes between bouts. First, subjects walked in the exoskeletons without any actuation. We will refer to this bout as the *unpowered* condition. Subjects then walked using the dynamic gain proportional myoelectric controller in order to re-familiarize themselves with the devices and to generate the data necessary to build the control signals for the timing-based mechanically intrinsic controller. This walking bout served purely as a warm up for subjects and a calibration for the timing-based controller. As such, no results from this bout are presented here. After the warm up session, subjects walked using the timing-based mechanically intrinsic controller and then walked using the dynamic gain proportional myoelectric controller. We will refer to these bouts as the *timing-based* and the *proportional myoelectric* controller conditions, respectively. All walking bouts took place at 1.2 m/s on an instrumented treadmill. We considered the final three minutes of each walking bout for respiratory analysis and the final 25 strides of each walking bout for all gait analyses. We normalized all stride-related data from heel-strike (0% gait cycle) to heel-strike (100% gait cycle) of the same leg.

Metabolic cost
We measured subjects' O_2 and CO_2 flow rates during walking using a portable open-circuit indirect calorimetry system (CareFusion Oxycon Mobile, Hoechberg, Germany). We converted these measurements to metabolic power using formulas from Brockway [23]. We recorded a three minute standing trial from each subject at the beginning of the testing session and averaged it to get subjects' standing metabolic work rate. This calculated standing metabolic work rate was then subtracted from each walking bout to calculate the net metabolic work rate [24]. We analyzed each walking bout by averaging the final three minutes of recorded walking metabolic data, and then normalized these averages by subjects' body mass. During all testing, subjects remained in the aerobic range of exertion as all respiratory exchange ratios were less than one [25].

Electromyography
We measured muscle activity from the soleus, tibialis anterior, medial gastrocnemius, biceps femoris long head, vastus lateralis, rectus femoris, and gluteus maximus using electromyography (EMG). All EMG recordings and analysis, except for the soleus, came solely from the subjects' right leg. Soleus activity was recorded and analyzed from both the left and right legs since soleus activity was used as a control input for the proportional myoelectric controller. We recorded all muscle activity using bipolar surface electrodes (sample rate: 1000 Hz; Biometrics, Ladysmith, VA) with an inter-electrode distance of 2.0 cm and electrode diameter of 1.0 cm. The EMG amplifier had

a bandwidth of 20-460 Hz. We placed all electrodes on subjects' legs in accordance to the procedures of Winter and Yack [26].

During post processing, we high-pass filtered all raw EMG signals with a 35 Hz cut-off frequency (3rd order Butterworth filter, zero-lag) and then full-wave rectified the filtered signals. To compute the signals' linear envelopes, we low-pass filtered the rectified signals with a 10 Hz cut-off frequency (3rd order Butterworth filter, zero lag). Each linear envelope was then parsed by stride (heel-strike to heel-strike), normalized to stride cycle, and averaged. We normalized each muscle's linear envelope amplitude by its corresponding average peak voltage from the unpowered walking bout on a subject-specific basis [26]. In addition to the linear envelopes, we calculated the root mean square (r.m.s.) stride average for the rectified EMG signals. We normalized each muscle's r.m.s. stride average by its corresponding average from the unpowered walking bout on a subject-specific basis. All EMG normalization was done prior to averaging.

Kinematics
All subjects wore a 39 reflective marker set during testing (34 on the pelvis and lower limbs, 4 on the torso, and 1 on the head). We tracked all marker positions using a 10-camera motion capture system (sample rate: 100 Hz; Vicon, Oxford, UK). We calculated joint kinematics from the raw marker data using OpenSim 3.2 [27]. In OpenSim we scaled a generic 23 degree of freedom, 54 actuator model to subject specific marker placements. During processing, we ensured that all subject model scaling and inverse kinematic root mean square values were within the range recommend by OpenSim documentation [28].

We calculated the Pearson product moment correlations between different joint kinematic measurements across different walking bouts. We assessed similarities in joint kinematics by the coefficient of determination (R^2) of these correlations [22]. R^2 values approaching 1 indicate strong similarities in joint trajectories as an R^2 value equal to 1 indicates a perfect match in trajectories. R^2 values close to 0 indicate strong differences in trajectories.

We calculated all gait kinematic measures (step length, step width, step period, double support period) using motion capture data from the left and right calcaneus markers. All gait events were sensed using ground reaction force data from the instrumented treadmill. All raw motion data was first low-pass filtered using a 5 Hz cut-off frequency (3rd order Butterworth filter, zero-lag) to remove any motion artifact. Step length and step width were defined as the fore-aft and lateral distances, respectively, between the calcaneus markers at the time of detected heel strike. Step period was defined as the time between heel strikes of opposite feet, and double support period was defined as the time between heel strike of one foot and the toe off of the other.

Joint mechanics

To perform inverse dynamics, we imported all ground reaction force data into OpenSim 3.2 and used it in conjunction with the calculated joint kinematics. Each subject model's mass was scaled anthropomorphically with the manual addition of the mass at the shank and foot to account for the exoskeletons. We removed as much of the residual forces and moments of the inverse dynamics as possible by iteratively adjusting the model using OpenSim's residual reduction algorithm (RRA). All of the final residuals after using the RRA were within OpenSim's recommended ranges. They are presented in Table 1 [28].

We took the numerical derivative of the joint positions to calculate the joint angular velocities. We filtered these velocities with a 25 Hz cut-off frequency (3rd order Butterworth, zero-lag) to remove any amplified noise that may have resulted from the numerical differentiation. We then multiplied these calculated joint angular velocities by the joint torques resulting from the inverse dynamics to calculate joint power. Exoskeleton power was calculated in a similar fashion, using the calculated ankle angular velocity and the measured actuation torque from the load cell. We subtracted the exoskeleton power from the total ankle power at each time instance to calculate the biological ankle power. Average net joint power was computed by taking the time integral of the power time series data and dividing it by corresponding stride periods [29, 30]. We computed average positive and negative power values in the same way, but by separating out the time integrals to periods of positive and negative power, respectively.

Exoskeleton mechanics

We measured the distance of the exoskeleton joint center to the actuator attachment point as 10.07 cm. We were able to calculate the moment arm of the actuator at each time instance of collection from this distance measure and the calculated ankle kinematics. We filtered all load cell data with a 25 Hz cut-off frequency (3rd order Butterworth filter, zero-lag) and then multiplied it by this calculated moment arm to compute the exoskeleton torques. To calculate exoskeleton power, we multiplied these torques by the ankle angular velocity. We calculated

average exoskeleton power values in the same way as the average joint power values. We calculated exoskeleton mechanics from the left exoskeleton for half of the subjects and the right exoskeleton for the other half due to hardware capabilities during testing.

Statistical analyses

For all statistical comparisons we performed a paired t-test ($\alpha = 0.05$) between walking conditions with the timing-based controller and the proportional myoelectric controller. All tested data was confirmed to be of a normal distribution using a Jarque-Bera test. All reported values and measurements from here forward are presented as the mean $\pm$ the standard error of the mean (s.e.m.).

Results
Metabolic work rate

Walking with the exoskeletons powered, regardless of controller used, resulted in large decreases in metabolic work rate compared with the unpowered condition (Fig. 3). Net metabolic work rate of walking in the exoskeletons unpowered was 3.68 ± 0.23 W kg^{-1} (mean±s.e.m.). Net metabolic work rate of walking with the timing-based mechanically intrinsic controller was 2.95 ± 0.14 W kg^{-1}, or a $19.2 \pm 2.5\%$, decrease compared to the unpowered condition. Net metabolic work rate of walking with the dynamic gain proportional myoelectric controller was 2.95 ± 0.12 W kg^{-1}, or a $19.0 \pm 2.5\%$, decrease compared to the unpowered condition. There was no significant difference in metabolic work rates between the timing-based controller and the proportional myoelectric controller ($P = 0.966$).

Electromyography

The largest change in muscle activity was observed at subjects' soleus muscle (Fig. 4). When walking with the timing-based controller, subjects achieved a soleus r.m.s. EMG reduction of $28.2 \pm 1.0\%$ and a peak linear envelope reduction of $37.5 \pm 3.1\%$ compared to the unpowered condition. When walking with the proportional myoelectric controller, subjects achieved a soleus r.m.s. EMG reduction of $18.6 \pm 6.2\%$ and a peak linear envelope reduction of $28.8 \pm 4.7\%$ compared to the unpowered condition. Subjects soleus r.m.s. EMG was less when using the timing-based controller than when using the proportional

Table 1 Average residual values after final run of the RRA in OpenSim

	F_x (N)	F_y (N)	F_z (N)	M_x (Nm)	M_y (Nm)	M_z (Nm)	pErr$_x$ (cm)	pErr$_y$ (cm)	pErr$_z$ (cm)
Maximum	9.7	9.4	12.5	27.0	43.4	34.7	2.8	1.8	0.6
Root Mean Square	5.3	2.8	7.4	8.6	21.2	9.7	1.9	1.1	0.3

F_x, F_y, and F_z refer to the residual forces at the pelvis, and M_x, M_y, and M_z refer to the residual moments at the pelvis. pErr$_x$, pErr$_y$, and pErr$_z$ refer to the translational position error of the markers

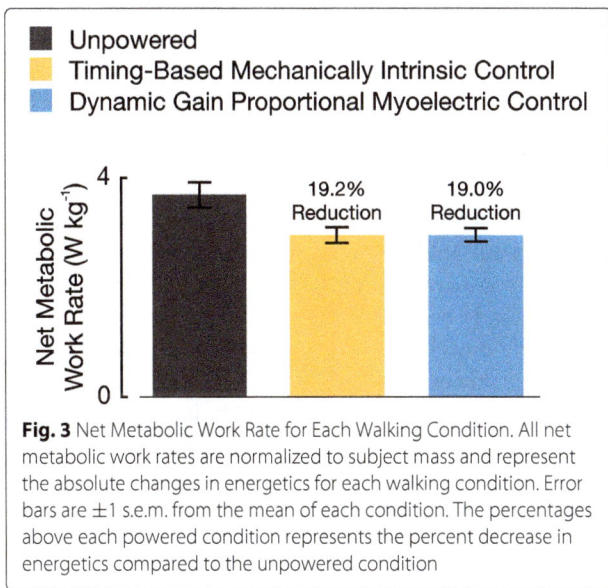

Fig. 3 Net Metabolic Work Rate for Each Walking Condition. All net metabolic work rates are normalized to subject mass and represent the absolute changes in energetics for each walking condition. Error bars are ±1 s.e.m. from the mean of each condition. The percentages above each powered condition represents the percent decrease in energetics compared to the unpowered condition

myoelectric controller, yet it was not a statistically significant difference ($P = 0.132$). There was a distinct qualitative difference in the shape of the two powered walking conditions' resulting linear envelopes (Fig. 4a). Subjects exhibited a significantly lower peak soleus linear envelope value when using the timing-based controller compared to the proportional myoelectric controller ($P = 0.026$). Also, on average subjects showed $11.0 \pm 4.9\%$ less muscle

activity with the timing-based controller compared to the proportional myoelectric controller during the mid and late stance phases of gait (30-50% gait cycle).

Subjects also experienced large reductions in rectus femoris activity during the powered walking conditions compared to the unpowered condition. When walking with the timing-based controller, subjects achieved a rectus femoris r.m.s. EMG reduction of $8.8 \pm 7.5\%$ and a peak linear envelope reduction of $35.2 \pm 20.3\%$ compared to the unpowered condition. When walking with the proportional myoelectric controllers, subjects achieved a rectus femoris r.m.s. EMG reduction of $13.0 \pm 8.9\%$ and a peak linear envelope reduction of $38.6 \pm 15.0\%$ compared to the unpowered condition. There was little to no difference in the resulting average rectus femoris linear envelopes between the two controllers (Fig. 4a). No statistically significant differences were observed between the two powered conditions resulting r.m.s. EMG values at the tibialis anterior, medial gastrocnemius, biceps femoris long head, vastus lateralis, and gluteus maximus (all $P > 0.05$). These additional muscle r.m.s. EMG values and their corresponding statistics are presented in the Additional file 1: Table S1.

Gait kinematics

There were slight differences between walking conditions' mean gait kinematics (Table 2). Subjects exhibited slightly larger mean step lengths and step widths when using the

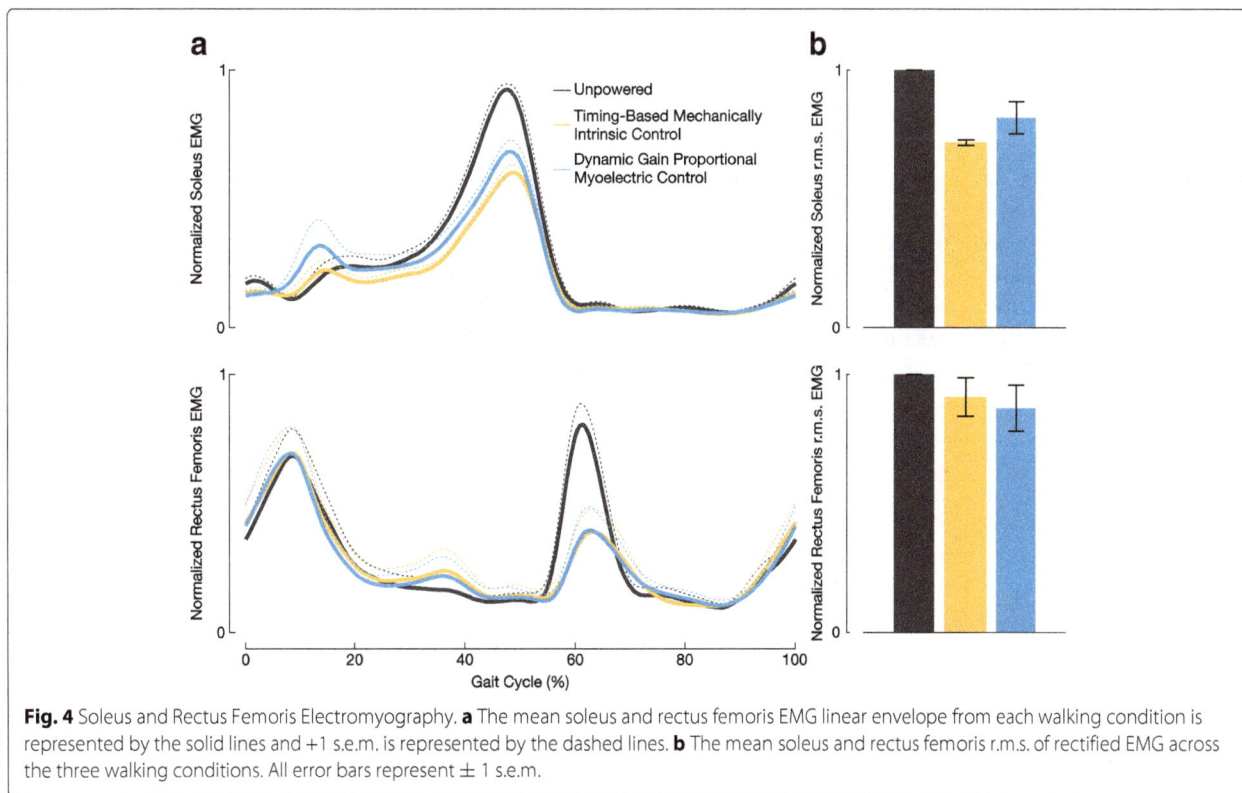

Fig. 4 Soleus and Rectus Femoris Electromyography. **a** The mean soleus and rectus femoris EMG linear envelope from each walking condition is represented by the solid lines and +1 s.e.m. is represented by the dashed lines. **b** The mean soleus and rectus femoris r.m.s. of rectified EMG across the three walking conditions. All error bars represent ± 1 s.e.m.

timing-based controller than when using the proportional myoelectric controller ($P = 0.004$ and $P = 0.030$, respectively). There was no statistically significant differences in gait kinematic variability between the two powered conditions (Table 3).

Joint kinematics

During powered conditions, subjects experienced the largest deviations from unpowered walking kinematics at the ankle. Subjects increased plantar flexion by an average $\sim14°$ during the mid-to-late stance phase of gait when using both the timing-based and the proportional myoelectric controllers compared to the unpowered condition (Fig. 5). A linear regression between ankle kinematics of the timing-based controller and of the unpowered condition resulted in an R^2 value of 0.73 ± 0.05. A linear regression between ankle kinematics of the proportional myoelectric controller and of the unpowered condition resulted in an R^2 value of 0.71 ± 0.08. A linear regression between ankle kinematics of the timing-based controller and the proportional myoelectric controller resulted in an R^2 value of 0.98 ± 0.01.

There were little to no changes in joint kinematics at every other joint between conditions. Linear regressions of knee and hip kinematics between powered and unpowered conditions all resulted in R^2 values greater than 0.98. Linear regressions of knee and hip kinematics between the two controllers all resulted in R^2 values greater than 0.99.

Joint kinetics

Subjects increased their mean total moment at the ankle (biological and exoskeleton) by ~0.14 Nm kg^{-1} during the early-to-mid stance phase (0-30% gait cycle) when comparing either of the powered conditions to the unpowered condition (an increase of $\sim48.9\%$, Fig. 5). The observed increase in total ankle plantar flexion moment during the early to mid stance phase corresponds with a decrease in hip flexion moment. Subjects decreased their mean hip flexion moment ~0.12-0.15 Nm kg^{-1} during this phase of the gait cycle when comparing either of the powered conditions to the

unpowered conditions (a decrease of ~25-31%). Subjects also decreased their mean knee extension moment ~0.08-0.10 Nm kg^{-1} during the mid and late stance phase (30-50% gait cycle) when comparing the powered conditions to the unpowered condition (a decrease of ~31-42%).

Subjects showed large increases in positive and net average total ankle power when the exoskeletons were powered compared to unpowered (Fig. 6). When using the timing-based controller, subjects had an average positive total ankle power 0.13 ± 0.01 W kg^{-1} and an average net total ankle power 0.15 ± 0.01 W kg^{-1} larger than that when walking in the devices unpowered (an increase of $55.2 \pm 4.0\%$ and $213.0 \pm 38.5\%$, respectively). When using the proportional myoelectric controller, subjects had an average positive total ankle power 0.15 ± 0.01 W kg^{-1} and an average net total ankle power 0.16 ± 0.01 W kg^{-1} larger than that when walking in the devices unpowered (an increase of $64.0 \pm 3.8\%$ and $222.9 \pm 42.3\%$, respectively). Subjects showed significantly larger average positive and negative total ankle power when using the proportional myoelectric controller compared to when using the timing-based controller ($P = 0.005$ and $P = 0.001$, respectively). There was no statistically significant difference in average positive, negative, or net exoskeleton power output between the two controllers ($P = 0.124$, $P = 0.313$, and $P = 0.138$, respectively). There was also no statistically significant difference in average positive, negative, or net biological ankle power output between the two controllers ($P = 0.056$, $P = 0.102$, and $P = 0.057$, respectively); however, the difference in average positive and net biological ankle power were near significant. Subjects on average achieved ~0.18 W kg^{-1} greater exoskeleton peak power when using the timing-based controller than when using the proportional myoelectric controller (an increase of $\sim11.1\%$). There was a statistically significant difference between these peak power values ($P = 0.048$). This increase in peak exoskeleton power corresponded with an average decrease in peak biological ankle power of ~0.11 W kg^{-1} when using the timing-based controller compared to the proportional myoelectric controller (a decrease of $\sim8.3\%$).

Table 2 Resulting mean gait kinematics of each walking bout

Walking condition	Step length (Normalized)	Step width (Normalized)	Step period (ms)	Double support period (ms)
Unpowered	0.713 ± 0.010	0.173 ± 0.011	586.3 ± 5.6	161.7 ± 5.0
Timing-Based	0.704 ± 0.007	0.190 ± 0.016	591.6 ± 6.9	167.2 ± 2.8
Proportional Myoelectric	0.692 ± 0.008	0.182 ± 0.014	586.5 ± 6.6	169.0 ± 2.2
P-Value	0.004	0.030	0.095	0.256

All values are reported as mean±s.e.m. across subjects. All distance measurements have been normalized by leg length. $P<0.05$ represents a statistically significant difference between the proportional myoelectric controller and the timing-based controller

Table 3 Resulting gait kinematic variability of each walking bout

Walking condition	Step length (Normalized)	Step width (Normalized)	Step period (ms)	Double support period (ms)
Unpowered	0.021 ± 0.002	0.018 ± 0.002	14.1 ± 1.2	7.5 ± 0.6
Timing-Based	0.023 ± 0.002	0.021 ± 0.002	17.6 ± 1.5	9.2 ± 0.7
Proportional Myoelectric	0.026 ± 0.004	0.021 ± 0.001	17.1 ± 2.2	11.2 ± 1.1
P-Value	0.231	0.970	0.615	0.210

Variability has been defined as the average standard deviation across subjects. All values are reported as mean±s.e.m. across subjects. All distance measurements have been normalized by leg length. $P<0.05$ represents a statistically significant difference between the proportional myoelectric controller and the timing-based controller

Due to large variability in subject data, this observation was not of a statistically significant difference ($P = 0.439$).

Subjects put forth significantly greater positive average knee power when using the proportional myoelectric controller than when using the timing-based controller ($P = 0.003$, Fig. 7). There were no statistically significant differences in negative or net positive power at the knee between the two controllers ($P = 0.851$ and $P = 0.063$, respectively). Subjects showed large differences in average negative and net power at the hip between powered and unpowered conditions. When using the timing-based controller, subjects had an average negative hip power 0.04 ± 0.01 W kg^{-1} and an average net hip power 0.09 ± 0.02 W kg^{-1} larger than that when walking in the devices unpowered (an increase of $52.3 \pm 5.0\%$ and $28.1 \pm 4.1\%$, respectively). When using the proportional myoelectric controller, subjects had an average negative hip power 0.05 ± 0.01 W kg^{-1} and an average net hip power 0.09 ± 0.01 W kg^{-1} larger than that when walking in the devices unpowered (an increase of $66.4 \pm 9.8\%$ and

$28.0 \pm 2.5\%$, respectively). There was no statistically significant difference in average positive, negative, or net hip power between controllers ($P = 0.232$, $P = 0.057$, and $P = 0.934$, respectively).

Discussion

Our primary hypothesis was that metabolic work rate would differ between walking with the timing-based mechanically intrinsic controller and the dynamic gain proportional myoelectric controller. However, we found quite the opposite. Results show that there was no statistically significant difference in metabolic work rate between the two control strategies in this experiment (Fig. 3). The reasoning for why we expected a different metabolic work rate between controllers was that we expected subjects to use each controller in a unique way due to the fact that one control strategy was dependent on muscle recruitment and the other was not. Although we did not observe a difference in metabolic work rate, we did observe differences in other biomechanical measures.

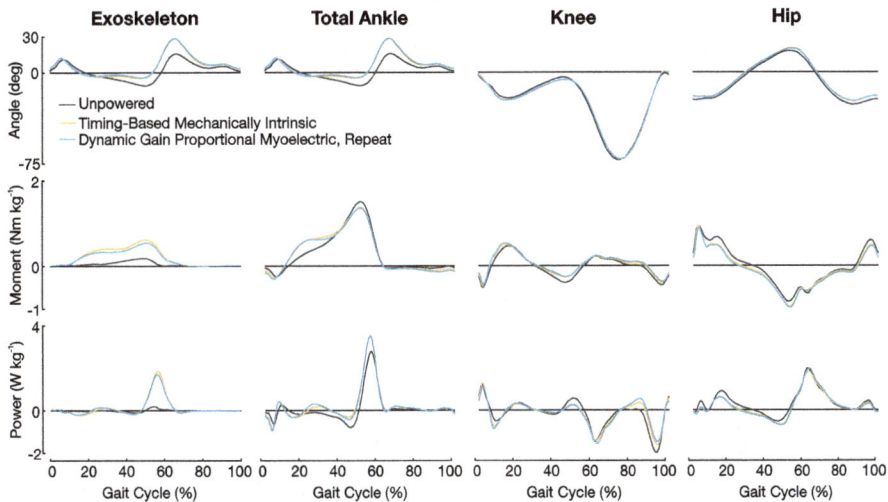

Fig. 5 Joint Kinematics, Dynamics, and Power. The mean joint angles, moments, and powers from the unpowered, timing-based mechanically intrinsic control, and second bout with the dynamic gain proportional myoelectric control conditions. Joint dynamics and power have been normalized by subject mass. In the kinematics and dynamics subplots all positive numbers represent extension while all negative numbers represent flexion

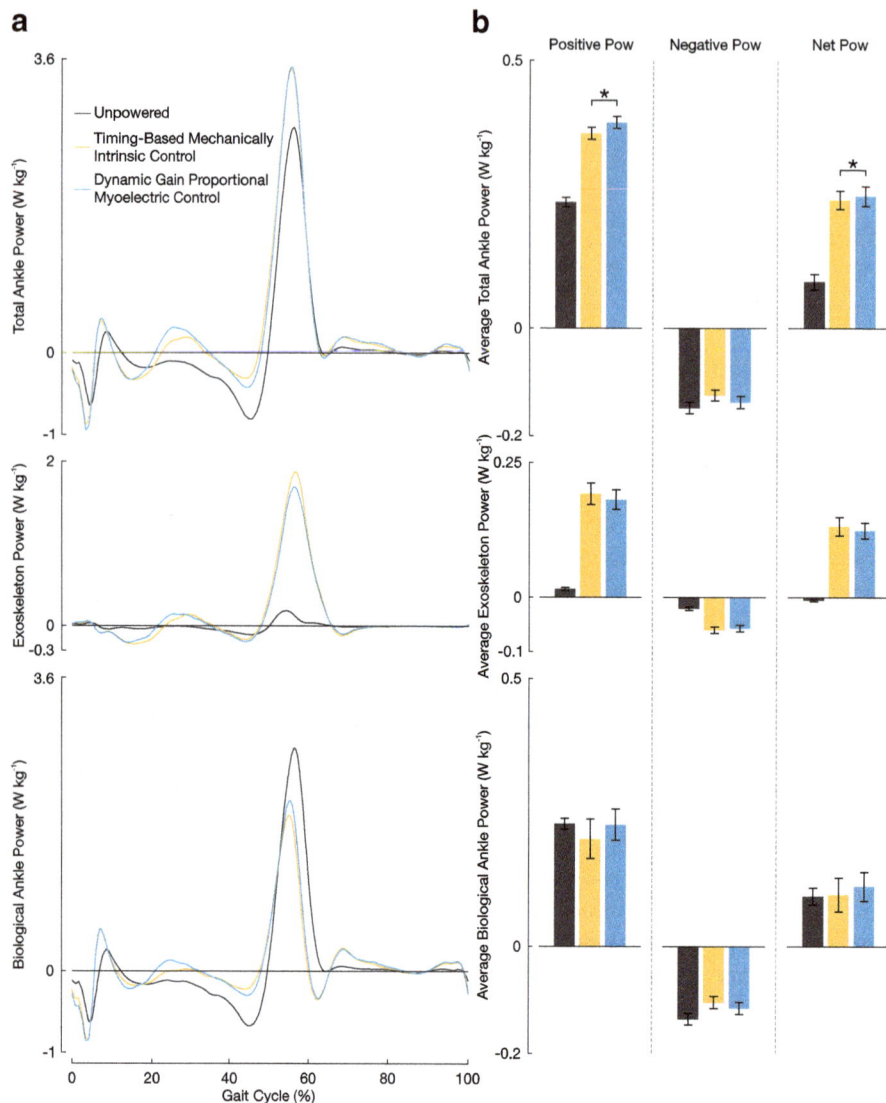

Fig. 6 Ankle Power Contributions. **a** Mean total ankle power, exoskeleton power, and biological ankle power across the three walking conditions. The exoskeleton power was calculated from ankle kinematics and force outputs recorded using the exoskeletons' load cells. The biological power was calculated by subtracting the exoskeleton power from the total ankle power. **b** Average power plots of positive, negative, and net power for total ankle power, exoskeleton power, and biological ankle power. All error bars represent ±1 s.e.m. An asterisk above the plots represents a significant difference between the two powered walking conditions ($P < 0.05$)

Soleus muscle recruitment differed between walking with the proportional myoelectric controller and with the timing-based controller. Although there was not a statistically significant difference in soleus r.m.s. EMG values between the two walking conditions, there was a strong trend in subjects using less soleus muscle recruitment when using the timing-based controller than when using the proportional myoelectric controller. This was made evident by the absolute values of the r.m.s. EMG calculations and the fact that subjects' resulting soleus linear envelopes when using the timing-based controller were 11% less than that of the proportional myoelectric

controller during the mid and late stance phases of gait (Fig. 4a). Additionally, the peak value of subjects' soleus linear envelopes when using the timing-based controller was significantly less than that when using the proportional myoelectric controller. Similar trends were observed in medial gastrocnemius r.m.s. EMG calculations as well (Additional file 1: Table S1). We believe the reason we did not observe differences in metabolic work rate in this study despite this difference in muscle recruitment was that these devices targeted a relatively small muscle group. If repeated with an exoskeleton that targeted larger muscle groups, such as with a hip

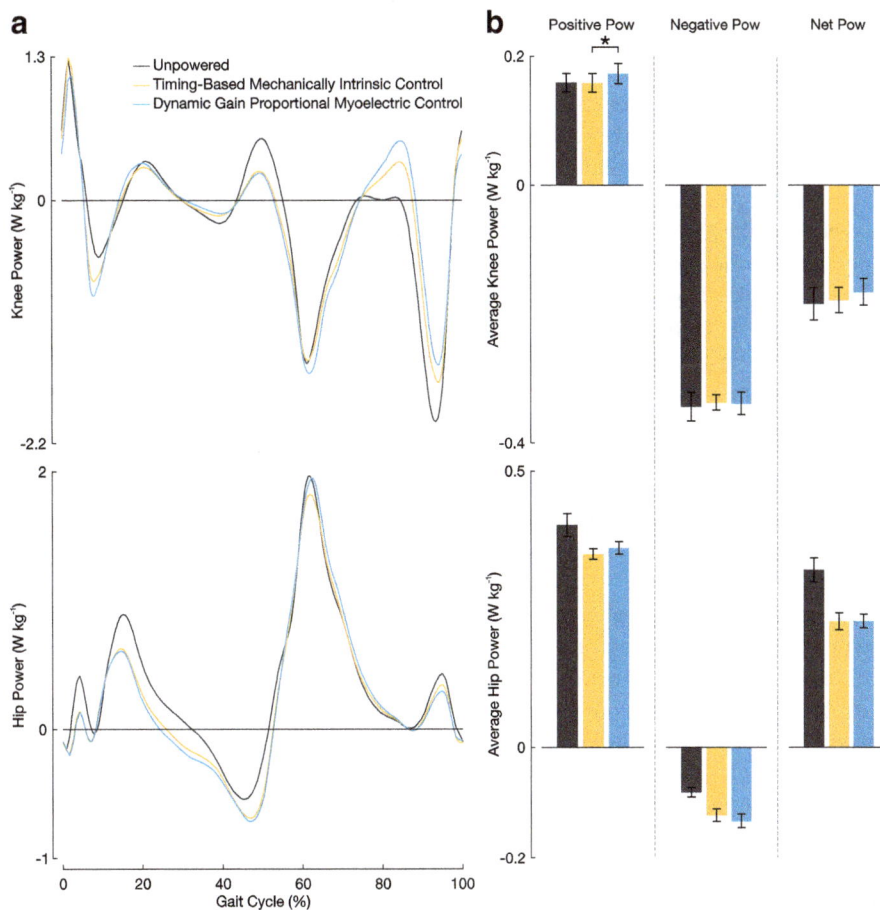

Fig. 7 Knee and Hip Power Contributions. **a** Mean knee power and mean hip power across the three walking conditions. **b** Average power plots of positive, negative, and net power at the knee and hip. All error bars represent ± 1 s.e.m. An asterisk above the plots represents a significant difference between the two powered walking conditions (P < 0.05)

exoskeleton [31–33], it might be expected to see differences in metabolic work rate; however, further research is needed to make this conclusion.

The observed differences in recruitment of plantar flexor muscles had a direct effect on resulting ankle mechanics. We observed that subjects walked with significantly larger average positive and negative total ankle power when using the proportional myoelectric controller than when using the timing-based controller (Fig. 6). This increase in power magnitude at the ankle is due to the very slight differences in total ankle moment of the two controller conditions (Fig. 5). In looking at the breakdown of total ankle power contributions we see that subjects trended toward significantly larger peak exoskeleton power output when using the timing-based controller than the proportional myoelectric controller (an increase of 11.1%) . This corresponded with a trend in decreased peak biological ankle power output (a decrease of 8.3%). Additionally, subjects used less average positive and net biological ankle power when walking with the timing-

based controller than with the proportional myoelectric controller. These differences in average positive and net biological ankle power were near statistical significance (P = 0.056 and P = 0.057, respectively). These ankle power results suggest that when using the timing-based controller subjects were contributing less to locomotion at the biological ankle and are more so 'along for the ride' [34]. This makes sense given that active engagement and involvement at the ankle is not necessarily required when using the timing-based controller. So long as heel strike occurs, subjects will receive actuation. When using the proportional myoelectric controller, active involvement on a muscular level is necessary to directly control the actuation of the device. Additionally, these changes in ankle dynamics seemed to have had an effect on subjects average positive knee power as subjects walked with significantly more positive knee power when using with the proportional myoelectric controller than when using with the timing-based controller.

We attribute these differences in muscle recruitment, and thus the resulting observed differences in ankle power, to the theory of slacking. The idea behind slacking is that the human motor system is always trying to minimize its levels of muscle activation during repetitive tasks where movement error is small, such as walking [34, 35]. One hypothesis for interpreting the differences in soleus muscle recruitment between the two controllers is that when using the proportional myoelectric controller, users can only slack so far before signal quality affects walking stability. This is an inherent technical limitation of using measures of muscle activity to drive a controller. As mentioned prior, neural signals, such as muscle activity, often have large noise content. Therefore as subjects decrease their muscle activity, the signal-to-noise ratio of the measurement decreases making it difficult to separate the signal from the noise. In this specific experiment, the dynamically adjusting gain of the proportional myoelectric controller increases to compensate for decreases in muscle activity. This larger gain will amplify any noise that makes it through the filtering process along with the intended control signal. This amplified noise could then make control of the device difficult and potentially cause for instability with walking. Given this argument, we believe there is a maximum level of slacking that can be obtained with the proportional myoelectric controller presented here. When using the timing-based controller, the actuation is consistently the same for each step regardless of muscle activity. Because of this, users can potentially slack their muscle activity further than with the proportional myoelectric controller without any change to actuation.

Another hypothesis for interpreting the differences in soleus muscle recruitment between the two controllers is that when using the proportional myoelectric controller, users can only slack so far due to the means in which the controller is triggered. No matter what, subjects must use some amount of muscle recruitment to actuate the proportional myoelectric controller. Due to the fact that this controller inherently guarantees synchronous actuation with the user, the user is always moving with the device during actuation. When using the timing-based controller, subjects do not necessarily need to move with the device. They could potentially lean into the actuation and let it propel them forward in a way that is not possible with the proportional myoelectric controller. This could potentially explain the observed increases in peak exoskeleton power and decreases in biological ankle power. Once figuring out this strategy, subjects can exploit it and become disengaged at a muscle level during walking. Thus, subjects are able to slack further when using the timing-based controller.

Equally interesting to the resulting differences in these two control strategies are how in which the two were similar. The results from this study show that regardless of the control strategy being used, the actuation from the exoskeletons resulted in large reductions the user's metabolic work rate compared to walking unpowered in the devices. The absolute value of these reductions is comparable to previous work in the field [1, 3, 4, 19]. Although it is not a novel finding to show that actuation of an exoskeleton can reduce the metabolic work rate compared to unpowered walking, it is a good proof that both control strategies were able to work in parallel with user to offload some of the energetic requirements of walking. Additionally, gait kinematics between the two controllers were relatively unchanged (Tables 2 and 3). We found that all lower extremity joint kinematics were largely unchanged from one controller to the other, as evident that all regressions between the two controllers resulted in R^2 values greater than 0.98 (Fig. 5). We also observed that regardless of the controller being used, subjects adapted to large increases in total ankle powered compared to the unpowered walking condition. This large increase in total ankle power corresponded with large reductions in power at the hip. These reductions in hip power were congruent with reductions in EMG activity at the rectus femoris (Fig. 4b). This trade off in joint power and muscle activity between the ankle and hip is consistent with previous work by our research group and that observed by others with different devices and controllers [4, 19, 36]. We find all of these resulting similarities between the two controllers an interesting finding as they show that if a timing-based controller is designed properly and used under the appropriate walking constraints, the resulting biomechanical and energetic adaptations mimic that of the proportional myoelectric controller. With the correct design, a researcher could potentially use either type of control scheme with an ankle exoskeleton and achieve largely the same results for steady-state walking; the major differences being in the resulting ankle muscle recruitment and ankle mechanics.

It is difficult to pinpoint the reasons behind the biomechanical differences observed between the two controllers, but the fact that they exist lend insight to when one controller may be better suited than another. For example, if a device is targeted toward therapeutic rehabilitation of neurological injuries [37], a controller driven by neural signals may be more beneficial than one driven by mechanically intrinsic signals due to users being more engaged at a muscle level when using a controller driven by neural signals. This suggestion is drawn from the success of gait training with human therapists being more successful than that with robotic devices in patients with chronic stroke [38]. This difference is attributed to patients' active involvement when working with a therapist over a robotic device. As this study has only considered testing with healthy subjects, further research would need to be conducted with a clinical population to draw definitive conclusions on this. Additionally, the results from this study suggest that if a metabolic reduction is of interest, it appears that either type of control strategy could be employed.

We acknowledge that this study is a comparison of a single controller driven by neural signals and a single controller driven by mechanically intrinsic signals. There are an infinite number of possible controllers for each that could be compared; however, we believe this is a strong starting point for future work in better understanding controller design for specific applications. Seeing as each control strategy lends itself to different pros and cons, a hybrid of the two approaches may be advantageous, an area of research many have already begun exploring [39–42]. We also acknowledge that this experiment was performed with a young, able-bodied population walking in a straight line at a constant velocity with a hardware platform that was limited in torque output. Further research would need to be performed to show how these principles hold with different populations, devices, and walking scenarios.

Conclusion

This study aimed to compare the differences between walking in bilateral ankle exoskeletons using a dynamic gain proportional myoelectric controller and using a timing-based mechanically intrinsic controller. We hypothesized that these two controllers would result in different measures of metabolic work rate due to expected differences in biomechanical measures. We observed no differences in metabolic work rate, small changes in joint kinetics at the knee and hip, and virtually no difference on all leg joint kinematics between the two controllers. As such, we can conclude that if designed properly and under the appropriate walking constraints, the timing-based controller can adequately mimic the proportional myoelectric controller. The major differences between these two controllers that we did observe were at the ankle. Subjects showed increased soleus muscle activity when using the proportional myoelectric controller than when using the timing-based controller. This corresponded with significantly larger positive and net total ankle power when using the proportional myoelectric controller than when using the timing-based controller. These findings suggest that a controller driven by neural signals may be better suited for therapeutic rehabilitation applications while either controller is well suited for human augmentation purposes.

Acknowledgements
The authors would like to acknowledge Sandy Mouch and Reilley Jones for their help with data collections and data processing. Additionally, the authors would like to acknowledge and thank Daniel Jacobs for his support with the hardware used in these experiments.

Funding
This work was financially supported by funds from a U.S. Department of Defense Grant (W81XWH-09-2-0142). Additionally, a University of Michigan Rackham Graduate Student Research Grant helped support this study.

Authors' contributions
All authors took part in conceptualizing the study. JK conducted the experiments and analyzed the data while all authors interpreted the results. All authors participated in writing, editing, and approving the final manuscript.

Competing interests
The authors declare that they have no competing interests.

Author details
[1] Department of Mechanical Engineering, University of Michigan, 2350 Hayward, 48109 Ann Arbor, MI, USA. [2] J. Crayton Pruitt Family Department of Biomedical Engineering, University of Florida, 1275 Center Drive, 32611 Gainesville, FL, USA. [3] Department of Mechanical Engineering, University of Florida, 1275 Center Drive, 32611 Gainesville, FL, USA.

References
1. Malcolm P, Derave W, Galle S, De Clercq D. A simple exoskeleton that assists plantarflexion can reduce the metabolic cost of human walking. PloS ONE. 2013;8:56137.
2. Mooney LM, Rouse EJ, Herr HM. Autonomous exoskeleton reduces metabolic cost of human walking during load carriage. J Neuroeng Rehabil. 2014;11:0003–11.
3. Jackson RW, Collins SH. An experimental comparison of the relative benefits of work and torque assistance in ankle exoskeletons. J Appl Physiol. 2015;119(5):541–57.
4. Quinlivan B, Lee S, Malcolm P, Rossi D, Grimmer M, Siviy C, Karavas N, Wagner D, Asbeck A, Galiana I, et al. Assistance magnitude versus metabolic cost reductions for a tethered multiarticular soft exosuit. Sci Robot. 2017;2(2):4416.
5. Zhang J, Fiers P, Witte KA, Jackson RW, Poggensee KL, Atkeson CG, Collins SH. Human-in-the-loop optimization of exoskeleton assistance during walking. Science. 2017;356(6344):1280–4.
6. Kilicarslan A, Prasad S, Grossman RG, Contreras-Vidal JL. High accuracy decoding of user intentions using eeg to control a lower-body exoskeleton. In: 2013 35th Annual International Conference of the IEEE Engineering in Medicine and Biology Society (EMBC). Osaka: IEEE; 2013. p. 5606–9.
7. Hogan N. A review of the methods of processing emg for use as a proportional control signal. Biomed Eng. 1976;11:81–6.
8. Sawicki GS, Ferris DP. Mechanics and energetics of level walking with powered ankle exoskeletons. J Exp Biol. 2008;211:1402–13.
9. Li D, Becker A, Shorter KA, Bretl T, Hsiao-Wecksler E. Estimating system state during human walking with a powered ankle-foot orthosis. Mechatron IEEE/ASME Trans. 2011;16:835–44.
10. Jimenez-Fabian R, Verlinden O. Review of control algorithms for robotic ankle systems in lower-limb orthoses, prostheses, and exoskeletons. Med Eng Phys. 2012;34:397–408.
11. Asbeck AT, De Rossi SM, Holt KG, Walsh CJ. A biologically inspired soft exosuit for walking assistance. Int J Robot Res. 2015;34(6):744–62.
12. Galle S, Malcolm P, Collins SH, De Clercq D. Reducing the metabolic cost

of walking with an ankle exoskeleton: interaction between actuation timing and power. J Neuroeng Rehabil. 2017;14(1):35.

13. Quintero D, Villarreal DJ, Gregg RD. Preliminary experiments with a unified controller for a powered knee-ankle prosthetic leg across walking speeds. In: Intelligent Robots and Systems (IROS), 2016 IEEE/RSJ International Conference On. Daejeon: IEEE; 2016. p. 5427–33.

14. Young AJ, Ferris DF. State of the art and future directions for lower limb robotic exoskeletons. IEEE Transact Neural Syst Rehab Eng. 2017;25.2: 171–82.

15. Cavanagh P, Komi P. Electromechanical delay in human skeletal muscle under concentric and eccentric contractions. Eur J Appl Physiol Occup Physiol. 1979;42(3):159–63.

16. Zhang J, Cheah CC, Collins SH. Experimental comparison of torque control methods on an ankle exoskeleton during human walking. In: Robotics and Automation (ICRA), 2015 IEEE International Conference On. Seattle: IEEE; 2015. p. 5584–9.

17. Ding Y, Galiana I, Siviy C, Panizzolo FA, Walsh C. Imu-based iterative control for hip extension assistance with a soft exosuit. In: Robotics and Automation (ICRA), 2016 IEEE International Conference On. Stockholm: IEEE; 2016. p. 3501–8.

18. Cain SM, Gordon KE, Ferris DP. Locomotor adaptation to a powered ankle-foot orthosis depends on control method. J NeuroEng Rehabil. 2007;4(1):1.

19. Koller JR, Jacobs DA, Ferris DP, Remy CD. Learning to walk with an adaptive gain proportional myoelectric controller for a robotic ankle exoskeleton. J Neuroeng Rehabil. 2015;12(1):97.

20. Ferris DP, Czerniecki JM, Hannaford B. An ankle-foot orthosis powered by artificial pneumatic muscles. J Appl Biomech. 2005;21:189.

21. Ferris DP, Gordon KE, Sawicki GS, Peethambaran A. An improved powered ankle–foot orthosis using proportional myoelectric control. Gait Posture. 2006;23:425–8.

22. Gordon KE, Ferris DP. Learning to walk with a robotic ankle exoskeleton. J Biomech. 2007;40:2636–44.

23. Brockway J. Derivation of formulae used to calculate energy expenditure in man. Hum Nutr Clin Nutr. 1987;41:463–71.

24. Griffin TM, Roberts TJ, Kram R. Metabolic cost of generating muscular force in human walking: insights from load-carrying and speed experiments. J Appl Physiol. 2003;95:172–83.

25. Brooks GA, Fahey TD, White TP, et al. Exercise Physiology: Human Bioenergetics and Its Applications. Mountain View: Mayfield Publishing Company; 1996.

26. Winter D, Yack H. Emg profiles during normal human walking: stride-to-stride and inter-subject variability. Electroencephalogr Clin Neurophysiol. 1987;67:402–11.

27. Delp SL, Anderson FC, Arnold AS, Loan P, Habib A, John CT, Guendelman E, Thelen DG. Opensim: open-source software to create and analyze dynamic simulations of movement. Biomed Eng IEEE Trans. 2007;54:1940–50.

28. Hicks J, Seth A, Hamner S, Demers M. Simulation with OpenSim - Best Practices. https://simtk-confluence.stanford.edu/display/OpenSim/Simulation+with+OpenSim+-+Best+Practices. Accessed Jan 2017.

29. Farris DJ, Sawicki GS. The mechanics and energetics of human walking and running: a joint level perspective. J R Soc Interface. 2011;9:110–8.

30. Collins SH, Wiggin MB, Sawicki GS. Reducing the energy cost of human walking using an unpowered exoskeleton. Nature. 2015;522.7555:212.

31. Lewis CL, Ferris DP. Invariant hip moment pattern while walking with a robotic hip exoskeleton. J Biomech. 2011;44(5):789–93.

32. Asbeck AT, Schmidt K, Walsh CJ. Soft exosuit for hip assistance. Robot Auton Syst. 2015;73:102–10.

33. Seo K, Lee J, Lee Y, Ha T, Shim Y. Fully autonomous hip exoskeleton saves metabolic cost of walking. In: Robotics and Automation (ICRA), 2016 IEEE International Conference On. Stockholm: IEEE; 2016. p. 4628–35.

34. Wolbrecht ET, Chan V, Reinkensmeyer DJ, Bobrow JE. Optimizing compliant, model-based robotic assistance to promote neurorehabilitation. IEEE Trans Neural Syst Rehabil Eng. 2008;16(3):286–97.

35. Reinkensmeyer DJ, Akoner OM, Ferris DP, Gordon KE. Slacking by the human motor system: computational models and implications for robotic orthoses. In: Annual International Conference of the IEEE Engineering in Medicine and Biology Society. Minneapolis: IEEE; 2009. p. 2129–32.

36. Mooney LM, Herr HM. Biomechanical walking mechanisms underlying the metabolic reduction caused by an autonomous exoskeleton. J Neuroeng Rehabil. 2016;13(1):4.

37. Awad LN, Bae J, O'Donnell K, De Rossi SM, Hendron K, Sloot LH, Kudzia P, Allen S, Holt KG, Ellis TD, et al. A soft robotic exosuit improves walking in patients after stroke. Sci Transl Med. 2017;9(400):9084.

38. Hornby TG, Campbell DD, Kahn JH, Demott T, Moore JL, Roth HR. Enhanced gait-related improvements after therapist-versus robotic-assisted locomotor training in subjects with chronic stroke. Stroke. 2008;39(6):1786–92.

39. Lee S, Sankai Y. Power assist control for walking aid with hal-3 based on emg and impedance adjustment around knee joint. In: Intelligent Robots and Systems, 2002. IEEE/RSJ International Conference On. Lausanne: IEEE; 2002. p. 1499–504.

40. Au S, Berniker M, Herr H. Powered ankle-foot prosthesis to assist level-ground and stair-descent gaits. Neural Netw. 2008;21(4):654–66.

41. Young A, Kuiken T, Hargrove L. Analysis of using emg and mechanical sensors to enhance intent recognition in powered lower limb prostheses. J Neural Eng. 2014;11(5):056021.

42. Takahashi KZ, Lewek MD, Sawicki GS. A neuromechanics-based powered ankle exoskeleton to assist walking post-stroke: a feasibility study. J Neuroeng Rehabil. 2015;12(1):23.

2

Energy storing and return prosthetic feet improve step length symmetry while preserving margins of stability in persons with transtibial amputation

Han Houdijk[1,2*], Daphne Wezenberg[3], Laura Hak[1] and Andrea Giovanni Cutti[4]

From Second World Congress hosted by the American Orthotic & Prosthetic Association (AOPA)
Las Vegas, NV, USA. 06-09 September 2017

Abstract

Background: Energy storing and return (ESAR) feet are generally preferred over solid ankle cushioned heel (SACH) feet by people with a lower limb amputation. While ESAR feet have been shown to have only limited effect on gait economy, other functional benefits should account for this preference. A simple biomechanical model suggests that enhanced gait stability and gait symmetry could prove to explain part of the difference in the subjective preference between both feet.

Aim: To investigate whether increased push-off power with ESAR feet increases center of mass velocity at push off and enhance intact step length and step length symmetry while preserving the margin of stability during walking in people with a transtibial prosthesis.

Methods: Fifteen people with a unilateral transtibial amputation walked with their prescribed ESAR foot and a SACH foot at a fixed walking speed (1.2 m/s) over a level walkway while kinematic and kinetic data were collected. Push-off work generated by the foot, center of mass velocity, step length, step length symmetry and backward margin of stability were assessed and compared between feet.

Results: Push-off work was significantly higher when using the ESAR foot compared to the SACH foot. Simultaneously, center of mass velocity at toe-off was higher with ESAR compared to SACH, and intact step length and step length symmetry increased without reducing the backward margin of stability.

Conclusion: Compared to the SACH foot, the ESAR foot allowed an improvement of step length symmetry while preserving the backward margin of stability at community ambulation speed. These benefits may possibly contribute to the subjective preference for ESAR feet in people with a lower limb amputation.

Keywords: Amputation, Prosthesis, Stability, Symmetry, Gait, Rehabilitation

* Correspondence: h.houdijk@vu.nl
[1]Department of Human Movement Sciences, Faculty of Behavioral and
Movement Sciences, Vrije Universiteit Amsterdam, Van der Boechorststraat 9,
1081 BT Amsterdam, The Netherlands
[2]Department of Research and Development, Heliomare Rehabilitation, Wijk
aan Zee, the Netherlands
Full list of author information is available at the end of the article

Background

Energy storing and return prosthetic (ESAR) feet have been available for decades. These prosthetic feet include carbon fiber components, or other spring-like material, that allow storing of mechanical energy during stance and releasing this energy during push-off [1]. This property has long been claimed to reduce the metabolic energy required for walking and hence improve walking economy. However limited scientific evidence has been found to corroborate this hypothesis [2–7]. Biomechanical studies have demonstrated enhanced mechanical energy storage in early stance and a considerable increase in positive power during push-off while using ESAR feet compared to conventional rigid feet [8–11]. In addition, studies have demonstrated that the increased external mechanical work during prosthetic walking seems to depend on a reduced push-off power [12] and that this is mitigated when walking with ESAR feet [9, 13]. Nevertheless these effects on mechanical energy transfers during walking, do not clearly translate into positive effects on metabolic energy expenditure and gait economy [14, 15]. It has been suggested that positive effects of increased mechanical ankle push-off power, are negated by an increased muscle activation required for body support or to control power transfer across residual joints in the prosthetic leg [16–18].

Despite the apparent absence of increased walking economy, ESAR feet remain the feet of preference for most people using lower limb prostheses [19, 20]. This gives rise to the consideration that other functional benefits, beyond economy, should exist. It has previously been shown that ESAR feet could reduce mechanical load, and therefore potentially prevent overload injuries in prosthetic or intact leg [21]. Alternatively, recent insights in the gait pattern of people with a lower limb amputation suggest that the enhanced ankle push-off power with an ESAR foot might enhance gait stability and improve gait symmetry [22].

A stable gait requires that the body's center of mass is controlled relative to the continuously changing base of support, i.e. the stance foot. In the fore-aft direction, this entails that the body's center of mass needs to pass the leading foot during each stance phase, otherwise an interrupted forward progression or backward fall will occur [23]. The likelihood for the center of mass to successfully pass the leading foot can be assessed using the 'margin of stability concept' postulated by Hof et al. [24, 25]. Based on the inverted pendulum characteristics of human gait the position of the center of mass over time can be predicted based on its initial position, its velocity and the natural frequency of the inverted pendulum. Using these parameters, the so-called extrapolated center of mass can be calculated (Fig. 1). To maintain forward progression and make a subsequent step, the extrapolated center of mass needs to project anterior to the posterior border of the leading foot at the instant of toe-off of the trailing leg. The distance between the extrapolated center of mass and posterior border of the foot indicates the backward margin of stability. The smaller the backward margin of stability, the bigger the chance that the center of mass will not pass the foot in the presence of perturbations during single leg stance.

Recently, we have [22] demonstrated the effect of a reduced ankle push-off power on regulating the backward margin of stability during the intact step in people with a lower limb prosthesis. It was shown that due to a reduced ankle push-off power the center of mass velocity at toe-off of the prosthetic leg is lower compared to the contralateral step. This results in a reduction in the forward projection of the extrapolated center of mass and hence a potentially reduced backward margin of stability. To preserve sufficient backward margin of stability, people walking with a lower limb prosthesis appear to reduce intact leg step length, even though this inevitably leads to step length asymmetry (Fig. 1). From this mechanism, it can be derived that a prosthetic foot and ankle that increases push-off power might be beneficial as it would allow the user to improve gait symmetry without reducing the backward margin of stability.

In this study, we investigated the potential effect of energy storing and return feet on gait symmetry and backward margins of stability in a group of people with a transtibial amputation. We compared level ground walking using an ESAR foot and a SACH foot and hypothesized that the higher push-off power of the ESAR foot compared to the SACH foot will increase center of mass velocity at toe-off, increase intact step length and step length symmetry without reducing the backward margins of stability.

Methods

Data used for this study was previously collected and published to assess differences in external work during walking with ESAR and SACH feet [9]. The specific details on data collection and analysis relevant for the current study are outlined below.

Participants

Fifteen male participants with a transtibial prosthesis (age 55.8 ± 11.1 yr., weight 86.0 ± 12.6 kg, height 1.74 ± 0.04 m) were included in this study. All participants underwent amputation due to trauma, were classified at K3 level, and were free from other musculoskeletal, neurological or cardiovascular co-morbidities. All participants had walked with an ESAR prosthetic foot for at least two years before inclusion in the study. They were all informed on the study aim and procedure and provided written informed consent. The study was approved by the INAIL research board (Commissione Tecnico Scientifica, Budrio, Italy), and performed in accordance with the declaration of Helsinki.

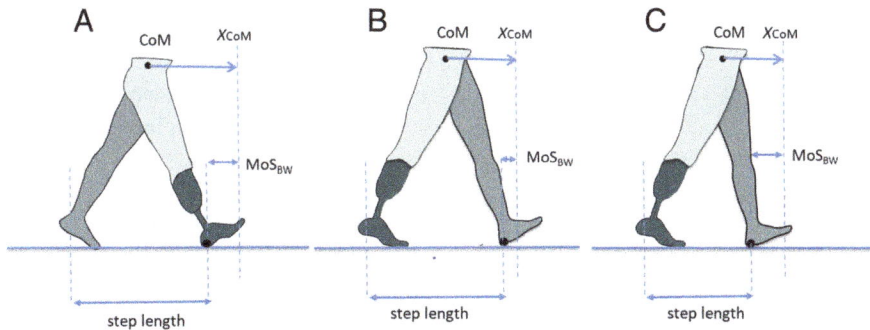

Fig. 1 During walking, forward progression is maintained when the extrapolated center of mass (X$_{CoM}$) projects anterior to the posterior border of the base of support at toe-off, i.e. when the backward margin of stability (MoS$_{BW}$) at toe off is positive. In prosthetic gait, control of MoS$_{BW}$ is affected by reduced push-off power of the prosthetic foot. **a** Depicts the prosthetic step for which no problem occurs. **b** Depicts the intact step. Due to the reduced push-off power of the prosthetic foot the center of mass velocity is reduced and hence X$_{CoM}$ projects less far anteriorly. With normal step length, the MoS$_{BW}$ would be reduced causing a treat for a loss of progression or a backward fall. **c** When the intact leg step length is reduced, MoS$_{BW}$ is restored but at the expense of step length asymmetry (i.e intact step is shorter compared to the prosthetic step)

Procedure

Participants visited the prosthetic center on two separate days to assess their gait pattern while using their pre-scribed ESAR foot (for all participants this was the Vari-Flex, Össur, Iceland) and a SACH foot (1D10, Ottobock, Germany). On the first day gait analysis was performed while participants walked with their prescribed ESAR foot to which they were already accustomed. At the end of this measurement session participants were fitted with the SACH foot below their existing socket, which was aligned by a certified prosthetist. Participants used this foot in their daily life during the next 24 h to get accustomed to it, before returning to the clinic for a subsequent gait analysis using this SACH foot.

During the gait analysis participants walked up and down a 10-m walkway at a fixed walking speed of 1.2 m·s^{-1}, which was controlled online using photocells (Microgate RaceTime2, Italy). A fixed speed over all participants and conditions was selected, since the outcome measures of this study are highly affected by walking speed, and potential speed differences between conditions would obscure the direct dependence of the analyzed gait parameters on foot type. The speed of 1.2 m·s^{-1} was selected as it was expected that participants would be able to walk comfortably at this speed with both types of feet. Self-selected walking speed of the participants was measured before the experiment with the ESAR foot as a reference. This self-selected speed appeared on average to be slightly but significantly higher (1.27 m·s^{-1}, $p = 0.03$). Data from a minimum of 3 strides were collected for both intact and prosthetic leg while walking with the two different prosthetic feet.

Data collection

Kinematic data was collected using a 10-camera opto-electronic system at 100 Hz (VICON; Oxford,

United Kingdom). Markers were attached bilaterally on the anterior and posterior iliac spines, lateral epicondyles of the femur, lateral malleolus of the fibula. For the prosthetic side, lateral malleolus location was approximated as the distal end of the rigid pylon. Ground reaction forces were measured at 1000 Hz using two force plates (0.60 × 0.40 m. Kistler: Winterthur, Switzerland) embedded in the middle of the walkway. Gait speed while crossing the force plates was monitored using two photocells (Microgate Racetime 2; Bolzano, Italy).

Data analysis

Force plate data was filtered at 100 Hz using a fourth order zero lag Butterworth low pass filter. All analyses were performed in the sagittal plane of progression. Force plate data was used to identify initial contact and toe-off based on a threshold vertical force of 25 N. Prosthetic step length (SL$_{prosthetic}$) was calculated as the distance between the malleolus marker of the prosthetic leading and intact trailing leg at the moment of initial contact. Intact step length (SL$_{intact}$) was calculated in a similar method at the time of initial contact of the intact leg. Step length symmetry (SL$_{symm}$) was defined as the difference between prosthetic step length and intact step length:

$$SL_{symm} = SL_{prosthetic} - SL_{intact} \tag{1}$$

Power generated by the prosthetic foot and ankle during stance was calculated using the method outlined by Prince et al. [8, 26], summing both the translational power and rotational power transferred from the foot to the shank:

$$P_{ankle} = \boldsymbol{F}_{dist} \cdot \boldsymbol{v}_{dist} + \boldsymbol{M}_{dist} \cdot \boldsymbol{\omega}_{shank} \tag{2}$$

where the subscript '$dist$' represents the distal point of

the rigid part of the prosthetic leg at approximately the level of the malleoli of the intact leg. F_{dist} and v_{dist} are the reaction forces and linear velocity of this distal point, M_{dist} represent the net moment at the distal point and ω_{shank} the angular velocity of the shank. Ankle push-off work (W_{ankle}, J·kg^{-1}) was determined as the time integral of the positive power burst prior to toe-off.

Center of mass position (CoM) was calculated from the average of the four iliac markers. Center of mass velocity (v_{CoM}) was calculated as the time derivative of the CoM position. Following the description of Hof et al. (2005, 2008) the extrapolated center of mass (X_{CoM}), represents the predicted position of the center of mass after the natural cycle time of the pendular motion of the leg, and was calculated as:

$$X_{CoM} = CoM + v_{CoM}\sqrt{l/g} \qquad (3)$$

with l representing leg length (distance from floor to trochanter major), g representing gravitational acceleration and $\sqrt{l/g}$ representing the natural frequency of the leg pendulum.

The backward margin of stability was defined according to Hak et al. [23]:

$$MoS_{BW} = X_{CoM} - BoS \qquad (4)$$

with the posterior border of the base of support (BoS) of the leading leg represented by the malleolus. Hence, a positive MoS_{BW} indicates a stable condition in which the CoM passes the leading stance foot. This definition is in line with previous studies of Hak et al. [22, 27]. However, it is the reverse from the original definition of Hof et al. [25], which was postulated for upright standing during which X_{CoM} should not pass the border of the base of support. Therefore, contrary to the current definition, Hof et al. defined MoS positive when it did not exceed the border of the BoS.

All primary outcomes were assessed at the instant of toe-off of the trailing prosthetic leg, as this is the instant that the trailing leg can no longer generate push-off power to accelerate CoM. Hence, at toe-off the condition for dynamic stability (i.e $MoS_{BW} > 0$) needs to be satisfied. However, v_{CoM} and MoS_{BW} were also analyzed at heel strike of the intact leading leg (occurring prior to toe-off), to test whether differences in these parameters between feet originate primarily during the double support phase, during which push off power is predominantly generated.

Except from step length and step length symmetry, outcomes were only analyzed for the step in which the prosthetic leg is the trailing push-off leg and the intact leg is the leading leg (i.e. the intact step). All parameters were separately analyzed for each of the three strides collected, after which outcomes were averaged to obtain a mean score for each subject and prosthetic foot type.

Statistics

The differences in push-off work of the prosthetic foot, step length, step length symmetry, v_{CoM} and MoS_{BW} at toe-off between walking with ESAR and SACH foot were analyzed using paired samples t-tests. Differences in the changes in v_{CoM} and MoS_{BW} during double support, from heel contact to toe-off, between ESAR and SACH were analyzed using two-way ANOVA. Significance level was set a-priori at p-value < 0.05.

Results

All participants succeeded to walk comfortably on both ESAR and SACH foot. Walking speed in both foot conditions was on average 1.22 ± 0.02 m·s^{-1}. Stride length did not differ between condition (1.38 ± 0.06 vs. 1.37 ± 0.07 for ESAR vs. SACH).

Push-off power of the prosthetic foot was significantly higher while walking with the an ESAR foot compared to a SACH foot (Fig. 2). This resulted in an increase of push-off work of 120% when walking with the ESAR foot compared to SACH (0.11 ± 0.03 vs. 0.05 ± 0.02 J·kg^{-1} for ESAR and SACH resp., $p < 0.001$)(Fig. 3), as was previously reported by Wezenberg et al. [9].

Step length of the intact step was larger when walking with the ESAR foot compared to the SACH foot (0.68 ± 0.03 vs. 0.66 ± 0.04 m, $p = 0.004$) (Fig. 3). This increase in intact

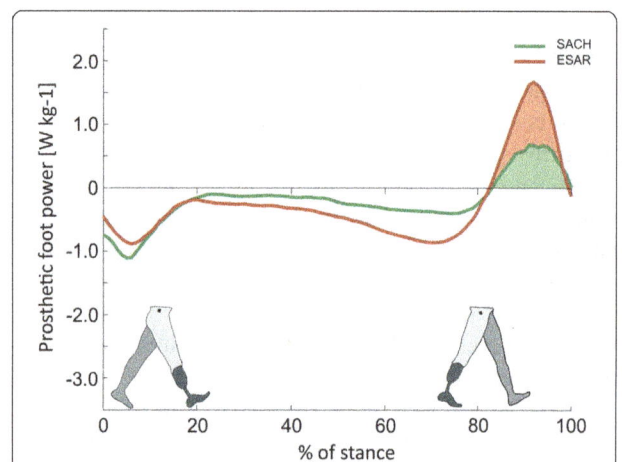

Fig. 2 Push-off power of the prosthetic foot as a function of normalized stance time. The ESAR foot (red) generates negative power, storing elastic energy, in midstance and generates a higher positive push-off power, returning, more elastic energy during push-off compared to the SACH foot (green). The coloured surface below the power profile indicates the amount of work delivered during push-off (Figure amended from Wezenberg et al. 2014 [9])

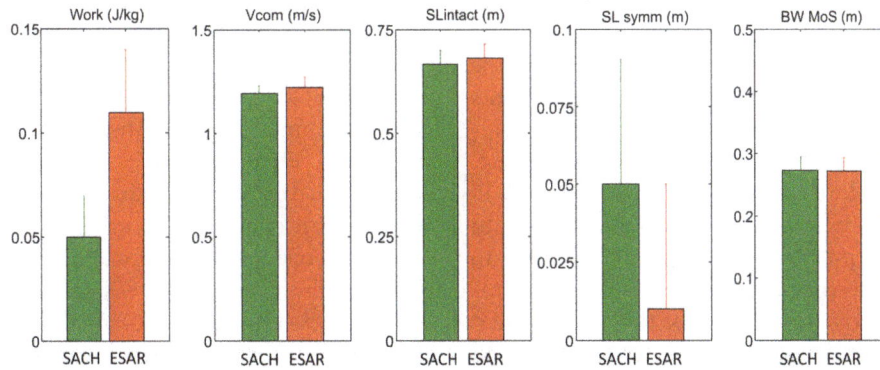

Fig. 3 Difference in push-off work of the prosthetic foot (Work), center of mass velocity (v_{com}), intact step length (SLintact), step length symmetry (SLsymm) and backward margin of stability (MOS_{BW}) between walking with the SACH foot (green) and ESAR foot (red). * denotes significant difference between foot conditions

step length improved step length symmetry ($p < 0.001$). The difference in step length between the intact and prosthetic step, reduced from 0.05 ± 0.04 m while walking with the SACH foot, to only 0.01 ± 0.04 m while walking with the ESAR foot.

Center of mass velocity decreased significantly more during the double support phase when walking with the SACH foot compared to walking with the ESAR foot (interaction effect foot x time $p < 0.000$) (Fig. 4). At the instant of toe-off, center of mass velocity was higher when walking with the ESAR foot compared to the SACH foot (1.22 ± 0.05 vs 1.19 ± 0.04 m·s^{-1}, $p = 0.03$, Fig. 3), while there was no difference at heel strike.

Concurrently, backward margin of stability was lower at heel strike when walking with ESAR compared to SACH (0.137 ± 0.022 vs 0.153 ± 0.023 m, $p = 0.001$), but showed a larger increase during double support (interaction effect foot x time p = 0.001) (Fig. 4). Hence, at toe off the backward margin of stability did not differ significantly between foot conditions (0.271 ± 0.022 vs 0.272 ± 0.022 m, $p = 0.36$) (Fig. 3).

Discussion

In this study, we investigated a potential functional benefit of energy storing and return (ESAR) prosthetic feet. Specifically, we investigated whether ESAR feet could preserve gait stability while restoring gait symmetry. Such benefit may possibly contribute to the general preference of people with a lower limb amputation for these types of prosthetic feet, considering the previously observed absence of improvements in gait economy. Both gait stability and symmetry are frequently mentioned objectives for people with a lower limb amputation who need to regain walking ability with a prosthesis.

Based on a simple biomechanical model of human gait (Fig. 1) and the known increase in push-off power, we

hypothesized that compared to the conventional SACH feet ESAR feet would increase center of mass velocity at toe-off, increase extrapolated center of mass forward projection and as such potentially enhance the backward margin of stability. This would allow the prosthetic user to increase intact step length and restore step length symmetry, without reducing the backward stability margin.

Conditional for this hypothesis is an increase in push-off power of ESAR feet relative to SACH feet. Indeed for the type of ESAR foot used in this study the

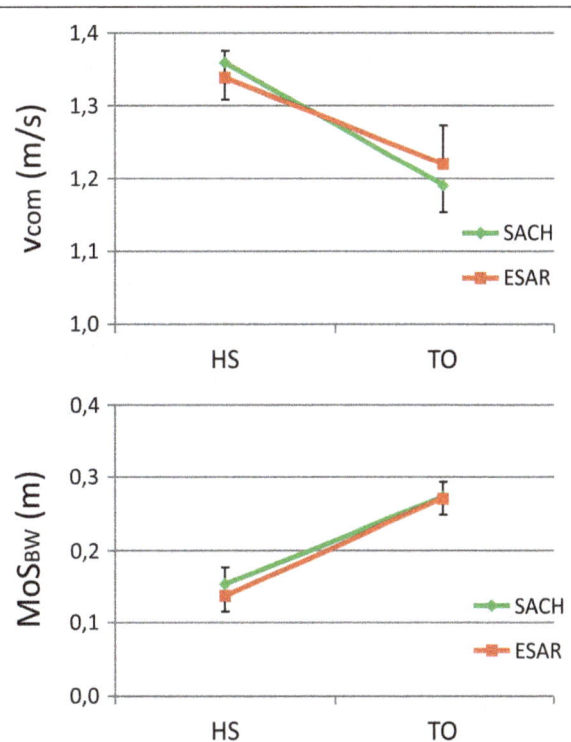

Fig. 4 Change in center of mass velocity (v_{com}) and backward margin of stability (MoS_{BW}) during the double support phase, from heel strike (HS) of the intact leg until toe-off (TO) of the prosthetic leg during walking with the SACH (green) and ESAR (red) foot

positive work performed by the foot and ankle unit was on average 2.2 times higher compared to work performed by the SACH foot, but remains about half of the intact leg ankle foot and ankle power [9]. Similar results have been found in previous studies into the energy return of ESAR and SACH feet [28, 29], although the magnitude of energy return of prosthetic feet reported in literature varies considerably. This is not only due to differences between prosthetic feet type, but also due to methodological differences. Specifically, the way researchers deal with the non-rigidity of the foot segment and the lack of a well-defined ankle center of rotation in the calculation of power generated by the compliant prosthetic foot and ankle system [8, 30]. These issues obscure the comparison of energetic properties between different feet presented in literature.

The increased push-off power of the ESAR foot likely results in a higher velocity of the center of mass at toe-off. In fact, center of mass velocity decreased during the double support phase for both prosthetic feet, but this decrease was attenuated more in the ESAR condition compared to the SACH condition. This difference in the change of center of mass velocity during the specific phase of double support indicates that increased push-off power with ESAR likely accounts for the observed effects, as push off power is predominantly generated during this double support phase. This relation between ankle push-off power and center of mass propulsion is corroborated by previous simulation studies, which mathematically showed a direct relation between the amount of energy return of prosthetic feet and the propulsion of the body's center of mass [31, 32]. Alternatively, it might be argued that the difference in roll-over shape [33] between the two types feet, might contribute to the difference in center of mass velocity at toe off. It has been demonstrated previously that the roll-over shape of the ESAR foot used in this study has a larger arc length, providing a longer lever to the foot segment [9]. In passive feet a proper roll-over shape could also enhance the step-to-step transition, apart from ankle push off power, and attenuate deceleration of the center of mass double support [34]. It is however not known how roll-over shape and push off power interact in dynamic ESAR feet, and how the effect on center of mass velocity could be partitioned over both. This should be explored in the future studies.

Because of the larger center of mass velocity at toe-off with the ESAR foot, the extrapolated center of mass projects more anterior compared to the SACH condition. This allows the prosthetic user to make a larger step with the intact leg, without compromising the backward margin of stability. This increase in intact step length, observed with the ESAR foot, resulted in increased step length symmetry when walking with the ESAR foot.

Although step length symmetry, on its own, is not necessarily a functional benefit [22], often gait symmetry is considered a goal in gait training [35, 36]. From a cosmetic point of view patients might prefer a close to normal symmetric gait pattern as to not stand out in the crowd. Furthermore, it has been speculated that gait symmetry might indirectly provide functional benefits as it could reduce mechanical overload on the intact and residual leg and on the low back, which are both common co-morbidities in people with a lower limb amputation [21, 37]. This difference in mechanical loading of the intact leg has indeed been presented previously (in terms of external mechanical work) for this data set [9]. Hence, improving gait symmetry might be considered a relevant functional benefit of ESAR feet.

The backward margin of stability at toe off was similar between foot condition. Nevertheless, this can be interpreted as a positive effect of the ESAR foot. Without the additional push off power of the ESAR foot, as in the SACH foot, an increased intact step length would have resulted in reduced margins of stability given the constraints outlined in Fig. 1. This can further be substantiated when analyzing the change in backward margin of stability during double support (Fig. 4), the phase during which push-off occurs. At heel strike of the intact leg margin of stability is smaller in the ESAR condition compared to the SACH condition. This is due to the fact that participants walk with a larger intact step length with the ESAR foot, while center off mass velocity at heel strike is similar between conditions. During double support the center of mass velocity decreases in both conditions but this decrease is smaller with the ESAR foot. The concomitant higher center of mass velocity at toe off with the ESAR foot results in similar margins of stability between feet, making up for the initial negative effect of increased step length. A similar effect of ankle push-off on the control of the backward margin of stability can also be seen when comparing the intact and prosthetic step in prosthetic gait [22]. Such enhanced control over the backward margin of stability might affect balance confidence of the prosthetic user, which has been indicated as an important predictor of self-reported mobility performance and social activity [38, 39]. When the prosthetic user is perceptive to this change in control over the backward margin of stability, this effect might contribute to the preference of many users for energy storing and return prosthetic feet over solid feet.

This study, designed to investigate a specific mechanical consequence of the constraints of prosthetic feet, is subject to several limitations. The experiments were performed at a fixed walking speed between conditions (prosthetic foot). This was done to avoid the confounding effect of walking speed on the outcome parameters, which would obscure interpretation of the underlying mechanics. Although strong evidence is lacking [15], it has been suggested that people tend to walk slower with SACH feet compared to ESAR feet. Such a reduction in walking speed could be a strategy to cope with the indicated constraint on gait stability. While in this study we demonstrate that this specific constraint of SACH feet on step length symmetry and margin of stability exists at equivalent speeds, it should be explored in the future how differences in walking speed influence this constraint. A second limitation is the fact that we included participants that were all currently using the ESAR Variflex foot. The SACH foot was provided to them for the purpose of this experiment. They were allowed a 24-h accommodation period at home to get used to the SACH foot. Moreover, they all had some previous experience with SACH and most of them use a SACH foot in their current bathing/in-house prosthesis. Nevertheless, we cannot rule out if a lack of acclimation on the SACH foot influenced our results. However, the effects found in our study agreed very well with the hypothesized differences between feet. This provides some confidence to the fact that hypothesized mechanical constraints indeed exist in prosthetic walking, although with more practice people might find smart strategies to cope with these constraints. Next to the effect of practice other factors might have influence the observed effects. Imperfect socket fit or alignment could affect step length and symmetry. We tried to minimize this effect by allowing participants to use their own socket with both feet, and by having a certified prosthetist optimize alignment of the SACH foot before the experiment. No participant indicated stump problems during the experiments. Another limitation of this study is that we only investigated one type of ESAR feet, i.e. Variflex (Össur, Iceland). In general, all ESAR feet do provide increased push power and are expected to allow for the improved control over the backward margin of stability and step length symmetry as found in this study. However, this general effect should be confirmed in other feet. Moreover, assessing these parameters could be used as a benchmark test for different prosthetic feet. Finally, results of this study were obtained in a group of relatively active persons with a transtibial amputation as a result of trauma. Generalization of the results to less active persons or different amputation causes or levels should be done with caution. For instance, within the population of people with transfemoral prosthesis, step length asymmetry is less consistently directed towards a shorter intact step length [36, 40]. Given the limitations presented above, generalization of the results to less controlled conditions and their contribution to the experienced benefits of ESAR feet in daily life should be interpreted with care. However, we believe that this study design does reflect a basic mechanical constraint of prosthetic feet and the related effect on step length symmetry and margin of stability.

Conclusion
In conclusion, this study showed that the energy storing and return (ESAR) prosthetic foot can enhance center of mass propulsion, thereby allowing a symmetric gait pattern while preserving the backward margin of stability. These benefits on gait stability and symmetry might possibly contribute to the general preference of people with a transtibial amputation for these dynamic prosthetic feet. Current findings can prove to be helpful in the design, prescription and evaluation of future prosthetic feet.

Acknowledgements
The authors would like to acknowledge the contribution of Leonardo Cavrini and Fausto Caprara (certified prosthetists/orthotists) for their help during the measurements and Davide Veronesi for the help in recruiting the participants for the measurements. Finally we would like the reviewers of this manuscript for their valuable comments and suggestions.

Funding
This study was unfunded. The publication cost of this article was funded by the American Orthotic & Prosthetic Association (AOPA).

Authors' contributions
All authors have read and approved the final version of the manuscript.

Competing interests
The authors declare that they have no competing interests.

Author details
[1]Department of Human Movement Sciences, Faculty of Behavioral and Movement Sciences, Vrije Universiteit Amsterdam, Van der Boechorststraat 9, 1081 BT Amsterdam, The Netherlands. [2]Department of Research and Development, Heliomare Rehabilitation, Wijk aan Zee, the Netherlands. [3]Department of Health & Technology | Human Kinetic Technology, The Hague University of Applied Sciences, The Hague, The Netherlands. [4]Production Directorate, Applied Research, INAIL Prosthesis Center, Vigorso di Budrio, Bologna, Italy.

References
1. Ehara Y, Beppu M, Nomura S, Kunimi Y, Takahashi S. Energy storing property of so-called energy-storing prosthetic feet. Arch Phys Med Rehabil. 1993;74(1):68–72.
2. Lehmann JF, Price R, Boswell-Bessette S, Dralle A, Questad K. Comprehensive analysis of dynamic elastic response feet: Seattle ankle/lite foot versus SACH foot. Arch Phys Med Rehabil. 1993;74(8):853–61.
3. Torburn L, Powers CM, Guiterrez R, Perry J. Energy expenditure during ambulation in dysvascular and traumatic below-knee amputees: a comparison of five prosthetic feet. J Rehabil Res Dev. 1995;32(2):111–9.

4.   Klodd E, Hansen A, Fatone S, Edwards M. Effects of prosthetic foot forefoot flexibility on oxygen cost and subjective preference rankings of unilateral transtibial prosthesis users. J Rehabil Res Dev. 2010;47(6):543–52.

5.   Graham LE, Datta D, Heller B, Howitt J. A comparative study of oxygen consumption for conventional and energy-storing prosthetic feet in transfemoral amputees. Clin Rehabil. 2008;22(10–11):896–901.

6.   Hsu MJ, Nielsen DH, Lin-Chan SJ, Shurr D. The effects of prosthetic foot design on physiologic measurements, self-selected walking velocity, and physical activity in people with transtibial amputation. Arch Phys Med Rehabil. 2006;87(1):123–9.

7.   Casillas JM, Dulieu V, Cohen M, Marcer I, Didier JP. Bioenergetic comparison of a new energy-storing foot and SACH foot in traumatic below-knee vascular amputations. Arch Phys Med Rehabil. 1995;76(1):39–44.

8.   Prince F, Winter DA, Sjonnensen G, Powell C, Wheeldon RK. Mechanical efficiency during gait of adults with transtibial amputation: a pilot study comparing the SACH, Seattle, and golden-ankle prosthetic feet. J Rehabil Res Dev. 1998;35(2):177–85.

9.   Wezenberg D, Cutti AG, Bruno A, Houdijk H. Differentiation between solid-ankle cushioned heel and energy storage and return prosthetic foot based on step-to-step transition cost. J Rehabil Res Dev. 2014;51(10):1579–89.

10. Geil MD, Parnianpour M, Quesada P, Berme N, Simon S. Comparison of methods for the calculation of energy storage and return in a dynamic elastic response prosthesis. J Biomech. 2000;33(12):1745–50.

11. Gitter A, Czerniecki JM, DeGroot DM. Biomechanical analysis of the influence of prosthetic feet on below-knee amputee walking. Am J Phys Med Rehabil. 1991;70(3):142–8.

12. Houdijk H, Pollmann E, Groenewold M, Wiggerts H, Polomski W. The energy cost for the step-to-step transition in amputee walking. Gait & Posture. 2009;30(1):35–40.

13. Segal AD, Zelik KE, Klute GK, Morgenroth DC, Hahn ME, Orendurff MS, Adamczyk PG, Collins SH, Kuo AD, Czerniecki JM. The effects of a controlled energy storage and return prototype prosthetic foot on transtibial amputee ambulation. Hum Mov Sci. 2012;31(4):918–31.

14. Versluys R, Beyl P, Van Damme M, Desomer A, Van Ham R, Lefeber D. Prosthetic feet: state-of-the-art review and the importance of mimicking human ankle-foot biomechanics. Disabil Rehabil Assist Technol. 2009;4(2):65–75.

15. Hofstad CJ, van der Linde H, van Limbeek J, Postema K. Prescription of prosthetic ankle-foot mechanisms after lower limb amputation. Cochrane Database Syst Rev. 2004;(1). Art. No.: CD003978. https://doi.org/10.1002/14651858.CD003978.pub2.

16. Fey NP, Klute GK, Neptune RR. The influence of energy storage and return foot stiffness on walking mechanics and muscle activity in below-knee amputees. Clin Biomech. 2011;26(10):1025–32.

17. Fey NP, Klute GK, Neptune RR. Altering prosthetic foot stiffness influences foot and muscle function during below-knee amputee walking: a modeling and simulation analysis. J Biomech. 2013;46(4):637–44.

18. Ventura JD, Klute GK, Neptune RR. The effect of prosthetic ankle energy storage and return properties on muscle activity in below-knee amputee walking. Gait & Posture. 2011;33(2):220–6.

19. Hafner BJ, Sanders JE, Czerniecki J, Fergason J. Energy storage and return prostheses: does patient perception correlate with biomechanical analysis? Clin Biomech. 2002;17(5):325–44.

20. Postema K, Hermens HJ, de Vries J, Koopman HF, Eisma WH. Energy storage and release of prosthetic feet. Part 2: subjective ratings of 2 energy storing and 2 conventional feet, user choice of foot and deciding factor. Prosthetics Orthot Int. 1997;21(1):28–34.

21. Morgenroth DC, Segal AD, Zelik KE, Czerniecki JM, Klute GK, Adamczyk PG, Orendurff MS, Hahn ME, Collins SH, Kuo AD. The effect of prosthetic foot push-off on mechanical loading associated with knee osteoarthritis in lower extremity amputees. Gait Posture. 2011;34(4):502–7.

22. Hak L, van Dieen JH, van der Wurff P, Houdijk H. Stepping asymmetry among individuals with unilateral Transtibial limb loss might be functional in terms of gait stability. Phys Ther. 2014;94(10):1480–8.

23. Hak L, Houdijk H, Beek PJ, van Dieën JH. Steps to take to enhance gait stability: The effect of stride frequency, stride length, and walking speed on local dynamic stability and margins of stability. PLoS ONE. 2013;8(12): e82842.

24. Hof AL. The 'extrapolated center of mass' concept suggests a simple control of balance in walking. Hum Mov Sci. 2008;27(1):112–25.

25. Hof AL, Gazendam MG, Sinke WE. The condition for dynamic stability. J Biomech. 2005;38(1):1–8.

26. Prince F, Winter DA, Sjonnesen G, Wheeldon RK. A new technique for the calculation of the energy stored, dissipated, and recovered in different ankle-foot prostheses. IEEE Trans Rehabil Eng. 1994;2(4):247–55.

27. Hak L, Houdijk H, Steenbrink F, Mert A, van der Wurff P, Beek PJ, van Dieen JH. Stepping strategies for regulating gait adaptability and stability. J Biomech. 2013;46(5):905–11.

28. Barr AE, Siegel KL, Danoff JV, McGarvey CL 3rd, Tomasko A, Sable I, Stanhope SJ. Biomechanical comparison of the energy-storing capabilities of SACH and carbon copy II prosthetic feet during the stance phase of gait in a person with below-knee amputation. Phys Ther. 1992;72(5):344–54.

29. van der Linden ML, Solomonidis SE, Spence WD, Li N, Paul JP. A methodology for studying the effects of various types of prosthetic feet on the biomechanics of trans-femoral amputee gait. J Biomech. 1999;32(9):877–89.

30. Takahashi KZ, Stanhope SJ. Mechanical energy profiles of the combined ankle-foot system in normal gait: insights for prosthetic designs. Gait Posture. 2013;38(4):818–23.

31. Zmitrewicz RJ, Neptune RR, Sasaki K. Mechanical energetic contributions from individual muscles and elastic prosthetic feet during symmetric unilateral transtibial amputee walking: a theoretical study. J Biomech. 2007;40(8):1824–31.

32. Silverman AK, Neptune RR. Muscle and prosthesis contributions to amputee walking mechanics: a modeling study. J Biomech. 2012;45(13):2271–8.

33. Hansen AH, Childress DS. Investigations of roll-over shape: implications for design, alignment, and evaluation of ankle-foot prostheses and orthoses. Disabil Rehabil. 2010;32(26):2201–9.

34. Adamczyk PG, Collins SH, Kuo AD. The advantages of a rolling foot in human walking. J Exp Biol. 2006;209(20):3953–63.

35. Agrawal V, Gailey R, O'Toole C, Gaunaurd I, Finnieston A. Influence of gait training and prosthetic foot category on external work symmetry during unilateral transtibial amputee gait. Prosthetics Orthot Int. 2013;37(5):396–403.

36. Darter BJ, Nielsen DH, Yack HJ, Janz KF. Home-based treadmill training to improve gait performance in persons with a chronic transfemoral amputation. Arch Phys Med Rehabil. 2013;94(12):2440–7.

37. Gailey R, Allen K, Castles J, Kucharik J, Roeder M. Review of secondary physical conditions associated with lower-limb amputation and long-term prosthesis use. J Rehabil Res Dev. 2008;45(1):15–29.

38. Miller WC, Deathe AB, Speechley M, Koval J. The influence of falling, fear of falling, and balance confidence on prosthetic mobility and social activity among individuals with a lower extremity amputation. Arch Phys Med Rehabil. 2001;82(9):1238–44.

39. Miller WC, Speechley M, Deathe AB. Balance confidence among people with lower-limb amputations. Phys Ther. 2002;82(9):856–65.

40. Prinsen EC, Nederhand MJ, Sveinsdottir HS, Prins MR, van der Meer F, Koopman HF, Rietman JS. The influence of a user-adaptive prosthetic knee across varying walking speeds: a randomized cross-over trial. Gait Posture. 2017;51:254–60.

3

Economic benefits of microprocessor controlled prosthetic knees

Christine Chen[1], Mark Hanson[1], Ritika Chaturvedi[2], Soeren Mattke[3], Richard Hillestad[1] and Harry H. Liu[3*]

From Second World Congress hosted by the American Orthotic & Prosthetic Association (AOPA)
Las Vegas, NV, USA. 06-09 September 2017

Abstract

Background: Advanced prosthetic knees allow for more dynamic movements and improved quality of life, but payers have recently started questioning their value. To answer this question, the differential clinical outcomes and cost of microprocessor-controlled knees (MPK) compared to non-microprocessor controlled knees (NMPK) were assessed.

Methods: We conducted a literature review of the clinical and economic impacts of prosthetic knees, convened technical expert panel meetings, and implemented a simulation model over a 10-year time period for unilateral transfemoral Medicare amputees with a Medicare Functional Classification Level of 3 and 4 using estimates from the published literature and expert input. The results are summarized as an incremental cost effectiveness ratio (ICER) from a societal perspective, i.e., the incremental cost of MPK compared to NMPK for each quality-adjusted life-year gained. All costs were adjusted to 2016 U.S. dollars and discounted using a 3% rate to the present time.

Results: The results demonstrated that compared to NMPK over a 10-year time period: for every 100 persons, MPK results in 82 fewer major injurious falls, 62 fewer minor injurious falls, 16 fewer incidences of osteoarthritis, and 11 lives saved; on a per person per year basis, MPK reduces direct healthcare cost by $3676 and indirect cost by $909, but increases device acquisition and repair cost by $6287 and total cost by $1702; on a per person basis, MPK is associated with an incremental total cost of $10,604 and increases the number of life years by 0.11 and quality adjusted life years by 0.91. MPK has an ICER ratio of $11,606 per quality adjusted life year, and the economic benefits of MPK are robust in various sensitivity analyses.

Conclusions: Advanced prosthetics for transfemoral amputees, specifically MPKs, are associated with improved clinical benefits compared to non-MPKs. The economic benefits of MPKs are similar to or even greater than those of other medical technologies currently reimbursed by U.S. payers.

Keywords: Amputee, Microprocessor controlled knee, Economic analysis, Incremental cost effectiveness ratio, Transfemoral amputation

* Correspondence: hliu@rand.org
[3]RAND Corporation, 20 Park Plaza, Suite 920, Boston, MA 02116, USA
Full list of author information is available at the end of the article

Background

There are about 185,000 amputations conducted per year in the U.S. [1]. Currently, approximately 1.9 million individuals are living with limb loss according to the Centers for Disease Control and Prevention [2], a figure expected to rise to 3.6 million by 2050 [1]. Of this number, it is estimated that 18.5 to 21.0% are transfemoral amputees [3, 4]. Transfemoral amputation, or the removal of a limb above the knee joint, is performed to remove ischemic, infected, or irreversibly damaged tissue and is generally a life-saving procedure. About 82% of transfemoral amputations are due to peripheral artery disease and/or diabetes, followed by trauma, cancer, infection, and congenital defects [5, 6].

Advanced technologies can help transfemoral amputees improve functional mobility and as a result, quality of life. A transfemoral amputee often has difficulty in regaining normal movement. For example, transfemoral amputees must use 35–65% more energy [7–10] to walk than a person with two legs due to complexities in the knee joint. Over the last decade, major technological advancements such as microprocessors, and their associated load and position sensors have catalyzed the modernization of prosthetics [11]. Such advanced prosthetic knees and feet were developed to allow for safer movements across a range of walking environments and improving user quality of life [11–13].

Despite the rapid progress in advanced technologies, our healthcare payment system, however, has not yet evolved simultaneously, treating prosthetics as commodity products and emphasizing cost-cutting rather than good value for the money. Currently, the Centers for Medicare and Medicaid Services (CMS), the Department of Veterans Affairs, and private insurance companies restrict reimbursement of prosthetics based on the Medicare Functional Classification Level, an index for classifying the functional mobility and productivity potential of individuals with lower limb loss [14, 15]. Within Medicare, amputees often have to pay about 20% of the device cost out-of-pocket when they purchase a new device; if a prosthetic device is not covered, amputees have to pay for the entire device out of pocket. Consequently, patients often choose low-cost prosthetic devices and may not realize their potential in functional mobility [16]. With increasing cost-cutting pressure in recent years, payers have shifted part of such pressure onto the prosthetics industry. For example, citing a 2011 report by the Office of Inspector General [17], the CMS issued new local coverage rules in 2015 to tighten the rules for reimbursing lower-limb prosthetics.

An open and candid dialog among stakeholders would help us strike the right balance between improving clinical outcomes and controlling healthcare cost, and this is where robust evidence should play a critical role, such as evidence for the incremental value of advanced prosthetics in comparison to conventional prosthetics. On the one hand, payers should ensure patient access to advanced technologies with proven health benefits, but on the other hand, they have the fiduciary obligation to contain ever-expanding healthcare costs. To address this, quality clinical and economic data, as well as rigorous studies, are required to demonstrate the value of prosthetics and associated services. In the absence of head-to-head clinical trial data, a modeling study was conducted to leverage existing evidence to assess the cost-effectiveness of advanced prosthetics such as microprocessor-controlled prosthetic knees compared to non-microprocessor alternatives from the societal perspective.

Methods

The clinical and economic benefits of microprocessor-controlled prosthetic knees (MPK) were compared with those of non-microprocessor controlled prosthetic knees (NMPKs) from a societal perspective, and the results are summarized as an incremental cost-effectiveness ratio (ICER) — a commonly accepted measure for cost-effectiveness or value for money. ICER is defined as the additional resource requirements per unit of additional health gained, which is typically measured by quality-adjusted-life-years (QALY). The analysis assessed various clinical and economic endpoints, including physical function, quality of life, direct healthcare costs, and indirect costs such as the impact on caregiving expenses, transportation expenses, and work productivity.

All costs were inflated to 2016 U.S. dollars using the medical care component of the Consumer Price Index [18] and, when applicable, were converted to U.S. dollars using the exchange rate at the time the study was conducted [19]. This study was approved by RAND's Human Subjects Protection Committee.

Target population

The analysis focuses on the Medicare population, which includes a diversely aged patient group, because CMS not only represents the largest payer for prosthetic devices in the country but also sets the market standard for reimbursement levels against which commercial payers and the Department of Veterans Affairs often benchmark. Besides, since unilateral K3 and K4 transfemoral amputees have historically been the primary users of advanced prosthetics, they are the target population of the main analysis. Unilateral K1 and K2 transfemoral amputees were examined in the sensitivity analysis. Dobson and DeVanzo LLC provided basic characteristics of the target populations for the simulation model based on the 2011–2014 Medicare claims data (see Additional file 1: Table S1).

Data sources

Literature review

PubMed, Embase, CINAHL, PsycINFO, Web of Science, and Google Scholar were searched for relevant peer-reviewed articles. References of the identified literature were manually searched for additional publications. Non-peer reviewed literature such as technical reports produced by government agencies or industry associations was also examined. For each input parameter, a range of estimates was compiled from the literature whenever possible, where the median value served as the base case in the simulation model, while the upper and lower bounds were used in the sensitivity analysis.

Expert panel process

An expert panel was convened to supplement the literature review, to validate the assumptions made, to ensure adequate and complete understanding of the prosthetics literature, and to ensure appropriate model development and construction. In addition, when the model parameters were not available in the published literature, experts were asked to provide estimates for such parameters. Fifteen experts were selected based on their publication record in the various topics that informed the simulation model. Telephone-based panel discussions and one-on-one interviews were conducted on an as-needed basis.

Cost of device acquisition

The cost of device acquisition is approximated using the current Medicare payment amount. Therefore, it does not necessarily represent the manufacturer list price. The base case value was based on expert input and the upper and lower bounds were derived from the 2016 Medicare fee schedule allowed payments [20] for the two most frequent combinations of L codes, which were identified among the new unilateral transfemoral amputees in the 2011–2014 Medicare claims data. The median of the Medicare allowed payments in the 2 years after the device fitting in the same Medicare population was used as the cost of device repair and physical therapy. Dobson & DaVanzo LLC conducted all the Medicare claims data analyses.

Simulation model

A cohort-level Markov model [21, 22] was developed to simulate the clinical and economic outcomes for a unilateral transfemoral amputee population. This hypothetical cohort was assigned to two different treatment strategies, NMPK or MPK, with all other prosthetic components being the same. The simulation was limited to 10 years because the existing evidence comes from relatively short-term studies, meaning that longer-term predictions can be subject to large uncertainty. All

health and cost outcomes were discounted to the present time using a 3% discount rate.

Because the data available from the literature permitted the conversion of only two clinical conditions, falls and osteoarthritis, into economic benefits, two modules were constructed for the model respectively. The lack of data, however, prevented the quantification of potential benefit derived from other medical conditions, such as obesity and cardiovascular diseases.

In the fall module, patients can experience three health states: fall, no fall, and death. Falls can be either medical, i.e., require medical attention, or non-medical. Medical falls can be minor, major, or fatal. Major injurious falls are associated with an admission to a medical facility. A patient may enter the "death" state from the "no fall" state due to causes other than falling. While Markov models are "memoryless," meaning the health state at a subsequent step depends only on the state at the previous step, the model updates the annual probability of falling to simulate the effect of learning. The osteoarthritis module has three states as well: no osteoarthritis, osteoarthritis, and death. Patients can move from one state to another until the end of the 10-year time period or death.

After implementing the model, validation testing was performed to assure that the computations were done correctly, and the outputs responded as expected to changes in key parameter input values. The model was programmed in Visual Basic for Applications for Microsoft Excel and followed the modeling guidelines of the International Society for Pharmacoeconomics and Outcomes Research [23].

Model parameters were compiled from the literature review, expert consultation, and the analysis of Medicare claims data. When parameters were not available from the published literature, expert opinion was used and, if needed, assumptions were made. The model parameters, assumptions, and data sources are listed in Table 1.

One-way sensitivity analyses were conducted where one input parameter was changed at a time to inspect the sensitivity of model results to changes in key input parameter values as they were varied individually. Probabilistic sensitivity analyses on model inputs with 1000 replications, assuming uniform distributions for all variables, were also conducted.

Results

Clinical benefits

Physical function

A number of studies assessed the effects of advanced prosthetics by measuring biomechanical and physical performances when subjects wore NMPK and after subjects were fitted with MPK. Overall, there is strong

Table 1 Model parameters, assumptions and data sources

Model parameter	Base case	Range	Data sources
Probability of falling per year			[26, 60]
MPK	26.00%	22.20–32.00%	
NMPK	82.00%	75.00–87.50%	
Proportion of medical falls	10.40%	6.20–19.60%	[61–63]
Proportion of fatal medical falls	7.00%	6.30–7.70%[a]	[64]
Proportion of major injury falls	40.00%	32.60–40.00%	[65, 66]
Proportion of minor injury falls	53.00%	53.00–60.50%	
Average number of falls per faller per year			[26, 59]
MPK	3.20	2.00–3.20	
NMPK	3.87	1.86–3.87	
Odds ratio of falling in year 4 vs. year 1	0.53	0.48–0.58[a]	[67]
Medical cost per major injurious fall	$24,844.52	$16,978.61 - $31,707.24	[65, 66, 68]
Medical cost per minor injurious fall	$1332.47	$620.69 - $6005.62	
Medical cost of fall-related death	$27,337.76	$27,337.76 - $29,578.20	[68, 69]
Caregiving expenses per person per year			[39, 70–72]
MPK	$2754.29	$2478.86 - $3029.72[a]	
NMPK	$3477.60	$3129.84 - $3825.36[a]	
Lost wages per person per year			
MPK	$1669.11	$1502.20 - $1836.02[a]	
NMPK	$2144.06	$1929.65 - $2358.47[a]	
Transportation expenses per person per year			
MPK	$463.46	$417.11 - $509.81[a]	
NMPK	$300.36	$270.32 - $330.40[a]	
Baseline prevalence of osteoarthritis (knee)			Medicare claims data 2011–2014
K1/K2	16.30%	14.67–17.93%[a]	
K3/K4	19.10%	17.19–21.01%[a]	
Probability of developing osteoarthritis per year			[34]; Expert opinion
MPK	1.50%	1.35–1.65%[a]	
NMPK	2.21%	1.99 - 2.43%[a]	
Osteoarthritis-related medical cost per year	$6639.72	$996.41 - $14,682.92	[73]
Osteoarthritis-related indirect cost per year	$1084.21	$606.89 - $1192.63	[74, 75]
Baseline mortality rate			Medicare claims data 2011–2014
K1/K2	18.00%	16.20–19.80%[a]	
K3/K4	9.31%	8.38–10.24%[a]	
Device acquisition cost in 10 years			2016 Medicare fee schedule; Medicare claims data 2011–2014; Expert opinion
MPK (plus 1 replacement)	$56,000.00	$44,750.00 - $58,118.00	
NMPK (plus 2 replacements)	$16,500.00	$7785.00 - $22,101.00	
Device repair cost per year			
MPK	$192.23	$173.01 - $211.45[a]	
NMPK	$135.95	$122.36 - $149.55[a]	
Physical therapy cost in year 1			
MPK	$1986.68	$1788.01 - $2185.35[a]	
NMPK	$1648.62	$1483.76 - $1813.48[a]	

Table 1 Model parameters, assumptions and data sources *(Continued)*

Model parameter	Base case	Range	Data sources
Physical therapy cost in year 2			
MPK	$1621.68	$1459.51 - $1783.85[a]	
NMPK	$1347.47	$1212.72 - $1482.21[a]	
Health utilities			[37–40]
MPK	0.82	0.75–0.83	
NMPK	0.66	0.60–0.92	
Discount rate	3.00%	2.00–5.00%	[76]

MPK microprocessor-controlled knees, *NMPK* non-microprocessor controlled knees. K1-K4: Medicare Functional Classification Level 1 to 4, respectively
[a]There are no range values directly from the literature; in the sensitivity analyses, they were derived through varying the base case value up and down by 10%. The design of the studies comparing the effectiveness of MPK to NMPK: Prospective cohort study [26, 39, 59, 60]; Retrospective cohort study [37, 40]; Cross-sectional study [38])

evidence suggesting that compared to NMPK, MPK is associated with improvements in walking speed [24–26], gait symmetry [13, 27], the ability to negotiate obstacles in the environment [11, 15, 26, 28], and safety in terms of reduced stumbles and falls. However, while there is some evidence suggesting improvement in other dimensions such as energy efficiency [11, 24, 29–32] and physical activity [28, 30, 33], the results are inconclusive.

Falls and fall-related mortality

Based on the simulation results, the risk of major injurious falls is reduced by 79% in MPK users compared to NMPK users, as the incidence rate decreases from 104 to 22 per 1000 person-years, and the incidence rate of minor injurious falls decreases from 78 to 16 per 1000 person-years (Fig. 1). Meanwhile, the incidence rate of fall-related deaths is 3 and 14 per 1000 person-years in MPK and NMPK users, respectively. That is, 11 lives would be saved by MPK if we observed 1000 amputees for 1 year.

Incidence of osteoarthritis

Kaufman and colleagues [34] observed that, compared to NMPK, MPK reduces the moment about the knee–an indirect measure of the force absorbed by the knee–of

the prosthetic limb by 30%. Thus, based on expert opinion, it was assumed that MPK would reduce the onset of osteoarthritis from 20 to 14 per 100 persons in a 10-year period. Incorporating these estimates into the simulation model resulted in 16 fewer incidences of osteoarthritis per 100 persons attributable to MPK over the ten-year model period.

Quality of life

On average, subjects experienced a 10% improvement in quality of life when using MPK compared to NMPK, measured by the Prosthesis Evaluation Questionnaire (PEQ) summary score [15, 28, 30, 35, 36]. Seelen [37] reports a 37% higher score in the 36-Item Short Form Health Survey (SF-36) in all amputees as well as recent amputees when they wore MPK compared to NMPK (Fig. 2). The EuroQol five dimensions questionnaire (EQ-5D) scores converted from SF-36 were 0.92 and 0.71 for MPK and NMPK users, respectively, which is consistent with the literature where the MPK group scored 21% higher in EQ-5D than the NMPK group [38–40].

According to the simulation results, the total number of life years in MPK users is 8.8 years greater than in NMPK users (554.4 vs. 545.7) if we observed 100 MPK users and 100 NMPK users over 10 years. Adjusting for

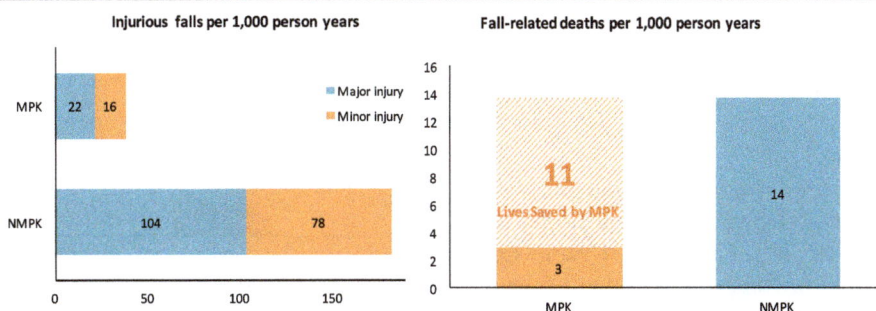

Fig. 1 Injurious Falls and Fall-related Deaths Among MPK and NMPK Users, Note: MPK: microprocessor-controlled knees; NMPK: non-microprocessor controlled knees

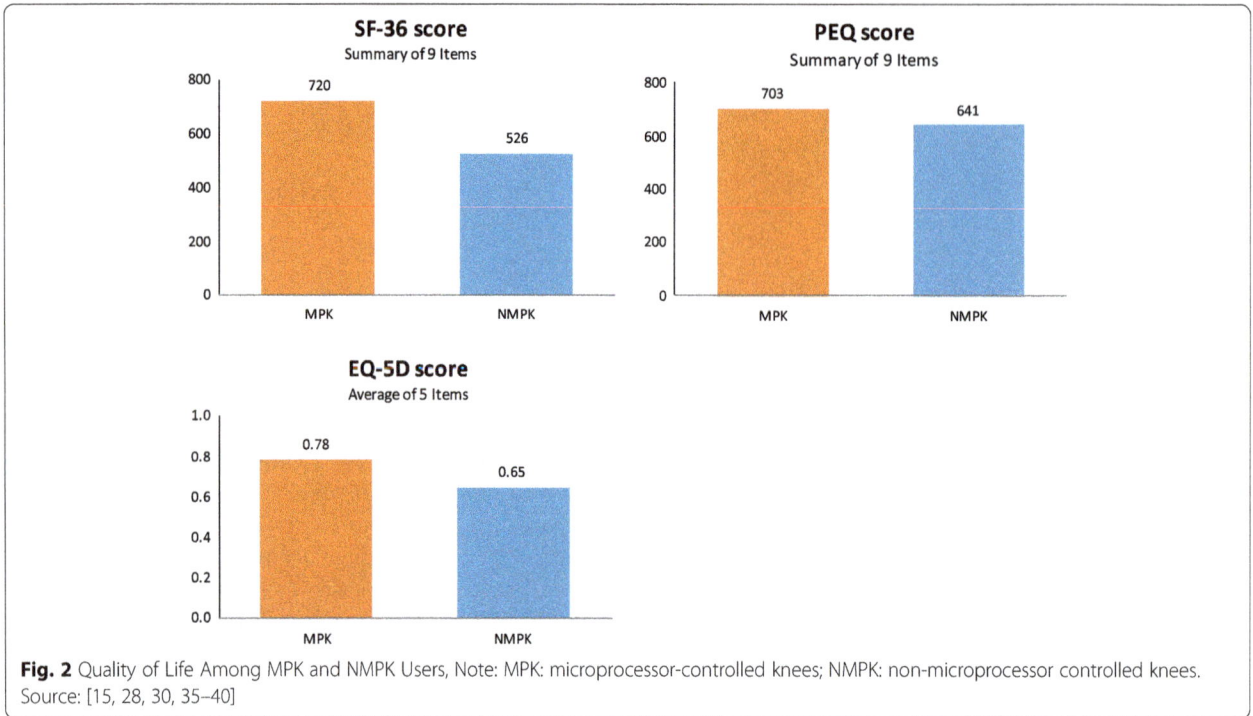

Fig. 2 Quality of Life Among MPK and NMPK Users, Note: MPK: microprocessor-controlled knees; NMPK: non-microprocessor controlled knees. Source: [15, 28, 30, 35–40]

quality of life, this leads to 91.4 more QALYs in MPK users compared to NMPK users (453.3 vs. 361.9). The probabilistic sensitivity analysis supports the same conclusions: on average, the number of life years increases by14 years, ranging from 5 to 25 years per 100 MPK users, and the discounted QALYs gained average 102 years, ranging from 82 to 125 years per 100 MPK users.

Economic benefits
Direct healthcare cost and indirect cost
The simulation for a 10-year period shows reductions in falls and incident osteoarthritis of the intact knees correspond to savings in direct healthcare cost of $3496 and $180 per person per year, respectively. Overall, on a per person per year basis, MPK users have a lower direct healthcare cost than NMPK users, $2890 vs. $6566 (Fig. 3). Moreover, MPK is associated with a reduction of $909 ($4268 vs. $5177) in indirect cost, which includes lost wages, caregiving expenses, and transportation expenses.

Cost of device acquisition
Over a 10-year time period, MPK acquisition and repair cost amounts to $7925 per person per year taking into account the effect of survival. The estimate varies from $6054 to $8379 in the probabilistic sensitivity analysis. Similarly, on a per person per year basis, the acquisition and repair of NMPK cost $1638, varying from $785 to $2183 according to the probabilistic sensitivity analysis.

Total cost
The resulting total cost in the simulation, defined as the sum of direct ($2890 vs. $6566), indirect ($4268 vs. $5177), and device acquisition and repair cost ($7925 vs. $1638), is $15,083 and $13,382 per person per year for MPK and NMPK users, respectively. The total cost estimates for both MPK and NMPK users are sensitive to the proportion of medical falls among all falls, the average number of falls per faller per year, medical cost per major or minor injury fall, osteoarthritis-related medical cost, and discount rate, as indicated in the one-way sensitivity analyses. In the best scenario, the total cost per person per year for MPK users is $5042 lower than that of NMPK users; in the worst scenario, MPK users cost

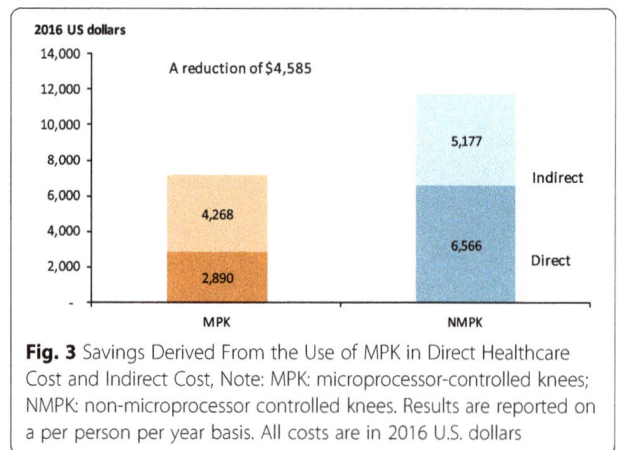

Fig. 3 Savings Derived From the Use of MPK in Direct Healthcare Cost and Indirect Cost, Note: MPK: microprocessor-controlled knees; NMPK: non-microprocessor controlled knees. Results are reported on a per person per year basis. All costs are in 2016 U.S. dollars

$5268 more per person per year compared to NMPK users.

In the K1 and K2 population, MPK is associated with a reduction of $4237 per person per year in direct cost and $928 in indirect cost. The total cost associated with MPK is $2022 higher per person per year compared to NMPK. In the best scenario, the total cost of MPK is $5671 less, and in the worst scenario, $6074 more expensive than NMPK.

Combining economic and clinical benefits

When the base case input values were used, for a 10-year time period, MPK resulted in an increase of 0.91 QALY per person and an increase of $10,604 in total cost per person, as illustrated by the orange-red dot in Fig. 4. The corresponding base case ICER is $11,606 per QALY. The blue dots in Fig. 4 were generated from the probabilistic sensitivity analysis. In summary, MPK devices are more effective in all of the simulated scenarios, but also more costly in 83% of the simulated scenarios. The probabilistic sensitivity analysis results in ICERs ranging from -$25,355 to $36,357 per QALY.

In the K1 and K2 population, MPK has an ICER of $13,568 per QALY. MPK may dominate NMPK as suggested in the probabilistic analysis, with an ICER of -$28,302 per QALY, meaning that it incurs lower total cost while leads to higher health status than does NMPK. The highest ICER is $41,498 per QALY in the probabilistic sensitivity analysis.

Discussion

This study is the first of its kind in the prosthetics literature in the U.S. that integrates both clinical and economic data to assess the cost-effectiveness of advanced prosthetics for transfemoral amputees, specifically MPK.

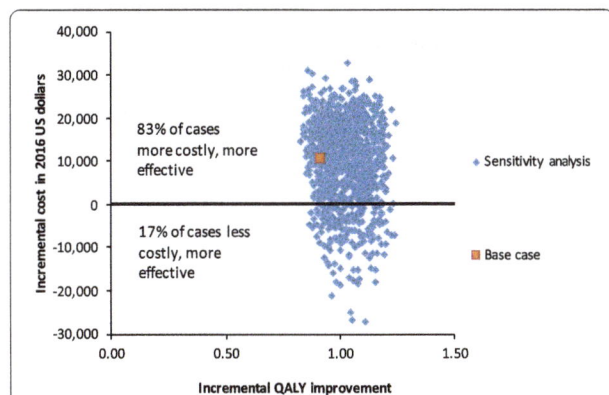

Fig. 4 Incremental Cost and Effectiveness of MPK in Comparison to NMPK in K3/K4 Amputees, Note: MPK: microprocessor-controlled knees; NMPK: non-microprocessor controlled knees. QALY: quality adjusted life year. All costs are in 2016 U.S. dollars

The results suggest that MPK is associated with substantial clinical benefits and cost-effectiveness compared to NMPK. It has been consistently demonstrated in the published literature that MPK leads to clinical improvements, such as improved walking speed, gait symmetry, and obstacle assessment. These clinical improvements, in turn, are associated with sizeable reductions in injurious falls and incident osteoarthritis and as a result, lower mortality rates.

The substantial clinical benefits of MPK can be largely attributed to reductions of falls with injuries and osteoarthritis incidences. This is plausible from a clinical perspective. For example, the computer software in MPK allows for the knee to dynamically adjust to uneven terrain, leading to improved stability and user confidence. The increased stability is thought to reduce cognitive burden and energy expenditure [41]. Increased stability, improved user confidence, and reduced cognitive burden and energy expenditures could all contribute to reductions in the risk of falls [15, 42].

The reduction in the knee moment associated with MPK likely eases the burden on the intact limb and therefore, reduces the probability of developing osteoarthritis in the intact knee. The knee moment is a surrogate for the force an individual absorbs when striking the ground during walking. Because of MPK's ability to adjust dynamically to uneven ground, MPK users are exposed to weaker forces when striking the ground, or smaller knee moment, than NMPK users. Due to the need for compensation, such forces are absorbed by the lower limb joints of the intact limb, and increase the burden on the healthy knee, hip and ankle, which is the expected mechanism through which osteoarthritis develops in the healthy limb [43].

When examining the life years gained, on average, an MPK user lives 0.09 year longer than an NMPK user over a 10-year time period; but when life years are adjusted by quality, an MPK user gains 0.91 QALYs over an NMPK user. The difference between the number of life years gained and the number of QALYs gained is attributed to the substantial improvement in the quality of life, ranging from 10% to 37%. This finding is consistent with prior evidence that MPK is associated with improved mobility, safety, user confidence, activities of daily living, the ability of living independently, and satisfaction [44–48], and thus substantially the better quality of life for amputees.

While there are some cases where a medical innovation leads to net cost savings, a majority of medical innovations would result in a positive ICER, where a new technology leads to better health but costs more than conventional technologies. The commonly accepted thresholds of fiscal costs for value varies from $50,000 to $150,000 [49–51]. In other words, if a new technology increases the cost by $50,000 or less for every QALY gained, it is considered having good value for the money. MPK has an ICER of $11,606 per QALY, well below the commonly accepted threshold, and thus provides good value for the money. In addition, even when compared to technologies commonly reimbursed by payers in the U.S., MPK fares better. For example, total knee arthroplasty and prophylactic cardioverter defibrillator implantation have an ICER of $14,572 and $76,396 per QALY, respectively [52–56], both of which are higher than that of MPK.

Because the payment system lags behind the advancement in technologies and focuses on cost-cutting rather than value, there is a need to shift the dialogue from a cost-driven payment approach to a value-based payment approach. And this is exactly where the U.S. health care system is headed [57]. However, sophisticated payment approaches such as outcome-based contracts or risk-sharing arrangements require the industry to develop sophisticated methodologies and robust evidence for the economic value of new technologies. As reflected in AOPA's Prosthetics 2020 Initiative, the industry is aiming to build the infrastructure needed for evidence generation, such as establishing patient registries and collecting clinical and economic data [58]. The initiative will help facilitate such a transition, while this analysis and the research gaps identified could serve as a good starting point.

Limitations

There is a limited number of studies that directly compare MPK to NMPK, and some model parameters had to come from studies examining a non-amputee population. For example, the proportion of medical falls out of all falls came from the non-amputee literature. The model assumes that parameters are generalizable from a non-amputee population to an amputee population.

The quality of the studies used to extract model parameters is suboptimal. For the parameters needed in the model, there are no published randomized clinical trials that compare MPK to NMPK. In addition, studies cited often have small sample sizes that could lead to large uncertainty in the estimates of MPK's impact [26, 59]. Also, studies comparing MPK to NMPK often collected data for a limited time period varying from several weeks to a year. For the studies with less than one-year observation period, findings beyond the study period had to be extrapolated for modeling purposes. No studies have examined long-term health outcomes such as obesity, diabetes, and cardiovascular diseases. The lack of studies on these long-term outcomes could potentially lead to an under-estimation of the economic impact of MPK.

Existing studies also have a narrow focus in terms of the amputee population, with an average age of between 38 and 62 and a functional level of K3 or K4. As a result, the effects of MPK on various outcomes might not be generalizable to the Medicare population although the Medicare population does contain numerous younger constituents, for example, dual-eligible combat injured Veterans and others. For the same reason, the modeling results for the K1 and K2 population may not be reliable because most model parameters were extracted from studies for K3 and K4 amputees.

No prior studies examined directly MPK's impact on incident osteoarthritis and the model relies on expert opinion. While it is generally accepted that differences in gait mechanics manifest in the development of osteoarthritis, there are no studies that demonstrate the causality. Expert consultation suggested that knee moments may represent a reasonable surrogate for the development of osteoarthritis; however, in the absence of long-term studies, it is a limitation.

Finally, the current Medicare payments were used as the numerator of the ICER. Since payment levels are different from the cost of manufacturing MPKs or NMPKs, the estimated numerators of ICERs may not represent the true cost differences between MPKs and NMPKs. If payment levels of MPK and NMPK change in the future, ICER ratios will change accordingly.

Conclusions

Prior studies have demonstrated that for transfemoral amputees, MPK is superior to NMPK in improving physical function and is associated with sizeable reductions in injurious falls and incident osteoarthritis in the intact limb. Once converted to economic benefits, MPK has an ICER of $11,606 per QALY gained and therefore provides good value for the money compared to NMPK. MPK's economic benefits are comparable to or even greater than widely reimbursed technologies such as total knee replacement and implantable cardioverter defibrillator.

Abbreviations
AOPA: American orthotic and prosthetic association; CMS: Centers for medicare and medicaid services; EQ-5D: EuroQol five dimensions questionnaire; ICER: Incremental cost-effectiveness ratio; K1: Medicare functional classification level 1; K2: Medicare functional classification level 2; K3: Medicare functional classification level 3; K4: Medicare functional classification level 4; MPK: Microprocessor-controlled prosthetic knee; NMPK: Non–microprocessor-controlled prosthetic knee; PEQ: Prosthesis Evaluation Questionnaire; QALY: Quality-adjusted life year; SF-36: 36-Item Short Form Health Survey

Acknowledgments
We would like to acknowledge the current and past Presidents the AOPA, including Charles Dankmeyer, James Campbell, and Michael Oros, who together with the Prosthetics 2020 Medical Advisory Board, the Steering Committee, and all the members of the Technical Advisory Committee for their knowledge and expertise. Thanks also go to the AOPA staff, in particular, Tom Fise, Joe McTernan, and Ashlie White for their support and guidance. We want to express our gratitude to our panel of experts who helped facilitate discussions and refine our methodology, literature review, and analysis, including Andreas Kannenberg, M.D., Ph.D. (Otto Bock Healthcare LP); Kenton Kaufman, Ph.D. (Mayo Clinic); Stephen Blatchford, M.Sc., M.B.A. (Chas A. Blatchford and Sons, Ltd.); Kim De Roy, M.Ed., M.Sc. (Ossur); Michael Oros, Certified Prosthetist and Orthotist, Fellow of the American Academy of Orthotists and Prosthetists (Scheck and Siress); Sam Liang, B.S.E., M.B.A. (Hanger Clinic); Jim Campbell, Ph.D. (Hanger Clinic); Michael Jason Highsmith, Ph.D. (Department of Veterans Affairs); David Moser, Ph.D. (Blatchford Group); Mike McGrath, Ph.D. (Blatchford Group); Saeed Zahedi, Ph.D. (Chas A. Blatchford and Sons, Ltd.); Maynard Carkhuff, B.S., M.B.A. (Freedom Innovations); Jim Colvin, B.S.E, M.S.E. (The Ohio Willow Wood Company); Robert Gailey, Ph.D. (University of Miami); and Brian Kaluf, B.S.E., Certified Prosthetist (Ability Prosthetics and Orthotics). In addition, special thanks go to David Felson, Ph.D., with the University of Manchester for his expert guidance on osteoarthritis and David Ganz, Ph.D., at the RAND Corporation for his help with the modeling of falls. We are grateful to Audrey El-Gamil and Nikolay Manolov at Dobson and DaVanzo, LLC, for their expertise and for providing information from Medicare claims data.

Funding
The publication cost of this article was funded by the American Orthotic and Prosthetic Association (AOPA). The sponsor helped the authors identify experts in the field to convene a technical panel but did not influence the study design, data collection, analysis, and the interpretation of findings.

Authors' contributions
HL managed the study and wrote the manuscript. RC and CC convened expert panel discussions, collected data, compiled the data into a format that could be utilized for the modeling, and were major contributors to the manuscript writing. MH conducted the simulation model, helped interpreted the simulation results, and contributed to the writing of the method section. SM provided guidance during the study and was a major contributor in writing the manuscript. RH provided guidance to the development and use of the simulation and critiqued the manuscript. All authors read and approved the final manuscript.

Authors' information
The manuscript was adapted from a RAND report, which can be downloaded here: https://www.rand.org/content/dam/rand/pubs/research_reports/RR2000/RR2096/RAND_RR2096.pdf.

Competing interests
The authors declare that they have no competing interests.

Author details
[1]RAND Corporation, 1776 Main Street, Santa Monica, CA 90401, USA. [2]RAND Corporation, 1200 South Hayes Street, Arlington, VA 22202-5050, USA. [3]RAND Corporation, 20 Park Plaza, Suite 920, Boston, MA 02116, USA.

References
1. Ziegler-Graham K, MacKenzie EJ, Ephraim PL, Travison TG, Brookmeyer R. Estimating the prevalence of limb loss in the United States: 2005 to 2050. Arch Phys Med Rehabil. 2008;89(3):422–9.
2. Centers for Disease Control and Prevention: Limb Loss Awareness. 2015.
3. National Center for Health Statistics. Health, United States. In: 2004: with chartbook on trends in the health of Americans; 2004.
4. Adams PF, Hendershot GE, Marano MA. Current estimates from the National Health Interview Survey. Vital Health Stat 10. 1996;1999(200):1–203.
5. Remes L, Isoaho R, Vahlberg T, Hiekkanen H, Korhonen K, Viitanen M, Rautava P. Major lower extremity amputation in elderly patients with peripheral arterial disease: incidence and survival rates. Aging Clin Exp Res. 2008;20(5):385–93.
6. Dillingham TR, Pezzin LE. Postacute care services use for dysvascular amputees: a population-based study of Massachusetts. Am J Phys Med Rehabil. 2005;84(3):147–52.
7. Traugh G, Corcoran P, Reyes R. Energy expenditure of ambulation in patients with above-knee amputations. Arch Phys Med Rehabil. 1975; 56(2):67–71.
8. Gjovaag T, Starholm IM, Mirtaheri P, Hegge FW, Skjetne K. Assessment of aerobic capacity and walking economy of unilateral transfemoral amputees. Prosthetics Orthot Int. 2014;38(2):140–7.
9. Starholm IM, Mirtaheri P, Kapetanovic N, Versto T, Skyttemyr G, Westby FT, Gjovaag T. Energy expenditure of transfemoral amputees during floor and treadmill walking with different speeds. Prosthetics Orthot Int. 2016;40(3):336–42.
10. Russell Esposito E, Rabago CA, Wilken J. The influence of traumatic transfemoral amputation on metabolic cost across walking speeds. Prosthetics Orthot Int. 2017; https://doi.org/10.1177/0309364617708649.
11. Seymour R, Engbretson B, Kott K, Ordway N, Brooks G, Crannell J, Hickernell E, Wheeler K. Comparison between the C-leg® microprocessor-controlled prosthetic knee and non-microprocessor control prosthetic knees: a preliminary study of energy expenditure, obstacle course performance, and quality of life survey. Prosthetics Orthot Int. 2007;31(1):51–61.
12. Bellmann M, Schmalz T, Blumentritt S. Comparative biomechanical analysis of current microprocessor-controlled prosthetic knee joints. Arch Phys Med Rehabil. 2010;91(4):644–52.
13. Kaufman KR, Frittoli S, Frigo CA. Gait asymmetry of transfemoral amputees using mechanical and microprocessor-controlled prosthetic knees. Clin Biomech. 2012;27(5):460–5.
14. Gailey RS, Roach KE, Applegate EB, Cho B, Cunniffe B, Licht S, Maguire M, Nash MS. The amputee mobility predictor: an instrument to assess determinants of the lower-limb amputee's ability to ambulate. Arch Phys Med Rehabil. 2002;83(5):613–27.
15. Hafner BJ, Smith DG. Differences in function and safety between Medicare functional classification Level-2 and -3 transfemoral amputees and influence of prosthetic knee joint control. J Rehabil Res Dev. 2009;46(3):417–33.
16. Rice T, Matsuoka KY. The Impact of Cost-Sharing on Appropriate Utilization and Health Status: A Review of the Literature on Seniors (2004). Med Care Res Rev. 2003;61:415–20. 427–428
17. AOPA: Breaking News: DME MACs Issue Draft Policy Revision for Lower Limb Prostheses. 2015.
18. Bureau of Labor Statistics. Consumer Price Index - All Items & Medical Care (2000–2016). In: United States Department of Labor, Bureau of Labor Statistics; 2017.
19. OANDA Corporation. Average Exchange Rates. In: OANDA; 2017.
20. Medicare Payment Advisory Commission. Medicare payment advisory commission report to the congress, march 2010. J Pain Palliat Care Pharmacother. 2010;24(3):302–5.
21. Hazen G. Cohort decomposition for Markov cost-effectiveness models. Med Decis Mak. 2011;31(1):19–34.
22. Sonnenberg FA, Beck JR. Markov models in medical decision making: a practical guide. Med Decis Mak. 1993;13(4):322–38.
23. Weinstein MC, O'brien B, Hornberger J, Jackson J, Johannesson M, McCabe C, Luce BR. Principles of good practice for decision analytic modeling in health-care evaluation: report of the ISPOR task force on good research practices—modeling studies. Value Health. 2003;6(1):9–17.
24. Orendurff MS, Segal AD, Klute GK, McDowell ML, Pecoraro JA, Czerniecki JM. Gait efficiency using the C-leg. J Rehabil Res Dev. 2006; 43(2):239–46.
25. Segal AD, Orendurff MS, Klute GK, McDowell ML, Pecoraro JA, Shofer J,

Czerniecki JM. Kinematic and kinetic comparisons of transfemoral amputee gait using C-LEG and MAUCH SNS prosthetic knees. J Rehabil Res Dev. 2006;43(7):857–69.

26. Kahle JT, Highsmith MJ, Hubbard SL. Comparison of nonmicroprocessor knee mechanism versus C-leg on prosthesis evaluation questionnaire, stumbles, falls, walking tests, stair descent, and knee preference. J Rehabil Res Dev. 2008;45(1):1–13.

27. Morgenroth DC, Gellhorn AC, Suri P. Osteoarthritis in the disabled population: a mechanical perspective. PM&R. 2012;4(5):S20–7.

28. Hafner BJ, Willingham LL, Buell NC, Allyn KJ, Smith DG. Evaluation of function, performance, and preference as transfemoral amputees transition from mechanical to microprocessor control of the prosthetic knee. Arch Phys Med Rehabil. 2007;88(2):207–17.

29. Schmalz T, Blumentritt S, Jarasch R. Energy expenditure and biomechanical characteristics of lower limb amputee gait: the influence of prosthetic alignment and different prosthetic components. Gait Posture. 2002;16(3):255–63.

30. Kaufman KR, Levine JA, Brey RH, McCrady SK, Padgett DJ, Joyner MJ. Energy expenditure and activity of transfemoral amputees using mechanical and microprocessor-controlled prosthetic knees. Arch Phys Med Rehabil. 2008; 89(7):1380–5.

31. Datta D, Heller B, Howitt J. A comparative evaluation of oxygen consumption and gait pattern in amputees using intelligent prostheses and conventionally damped knee swing-phase control. Clin Rehabil. 2005;19(4):398–403.

32. Johansson JL, Sherrill DM, Riley PO, Bonato P, Herr H. A clinical comparison of variable-damping and mechanically passive prosthetic knee devices. Am J Phys Med Rehabil. 2005;84(8):563–75.

33. Klute GK, Berge JS, Orendurff MS, Williams RM, Czerniecki JM. Prosthetic intervention effects on activity of lower-extremity amputees. Arch Phys Med Rehabil. 2006;87(5):717–22.

34. Kaufman KR, Levine JA, Brey RH, Iverson BK, McCrady SK, Padgett DJ, Joyner MJ. Gait and balance of transfemoral amputees using passive mechanical and microprocessor-controlled prosthetic knees. Gait Posture. 2007;26(4): 489–93.

35. Prinsen EC, Nederhand MJ, Olsman J, Rietman JS. Influence of a user-adaptive prosthetic knee on quality of life, balance confidence, and measures of mobility: a randomised cross-over trial. Clin Rehabil. 2015; 29(6):581–91.

36. William D, Beasley E, Shaw A. Investigation of the quality of life of persons with a Transfemoral amputation who use a C-leg® prosthetic device. Journal of Prosthetics & Orthotics (JPO). 2013;25(3):100–9.

37. Seelen HAM, Hemmen B, Schmeets AJ, Ament AJH, Evers SMA. Costs and consequences of a prosthesis with an electronically controlled stance and swing phase controlled knee joint. Technol Disabil. 2009;21(1/2):25–34.

38. Brodtkorb T-H, Henriksson M, Johannesen-Munk K, Thidell F. Cost-effectiveness of C-leg compared with non–microprocessor-controlled knees: a modeling approach. Arch Phys Med Rehabil. 2008;89(1):24–30.

39. Gerzeli S, Torbica A, Fattore G. Cost utility analysis of knee prosthesis with complete microprocessor control (C-leg) compared with mechanical technology in trans-femoral amputees. Eur J Health Econ. 2009;10(1):47–55.

40. Cutti AG, Lettieri E, Del Maestro M, Radaelli G, Luchetti M, Verni G, Masella C. Stratified cost-utility analysis of C-leg versus mechanical knees: findings from an Italian sample of transfemoral amputees. Prosthetics Orthot Int. 2017;41(3):227–36.

41. Highsmith MJ, Kahle JT, Bongiorni DR, Sutton BS, Groer S, Kaufman KR. Safety, energy efficiency, and cost efficacy of the C-leg for transfemoral amputees: a review of the literature. Prosthetics Orthot Int. 2010;34(4): 362–77.

42. Hafner BJ, Askew RL. Physical performance and self-report outcomes associated with use of passive, adaptive, and active prosthetic knees in persons with unilateral, transfemoral amputation: randomized crossover trial. J Rehabil Res Dev. 2015;52(6):677–99.

43. Felson DT. Osteoarthritis as a disease of mechanics. Osteoarthr Cartil. 2013; 21(1):10–5.

44. Berry D, Olson MD, Larntz K. Perceived stability, function, and satisfaction among transfemoral amputees using microprocessor and nonmicroprocessor controlled prosthetic knees: a multicenter survey. J Prosthet Orthot. 2009;21(1):32–42.

45. Theeven P, Hemmen B, Rings F, Meys G, Brink P, Smeets R, Seelen H. Functional added value of microprocessor-controlled knee joints in daily life

46. Theeven PJ, Hemmen B, Geers RP, Smeets RJ, Brink PR, Seelen HA. Influence of advanced prosthetic knee joints on perceived performance and everyday life activity level of low-functional persons with a transfemoral amputation or knee disarticulation. J Rehabil Med. 2012;44(5):454–61.

47. Sawers AB, Hafner BJ. Outcomes associated with the use of microprocessor-controlled prosthetic knees among individuals with unilateral transfemoral limb loss: a systematic review. J Rehabil Res Dev. 2013;50(3):273–314.

48. Kannenberg A, Zacharias B, Probsting E. Benefits of microprocessor-controlled prosthetic knees to limited community ambulators: systematic review. J Rehabil Res Dev. 2014;51(10):1469–96.

49. Institute for Clinical and Economic Review. Final Value Assessment Framework: Updates for 2017–2019. Boston: Institute for Clinical and Economic Review; 2017.

50. Weinstein MC. How much are Americans willing to pay for a quality-adjusted life year? Med Care. 2008;46(4):343–5.

51. Neumann PJ, Cohen JT, Weinstein MC. Updating cost-effectiveness–the curious resilience of the $50,000-per-QALY threshold. N Engl J Med. 2014; 371(9):796–7.

52. Losina E, Walensky RP, Kessler CL, Emrani PS, Reichmann WM, Wright EA, Holt HL, Solomon DH, Yelin E, Paltiel AD, et al. Cost-effectiveness of total knee arthroplasty in the United States: patient risk and hospital volume. Arch Intern Med. 2009;169(12):1113–21. discussion 1121-1112

53. Waimann CA, Fernandez-Mazarambroz RJ, Cantor SB, Lopez-Olivo MA, Zhang H, Landon GC, Siff SJ, Suarez-Almazor ME. Cost-effectiveness of total knee replacement: a prospective cohort study. Arthritis Care Res. 2014;66(4):592–9.

54. Ruiz D, Koenig L, Dall TM, Gallo P, Narzikul A, Parvizi J, Tongue J. The direct and indirect costs to society of treatment for end-stage knee osteoarthritis. J Bone Joint Surg Am. 2013;95(16):1473–80.

55. Elmallah RK, Chughtai M, Khlopas A, Bhowmik-Stoker M, Bozic KJ, Kurtz SM, Mont MA. Determining cost-effectiveness of total hip and knee arthroplasty using the short form-6D utility measure. J Arthroplast. 2017;32(2):351–4.

56. Garcia-Perez L, Pinilla-Dominguez P, Garcia-Quintana A, Caballero-Dorta E, Garcia-Garcia FJ, Linertova R, Imaz-Iglesia I. Economic evaluations of implantable cardioverter defibrillators: a systematic review. Eur J Health Econ. 2015;16(8):879–93.

57. Centers for Medicare and Medicaid Services. Better care. Smarter spending. Healthier people: improving quality and paying for what works. CMS Fact Sheet Accessed. 2016;25:2016.

58. The American Orthotic and Prosthetic Association. Prosthetics 2020 and Orthotics 2020. Alexandria: The American Orthotic and Prosthetic Association; 2017.

59. Wong CK, Rheinstein J, Stern MA. Benefits for adults with Transfemoral amputations and peripheral artery disease using microprocessor compared with nonmicroprocessor prosthetic knees. Am J Phys Med Rehabil. 2015; 94(10):804–10.

60. Dederer L. Quality of life of amputee patients after supply with the electronically controlled knee pass part "C-leg": Prospective consultation of patients with care. Dissertation (in German): Westfälische Wilhelms-Universität Münster, Germany; 2013.

61. Kelsey JL, Berry SD, Procter-Gray E, Quach L, Nguyen US, Li W, Kiel DP, Lipsitz LA, Hannan MT. Indoor and outdoor falls in older adults are different: the maintenance of balance, independent living, intellect, and zest in the elderly of Boston study. J Am Geriatr Soc. 2010;58(11):2135–41.

62. Schiller JS, Kramarow EA, Dey AN. Fall injury episodes among noninstitutionalized older adults: United States, 2001-2003. Adv Data. 2007; 21(392):1–16. https://www.ncbi.nlm.nih.gov/pubmed/17953135.

63. Verma SK, Willetts JL, Corns HL, Marucci-Wellman HR, Lombardi DA, Courtney TK. Falls and fall-related injuries among community-dwelling adults in the United States. PLoS One. 2016;11(3):e0150939.

64. Sterling DA, O'Connor JA, Bonadies J. Geriatric falls: injury severity is high and disproportionate to mechanism. J Trauma. 2001;50(1):116–9.

65. Kim SB, Zingmond DS, Keeler EB, Jennings LA, Wenger NS, Reuben DB, Ganz DA. Development of an algorithm to identify fall-related injuries and costs in Medicare data. Inj Epidemiol. 2016;3(1):1–11.

66. Mundell B, Maradit Kremers H, Visscher S, Hoppe K, Kaufman K. Direct medical costs of accidental falls for adults with transfemoral amputations. Prosthetics Orthot Int. 2017; https://doi.org/10.1177/0309364617704804.

67. Miller WC, Deathe AB, Speechley M, Koval J. The influence of falling, fear of

falling, and balance confidence on prosthetic mobility and social activity among individuals with a lower extremity amputation. Arch Phys Med Rehabil. 2001;82(9):1238–44.

68. Burns ER, Stevens JA, Lee R. The direct costs of fatal and non-fatal falls among older adults - United States. J Saf Res. 2016;58:99–103.

69. Stevens JA, Corso PS, Finkelstein EA, Miller TR. The costs of fatal and non-fatal falls among older adults. Injury Prev. 2006;12(5):290–5.

70. Pension Rights Center. Sources for income of older adults: US Department of Labor, Bureau of Labor Statistics; 2016.

71. Bureau of Labor Statistics. May 2015 National Occupational Employment and Wage Estimates. Washington, DC: Division of Occupational Employment Statistics; 2015.

72. Bureau of Labor Statistics: Labor Force Statistics from the Current Population Survey - Employment status of the civilian noninstitutional population by age, sex, and race. 2015.

73. Xie F, Kovic B, Jin X, He X, Wang M, Silvestre C. Economic and humanistic burden of osteoarthritis: a systematic review of large sample studies. PharmacoEconomics. 2016;34(11):1087–100.

74. Berger A, Hartrick C, Edelsberg J, Sadosky A, Oster G. Direct and indirect economic costs among private-sector employees with osteoarthritis. J Occup Environ Med. 2011;53(11):1228–35.

75. Dibonaventura M, Gupta S, McDonald M, Sadosky A. Evaluating the health and economic impact of osteoarthritis pain in the workforce: results from the National Health and wellness survey. BMC Musculoskelet Disord. 2011; 12(83):1–9.

76. Sanders GD, Neumann PJ, Basu A, Brock DW, Feeny D, Krahn M, Kuntz KM, Meltzer DO, Owens DK, Prosser LA. Recommendations for conduct, methodological practices, and reporting of cost-effectiveness analyses: second panel on cost-effectiveness in health and medicine. JAMA. 2016; 316(10):1093–103.

Economic value of orthotic and prosthetic services among medicare beneficiaries

Allen Dobson, Kennan Murray[*], Nikolay Manolov and Joan E. DaVanzo

From Second World Congress hosted by the American Orthotic & Prosthetic Association (AOPA)
Las Vegas, NV, USA. 06-09 September 2017

Abstract

Background: There are few studies of the economic value of orthotic and prosthetic services. A prior cohort study of orthotic and prosthetic Medicare beneficiaries based on Medicare Parts A and B claims from 2007 to 2010 concluded that patients who received timely orthotic or prosthetic care had comparable or lower total health care costs than a comparison group of untreated patients. This follow-up study reports on a parallel analysis based on Medicare claims from 2011 to 2014 and includes Part D in addition to Parts A and B services and expenditures. Its purpose is to validate earlier findings on the extent to which Medicare patients who received select orthotic and prosthetic services had less health care utilization, lower Medicare payments, and potentially fewer negative outcomes compared to matched patients not receiving these services.

Methods: This is a retrospective cohort analysis of 78,707 matched pairs of Medicare beneficiaries with clinical need for orthotic and prosthetic services ($N = 157,414$) using 2011–2014 Medicare claims data. It uses propensity score matching techniques to control for observable selection bias. Economically, a cost-consequence evaluation over a four-year time horizon was performed.

Results: Patients who received lower extremity orthotics had 18-month episode costs that were $1939 lower than comparable patients who did not receive orthotic treatment ($22,734 vs $24,673). Patients who received spinal orthotic treatment had 18-month episode costs that were $2094 lower than comparable non-treated patients ($23,560 vs $25,655). Study group beneficiaries receiving both types of orthotics had significantly lower Part D spending than those not receiving treatment ($p < 0.05$). Patients who received lower extremity prostheses had comparable 15-month episode payments to matched beneficiaries not receiving prostheses ($68,877 vs $68,893) despite the relatively high cost of the prosthesis.

Conclusions: These results were consistent with those found in the prior study and suggest that orthotic and prosthetic services provide value to the Medicare program and to the patient.

Keywords: Amputation, Cost-effectiveness, Limb-loss, Medicare, Orthoses, Prostheses, Rehabilitation

* Correspondence: kennan.murray@dobsondavanzo.com
Dobson DaVanzo & Associates, LLC, 450 Maple Avenue East, Suite 303,
Vienna, VA 22180, USA

Background

Orthotic and lower extremity prosthetic devices and related clinical services are designed to provide patients with stability and mobility. While the literature contains considerable evidence of geographic variation in both major amputation rates and the use of orthotic and prosthetic (O&P) services [1–3], there are limited studies of the extent to which beneficiaries who receive O&P services experience a reduction in complications and/or costs with favorable outcomes [4].

While the variability in measures of quality and patient outcomes in research on O&P services can make comparisons difficult, studies have shown that the provision of O&P services led to measurable improvements in the quality of patient care and functional and psychosocial outcomes [5–7]. Beyond physical health, receipt of O&P services is associated with improved mental health status, in terms of social functioning, general health perception, and role limitation due to emotional problems [8]. The receipt of O&P services may also lead to societal gains including the return to work [9].

Additionally, O&P services can reduce health care spending via better patient outcomes, which in turn reduce other types of health care utilization [10, 11]. Long-term savings are thought to result when patients receive appropriate orthotic and prosthetic care. Without such care, individuals may live more sedentary lifestyles, which research has shown leads to secondary complications, such as diabetes and related comorbidities, as well as increases in health care utilization and spending [12]. Additionally, in some cases, the use of more sophisticated technology has been found to increase the quality of care and patient outcomes [13]. The beneficiary's quality of life may very well be improved as well through increased mobility [14].

Our prior custom cohort study of orthotic and prosthetic Medicare beneficiaries that was based on Medicare claims experience over the 2007–2010 period found that the study group of patients who received timely orthotic or prosthetic care had lower total health care costs than a comparison group of untreated patients [10]. This study reports on a parallel analysis based on Medicare claims from 2011 to 2014 and includes Part D in addition to Parts A and B. Its primary objective is to validate earlier conclusions on the extent to which Medicare patients who received select orthotic and prosthetic services had less total health care utilization, lower Medicare payments, and/or fewer negative outcomes compared to matched patients not receiving these services. While the data are from Medicare only, the results of this study can inform the value proposition of orthotics and prosthetics for other payers.

Methods

A retrospective cohort design of 78,707 one-to-one matched pairs of Medicare constituents ($N = 157,414$) was utilized. From an economic design type, a cost-consequence evaluation design was used with a total four-year time horizon. The payer's perspective was selected for study to gain an understanding of value as it relates to orthotic and prosthetic provision under the Medicare program as a primary member of the reimbursement community. Study procedures were administered in accordance with the Declaration of Helsinki.

This study focuses on three types of O&P services – lower extremity orthoses, spinal orthoses, and lower extremity prostheses. The analytic methodology consisted of three key activities, including: 1) developing patient cohorts of orthotic and prosthetic users and matched comparison groups using a propensity score approach; 2) developing clinical episodes of care for each individual beneficiary; and 3) calculating descriptive statistics and analyzing the impact associated with each O&P service on Medicare episode utilization and payments.

Developing patient cohorts

Analyses were conducted using Medicare claims from a custom database provided by the Centers for Medicare & Medicaid Services (CMS) (Data Use Agreement No. 28710). We requested a sample of beneficiaries with claims from 2011 to 2014 for patients with specified etiological diagnoses who received select lower extremity orthotic, spinal orthotic, or lower extremity prosthetic services. The etiological diagnosis related to the condition which ultimately led to the need for the lower extremity orthotic, spinal orthotic, or lower extremity prosthetic service (e.g., a functional diagnosis for a prosthetic device), not the diagnosis linked to the claims at the time of receipt of the service.[1] These beneficiaries represented the study group population for each O&P service.

CMS identified the comparison (i.e., control) group population by matching beneficiaries to the patients who received orthotic and/or prosthetic devices (study group) based on the presence of an etiological diagnosis, gender, age, and state of residence. CMS provided up to five comparison group patients, who did not receive the select O&P services of interest, preliminarily matched to each study group patient.

The sampling methodology utilized by CMS to extract the custom cohorts allowed the analyses to reflect those Medicare beneficiaries who received an appropriate etiological diagnosis after January 1, 2011.

Beneficiaries who died within three months of the etiological diagnosis were excluded from the cohorts. To be included in the study group, patients were required to have received specified orthotic or prosthetic services between January 1, 2012 and June 30, 2013. Beneficiaries in the prosthetic sample were required to have a relevant amputation documented in the claims during the study period. This sampling methodology ensured that the database included one year of claims prior to, and at least 18 months following, the receipt of the O&P service. Medicare health care claims across all care settings from 2011 to 2014 were obtained for the beneficiaries who met sampling specifications. Care settings included inpatient and outpatient hospitals, long-term care hospitals, skilled nursing facilities, inpatient rehabilitation facilities, home health agencies, hospice, physician/carrier visits, and durable medical equipment, prosthetics, orthotics, and supplies.

This database of study and comparison group beneficiaries served as the framework for the analytic sample selected using propensity score matching techniques. We used a one-to-one propensity score match across study and comparison group patients based on etiological diagnosis, comorbidities, patient sociodemographic characteristics (age, gender, race), and historical health care utilization. Additionally, because in the prosthetic analysis the clinical severity (and risk of imminent death) may have been a driver of whether or not the patient received a prosthesis, patients were also matched on the timing of death in relation to amputation, if applicable. As a result, mortality across the groups was excluded as a study outcome for the prosthetic analysis.

Propensity score matching techniques are widely used in observational studies when randomized controlled trials (RCTs) are not possible or are unethical or impractical to administer [15]. Literature suggests that applying these techniques to observational studies is an appropriate technique to remove observable selection bias among treatment and comparison groups and can result in findings that look like RCTs [16–19]. In addition, analyses based on administrative claims data are much less expensive than clinical trials.

Proper matching of the study and comparison group patients limited the number of episodes included in our study but helped to ensure that the study and comparison group patients were clinically and demographically similar [20]. Table 1 shows the number of study and comparison group patients included in each service group before and after matching. Propensity score matching resulted in 43,487 matched pairs of Medicare beneficiaries in the lower extremity orthotic model; 34,575 matched pairs in the spinal orthotic model; and 545 matched pairs of recent amputees in the prosthetic model. The number of orthotic patients in this current study is higher than in the 2007–2010 analysis, a designed increase in sample size resulting from the specifications of the custom cohort database. The relatively small number of beneficiaries included in the lower extremity prosthetic model was due to the requirement that amputation occur during the study window, which ensured the exclusion of long-term users who received replacement prosthetics during the study window, and also to the number of variables used in developing the propensity score match.

Developing episodes of care

Patient episodes were constructed to capture health care diagnoses, utilization, and expenditures prior to and after receipt of the orthotic or prosthetic device. Because actual costs were utilized in the analysis, and because at least one year of claims data prior to and after device provision was included, no additional discounting assumptions were incorporated. All patient episodes contained a pre-service window prior to the episode start, which allowed for the identification of comorbid conditions, patterns of institutional care, and other health care utilization used for risk-adjustment during the matching process. Episodes

Table 1 Distribution of Pairs (Study Group and Comparison Group Matches)

	Lower extremity orthotic analysis		Spinal orthotic analysis		Lower extremity prosthetic analysis	
	Study group	Comparison group	Study group	Comparison group	Study group	Comparison group
Number of patients with O&P service and etiological diagnosis included in custom cohort	239,655	255,156	224,994	240,609	13,823	5959
Number of pairs after propensity score match	43,487	43,487	34,573	34,573	545	545
Percent of patients represented in the effective sample	18.1%	17.0%	15.4%	14.4%	3.9%	9.1%

Source: Dobson | DaVanzo analysis of custom cohort Standard Analytic Files (2011–2014) for Medicare beneficiaries who received O&P services from January 1, 2012 through June 30, 2013 (and matched comparisons), according to custom cohort database definition

also contained a period of follow-up care, used to track trends in overall health care utilization, expenditures, and outcomes.

The episodes were structured similarly for the lower extremity and spinal orthotic analyses. For study group beneficiaries in these two service types, the post-service episode started upon receipt of the orthotic service, and the pre-service window comprised the 12 months prior to this date. The post-service period captured up to 18 months of Medicare claims after receiving the orthotic service. Because comparison group beneficiaries did not receive orthotic services, a proxy episode start date was established. To ensure the same post-service window for which health care utilization and expenditures were tracked and compared across cohorts, the length of time between etiological diagnosis and episode start, or "lag time," for the comparison group was set to the average of the length of time for study group participants of similar age and gender. This lag time was added to the date of etiological diagnosis to create an episode start date for each comparison group beneficiary. Similar to the study group, the pre-service window comprised the 12 months prior to the episode start date, and the post-service window comprised the 18 months following the start date.

This episode structure was modified for the prosthetic analysis. In the 2007–2010 study, analysis using a temporal autocorrelation function indicated that the optimal length of the post-period for the prosthetic analysis was 12 months following the episode start, which was approximately three months after amputation. However, the Affordable Care Act (ACA) was implemented since our prior analysis, requiring modifications to this 2011–2014 study. The ACA had a considerable impact on hospital inpatient and outpatient mix, stay duration, and re-admission policies, among other factors. To address this, we used a 15-month episode period starting with the date of hospital discharge associated with amputation for the 2011–2014

lower extremity prosthetic population, as contrasted to the 3-month waiting period post-amputation and an immediately subsequent 12-month episode period we had used for the 2007–2010 study. Thus, both study and comparison groups had a pre-service window comprising the 12 months prior to this hospital discharge and a 15-month post-service window immediately following it.

Calculating descriptive statistics and analyzing impact of orthotic/ prosthetic devices on overall patient Medicare expenditures

For each of the three analyses (lower extremity orthoses, spinal orthoses, and lower extremity prostheses), descriptive statistics were calculated for the study and comparison groups after the propensity score matching. The two groups were compared to each other based on the distribution of patient characteristics including but not limited to age, gender, race, and comorbidities. We then compared the total average episode Medicare payments of the study and comparison groups over the post-service period, as well as the distribution of payments by care settings, and a range of outcome measures, such as falls, hospitalizations, and days of rehabilitative/physical therapy.

Results

Demographic analysis

Table 2 presents the descriptive statistics of matched patients for each O&P service. Since the propensity score matching criteria included patient demographic characteristics and controlled for observable selection bias, the study and comparison group patients were highly similar within each O&P service type. No significant differences were found between the matched study and comparison groups for any variables used in the propensity score matching process, including age, gender, dual eligibility, and race, for any O&P service ($p < 0.05$).

Table 2 Descriptive Statistics across Matched Pairs (2011–2014)

Demographic characteristic	Lower extremity orthotic model		Spinal orthotic model		Lower extremity prosthetic model	
	Study group	Comparison group	Study group	Comparison group	Study group	Comparison group
Number of beneficiaries	43,487	43,487	34,575	34,575	545	545
Average age	68.6	68.7	67.2	67.2	65.9	65.9
Dual eligibility status	29.7%	29.7%	34.9%	34.9%	39.2%	39.2%
Gender: female	43.1%	43.1%	37.6%	37.6%	17.4%	17.4%
Race/Ethnicity: white	84.7%	84.7%	81.2%	81.2%	68.8%	68.8%
Race/Ethnicity: black or african american	8.3%	8.3%	11.8%	11.8%	24.8%	24.8%
Race/Ethnicity: hispanic	4.4%	4.4%	5.0%	4.4%	6.4%	6.4%

Differences were not significant at $\alpha = 0.05$
Source: Dobson | DaVanzo analysis of custom cohort Standard Analytic Files (2011–2014) for Medicare beneficiaries who received O&P services from January 1, 2012 through June 30, 2013 (and matched comparisons), according to custom cohort database definition

Table 3 presents the ten most common etiological diagnoses for each type of O&P service, representing over 95% of beneficiaries in each service type. Because all matched pairs were required to have the same etiological diagnoses, the percentages are

Table 3 Etiological Diagnoses across Matched Pairs (2011–2014)

Etiological diagnosis	Percent of matched pairs with diagnosis
Lower extremity orthoses	
Other connective tissue disease	32.4%
Spondylosis; intervertebral disc disorders; other back problems	17.9%
Other nervous system disorders	16.7%
Osteoarthritis	11.3%
Acute cerebrovascular disease	5.6%
Acquired foot deformities	3.8%
Fracture of lower limb	2.1%
Sprains and strains	2.1%
Multiple sclerosis	1.8%
Joint disorders and dislocations; trauma-related	1.5%
Spinal orthoses	
Spondylosis; intervertebral disc disorders; other back problems	40.1%
Other connective tissue disease	25.7%
Other nervous system disorders	15.6%
Osteoarthritis	7.7%
Other bone disease and musculoskeletal deformities	6.1%
Sprains and strains	2.0%
Other fractures	1.2%
Joint disorders and dislocations; trauma-related	0.7%
Other acquired deformities	0.4%
Other congenital anomalies	0.3%
Lower extremity prostheses	
Diabetes mellitus with complications	30.6%
Chronic ulcer of skin	18.0%
Peripheral and visceral atherosclerosis	17.8%
Other non-traumatic joint disorders	8.5%
Skin and subcutaneous tissue infections	7.9%
Other circulatory disease	4.9%
Complication of device; implant or graft	3.8%
Complications of surgical procedures or medical care	2.8%
Open wounds of extremities	2.7%
Infective arthritis and osteomyelitis	2.1%

Source: Dobson | DaVanzo analysis of custom cohort Standard Analytic Files (2011–2014) for Medicare beneficiaries who received O&P services from January 1, 2012 through June 30, 2013 (and matched comparisons), according to custom cohort database definition

identical among the study and comparison groups, and Table 3 therefore presents the percent of matched pairs with each diagnosis. The most common etiological diagnosis for beneficiaries in the lower extremity orthotic analysis was other connective tissue disease, followed by spondylosis. These were also the top two diagnoses for beneficiaries in the spinal orthotic analysis, although the hierarchy was reversed. The most common diagnosis for beneficiaries in the lower extremity prosthetic analysis was diabetes mellitus with complications, followed by chronic ulcer of skin.

Outcomes analysis: lower extremity orthoses

Table 4 presents the health care utilization and payments by care setting for those who received lower extremity orthotic services (study group) compared to those who did not (comparison group). It presents the results of the updated 2011–2014 analysis as well as the results of the initial 2007–2010 analysis for comparison.

Across the 18-month episode, in this updated analysis the study group patients had a total Medicare payment of $22,734 compared to $24,673 for the comparison group, so the episode payment was $1939 lower for the study group ($p < 0.05$). A main cause for this difference was significantly fewer admissions to acute care hospitals, as the study group patients were admitted 0.52 times during the episode, compared to 0.87 times for the comparison group ($p < 0.05$). This lower rate of utilization lowered the total episode payments by $572 for patients receiving orthoses.

In addition, similar to the 2007–2010 analysis, we again found that the lower extremity orthotic study group had significantly lower payments to physicians and outpatient hospitals. Study group beneficiaries also had lower overall Part D drug spending, a significant difference of $1044 ($p < 0.05$).

Despite having lower total episode payments, beneficiaries receiving the lower extremity orthoses demonstrated significantly higher expenditures in most post-acute care settings, including inpatient rehabilitation facilities ($641 vs $378), skilled nursing facilities ($1619 vs $1504), and home health ($1187 vs $908) ($p < 0.05$). These results are similar to those of the 2007–2010 analysis, with the exception of skilled nursing facilities. In the earlier analysis, expenditures in this care setting were $765 less than the comparison group across the 18-month episode. In addition, patients who received lower extremity orthoses received significantly more outpatient therapy than those who did not receive the orthotic (12.53 vs 4.93 visits, $p < 0.05$). As shown in Table 4, analysis of other outcomes revealed that study group patients

Table 4 Spending and Utilization for 18-Month Lower Extremity Orthotic Episode (2007–2010 and 2011–2014)

Care setting	2007–2010 analysis n = 34,864 Matched pairs			2011–2014 analysis n = 43,487 Matched pairs		
	Study	Comparison	Difference	Study	Comparison	Difference
Physician	$6482	$7171	-$688 *	$5629	$6078	-$449 *
DME	$2002	$966	$1036 *	$763	$602	$162 *
Acute Care Hospital / Other inpatient	$8392	$10,828	-$2436 *	$5640	$6212	-$572 *
Long Term Care Hospital	$366	$639	-$273 *	$239	$294	-$55
Inpatient Rehabilitation Facility (IRF)	$1178	$924	$255 *	$641	$378	$262 *
Outpatient	$3552	$3752	-$199 *	$2778	$3127	-$349 *
Skilled Nursing Facility	$2415	$3180	-$765 *	$1619	$1504	$115 *
Home health	$2231	$1912	$320 *	$1187	$908	$279 *
Hospice	$388	$556	-$168 *	$319	$607	-$288 *
Total Part D Drug Spending	–	–	–	$3920	$4964	-$1044 *
Total	$27,007	$29,927	-$2920 *	$22,734	$24,673	-$1939 *
Number of therapy visits	17.36	12.10	5.26 *	12.53	4.93	7.60 *
Number of fractures and falls	1.45	1.52	−0.07	0.38	0.48	−0.10 *
Number of inpatient admissions	–	–	–	0.52	0.87	−0.35 *
Length of stay for inpatient admissions (days)	–	–	–	2.64	4.77	−2.14 *
Number of emergency room admissions	1.08	1.20	−0.12 *	0.83	1.22	−0.39 *
Number of IRF admissions	–	–	–	0.03	0.04	0.00 *
Length of stay for IRF admissions (days)	0.72	0.52	0.20 *	0.42	0.47	−0.05 *
12-Month mortality rate	–	–	–	0.00	0.01	−0.01 *

* Difference is significant at $\alpha = 0.05$

Source: Dobson | DaVanzo analysis of custom cohort Standard Analytic Files (2007–2010 and 2011–2014) for Medicare beneficiaries who received O&P services from January 1, 2008 through June 30, 2009 or January 1, 2012 through June 30, 2013 (and matched comparisons), according to custom cohort database definition

experienced significantly fewer falls and fractures (0.38 compared to 0.48, $p < 0.05$) and significantly fewer emergency room (ER) admissions (0.83 vs 1.22, $p < 0.05$).

Figure 1 presents the cumulative episode payment for those who received the lower extremity orthoses compared to those who did not by episode month. Despite a period of higher spending in Months 7 to 12, the study group patients had lower Medicare episode payments than the comparison group. Thus, over the entire 18-month episode the cost of the orthotic was fully amortized through reduced utilization in other settings. These findings are consistent with those of the 2007–2010 analysis.

Outcomes analysis: spinal orthoses

Table 5 presents the health care utilization and payments by care setting for those patients who received spinal orthoses (study group) compared to those who did not (comparison group). Across the 18-month episode, the study group patients had significantly lower total episode payments across all care settings ($23,560 vs $25,655, $p < 0.05$). This result is different

than that found in the 2007–2010 analysis, which found a nonsignificant difference in total episode spending between the study and comparison groups.

In this updated analysis, a major contributor to the difference in total episode payments between the study and comparison groups was significantly lower payments for Part D drugs in the study group ($840 lower among Part D users only, $p < 0.05$). Study group patients had higher payments for DME services, inpatient rehabilitation facilities, and home health, but lower payments to acute care hospitals, long-term care hospitals and physician offices ($p < 0.05$). This is somewhat different than our earlier analysis, which found higher payments to physician offices and lower payments to inpatient rehabilitation facilities.

Despite higher payments for inpatient rehabilitation care in the study group, the average length of stay in inpatient rehabilitation facilities was significantly lower in this group (0.24 vs 0.32, $p < 0.05$). These patients appear more likely to return home faster and to receive follow up care in the home, as evidenced by higher payments to home health among the study group ($1100 vs $901, $p < 0.05$).

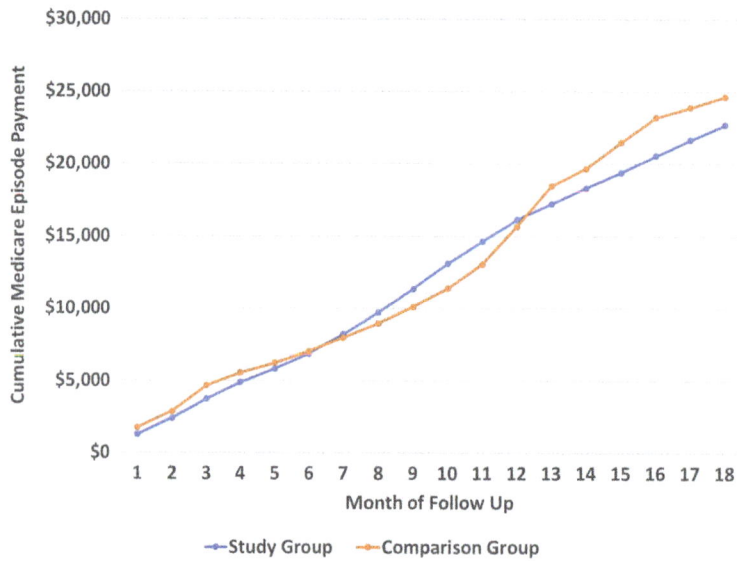

Fig. 1 Cumulative Lower Extremity Orthotic Episode Payment by Cohort

Study group patients who received spinal orthoses experienced the same number of fractures and falls compared to those who did not receive the orthoses, but a significantly lower number of emergency room admissions (0.81 admissions for the study group compared to 1.03 for the comparison group, $p < 0.05$).

Figure 2 presents the cumulative episode payment for those who received spinal orthoses compared to those who did not by episode month. Similar to the lower extremity orthotic analysis, this chart indicates that, despite a period of additional cost for the study group between months 7 to 12, the cost of the orthotic was fully amortized over the episode.

Outcomes analysis: lower extremity prostheses

Table 6 presents the health care payments by care setting for those who received lower extremity prostheses compared to those who did not. As discussed in the methodology, the results for lower extremity prostheses were compared across approximately 15 months post-service.

Across the 15-month episode, the study group patients had total Medicare payments that were slightly, but not significantly, lower than the comparison group ($68,877 for the study group compared to $68,893 for the comparison group). About 14% of the total episode payment for the study group patients is attributed to the prosthesis ($9694 of the total episode payment of $68,877). The prosthetic device represents an additional cost that was fully amortized within 15 months due to a reduction of care in other settings. This stands in contrast to the 2007–2010

analysis, which found higher total episode payments of $1015 among the study group.

The largest difference in payments between the study and comparison groups was for acute care hospitals. The study group patients had a significantly lower rate of hospitalization than the comparison group patients (1.23 admissions for the study group compared to 1.54 admissions for the comparison group, $p < 0.05$), resulting in lower episode Medicare payments for acute care hospitalizations ($15,529 for the study group compared to $19,851 for the comparison group, $p < 0.05$). These results are similar to those found in the 2007–2010 analysis.

Study group patients had significantly lower expenditures for facility-based long-term care and in-home hospice services than the comparison group patients ($p < 0.05$), but spending differences were not significantly different in other care settings. Expenditures were nominally lower among study group participants in physician offices, hospital outpatient departments, and skilled nursing facilities, but nominally higher among study group participants for inpatient rehabilitation facilities and home health. In addition, expenditures were lower for Part D drugs among the study group, although this difference was not significant.

Patients need to be trained and receive extensive therapy to properly use a prosthetic device, and study group patients had considerably higher utilization of outpatient therapy (26.86 visits vs 17.97 visits, $p < 0.05$). The number of fractures and falls and emergency room admissions were not significantly different between the study and comparison groups.

Figure 3 presents the cumulative episode payment for the study and comparison group by episode

Table 5 Spending and Utilization for 18-Month Spinal Orthotic Episode (2007–2010 and 2011–2014)

| Care setting | 2007–2010 analysis | | | 2011–2014 analysis update | | |
| | n = 6247 Matched pairs | | | n = 34,575 Matched pairs | | |
	Study	Comparison	Difference	Study	Comparison	Difference
Physician	$7907	$7439	$468*	$6291	$6570	-$279*
DME	$2605	$1288	$1317*	$722	$621	$101*
Acute Care Hospital / Other inpatient	$11,373	$11,830	-$457	$5913	$6294	-$381*
Long Term Care Hospital	$517	$837	-$320**	$190	$269	-$79*
Inpatient Rehabilitation Facility (IRF)	$990	$1188	-$198**	$433	$341	$92*
Outpatient	$3786	$4120	-$334	$2734	$3294	-$559*
Skilled Nursing Facility	$2188	$3175	-$987*	$1234	$1281	-$47*
Home Health	$2802	$2388	$414*	$1100	$901	$199*
Hospice	$431	$426	$5**	$234	$534	-$300*
Total Part D Drug Spending	–	–	–	$4709	$5550	-$840*
Total	$32,598	$32,691	-$93	$23,560	$25,655	-$2094*
Average number of therapy visits	14.95	12.91	2.04	6.14	2.06	4.08*
Average number of fractures and falls	2.05	1.56	0.50*	0.32	0.32	0.00
Average number of inpatient admissions	–	–	–	0.40	0.68	−0.28*
Length of Stay for inpatient admissions (days)	–	–	–	1.84	3.53	−1.69*
Average number of emergency room admissions	1.35	1.32	0.03	0.81	1.03	−0.23*
Average number of IRF Admissions	–	–	–	0.02	0.03	−0.01*
Length of Stay for IRF Admissions (days)	0.62	0.68	−0.06	0.24	0.32	−0.07*
12-Month Mortality Rate	–	–	–	0.00	0.01	−0.01*

* Difference is significant at $\alpha = 0.05$
** The difference in spending between the study and comparison groups for IRF, LTCH, Other Inpatient and Hospice settings combined was significant at $\alpha = 0.05$
Source: Dobson | DaVanzo analysis of custom cohort Standard Analytic Files (2007–2010 and 2011–2014) for Medicare beneficiaries who received O&P services from January 1, 2008 through June 30, 2009 or January 1, 2012 through June 30, 2013 (and matched comparisons), according to custom cohort database definition

month. This chart indicates that the cost of the prosthetic was slowly amortized over time; by the end of Month 15, the cumulative Medicare episode payment for the study group was similar to that of the comparison group, indicating that the cost of the prosthetic was fully amortized.

Discussion

The literature indicates that the receipt of orthotic and prosthetic services could increase a patient's mobility, ultimately reducing their health care utilization and increasing their quality of life. Based on this possibility, this study investigated the economic impact and value of lower extremity orthoses, spinal orthoses, and lower extremity prostheses. Propensity score matching techniques allowed for the comparison of clinically and demographically similar patients who received these services to those who did not, and thus for a determination of the economic impact of these services on the Medicare population. Because this study is based on Medicare claims data, it excludes some other sources of economic value and outcomes, such as the ability for patients with

prostheses to return to work or become more independent from social services. These are sources of economic impact from the societal and consumer's perspective, although they are not generally relevant to the largely nonworking Medicare population and were outside the scope of the current analysis.

Results indicated that over an 18-month period, patients who received lower extremity orthotics or spinal orthotics had reduced Medicare payments. Savings were in the range of $2000 for both types of orthotic services, or approximately 8% of total Medicare health costs in the follow-up period. Beneficiaries who received lower extremity prostheses had similar total episode payments over 15 months, despite the higher cost of the prosthetic device, due to lower expenditures in other care settings.

Within the lower extremity orthotics analysis, these results demonstrated lower payments to physicians, outpatient hospitals, and for Part D drugs. This may suggest overall lower morbidity or comorbidity in patients who receive the orthotic service. In addition, higher utilization of post-acute care may be an important reason why acute care hospital admissions

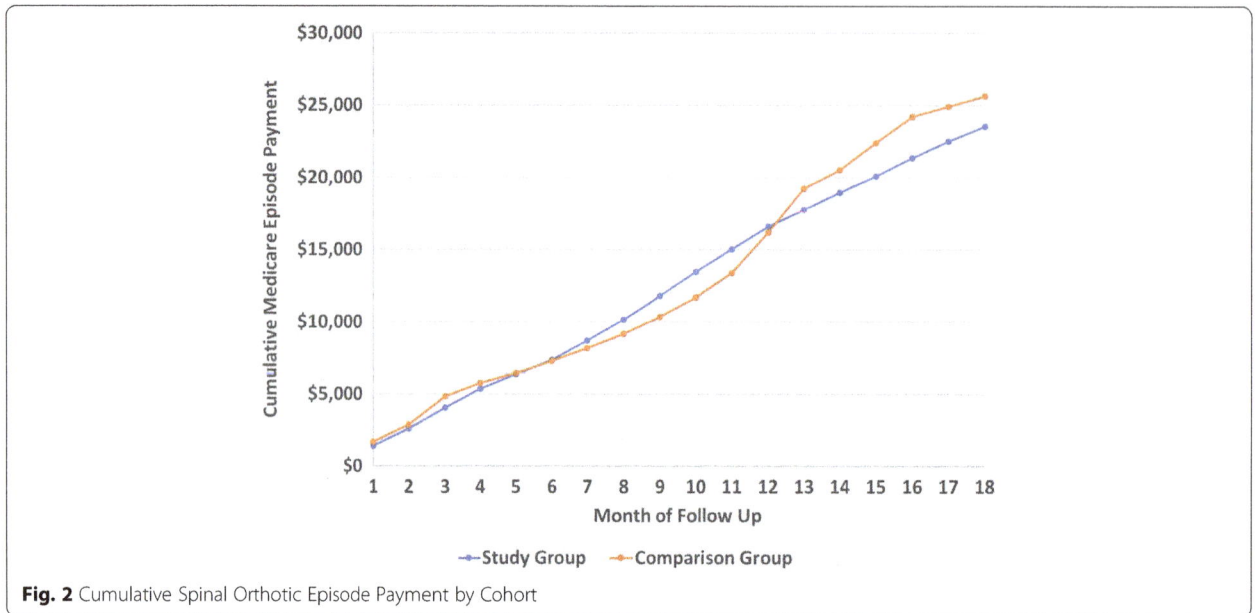

Fig. 2 Cumulative Spinal Orthotic Episode Payment by Cohort

and expenditures are significantly lower in the study group. That is, the higher use of post-acute care may eliminate the need for additional or subsequent admission to acute care hospitals, ultimately lowering total episode cost. The increased rate of outpatient therapy seen in the study group is consistent with Medicare's emphasis on restorative care for beneficiaries, when possible. It may be related to the lower rate of negative outcomes for patients who received O&P services, including fewer fractures and falls and emergency room visits. The results of this analysis suggest that with the receipt of the lower extremity orthotic, study group patients could withstand more intensive therapy that led to in increased standing stability, resulting in fewer emergency room admissions, hospitalizations, and lower Medicare payments.

In the spinal orthotic model, the lower payments for Part D drugs seen among study group beneficiaries could indicate lower prevalence of comorbid conditions and generally better health status among beneficiaries receiving spinal orthoses, compared to those who do not. Differences between this updated analysis and the previous one suggest that there may have been a different standard of care for patients receiving spinal orthotics in 2011–2014 than there was in 2007–2010. This updated analysis found higher payments for rehabilitation facilities among study group participants, which could indicate a shift toward more intensive facility-based rehabilitative care for beneficiaries receiving orthoses.

This analysis of lower extremity prosthetic services demonstrated that the cost of the prosthetic device and clinical prosthetic care was amortized within the

15-month follow-up period, offset by higher total costs for the untreated comparison group patients. Comparative efficacy trials and systematic reviews of components have found similar value concluding that some prosthetic components may be initially costlier but are ultimately worth funding due to lower fall risk, less work missed and improved quality of life [4, 14, 21]. In this study, through a reduction in acute care hospitalizations, physician visits, and facility-based care, patients experienced improved quality of life at a comparable Medicare episode payment.

Study and comparison group beneficiaries in this lower extremity prosthetic analysis had roughly a comparable number of fractures and falls, as well as comparable emergency room admission among lower extremity prosthetic users, compared to those who did not receive the service. Part of the savings due to reduced facility-based care was offset by more extensive physical therapy and rehabilitation presumably to teach patients how to properly use their prostheses, as amputees must learn balance and mobility with their new device. Additionally, the high use of therapy among beneficiaries in the study group may be associated with increased ambulation, which suggests that the study group patients with prostheses were less homebound than the comparison group. This increased level of independence among beneficiaries receiving prostheses may explain the similarity in the rate of falls and fractures and emergency room admissions among the study and comparison groups.

Much has changed in health care, and in orthotic and prosthetic care, since 2010. Despite research that suggests

Table 6 Spending and Utilization for 18-Month Lower Extremity Prosthetic Episode (2007–2010 and 2011–2014)

Care setting	2007–2010 analysis n = 428 Matched pairs			2011–2014 analysis update n = 545 Matched pairs		
	Study	Comparison	Difference	Study	Comparison	Difference
Physician	$7792	$11,883	-$4092*	$8270	$9920	-$1649
DME	$18,653	$2537	$16,116*	$15,323	$5018	$10,305*
Prosthetics Only: L5000 - L5999	–	–	–	$9694	$1782	$7912*
Acute Care Hospital / Other Inpatient	$18,080	$28,276	-$10196*	$15,529	$19,851	-$4321*
Long Term Care Hospital	$1408	$4102	-$2694**	$1445	$4017	-$2571*
Inpatient Rehabilitation Facility (IRF)	$2603	$2000	$603**	$3476	$3415	$61
Outpatient	$9373	$7291	$2082*	$8601	$8649	-$49
Skilled Nursing Facility	$8386	$8821	-$435	$5783	$6630	-$847
Home Health	$6181	$5692	$489	$5049	$4764	$285
Hospice	$715	$1572	-$857**	$104	$825	-$721*
Total Part D Drug Spending	–	–	–	$5297	$5806	-$508
Total	$73,191	$72,175	$1015	$68,877	$68,893	-$16
Average number of therapy visits	56.10	28.90	27.20*	26.86	17.97	8.89*
Average number of fractures and falls	0.90	0.72	0.18	0.46	0.41	0.05
Average number of inpatient admissions	1.18	1.51	−0.33	1.23	1.54	−0.31*
Length of stay for inpatient admissions (days)	–	–	–	7.53	11.44	−3.91*
Average number of emergency room admissions	1.55	2.10	−0.55*	2.14	2.03	0.11
Average number of IRF admissions	–	–	–	0.17	0.14	0.02
Length of stay for IRF admissions (days)	1.61	1.19	0.42	2.16	2.10	0.07

* Difference is significant at α = 0.05
** The difference in spending between the study and comparison groups for IRF, LTCH, Other Inpatient and Hospice settings combined was significant at α = 0.05
Source: Dobson | DaVanzo analysis of custom cohort Standard Analytic Files (2007–2010 and 2011–2014) for Medicare beneficiaries who received O&P services from January 1, 2008 through June 30, 2009 or January 1, 2012 through June 30, 2013 (and matched comparisons), according to custom cohort database definition

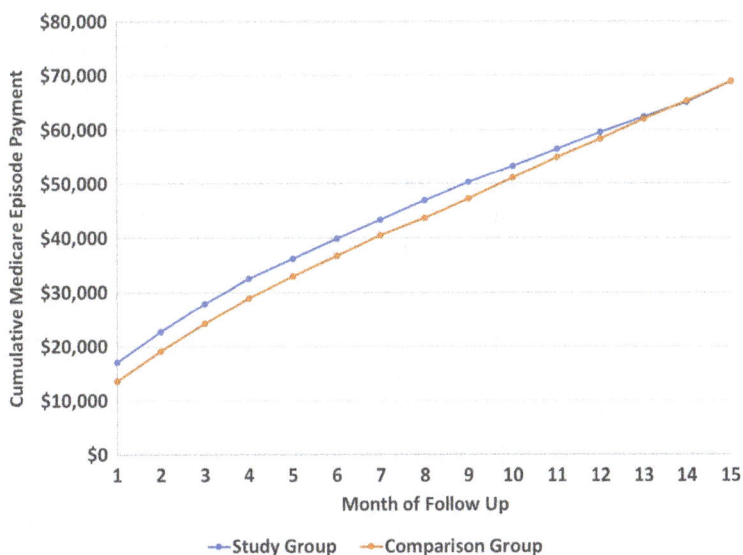

Fig. 3 Cumulative Lower Extremity Prosthetic Episode Payment by Cohort

that O&P services can prevent falls, reduce downstream clinical manifestations such as the development of diabetes, and lead to long-term savings in health care spending, patients can face significant barriers to access. Varying cost pressures caused Medicare prosthetic payments to decline by 6% between 2010 and 2014, and Medicare beneficiary access to more advanced prosthetics declined even more steeply, by approximately 36% over that same period [22]. In 2015, Medicare contractors proposed a new Local Coverage Determination (LCD) which would have further restricted access to more advanced devices, asserting, for example, that any Medicare beneficiary who had received a walker, wheel chair, crutches or cane would be automatically excluded from eligibility for more advanced devices. This proposed LCD prompted such controversy that the entire matter was referred to study, which has continued for nearly two years without any published conclusions. In the interim, the RAND Corporation has issued a new report underscoring the economic value of advanced technologies for amputees [23].

Our study suggest that lower extremity orthoses, spinal orthoses and lower extremity prostheses have the potential to increase quality of life and reduce facility-based care for applicable Medicare beneficiaries. Similarly, these results suggest that orthotic and prosthetic services provide value to the Medicare program, as well as to the patient. In orthotics, there is a clear savings margin for the treated study group patients. In prosthetics, the cost of the services, including the higher initial cost of the prosthesis itself, is completely amortized through reduced acute care hospitalizations and facility-based care. One clinical example of this is the situation where microprocessor knees have been shown to improve patient safety in patients with transfemoral amputation by reducing stumble and fall events [11].

Limitations
One limitation of the methodology was reliance on administrative data as opposed to clinical data recorded in the medical records. While the dataset included all fee-for-service health care utilization and payments, more detailed clinical indicators, such as functional status, were not available from the administrative data. Propensity score matching relied on all recorded patient demographic and clinical characteristics in an attempt to control for observable selection bias among those who received orthotic/prosthetic services compared to those who did not. More medical information could perhaps improve the selection of matched pairs.

Another limitation of the claims data was the lack of Medicare Advantage discharges and Medicaid long term care-related expenses for dually eligible patients. The

relationship of the Medicare to Medicaid payment systems is problematic for analyses that involve episodes of care, as the exclusion of Medicaid claims for dually eligible patients prohibits identification of patients who receive care in long-term care facilities as compared to the community. With additional data, reduction in long-term care facility use may have been determined to be another important outcome variable for the study group.

Conclusion
The results of this study generally echo those of the prior study, with some fluctuation in the cost difference between the study and comparison groups in specific subcategories of expenditures. Study group patients receiving lower extremity and spinal orthoses had significantly lower total episode spending than did the non-treated beneficiaries in the comparison group, despite having more therapy visits. Study group patients receiving lower extremity prostheses had average Medicare payments across all care settings that were slightly lower than the comparison group and the prosthetic cost was fully amortized within 15 months due to a reduction of care in other settings. Among other identified benefits to prosthetic use, prosthesis users had a significantly lower hospitalization rate than comparison group patients further resulting in lower Medicare payments for acute care hospitalizations. Across all analyses, the results cumulatively suggest that orthotic and prosthetic services provide value to the Medicare program, and potentially to other payers, as well as to the patient.

Endnotes
[1]Codes used to identify the etiological diagnoses of interest for the orthotic and prosthetic models are included in a separate technical methodology available from the authors.

Acknowledgements
The authors wish to acknowledge Tom Fise of the American Orthotics & Prosthetics association for his contribution to the design of the study and development of this manuscript.

Funding
The publication cost of this article was funded by the American Orthopedic & Prosthetic Association.

Authors' contributions
AD interpreted the patient data and was a major contributor in writing the manuscript. KM analyzed and interpreted the patient data and was a major contributor in writing the manuscript. NM analyzed the patient data and

was a major contributor in creating tables for the manuscript. JD interpreted the patient data and was a major contributor in writing the manuscript. All authors read and approved the final manuscript.

Competing interests
The authors declare that they have no competing interests.

References
1. Hubbard Winkler SL, Cowper Ripley DC, Wu S, Reker DM, Vogel B, Fitzgerald SG, Mann WC, Hoenig H. Demographic and clinical variation in veterans health administration provision of assistive technology devices to veterans poststroke. Arch Phys Med Rehabil. 2010;91(3):369–77.
2. Margolis DJ, Hoffstad O, Nafashi J, Leonard CE, Freeman CP, Hennessy S, Wiebe D. Location, location, location: geographic clustering of lower-extremity amputation among Medicare beneficiaries with diabetes. Diabetes Care. 2011;34:2363–7.
3. Wrobel JS, Mayfield JA, Reiber GE. Geographic variation of lower-extremity major amputation in individuals with and without diabetes in the Medicare population. Diabetes Care. 2011;24(5):860–4.
4. Highsmith MJ, Kahle JT, Lewandowski A, Klenow TD, Orriola JJ, Miro RM, Hill OT, Raschke SU, Orendurff MS, Highsmith JT, et al. Economic evaluations of interventions for transtibial amputees: a scoping review of comparative studies. Technol Innov. 2016;18:85–98.
5. Davies S, Gibby O, Phillips C, Price P, Tyrrell W. The health status of diabetic patients receiving orthotic therapy. Qual Life Res. 2000;9(2):233–40.
6. Leigh R, Barker S. The effect of specialist footwear on the quality of life of patients with lower leg ulcers. Wounds UK. 2007;3(4):19–23.
7. Price P. The diabetic foot: quality of life. Clinical Infectious Disease. 2004;39(2):129–31.
8. Samuelsson KAM, Toytari O, Salminen AL, Brandt A. Effects of lower limb prosthesis on activity, participation, and quality of life: a systematic review. Prosthetics Orthot Int. 2012;36(2):145–58.
9. Hebert JS, Burger H. Return to work following major limb loss. In: Schultz I, Gatchel R, editors. Handbook of return to work: from research to practice. 1st ed. Boston (MA): Springer; 2016. p. 505–18.
10. Dobson A, El-Gamil A, Manolov N, DaVanzo J. Economic value of orthotic and prosthetic services among Medicare beneficiaries: a claims-based retrospective cohort study. Mil Med. 2016;181(2S):18–24.
11. Highsmith MJ, Kahle JT, Bongiorni DR, Sutton BS, Groer S, Kaufman KR. Safety, energy efficiency, and cost efficacy of the C-leg for transfemoral amputees: a review of the literature. Prosthetics Orthot Int. 2010;34(4):362–77.
12. Novak D, Hooper M. Review and evaluation of LD20 an act to require insurance companies to cover the cost of prosthetics. Joint Standing Committee on Insurance and Financial Services of the 124th Maine Legislature; 2010. Available from: http://www.maine.gov/pfr/legislative/documents/LD020_Microprocessor_Prosthetic_Study_Final.doc. Accessed 15 Dec 2017.
13. California Technology Assessment Forum. Microprocessor-controlled prosthetic knees: a technology assessment. 2007. Available from: https://www.scribd.com/document/13027315/Microprocessor-Controlled-Prosthetic_Knees. Accessed 15 Dec 2017.
14. Highsmith MJ, Kahle J, Miro RM, Lura DJ, Dubey RV, Carey SL, Quillen WS, Mengelkoch LM. Perceived differences between the Genium and the C-leg microprocessor prosthetic knees in prosthetic-related function and quality of life. Technol Innov. 2014;15:369–75.
15. Trojano M, Pellegrini F, Paolicelli D, Fuiani A, Di Renzo V. Observational studies: propensity score analysis of non-randomized data. International MS Journal. 2009;16:90–7.
16. Austin PC. An introduction to propensity score methods for reducing the effects of confounding in observational studies. Multivar Behav Res. 2011;46:399–424.
17. Kuss O, Legler T, Borgermann J. Treatments effects from randomized trials and propensity score analyses were similar in similar populations in an example from cardiac surgery. J Clin Epidemiol. 2011;64(10):1076–84.
18. Dehejia R, Wahba S. Propensity score-matching methods for nonexperimental causal studies. Rev Econ Stat. 2002;84(1):151–61.
19. Rosenbaum PR, Rubin DB. The central role of the propensity score in observational studies for causal effects. Biometrika. 1983;70(1):41–55.
20. Austin PC. Optimal caliper widths for propensity-score matching when estimating differences in means and differences i proportions in observational studies. Pharm Stat. 2011;10:150–61.
21. Highsmith MJ, Klenow TD, Kahle JT, Wernke MM, Carey SL, Miro RM, Lura DJ, Sutton BS. Effects of the Genium knee system on functional level, stair ambulation, perceptive and economic outcomes in transfemoral amputees. Technol Innov. 2016;18:139–50.
22. Dobson A., DaVanzo J. Analysis of 2010-2014 Medicare Standard Analytic Files. 2017.
23. Liu H, Chen C, Hanson M, Chaturvedi R, Mattke S, Hillestad R. Economic value of advanced transfemoral prosthetics: Rand Corporation; 2017. Available from: https://www.rand.org/content/dam/rand/pubs/research_reports/RR2000/RR2096/RAND_RR2096.pdf. Accessed 15 Dec 2017

5

Improving internal model strength and performance of prosthetic hands using augmented feedback

Ahmed W. Shehata[1,2,3]* , Leonard F. Engels[4], Marco Controzzi[4], Christian Cipriani[4], Erik J. Scheme[1,2] and Jonathon W. Sensinger[1,2]

Abstract

Background: The loss of an arm presents a substantial challenge for upper limb amputees when performing activities of daily living. Myoelectric prosthetic devices partially replace lost hand functions; however, lack of sensory feedback and strong understanding of the myoelectric control system prevent prosthesis users from interacting with their environment effectively. Although most research in augmented sensory feedback has focused on real-time regulation, sensory feedback is also essential for enabling the development and correction of internal models, which in turn are used for planning movements and reacting to control variability faster than otherwise possible in the presence of sensory delays.

Methods: Our recent work has demonstrated that audio-augmented feedback can improve both performance and internal model strength for an abstract target acquisition task. Here we use this concept in controlling a robotic hand, which has inherent dynamics and variability, and apply it to a more functional grasp-and-lift task. We assessed internal model strength using psychophysical tests and used an instrumented Virtual Egg to assess performance.

Results: Results obtained from 14 able-bodied subjects show that a classifier-based controller augmented with audio feedback enabled stronger internal model ($p = 0.018$) and better performance ($p = 0.028$) than a controller without this feedback.

Conclusions: We extended our previous work and accomplished the first steps on a path towards bridging the gap between research and clinical usability of a hand prosthesis. The main goal was to assess whether the ability to decouple internal model strength and motion variability using the continuous audio-augmented feedback extended to real-world use, where the inherent mechanical variability and dynamics in the mechanisms may contribute to a more complicated interplay between internal model formation and motion variability. We concluded that benefits of using audio-augmented feedback for improving internal model strength of myoelectric controllers extend beyond a virtual target acquisition task to include control of a prosthetic hand.

Keywords: Prosthetics, Electromyography, Support vector machines, Internal model, Motor learning, Performance, Muscles, Real-time systems, Augmented feedback, Sensory feedback

* Correspondence: ahmed.shehata@unb.ca
[1]Institute of Biomedical Engineering, University of New Brunswick, Fredericton, NB E3B 5A3, Canada
[2]Department of Electrical and Computer Engineering, University of New Brunswick, Fredericton, NB E3B 5A3, Canada
Full list of author information is available at the end of the article

Background

The seemingly simple and seamless way adult humans use their hands to grasp and manipulate objects is in fact the result of years of training during childhood, and of a sophisticated blend of feedforward and feedback control mechanisms [1]. The function of such an elegant system may be corrupted when neurological injuries interrupt the connections between the central nervous system (CNS) and the periphery, as in the case of upper limb amputation. In this case, myoelectric prostheses provide a solution to restore hand function by partially restoring the feedforward control mechanism [2]. This mechanism is influenced by two key factors. The first factor is the way the user intentions are decoded, which affects the robustness of control signals driving the prosthesis' motors. The second factor is the human understanding of the system, which is modeled by the CNS and is known as the internal model [3]. The ability to accurately estimate the current state of the musculoskeletal system and properly integrate information from various sensory feedback forms to predict the future state is determined by the strength of the internal model developed [4]. For prosthesis users, this model is mismatched since their prosthetic device properties and control are very different from that of a normal limb, and therefore the need to develop a new internal model or adjust the current one is presumed.

For a representative motor task, such as grasp-and-lift, the brain refines and updates the internal model using multi-modal sensory feedback (tactile, visual, and auditory) during and after the movement [5]. Unlike unimpaired individuals, myoelectric prosthesis users have to rely more on visual feedback, which has been found to negatively affect performance, as users spend more time monitoring their prosthesis or the objects being manipulated [6]. This increased dependency on visual feedback is due to the lack of adequate sensory feedback from the prosthetic devices [7]. This deficiency contributes to an inability of users to fully adjust their internal model and is known to affect overall performance [8].

To address this deficiency, researchers have investigated ways of providing augmented sensory information using invasive and non-invasive methods [9, 10]. Several of the invasive methods show promise, including Targeted Sensory Reinnervation and stimulation of sensory peripheral nerves [11–15]. However, many prosthesis users prefer non-invasive methods that do not require surgical intervention [16, 17].

Researchers have correspondingly evaluated non-invasive sensory substitution methods to provide sensory information either through an alternate sensory channel or through the natural channel but in a different modality [9]. Vibro-tactile [18, 19], mechano-tactile [20], electrotactile [21–23], skin stretch [24], and auditory cues [25] are just some of the techniques that have been developed and assessed to provide prosthesis users with supplementary feedback. Although some studies have shown that augmented sensory feedback had little to no effect on performance [26], others have demonstrated the efficacy of augmented sensory feedback in enhancing motor control even for the same experimental procedure [9]. This conflict may arise in part because it is unclear how this augmented feedback affects internal model development and, ultimately, the performance.

One hypothesis is that feedback improves performance through the integration of feedback in a real-time manner during a movement, known as real-time regulation [27–29]. Many studies showed promising improvement in performance [30, 31], sense of embodiment [32], and prosthesis incorporation [33] when using feedback for real-time regulation; however the efficacy of the feedback methods used, such as resolution and latency, introduces a new challenge [34]. To overcome this challenge, Dosen et al. [35] proposed providing electromyography (EMG) biofeedback to the user through visual feedback. Their results showed that users were able to exploit the augmented visual biofeedback to improve their performance in a grasping task. In a follow-up study, Schweisfurth and colleagues [36] implemented the EMG biofeedback using a multichannel electrotactile interface to transmit discrete levels of myoelectric signals to users. They compared this feedback approach to classic force feedback and found that the electrotactile biofeedback allowed for more predictable control and improved performance. However, it is unclear whether this improvement is driven by the use of this feedback for real-time regulation or by the adjustments made to the internal model.

Our group has recently suggested a framework that demonstrates that the strength of the internal model is indeed affected by feedback [37]. In the field of myoelectric prosthesis control, we used this framework to assess the strength of the internal model developed for able-bodied subjects when using different myoelectric control strategies. A series of tests were conducted to extract parameters that are used in this framework to compute uncertainties in the developed internal model. One test quantified the ability of subjects to use feedback to adapt and modify their control signals. Other tests quantified variability in control signals for a given controller and variability in the provided feedback. These parameters were used in this framework to determine a weighted factor of the feedback that is assumed to be combined with the internal model based on the uncertainty of the feedback.

In a previous study [38], we noted that various types of control strategies, in the very act of filtering biological signals (i.e., movement classification and activation thresholds), provide inherently different levels of visual biofeedback to the user. For instance, classification-based control provides no visual feedback about any class except the one it deems to be the correct class, thus denying the user of any knowledge about partial activations of other classes [39]. Whereas most research has focused on the impact of those filters on the control (motor) performance of the prosthesis (see reviews [40, 41]), we demonstrated that it also affects the ability of the person to form an internal model. In that study, we assessed the internal model strength and performance when using two common myoelectric control strategies [39, 42] that differed in the inherent feedback provided to the user, namely: (a) regression-based control or (b) classification-based control.

For a two DOF task, a regression-based control provides users with proportional feedback about activations of both DOF while a classification-based control provides users with feedback about only one dominant DOF at a time. We showed that the inclusion of information about the smaller modulations in the secondary DOF in regression controllers (unfiltered control signals) provided valuable and rich information to improve the internal model, even though it resulted in worse short-term performance as measured using task accuracy and path efficiency. In contrast, the inherent filter in classification-based control, which limited the control signal variability and thus improved the smoothness of movements, also prevented the formation of a strong internal model. In other words, continuous feedback-rich control strategies may be used to improve internal model strength, but classification-based controllers enable better immediate performance. Intrigued by this outcome and attempting to incorporate the benefits of both control strategies, in our next study we combined a classification-based control with a regression-based audio-augmented sensory feedback in a virtual target acquisition task [43]. Our outcomes demonstrated that this combination enabled both the development of a stronger internal model than the regression-based controller and better performance than the classification-based controller.

In the present study, we extended our previous work by investigating the benefits of using audio-augmented feedback when controlling a prosthetic hand. The main goal was to assess whether the ability to decouple internal model strength and motion variability, using the continuous audio-augmented feedback, extended to real-world use, where the inherent mechanical variability and dynamics in the mechanisms as well as the user-socket interfaces may contribute to a more complicated interplay between internal model formation and motion variability. To accomplish this goal, we compared internal model strength and performance of a classifier-based myoelectric controller with and without audio-augmented feedback during a grasp-and-lift task using a multi-degree of freedom (DOF)

research prosthetic hand [44]. We assessed the internal model strength using psychophysical tests and used an instrumented Virtual Egg to assess the performance [38, 45]. Our results from 14 able-bodied subjects show that audio-augmented feedback may indeed be used to improve internal model strength and performance of a myoelectric prosthesis. These improvements may increase reliability and promote acceptance of prosthetic devices by powered prosthesis users.

Methods

Classifier-based myoelectric control is considered as one of the more advanced strategies of myocontrol [42] and may be implemented using various pattern recognition algorithms [46, 47]. In recent studies, we used a Support Vector Regression (SVR) algorithm, which has been proven to enable better performance than other algorithms, to implement a classifier-based myoelectric control strategy [38, 43]. This algorithm provided regression-based control signals that simultaneously activated more than 1 DOF at a time, which were subsequently gated to only allow the activation of 1 DOF at a time. In this work, we used these same gated, i.e., classifier-based control, signals to activate either hand open/close or thumb adduction/abduction of a prosthetic hand. Building on the classifier-based control, we implemented a novel control strategy, namely Audio-augmented Feedback control, which is able to effectively decouple internal model formation from control variability. We relayed information in the regression-based control signals through continuous auditory cues to augment the feedback from the classifier-based myoelectric control (Fig. 1). The amplitude of the audio feedback was directly proportional to the amplitude of the control signals. For each DOF, two distinct frequencies were assigned: open/close hand had 500/400 Hz assigned and thumb adduction/abduction had 900/800 Hz assigned.

Participants

14 healthy subjects (8 male, and 6 female; mean and standard deviation of age: 25 ± 4.5 years) participated in this study. All participants had either normal or corrected-to-normal vision, were right-handed, and none had earlier experience with myoelectric pattern recognition control. Written informed consent according to the University of New Brunswick Research and Ethics Board and to Scuola Superiore Sant'Anna Ethical Committee was obtained from subjects before conducting the experiment (UNB REB 2014–019 and SSSA 02/2017).

Setup

The experimental platform consisted of a robotic hand, an array of myoelectric sensors, a PC implementing the control strategy, headphones that conveyed audio feedback,

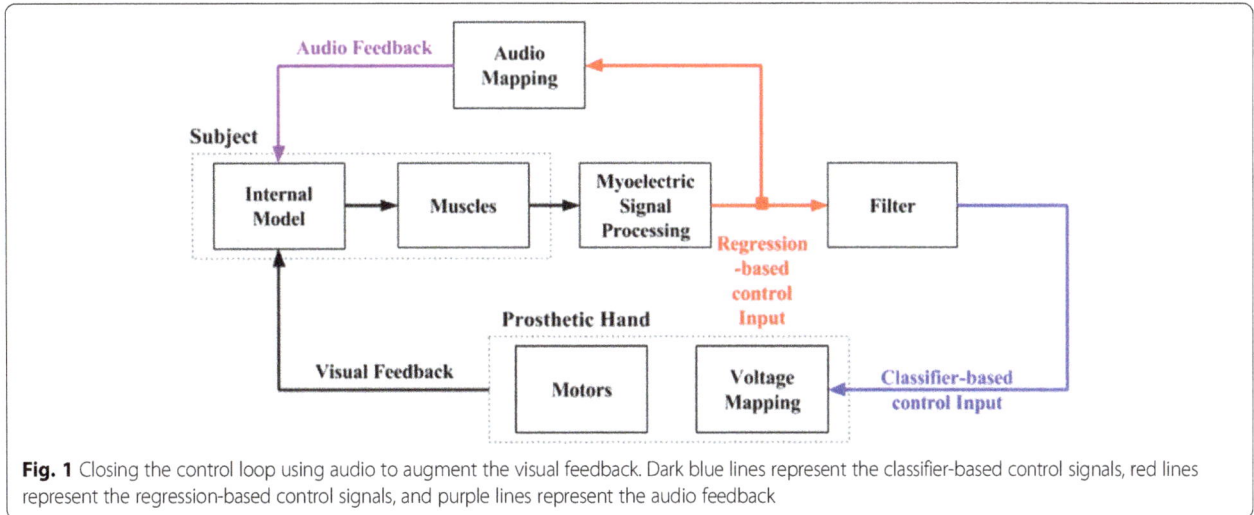

Fig. 1 Closing the control loop using audio to augment the visual feedback. Dark blue lines represent the classifier-based control signals, red lines represent the regression-based control signals, and purple lines represent the audio feedback

and a test object instrumented with force sensors (Fig. 2). The robotic hand was a right-handed version of the IH2 Azzurra Hand (Prensilia, IT) [44]. It consists of four fingers and a thumb actuated by five motors. In the present work, movements were limited to allow only flexion/extension of the thumb-index-middle digits and the abduction/adduction of the thumb. The hand included encoders on the motors, which were under position control based on commands sent over a serial bus from the PC. Subjects controlled the robotic hand using isometric muscle contractions sensed by an array of eight low power multi-channel operation electrodes (30 × 20 × 10 mm/electrode) placed around their forearm [48]. Seven subjects tested the classifier-based control without

augmented feedback (NF) and then retested with the audio-augmented feedback (AF). The remaining subjects tested the classifier-based control without augmented feedback (NF) twice to test for learning effects.

The test object was an *instrumented Virtual Egg* (iVE). The iVE is a rigid plastic test-object ($57 \times 57 \times 57$ mm^3; approximately 180 g) equipped with two strain gauge-based force sensors (Strain Measurement Devices, UK, model S215–53.3 N; each located at one of two parallel grasping sides), able to measure grip force exerted on the object. The iVE was programmed to virtually break whenever the grip force was larger than a preset threshold (approximately 3.1 N); this event was signaled to the subject through a colored light on the iVE [45].

Protocol

Participants were instructed to repeatedly grip, lift, replace, and release the iVE at a self-selected routine grasping speed. Specifically, their task consisted of (1) moving their right arm to reach the iVE with the robotic hand mounted on a bypass splint (Fig. 1), (2) contracting their own muscles to control the robotic hand so that it grasped the object, (3) lifting the iVE a few centimeters above the table, (4) putting the iVE back on the table, and, finally, (5) releasing the object by opening the hand.

During the experiment, subjects sat comfortably in front of a computer screen and wore a set of 1000 mW headphones (MDRZX100, Sony, JP) with the volume set to a maximum of 52.5 ± 3 dB (they could remove them during scheduled breaks between testing blocks). Subjects used each feedback method to complete a series of test blocks in a specific order after accomplishing a training and familiarization block. Before the start of each test block, subjects were given a two-minute break, in which they could stand up, remove the headset, unstrap the splint, and stretch if needed. The electrode

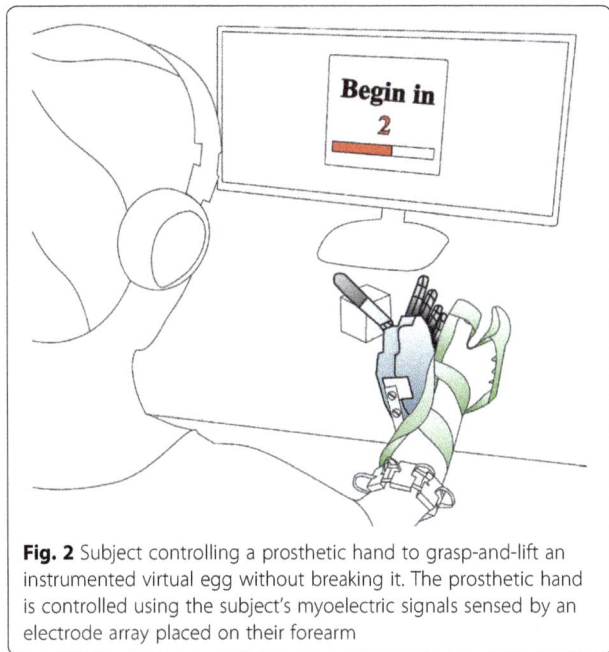

Fig. 2 Subject controlling a prosthetic hand to grasp-and-lift an instrumented virtual egg without breaking it. The prosthetic hand is controlled using the subject's myoelectric signals sensed by an electrode array placed on their forearm

array, however, was not removed for the duration of the experiment.

The training and familiarization block consisted of 40 grasp-and-lift trials. Subjects were given verbal instructions to complete the task without breaking the iVE in less than seven seconds after which a "Time out" text appeared on the computer screen and the artificial hand returned to a predetermined starting pose (Fig. 3). The training and familiarization starting pose was with the hand fully opened and thumb adducted (Fig. 3a). While in the first 25 trials, subjects were shown the feedback when the iVE broke (fragile mode), they were not given this feedback in the last 15 trials (rigid mode). This was done to keep subjects engaged with the task and not lose interest during the training block. Subjects were allowed to proceed to test blocks when they achieved at least 75% successful grasp-and-lift trials of the iVE in the training block.

The first test block was used to test adaptation to self-generated errors. In this block, subjects were asked to complete 40 grasp-and-lift trials in less than five seconds per trial. Adaptation rate was computed as how much subjects adjusted their grasp trajectory from one trial to the next based on error observed between their actual trajectory and activating only the hand close/open DOF, i.e., the optimal trajectory [49].

The second test block was used to measure the subject's perception threshold, i.e. a psychometric measure of sensory threshold for perception of a sensory stimulus. Subjects performed a series of two lift trials (fragile mode). In one of the two trials, a specific stimulus was added causing the hand to behave differently. The subjects were then asked to identify the changed trial by pressing the "1" or "2" key (for trial one or two) on a keyboard placed in front of them with their other hand. The magnitude of the added stimulus was calculated using an adaptive staircase as a rotation in the control space in degrees (Fig. 3 in [38]) with target probability set to 0.84 [50, 51]. For instance, if a subject was generating control signals for thumb abduction, a 90 degrees rotation in the control signal would switch activations from thumb abduction to hand close. Each trial lasted for four seconds and subjects were encouraged to take breaks between trials whenever they needed. The final noticeable stimulus reached was recorded when the number of reversals for this staircase reached 23 [38]. The starting pose of the prosthetic hand for the first and second block was similar to that of the training and familiarization block where subjects had to only activate the hand close/open DOF to achieve this task efficiently.

The third and last test block was used to measure performance. Subjects were given 20 trials to move the iVE (fragile mode) from one side of a barrier (H: 14.5 cm x W: 25 cm) to the other in less than 10 s per trial, similar to the Box and Blocks test [52]. The starting pose of the hand was adjusted to evaluate the subject's performance for a 2-DOF task in which subjects had to activate the thumb adduction/abduction DOF to lower the thumb and then activate the hand close/open DOF to grasp the iVE properly to lift it to the other side of the barrier (Fig. 3b). Table 1 summarizes the experimental protocol used in this study.

Outcome measures
Internal model parameters
Similar to our previous research [38, 43], we assessed human understanding of the myoelectric control strategy

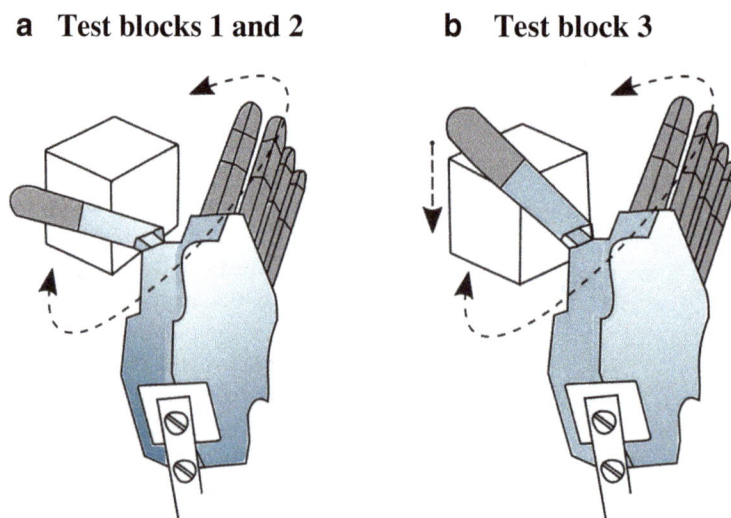

Fig. 3 Hand starting pose. **a** Starting pose for the training and familiarization, adaptation, and JND blocks. Subjects had to only activate the thumb and fingers flexion to grasp the object carefully without breaking it. **b** Starting pose for the performance test: fingers and thumb are extended, and the thumb is abducted. Subjects had to adduct the thumb and then close the hand to grasp the object and transfer it from one side of a barrier to the other

Table 1 Summary of the experimental protocol

Task	Description
Control Practice	Control the prosthetic hand for two minutes – a combination of close/open the prosthetic hand and abduct/adduct the thumb.
Training and Familiarization	25 trials of grasp-and-lift of the iVE with the breaking feedback and 15 grasp-and-lift trials without the breaking feedback. Each trial lasted for seven seconds.
Adaptation rate test	A total of 40 grasp-and-lift trials. Each trial lasted for five seconds.
Perception threshold test	Grasp-and-lift the iVE in less than four seconds and identify the trial with the added stimulus in a set of two trials, repeat this task until convergence of an adaptive staircase.
Performance test	Transfer the iVE from one side of a barrier to the other 20 times in less than 10 s per transfer.

for a grasp-and-lift task using the following psychometric measures:

- Adaptation rate $(-\beta_1)$ is a measure of feedforward modification of the control signal from one trial to the next [37]. For each trial in the adaptation rate test, control signal activations in both DOFs, i.e., flex/extend thumb-index-middle digits and adduct/abduct thumb, were recorded. To capture the subject's feedforward intent, the first 500 ms of the recorded activations for each trial were analyzed. The target control signal was the activation of the closing of the prosthetic hand only (i.e., flex/extend thumb-index-middle digits). Other activations were considered as self-generated errors, which subjects were instructed to minimize. The following equation was used to compute this adaptation rate.

$$error_{n+1} - error_n = \beta_1 \times error_n + \beta_0 \quad (1)$$

where $error$ is the angle formed between the closing of the hand activation trajectory, i.e., target, and the actual hand activation trajectory; n is the trial number; β_0 is the linear regression constant; and $-\beta_1$ is the adaptation rate. A unity value indicates perfect adaptation, i.e., internal model modified to perfectly compensate for errors.

- Just-noticeable-difference (JND) is a measure of the minimum perceivable stimulus in degrees identified by the subject when using each feedback method [50]. A lower threshold indicated better user ability to perceive small perturbations in the control strategy used. This parameter was extracted from the Perception threshold test block as the final noticeable stimulus when the number of reversals for an adaptive staircase reached 23.
- Internal model uncertainty (P_{param}) is a measure of the confidence of a user in the internal model they developed for a control strategy with a certain feedback method. This parameter was computed

using outcomes from both the first and second test blocks [38].

Performance parameters

- Completion Rate (CR) is the percentage of the successful transfers of the iVE from one side of the barrier to the other without breaking it (fragile mode). This parameter was extracted from the third test block.
- Mean Completion Time (MCT) is defined as the time taken to successfully transfer the iVE from one side of the barrier to the other without breaking it (fragile mode). This parameter was also extracted from the third test block.
- Trial submovements (TS) is the number of submovements per trial. This parameter is calculated as the number of zero-crossing pairs of the third derivative of the grasp force profile per trial [53]. The number of submovements served as an indicator of use of feedback for real-time regulation of the grasping force [54–56]. The higher this number, the greater the use of feedback in real-time regulation. This parameter was extracted from the adaptation test.

Statistical analysis

The Statistical Package for the Social Science software (SPSS v25.0, IBM, US) was used to run Levene's test on JND, adaptation rate, internal model uncertainty, and performance measure results to investigate homogeneity in variances of the data. If data variances were found to be homogenous, we ran two-sample paired t-tests to assess differences between these outcome measures at a significance criterion of $\alpha = 0.05$ for the two feedbacks tested. If data variances were found to be nonhomogeneous, a Wilcoxon signed-rank test was conducted. For the group of subjects who tested and retested the NF controller, repeated measures ANOVA was used to compute intraclass correlation coefficient (ICC) for internal model parameters and performance parameters using a two-way mixed effects model with absolute agreement at a 95% confidence interval to investigate the effect of prolonged exposure to a control strategy. The confidence interval was calculated using the standard deviation (95% CI = mean ± 1.97 × SD). If not denoted otherwise, all numbers in the text refer to mean ± SD.

Results

To confirm that the benefits of using audio-augmented feedback for improving internal model strength of myo-electric controllers extend beyond a virtual target acquisi-tion task [43], we assessed the internal model developed when using this audio-augmented controller and the no-augmented feedback controller to control a prosthetic hand for a grasp-and-lift task. In addition, short-term perform-ance when using both controllers was evaluated.

Internal model assessment

Two psychophysical experiments were employed to evalu-ate parameters that are used to assess internal model strength [38]. The first experiment tested the trial-by-trial adaptation to self-generated errors. The outcome from that test indicated how much the internal model was modified from one trial to the next based on error feedback.

Results from the adaptation test (first test block) proved a statistically significant difference between subjects using NF and AF control strategies (two paired-samples t-test (t (6) = – 4.6, p = 0.004)). In particular, the AF control strategy promoted a significantly higher adaptation rate (1.2 ± 0.25) than the NF control strategy (0.75 ± 0.15) (Fig. 4a).

The outcomes from the perception threshold test matched with those from the adaptation test. Audio-augmented feedback control strategy enabled a significantly lower perception threshold (44.6 ± 10 degrees) than the NF controller (58.5 ± 12.5 degrees) (paired samples t-test (t (6) = 3.4, p = 0.014)) (Fig. 4b).

The adaptation rate and the JND were used to compute the internal model uncertainty developed for each of the tested feedback conditions. Again, the AF control strategy promoted a lower internal model uncertainty (0.22 ± 0.11) compared to subjects using NF control strategy (1.8 ± 0.6) (related samples Wilcoxon signed-rank test; p = 0.018) (Fig. 4c).

Test-retest of NF controller: Results for internal model assessment parameters showed no significant within-subject effect of retesting NF controller with good reliabil-ity (ICC > 0.65). Table 2 summarizes the statistical analysis for these results.

All in all, these results align with previous studies [43] and confirm that audio-augmented feedback pro-motes: (1) high adaptation rate, (2) the user's ability to perceive low sensory threshold and, in turn (3) a strong internal model for a grasp-and-lift task using a pros-thetic hand.

Performance test

The completion rate (in the last test block) proved higher when using the AF control strategy (65 ± 12%) than when using the NF control strategy (37.34 ± 19%) (Two paired-sample t-test, (t (6) = – 2.87, p = 0.028) (Fig. 5). Notably, testing of the mean completion time did not exhibit a significant difference (MCT_{AF} = 8.3 ± 0.74 s; MCT_{NF} = 8.4 ± 0.65 s) (Fig. 6).

Test-retest of NF controller: Similar to the internal model assessment parameters results, results for perform-ance parameters showed no significant within-subject ef-fect of retesting the NF controller with very good reliability (ICC > 0.9, CR) and good reliability (ICC = 0.55, MCT) (Table 2).

Submovements analysis was performed on data recorded from only five subjects as the iVE failed to record data for the other two subjects due to a communication error. When using the NF control strategy, subjects changed their grasping force during the grasp-and-lift task, though not as much as when using AF control strategy (Fig. 7). Results show that subjects using AF control strategy had a sig-nificantly higher number of submovements (3.94 ± 0.12) than subjects using NF control strategy (3.26 ± 0.17) as de-termined by a two-sample independent t-test (t (90) = – 3.17, p = 0.002) (Fig. 8). These results suggest that audio-augmented feedback enables better short-term per-formance by enabling the development of a stronger in-ternal model.

Discussion

Many studies have focused on improving performance of myoelectric prosthesis control by providing feedback to the user, but only a few have investigated the effect of this feedback on the internal model, which is key to im-proving long-term performance [57]. Due to an inability to assess internal model strength, this effect remained unquantified. For the first time, we used a recently de-veloped psychophysical framework to assess the strength of the internal model developed when using different myoelectric prosthesis controllers [38]. In earlier work, we demonstrated that audio-augmented feedback improves internal model strength and the performance of myoelec-tric prosthesis control in a virtual target acquisition task [43]. We argued that these improvements may extend beyond a virtual target acquisition task. In this study, we tested the classifier-based control with and without audio-augmented feedback for a grasp-and-lift task when using a prosthetic hand. Our results confirm the hypoth-esis that audio-augmented feedback enables the develop-ment of a strong internal model and better short-term performance when controlling a prosthetic hand for a grasp-and-lift task.

Even when using different controllers, humans are able to incorporate previous knowledge and experience to

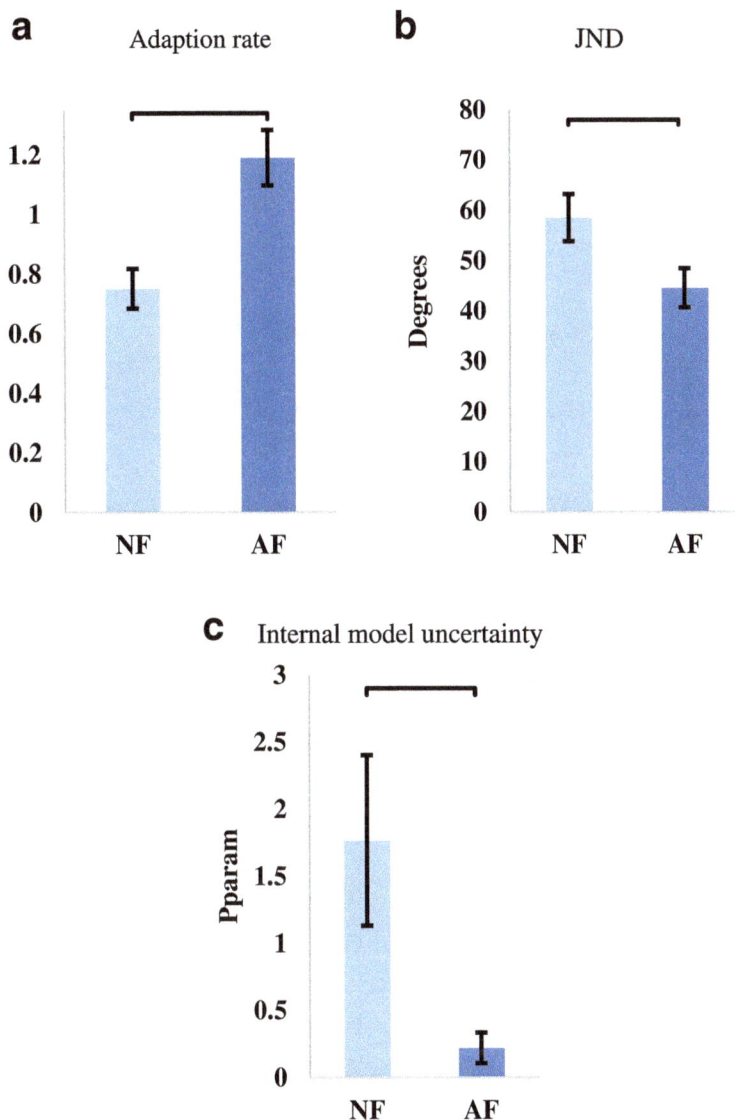

Fig. 4 Psychophysical test results. **a** Adaptation rate results showing audio-augmented feedback control strategy enabling higher adaptation to self-generated error than the no-augmented feedback control strategy. **b** Perception threshold test results showing low JND value when using the audio-augmented controller. **c** Internal model uncertainty (Pparam) results showing significant reduction in the internal model uncertainty when using the audio-augmented feedback control strategy. Horizontal bars indicate statistical significant difference. NF: No-augmented Feedback. AF: Audio-augmented Feedback

Table 2 Summary of test-retest for the Nf controller results

Outcome measure	ANOVA repeated measure p	ICC	SEM
Adaptationrate	0.86	0.65	0.102
Just-noticeable-difference	0.21	0.65	4.4
Internal model uncertainty	0.64	0.9	0.53
Completion Rate	0.57	0.9	1.2
Mean completion time	0.47	0.55	0.16

accomplish tasks [38]. To minimize this translation of stronger internal models, all subjects in this study tested the no-augmented feedback controller first, followed by the augmented audio feedback controller. It could be possible that the reduction in internal model uncertainty for the audio-augmented controller is due, in part, to the prolonged exposure to the control strategy and the experiment. This possibility, however, was addressed in this work when subjects were asked to test and re-test the same control strategy (no-augmented feedback) and it was concluded that there was no improvement in adaptation rate, JND, internal model strength, or

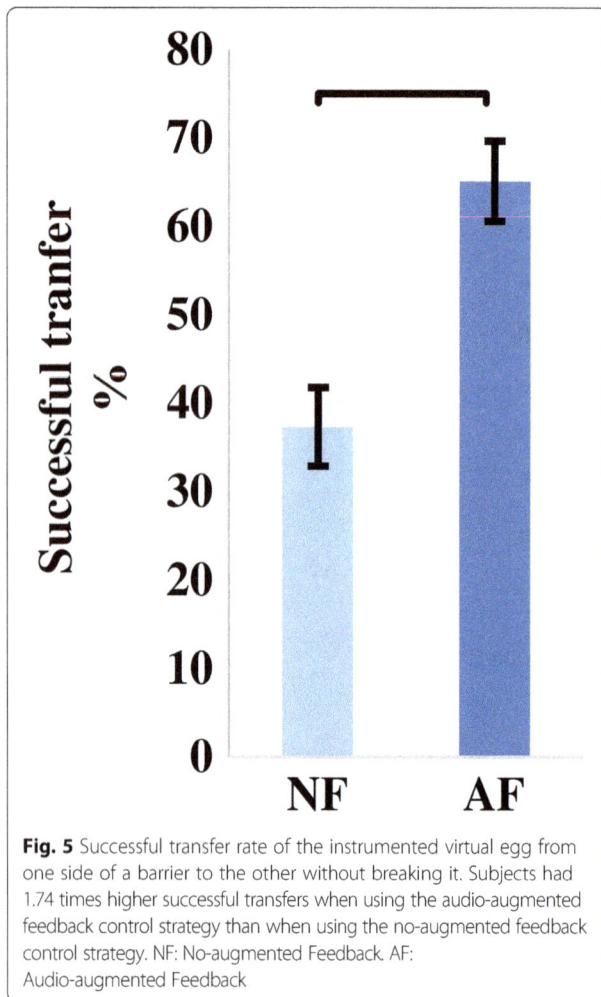

Fig. 5 Successful transfer rate of the instrumented virtual egg from one side of a barrier to the other without breaking it. Subjects had 1.74 times higher successful transfers when using the audio-augmented feedback control strategy than when using the no-augmented feedback control strategy. NF: No-augmented Feedback. AF: Audio-augmented Feedback

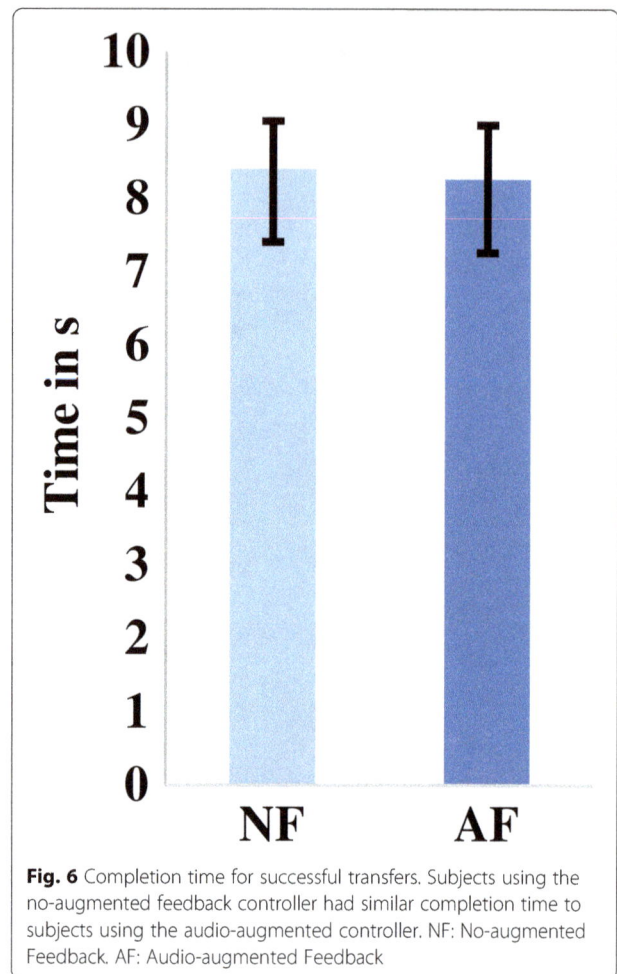

Fig. 6 Completion time for successful transfers. Subjects using the no-augmented feedback controller had similar completion time to subjects using the audio-augmented controller. NF: No-augmented Feedback. AF: Audio-augmented Feedback

performance due to the repetition of the test. Consequently, we argue that any improvement in those parameters is due to the control strategy used and not due to prolonged exposure.

To ensure that the continuous audio feedback was not a distraction to the user and, in turn, did not compromise short-term performance, we assessed the short-term performance by computing the completion rate (without breaking the object). Outcomes, in fact, showed a significantly better performance when subjects used the AF compared to the NF controller, albeit both controllers had similar completion time. The submovements analysis revealed that subjects adjusted their grasping forces more frequently when using the AF controller than when they used the NF controller. This finding suggests that augmented audio feedback may not only be used for developing internal models, but subjects' high confidence in the feedback lead to them using this feedback for real-time regulation too. Hence, regression-based augmented audio feedback improves both short-term performance through real-time regulation and long-term

performance through development of strong internal models.

Although we did not measure the cognitive load of using audio feedback in this work, other researchers have found that audio feedback may be used to alleviate the cognitive burden when combined with visual feedback [25]. Internal model assessment results from this study may be used to further explain how audio feedback reduces the cognitive load. To further support our findings, future work may include utilizing visual attention measures developed in [6] to quantitatively determine the effect of using controllers with and without feedback on visual attention.

Although the results found in this study providing compelling evidence that internal models can indeed be improved using augmented feedback, they must still be confirmed in the target population. Although we tested only able-bodied subjects, we suspect that similar internal model results may be found when testing amputees since internal model assessment parameters are measures of human behavior and understanding and not physical ability [39]. That said, performance results found here may be

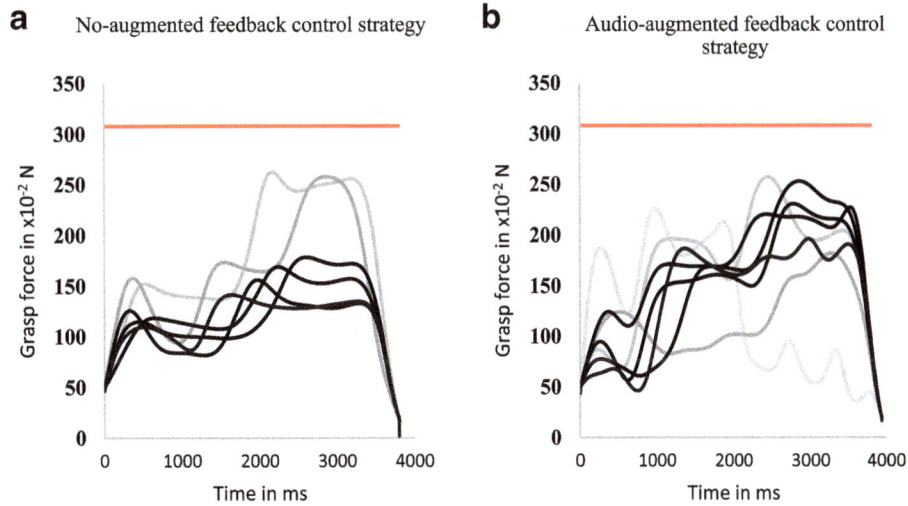

Fig. 7 Progression of grasp-and-lift trials ranging from the beginning of the task (light gray) to the end of the task (dark gray). Representative data from a single subject during adaptation rate test using (**a**) the no-augmented feedback control strategy (moderate grasp force changes per trial) and (**b**) the audio-augmented feedback control strategy (high grasp force changes per trial). The red line in both plots shows the preset breaking force

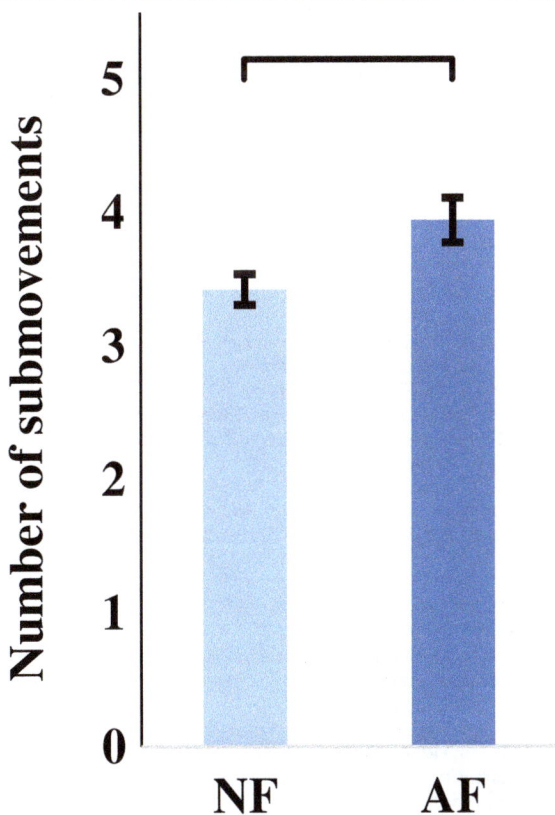

Fig. 8 Submovements computed from the grasp forces of successful trials from the adaptation rate test for a sample of five subjects. NF: No-augmented Feedback. AF: Audio-augmented Feedback

scaled when testing amputees due to differences in prosthesis attachment, i.e., bypass vs. socket, and placement of the surface electrode array. One might argue that the control strategy (model) trained and used by able-bodied subjects in this study will be very different than the one trained and used by an amputee. In fact, the control model trained for every individual and for every session is unique and tuned to that individual regardless of chosen location of the electrode array or muscle mass. This trained model is driven by how individuals contract their muscles for a given DOF model training. The length of the residual limb available for electrode placement and integration of sensory feedback in the socket are indeed challenges that are not faced when testing able-bodied subjects and must be addressed when testing amputees. It must be noted that the use of the audio feedback modality in this work reduces the challenges associated with integrating sensory feedback mechanisms within the socket.

In this study, we conducted psychophysical tests on one DOF, i.e., closing the hand to grasp-and-lift an object, to avoid fatigue and loss of motivation. However, we designed the performance test for a two-DOF task where subjects had to activate both DOFs, i.e., digits flexion/extension and thumb adduction/abduction, to ensure that they were able to fully control the device to achieve the task and to collect performance results that could be compared to previous studies [38, 42, 43]. During the performance test, we noticed that lifting the weight of the prosthetic hand affected users' ability to open the hand after grasping the object, which affected the performance for both control strategies tested equally. This weight effect could be avoided in future experiments by using a tool balancer [58].

Furthermore, some subjects reported that continuous audio feedback may be a distraction; however, our results show that, although subjects may not purposely focus on integrating this feedback, they unconsciously integrate it into their internal models. With this in mind, a new question arises: would a task specific discrete audio feedback, i.e., discrete beeps on contact and release of an object akin to the Discrete Event-driven Sensory feedback Control (DESC) principle [1, 59], be less irritating while potentially enabling similar integration? This question will be addressed in future research.

Although audio-augmented feedback showed promising results, the minimum quantity of feedback that is useful for developing strong internal models must still be identified, along with what quality is required for real-time regulation. Future work informed by this study includes: investigating the benefits of using audio feedback for limb-different individuals, exploring a combination of other augmented feedback that might enable an even stronger internal model, exploring the effect of augmenting other feedback modalities on the internal model strength, investigating the effect of audio-augmented feedback control strategy for a more complex task on the internal model strength and the performance, and, finally, investigating the retention of internal models developed while using the audio-augmented feedback control strategy.

Conclusions

We extended our previous work to investigate the benefits of using audio-augmented feedback by testing a classifier-based control with and without this feedback for a grasp-and-lift task when using a prosthetic hand. Results from psychophysical and performance tests showed that audio-augmented feedback enables the development of a strong internal model and better short-term performance. In addition, we concluded that audio feedback may be used in real-time regulation of grasping forces during a grasp-and-lift task.

Acknowledgments
The authors thank Adam Wilson for feedback on training procedures. Many thanks to Francesco Clemente and Michele Bacchereti for their maintenance of the IH2 Azzurra Hand and the instrumented virtual egg.

Funding
This work was supported by the Natural Sciences and Engineering Research Council of Canada (NSERC), the New Brunswick Health Research Foundation (NBHRF), and the European Commission (DeTOP - #687905). The work by C.C. was also funded by the European Research Council (MYKI - #679820).

Authors' contributions
AS, CC, ES, and JS planned the experiments. AS, LE, and MC prepared the experiments. AS and LE conducted the experiments. All authors analyzed the results, reviewed the manuscript, and approved the submitted version.

Competing interests
The authors declare that they have no competing interests.

Author details
[1]Institute of Biomedical Engineering, University of New Brunswick, Fredericton, NB E3B 5A3, Canada. [2]Department of Electrical and Computer Engineering, University of New Brunswick, Fredericton, NB E3B 5A3, Canada. [3]Division of Physical Medicine and Rehabilitation, Department of Medicine, University of Alberta, Edmonton, AB T6G 2E1, Canada. [4]Scuola Superiore Sant'Anna, The BioRobotics Institute, V.le R. Piaggio 34, 56025 Pontedera, PI, Italy.

References
1. Johansson RS, Cole KJ. Sensory-motor coordination during grasping and manipulative actions. Curr Opin Neurobiol. 1992;2:815–23.
2. Dromerick AW, Schabowsky CN, Holley RJ, Monroe B. Feedforward control strategies of subjects with transradial amputation in planar reaching. J Rehabil Res Dev. 2010;47(3):201.
3. Kawato M. Internal models for motor control and trajectory planning. Curr Opin Neurobiol. 1999;9:718–27.
4. Wolpert DM, Ghahramani Z, Jordan MI. An internal model for sensorimotor integration. Science (80-). 1995;269:1880–2. https://doi.org/10.1126/science.7569931.
5. Imamizu H, Miyauchi S, Tamada T, Sasaki Y, Takino R, Pu̇tz B, Yoshioka T, Kawato M. Human cerebellar activity reflecting an acquired internal model of a new tool. Nature. 2000;403(6766):192.
6. Parr JV, Vine SJ, Harrison NR, Wood G. Examining the spatiotemporal disruption to gaze when using a myoelectric prosthetic hand. J Mot Behav. 2018;50(4):416-25.
7. Atkins DJ, Heard DC, Donovan WH. Epidemiologic overview of individuals with upper-limb loss and their reported research priorities. J Prosthetics and Orthotics. 1996;8(1):2-11.
8. Lum PS, Black I, Holley RJ, Barth J, Dromerick AW. Internal models of upper limb prosthesis users when grasping and lifting a fragile object with their prosthetic limb. Exp Brain Res. 2014;232:3785–95.
9. Antfolk C, D'Alonzo M, Rosén B, Lundborg G, Sebelius F, Cipriani C. Sensory feedback in upper limb prosthetics. Expert Rev Med Devices. 2013;10:45–54. https://doi.org/10.1586/erd.12.68.
10. Childress DS. Closed-loop control in prosthetic systems - historical perspective. Ann Biomed Eng. 1980;8:293–303. http://hopper.library.northwestern.edu/sfx/?&atitle=CLOSED-LOOP+CONTROL+IN+PROSTHETIC+SYSTEMS+-+HISTORICAL-PERSPECTIVE&auinit=DS&aulast=CHILDRESS&date=1980&epage=303&issn=0090-6964&issue=4-6&sid=ISI:WoK&spage=293&title=ANN+BIOMED+ENG&title=ANNALS+OF+BIOM
11. Kuiken TA, Dumanian GA, Lipschutz RD, Miller LA, Stubblefield KA. The use of targeted muscle reinnervation for improved myoelectric prosthesis control in a bilateral shoulder disarticulation amputee. Prosthetics Orthot Int. 2004;28:245–53.
12. Hebert JS, Olson JL, Morhart MJ, Dawson MR, Marasco PD, Kuiken TA, et al. Novel targeted sensory Reinnervation technique to restore functional hand sensation after Transhumeral amputation. IEEE Trans neural Syst Rehabil Eng. 2014;22:765–73.
13. Tan DW, Schiefer MA, Keith MW, Anderson JR, Tyler J, Tyler DJ. A neural interface provides long-term stable natural touch perception. Sci Transl Med. 2014;6(257):257ra138-.
14. Davis TS, Wark HA, Hutchinson DT, Warren DJ, O'Neill K, Scheinblum T, Clark GA, Normann RA, Greger B. Restoring motor control and sensory feedback in people with upper extremity amputations using arrays of 96 microelectrodes implanted in the median and ulnar nerves. J Neural Eng. 2016;13(3):036001.
15. Delgado-Martínez I, Righi M, Santos D, Cutrone A, Bossi S, D'Amico S, Del Valle J, Micera S, Navarro X. Fascicular nerve stimulation and recording using a novel double-aisle regenerative electrode. Journal of a novel double-aisle regenerative electrode. J Neural Eng. 2017;14(4):046003.

16. Cordella F, Ciancio AL, Sacchetti R, Davalli A, Cutti AG, Guglielmelli E, et al. Literature Review on Needs of Upper Limb Prosthesis Users. Front Neurosci. 2016;10:1–14.

17. Engdahl SM, Christie BP, Kelly B, Davis A, Chestek CA, Gates DH. Surveying the interest of individuals with upper limb loss in novel prosthetic control techniques. J Neuroeng Rehabil. 2015;12(1):53.

18. Rombokas E, Stepp CE, Chang C, Malhotra M, Matsuoka Y. Vibrotactile sensory substitution for electromyographic control of object manipulation. IEEE Trans Biomed Eng. 2013;60:2226–32.

19. D'Alonzo M, Cipriani C. Vibrotactile sensory substitution elicits feeling of ownership of an alien hand. PLoS One. 2012;7

20. Antfolk C, D'Alonzo M, Controzzi M, Lundborg G, Rosen B, Sebelius F, et al. Artificial redirection of sensation from prosthetic fingers to the phantom hand map on transradial amputees: Vibrotactile versus mechanotactile sensory feedback. IEEE Trans Neural Syst Rehabil Eng. 2013;21:112–20.

21. Kaczmarek KA, Webster JG, Bach-y-Rita P, Tompkins WJ. Electrotactile and vibrotactile displays for sensory substitution systems. IEEE Trans Biomed Eng. 1991;38:1–16.

22. Green AM, Chapman CE, Kalaska JF, Lepore F. Sensory feedback for upper limb prostheses. Enhancing Perform Action Percept Multisensory Integr Neuroplast Neuroprosthetics. 2011;69

23. Gonzalez-Vargas J, Dosen S, Amsuess S, Yu W, Farina D. Human-machine interface for the control of multi-function systems based on electrocutaneous menu: application to multi-grasp prosthetic hands. PLoS One. 2015;10:e0127528.

24. Wheeler J, Bark K, Savall J, Cutkosky M. Investigation of rotational skin stretch for proprioceptive feedback with application to myoelectric systems. IEEE Trans Neural Syst Rehabil Eng. 2010;18:58–66.

25. Gonzalez J, Soma H, Sekine M, Yu W. Psycho-physiological assessment of a prosthetic hand sensory feedback system based on an auditory display: a preliminary study. J Neuroeng Rehabil. 2012;9:33. https://doi.org/10.1186/1743-0003-9-33.

26. Cipriani C, Zaccone F, Micera S, Carrozza MC. On the shared control of an EMG-controlled prosthetic Hand : analysis of user – prosthesis interaction. IEEE Trans Robot. 2008;24:170–84.

27. Chatterjee A, Chaubey P, Martin J, Thakor N. Testing a prosthetic haptic feedback simulator with an interactive force matching task. JPO J Prosthetics Orthot. 2008; 20:27–34.

28. Ninu A, Member S, Dosen S, Muceli S, Rattay F, Dietl H, et al. Closed-Loop Control of Grasping With a Myoelectric Hand Prosthesis : Which Are the Relevant Feedback Variables for Force Control ? 2014;:1041–52.

29. Raspopovic S, Capogrosso M, Petrini FM, Bonizzato M, Rigosa J, Di Pino G, et al. Restoring natural sensory feedback in real-time bidirectional hand prostheses. Sci Transl Med. 2014 6:222ra19–222ra19

30. Dosen S, Markovic M, Strbac M, Perovic M, Kojic V, Bijelic G, et al. Multichannel Electrotactile feedback with spatial and mixed coding for closed-loop control of grasping force in hand prostheses. IEEE Trans Neural Syst Rehabil Eng. 2016;4320:1–1. https://doi.org/10.1109/TNSRE.2016.2550864.

31. Markovic M, Karnal H, Graimann B, Farina D, Dosen S. GLIMPSE: Google Glass interface for sensory feedback in myoelectric hand prostheses. J Neural Eng. 2017;14(3):036007.

32. Marasco PD, Kim K, Colgate JE, Peshkin MA, Kuiken TA. Robotic touch shifts perception of embodiment to a prosthesis in targeted reinnervation amputees. Brain. 2011;134:747–58.

33. Sengul A, Shokur S, Bleuler H. Brain incorporation of artificial limbs and role of haptic feedback. In: Rodić A, Pisla D, Bleuler H, editors. New trends in medical and service robots: challenges and solutions. Cham: Springer International Publishing; 2014. p. 257–68.

34. Zafar M, Van Doren CL. Effectiveness of supplemental grasp-force feedback in the presence of vision. Med Biol Eng Comput. 2000;38:267–74.

35. Dosen S, Markovic M, Somer K, Graimann B, Farina D. EMG biofeedback for online predictive control of grasping force in a myoelectric prosthesis. J Neuroeng Rehabil. 2015;12:55.

36. Schweisfurth MA, Markovic M, Dosen S, Teich F, Graimann B, Farina D. Electrotactile EMG feedback improves the control of prosthesis grasping force. J Neural Eng. 2016;13:56010.

37. Johnson RE, Kording KP, Hargrove LJ, Sensinger JW. Adaptation to random and systematic errors : Comparison of amputee and non-amputee control interfaces with varying levels of process noise. PLoS One. 2017:1–19.

38. Shehata AW, Scheme EJ, Sensinger JW. Evaluating internal model strength and performance of myoelectric prosthesis control strategies. IEEE Trans Neural Syst Rehabil Eng. 2018;26:1046–55.

39. Shehata AW, Scheme EJ, Sensinger JW. The effect of myoelectric prosthesis control strategies and feedback level on adaptation rate for a target acquisition task. InRehabilitation Robotics (ICORR), 2017 International Conference. IEEE. 2017. pp 200-204.

40. Huang Y, Englehart KB, Member S, Hudgins B, Chan ADC. Scheme for Myoelectric Control of Powered Upper Limb Prostheses. 2005;52:1801–11.

41. Scheme E, Englehart K. Electromyogram pattern recognition for control of powered upper-limb prostheses: state of the art and challenges for clinical use. J Rehabil Res Dev. 2011;48:643–59.

42. Hahne JM, Markovic M, Farina D. User adaptation in myoelectric man-machine interfaces. Scientific reports. 2017;7(1):4437.

43. Shehata AW, Scheme EJ, Sensinger JW. Audible Feedback Improves Internal Model Strength and Performance of Myoelectric Prosthesis Control. Scientific reports. 2018;8(1):8541.

44. Cipriani C, Controzzi M, Carrozza MC. The SmartHand transradial prosthesis. J Neuroeng Rehabil. 2011;8(1):29.

45. Controzzi M, Clemente F, Pierotti N, Bacchereti M, Cipriani C. Evaluation of hand function trasporting fragile objects: the virtual eggs test. In: Myoelectric Control Symposium. 2017.

46. Hargrove L, Englehart K, Hudgins B. A comparison of surface and intramuscular myoelectric signal classification. IEEE Trans Biomed Eng. 2007;54:847–53.

47. Tenore F, Ramos A, Fahmy A, Acharya S, Etienne-Cummings R, Thakor NV. Towards the control of individual fingers of a prosthetic hand using surface EMG signals. Conf Proc IEEE Eng Med Biol Soc. 2007;2007:6146–9. https://doi.org/10.1109/IEMBS.2007.4353752.

48. Wilson AW, Losier YG, Parker PA, Lovely DF. A bus-based smart myoelectric electrode/amplifier — system requirements. IEEE Trans Instrum Meas. 2011;60:1–10.

49. Bastian AJ. Understanding sensorimotor adaptation and learning for rehabilitation. Curr Opin Neurol. 2008;21:628–33. https://doi.org/10.1097/WCO.0b013e328315a293.Understanding.

50. Faes L, Nollo G, Ravelli F, Ricci L, Vescovi M, Turatto M, et al. Small-sample characterization of stochastic approximation staircases in forced-choice adaptive threshold estimation. Percept {&} Psychophys. 2007;69:254–62.

51. Ernst MO, Banks MS. Humans integrate visual and haptic information in a statistically optimal fashion. Nature. 2002;415:429–33. https://doi.org/10.1038/415429a.

52. Mathiowetz V, Volland G, Kashman N, Weber K. Adult norms for the box and block test of manual dexterity. Am J Occup Ther. 1985;39:386–91.

53. Fishbach A, Roy SA, Bastianen C, Miller LE, Houk JC. Deciding when and how to correct a movement : discrete submovements as a decision making process. Exp Brain Res. 2007;177:45–63.

54. Doeringer JA, Hogan N. Intermittency in preplanned elbow movements persists in the absence of visual feedback. J Neurophysiol. 1998;80:1787–99.

55. Kositsky M, Barto AG. The emergence of multiple movement units in the presence of noise and feedback delay. Adv neural Inf process Syst 14, NIPS 2001. Proc. 2001;14:1–8.

56. Dipietro L, Krebs HI, Fasoli SE, Volpe BT, Hogan N. Submovement changes characterize generalization of motor recovery after stroke. Cortex. 2009;45:318–24.

57. Strbac M, Isakovic M, Belic M, Popovic I, Simanic I, Farina D, et al. Short- and Long-Term Learning of Feedforward Control of a Myoelectric Prosthesis with Sensory Feedback by Amputees. IEEE Trans Neural Syst Rehabil Eng. 2017:4320 c.

58. Wilson AW, Blustein DH, Sensinger JW. A third arm – design of a bypass prosthesis enabling incorporation: The International Conference on Rehabilitation Robotics; 2017. p. 1381–6

59. Clemente F, D'Alonzo M, Controzzi M, Edin BB, Cipriani C. Non-invasive, temporally discrete feedback of object contact and release improves grasp control of closed-loop myoelectric transradial prostheses. IEEE Trans Neural Syst Rehabil Eng. 2016;24:1314–22.

6

Bilateral reaching deficits after unilateral perinatal ischemic stroke

Andrea M. Kuczynski[1,2] (iD), Adam Kirton[1,2,3], Jennifer A. Semrau[1,3] and Sean P. Dukelow[1,3]*

Abstract

Background: Detailed kinematics of motor impairment of the contralesional ("affected") and ipsilesional ("unaffected") limbs in children with hemiparetic cerebral palsy are not well understood. We aimed to 1) quantify the kinematics of reaching in both arms of hemiparetic children with perinatal stroke using a robotic exoskeleton, and 2) assess the correlation of kinematic reaching parameters with clinical motor assessments.

Methods: This prospective, case-control study involved the Alberta Perinatal Stroke Project, a population-based research cohort, and the Foothills Medical Center Stroke Robotics Laboratory in Calgary, Alberta over a four year period. Prospective cases were collected through the Calgary Stroke Program and included term-born children with magnetic resonance imaging confirmed perinatal ischemic stroke and upper extremity deficits. Control participants were recruited from the community. Participants completed a visually guided reaching task in the KINARM robot with each arm separately, with 10 parameters quantifying motor function. Kinematic measures were compared to clinical assessments and stroke type.

Results: Fifty children with perinatal ischemic stroke (28 arterial, mean age: 12.5 ± 3.9 years; 22 venous, mean age: 11.5 ± 3.8 years) and upper extremity deficits were compared to healthy controls ($n = 147$, mean age: 12.7 ± 3.9 years). Perinatal stroke groups demonstrated contralesional motor impairments compared to controls when reaching out (arterial = 10/10, venous = 8/10), and back (arterial = 10/10, venous = 6/10) with largest errors in reaction time, initial direction error, movement length and time. Ipsilesional impairments were also found when reaching out (arterial = 7/10, venous = 1/10) and back (arterial = 6/10). The arterial group performed worse than venous on both contralesional and ipsilesional parameters. Contralesional reaching parameters showed modest correlations with clinical measures in the arterial group.

Conclusions: Robotic assessment of reaching behavior can quantify complex, upper limb dysfunction in children with perinatal ischemic stroke. The ipsilesional, "unaffected" limb is often abnormal and may be a target for therapeutic interventions in stroke-induced hemiparetic cerebral palsy.

Keywords: Perinatal stroke, Cerebral palsy, Motor control, Reaching, Robotics

* Correspondence: sean.dukelow@albertahealthservices.ca
[1]University of Calgary, Calgary, AB T2N 2T9, Canada
[3]Department of Clinical Neurosciences, Foothills Medical Centre, Hotchkiss Brain Institute, 1403 – 29th St. NW, Calgary, AB, Canada
Full list of author information is available at the end of the article

Background

Perinatal stroke is an early vascular brain injury that accounts for most hemiparetic cerebral palsy (HCP) [1]. The most common perinatal stroke types are large arterial ischemic strokes (AIS) in the middle cerebral artery territory and smaller fetal periventricular venous infarctions (PVI) of the subcortical white matter [2]. While both types of lesions can damage the sensory-motor system, children with PVI typically show milder impairments. These differences may be attributed to the purely subcortical nature of the venous infarctions compared to the cortical and subcortical injuries sustained within the middle cerebral artery in children with arterial stroke [3]. Differences in timing of the injury may also influence motor development, as PVI lesions are incurred before 32–34 weeks gestation and most arterial lesions are acquired near term.

Most children incur lifelong developmental deficits after perinatal stroke, with 80% having contralateral hemiparesis [3]. While motor impairments of the contralesional upper limb have been the primary focus in rehabilitation, studies have suggested that the "unaffected" ipsilesional limb also shows deficits in coordination, dexterity, strength, and movement speed [4–9]. Many activities of daily living depend on the input and coordination of both arms, therefore developing a better understanding of upper limb impairments may advance therapies and improve outcomes.

Our understanding of motor system development following perinatal stroke has improved markedly in the past decade [3, 10]. At birth, corticospinal tracts are bilateral, with ipsilateral projections withdrawing in the first years of development, resulting in predominantly contralateral limb control [11, 12]. Early perinatal stroke often results in persistent ipsilateral corticospinal projections from the non-lesioned hemisphere to the stroke-affected limbs [13]. Ipsilateral control is associated with poor clinical outcome and reduced hand function in HCP [8, 13, 14]. Much less is known about the development of the control mechanisms for the ipsilesional limb. Gaining a detailed understanding of the movement kinematics of both upper extremities will serve to advance understanding of development and application of potential therapeutic options in HCP.

Robotic technology has been used to objectively quantify complex, discrete sensorimotor functions in adult stroke [15–17] and sensory impairments in children with stroke [18, 19]. The current study aimed to evaluate motor function in hemiparetic children to: 1) characterize movement of the contralesional and ipsilesional upper limbs with a robotic assessment; 2) assess correlations between kinematic and clinical measures of movement. We hypothesized that motor performance, as measured by a visually guided reaching task, in both upper extremities would be more impaired in AIS compared to PVI, and that kinematic parameters would be moderately correlated with clinical motor assessments.

Methods

Participant criteria

This was a prospective, case-controlled study involving the Alberta Perinatal Stroke Project, a population-based research cohort [20], and the Foothills Medical Centre Stroke Robotics Laboratory (Calgary, AB) between September 2013 and August 2016. Inclusion criteria were: 1) age 6–19 years, 2) clinical and MRI confirmation of perinatal stroke (AIS, PVI), 3) symptomatic hemiparesis (Pediatric Stroke Outcome Measure [21] sensorimotor component > 0.5 and Manual Abilities Classification System [22] grades I-IV), 4) gestational age > 36 weeks, 5) visual acuity of at least 20/30, and 6) written informed consent/assent. Exclusion criteria were: 1) multifocal stroke, 2) other neurological disorders not attributable to perinatal stroke, 3) severe hemiparesis (Manual Abilities Classification System [22] grade V, indicating no voluntary contraction in the hemiparetic hand), 4) severe spasticity (Modified Ashworth Scale [23] > 3 in any muscle tested), 5) inability to comply with the study protocol, 6) upper limb surgery, botulinum toxin treatment, constraint or brain stimulation therapy within 6 months of study participation.

Typically developing children (6–19 years of age) without neurological impairment were recruited and completed the same evaluations. Written informed consent was obtained from all participants and their parents/guardians. This study was approved by the institutional University of Calgary Conjoint Health Research Ethics Board (CHREB), ID REB15–0136.

Robotic reaching assessment

The KINARM robotic exoskeleton (BKIN Technologies Ltd., Kingston, Ontario) quantified movement [24]. Participants were fit to the modified wheelchair base with each arm supported by the exoskeleton (Fig. 1a). The robotic device permits free movement of the participant's arms in the horizontal plane while monitoring the movement at the shoulder and/or elbow joint [25] and the device has been described in more detail elsewhere [15]. The spatial accuracy of the device in the current task was 0.7 mm with a sampling frequency of 1000 Hz.

A visually guided reaching task evaluated motor performance of both arms. Participants were instructed to move their hand quickly and accurately from a fixed central position to one of four peripheral targets located in the circumference of a circle, separated by 6 cm (Fig. 1). Each participant completed 40 trials with each arm (20 reaches out, 20 back). Peripheral target illumination order was pseudo-randomized. Subjects performed the task once with each arm. All participants performed the

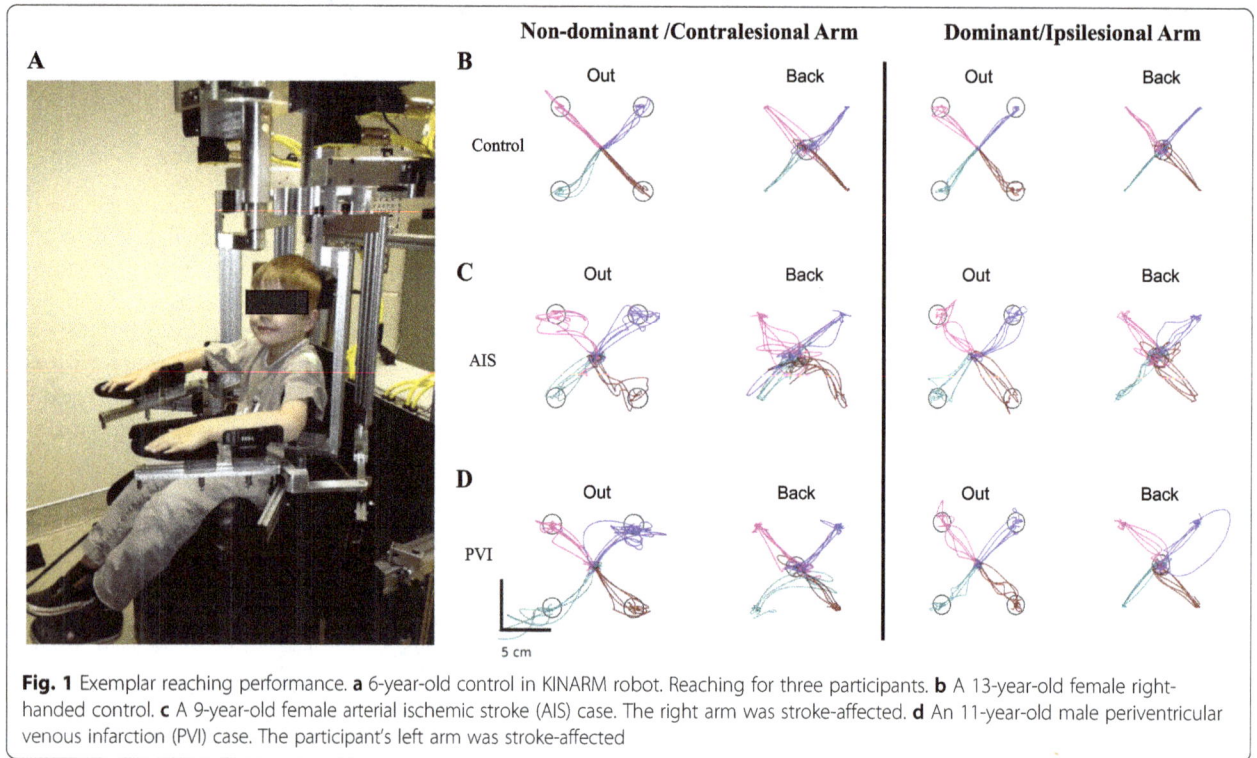

Fig. 1 Exemplar reaching performance. **a** 6-year-old control in KINARM robot. Reaching for three participants. **b** A 13-year-old female right-handed control. **c** A 9-year-old female arterial ischemic stroke (AIS) case. The right arm was stroke-affected. **d** An 11-year-old male periventricular venous infarction (PVI) case. The participant's left arm was stroke-affected

task with their dominant limb first. The arms of partici-pants with stroke are herein referred to as either con-tralesional or ipsilesional, whereas control participants' arms are either dominant or non-dominant.

Determination of movement onset/offset in robotic assessments

For each participant, movement onset was calculated during a 500 ms period prior to peripheral target ap-pearance, in which the subject held their hand position in the start target. During this period, two measures were calculated: maximum posture speed (PS_{max}) and minimum posture speed (PS_{min}). PS_{max} was calculated as the 95th percentile of hand speed in the 500 ms when the hand was positioned in the central target, prior to the illumination of the peripheral target across all trials, while PS_{min} was defined as the 50th percentile of hand speed during this time period [15]. Based on these two thresholds, movement onset was defined as the time when either a) a local minimum in hand speed below PS_{max} was found, or b) the hand speed fell below PS_{min}. Movement onset was not recorded if a participant's hand speed never dropped below PS_{max}, or if the participant's hand left the central target > 2000 ms after the illumin-ation of the peripheral target.

The same thresholds described above were used to de-fine movement offset as the time when the participant reached the peripheral target and a) the first local hand speed minima below PS_{max}, or b) hand speed below PS_{min}

was found. If a participant did not reach the peripheral target, movement offset was not recorded.

Description of robotic parameters

Ten parameters, which have been previously described [15], were used to describe different aspects of the reaching movements and calculated for movements reaching out and back:

1) *Postural speed (PS):* hand speed (in cm/s) while holding in the central target. One posture speed score was calculated for each arm.
2) *Reaction time (RT):* time (in seconds) from the peripheral target illumination to the onset of arm movement.
3) *Initial direction error (IDE):* angular deviation (in degrees) between a) a straight line from the hand position at movement onset to the peripheral target, and b) a vector from the hand position at movement onset to the position after the initial movement. The time between movement onset and the first minimum hand speed was defined as the initial stage of movement.
4) *Initial distance ratio (IDR):* the ratio of distance the hand moved during the initial movement to the distance the hand moved between movement onset and offset. A ratio of > 1 represents a distance moved greater than required to reach the peripheral target.

5) *Initial speed ratio (ISR):* the ratio of the maximum hand speed during initial movement to the global hand speed maximum of the trial. In typical reaching movements, healthy participants should move with ISR = 1 as the speed profile of their movements is typically a smooth bell-shaped curve.

6) *Speed maxima count (SMC):* the number of speed peaks associated with arm movement between movement onset and movement offset.

7) *Minimum-maximum speed difference (MMSD):* the difference between speed maxima and minima after the initial movement.

8) *Movement time (MT):* total time (in seconds) from movement onset to offset.

9) *Path length ratio (PLR):* total distance traveled by the hand between movement onset and offset compared to the shortest distance between targets.

10) *Maximum speed (MS):* maximum speed (in cm/s) achieved during the entire movement (40 trials).

Control performance was fit with a line of best fit (SigmaPlot, Systat Software Inc., San Jose) to account for age effects. Ninety-five percent prediction bands for controls were calculated from the mean curves to develop normative ranges. Participants that fell outside these prediction bands for a given parameter were considered to have failed that parameter relative to the control performance.

Clinical assessments

At the beginning of each session, an experienced therapist performed clinical assessments including:

A. *Muscle strength* of the shoulder, elbow, wrist, and finger was graded using the Medical Research Council scale bilaterally for all participants [26]. Scores ranged from 0 (no muscular contraction) to 5 (normal muscle strength) with a maximum score of 60/arm.

B. *Modified Ashworth Scale (MAS)* assessed tone of shoulders, elbows, and wrists in all children with perinatal stroke [23]. Scores ranged from 0 (no increase in tone) to 4 (rigidity) and were summed to give one total score.

C. *Chedoke-McMaster Stroke Assessment (CMSA)* assessed both contralesional and ipsilesional movement in the arms and hands of children with perinatal stroke [27]. Scores ranged from 0 (paralysis) to 7 (normal movement).

D. *Assisting Hand Assessment (AHA)* assessed 22 real-world activities and measured bimanual upper extremity motor function in hemiparetic children with perinatal stroke [28]. Scores were expressed as logit units, ranging from 0 (no use of the hand) to 100 (normal function).

E. *Melbourne Assessment Unilateral Upper Limb Function (MA)* assessed 16 tasks of reaching and grasping of different sized objects to evaluate finger dexterity and speed of movement in hemiparetic children with perinatal stroke [29]. Scores ranged from 0 (unable to perform) to 100 (no difficulty).

F. *Purdue pegboard test (PPB)* (LaFayette Instrument Co, LaFayette, IN) tested fine motor function of each hand separately in all participants. Participants picked up one peg at a time and successively filled them down a sequence of holes, as quickly as possible in 30 s. This test was repeated twice and the best score used in analysis.

G. *Modified Edinburgh Handedness Inventory* determined hand dominance using a 10-item assessment [30]. Right arm use for an item was scored + 10 while left arm use was scored – 10. Equal use of both limbs (ambidextrous) was scored 0. Completely right-hand dominant individuals scored + 100, while left-hand dominant individuals scored – 100. Subjects scoring between – 50 and + 50 (with the exception of 0) were classified as mixed handedness and were classified according to their self-reported handedness.

H. Visual fields were assessed using confrontation and scored as normal or abnormal (hemianopsia, quadrantanopsia).

I. The Behavioural Inattention Test (BIT) assessed visuospatial function using six conventional subtests (line bisection, line crossing, star cancellation, letter cancellation, figure and shape copying, representational drawing) for a total possible score of 146 with scores < 130 indicating hemispatial neglect [31].

Statistical analyses

Statistical analyses were performed using SigmaPlot and SPSS (IBM, Armonk, NY). Kolmogorov-Smirnov tests determined the normality of data distributions. A one-way ANCOVA was conducted using SPSS to determine whether differences existed between the three groups (AIS, PVI, controls) for each reaching parameter while controlling for age. Post-hoc pairwise comparisons were then conducted using Bonferroni corrections for multiple comparisons ($\alpha = 0.05$). Within each group, Mann-Whitney U-tests or paired t-tests compared performance between both upper limbs and between out and back performance of each limb. Partial Spearman's correlations controlling for age assessed the relationship of bilateral reaching parameters with clinical assessments (controlled for comparisons to 6 clinical measures, $\alpha = 0.05$, $p < 0.008$). In the case of missing clinical data, participants were removed from the analysis.

Results

Table 1 summarizes the demographic and clinical characteristics of the participants. Overall, 28 AIS, 22 PVI, and 147 healthy controls were included in the study. Examples of bilateral reaching performance are shown in Fig. 1. An exemplar control demonstrates normal reaching movements of both upper extremities. Typical AIS and PVI participants demonstrated impairments in performing the same reaching movements. The percentage of AIS and PVI participants that failed each robotic parameter is in Fig. 2. Table 2 describes the mean performance of the three groups across each reaching parameter.

Contralesional / non-dominant reaching

The AIS group showed impairments in all reaching parameters when reaching out with their contralesional arm compared to the non-dominant arm of controls (Table 2). PVI participants were impaired in 8 of 10 parameters. Both stroke groups had slower reaction times ($F(2,196) = 28.8$, $p < 0.001$), larger initial direction errors ($F(2,196) = 67.1$, $p < 0.001$), moved with longer initial movements ($F(2,196) = 43.5$, $p < 0.001$), and had greater movement time ($F(2,196) = 51.5$, $p < 0.001$; Fig. 3). The

AIS group had longer reaction times ($p < 0.01$), larger initial direction error ($p = 0.05$), and longer movement times ($p < 0.01$) with slower maximum speed ($p < 0.05$) compared to PVI when reaching out.

When reaching back to the central target with their contralesional arm, the AIS group again showed impairments in all 10 reaching parameters. Conversely, the PVI group showed impairments in 6 parameters (Table 2). Both stroke groups had slower reaction times ($F(2,196) = 22.8$, $p < 0.05$), larger initial direction errors ($F(2,196) = 55.3$, $p < 0.001$), and slower movement times ($F(2,196) = 49.0$, $p < 0.001$; Fig. 4) than controls. The AIS group differed from PVI on 7 parameters. AIS subjects had greater reaction time ($p < 0.05$) and initial direction error ($p < 0.05$), longer ($p < 0.01$) and slower ($p < 0.001$) initial movements, made more sub-movements ($p = 0.001$), and had slower ($p = 0.001$) and longer movements ($p < 0.01$).

Differences in contralesional / non-dominant reaches out and back

Comparing the reaching out to reaching back, controls had slower reaction times ($Z = -2.78$, $p < 0.01$), larger initial direction errors ($Z = -5.92$, $p < 0.001$), shorter initial movements ($Z = 5.58$, $p < 0.001$), moved slower initially ($Z = 2.34$, $p < 0.05$), made more sub-movements ($Z = -5.09$, $p < 0.001$), shorter movements ($t(146) = -2.03$, $p < 0.05$), and slower maximum speed ($t(146) = -6.57$, p

Table 1 Demographic information

	AIS		PVI		Controls	
Number of Subjects	28		22		147	
Age (years)	12.5 ± 3.9		11.5 ± 3.8		12.7 ± 3.9	
Sex (female, male)	10, 18		8, 14		71, 76	
Paretic Limb (L, R)	10, 18		11, 11		–	
Handedness (L, R, M)	18, 10, 0		8, 12, 2		8, 127, 12	
Logit AHA [0–100]	61.3 ± 19.9 (32–100)[a]		75.2 ± 16.0 (55–100)[c]		–	
MA [0–100]	69.1 ± 21.3 (31–100)[a]		89.4 ± 10.7 (64–100)[c]		–	
BIT [0–146]	129.5 ± 22.2 (56–145)[b]		138.5 ± 5.6 (122–146)[b]		–	
	Contralesional	Ipsilesional	Contralesional	Ipsilesional	Non-dominant	Dominant
Strength [0–60]	48.2 ± 8.7 (30–60)	59.9 ± 0.4 (58–60)[b]	55.6 ± 3.9 (47–60)	60.0 ± 0.0 (60)[b]	60.0 ± 0.2 (58–60)[d]	60.0 ± 0.09 (59–60)[b]
MAS [0–24]	3.64 ± 3.1 (0–15)	0.0 ± 0.0	1.91 ± 2.6 (0–10)	0.0 ± 0.0	–	–
CMSA Arm [1–7]	[0, 0, 13, 2, 5, 3, 5]	[0, 0, 0, 0, 0, 4, 24]	[0, 0, 3, 1, 4, 4, 10]	[0, 0, 0, 0, 0, 5, 17]	–	–
CMSA Hand [1–7]	[0, 5, 12, 5, 3, 2, 1]	[0, 0, 0, 0, 1, 5, 22]	[0, 1, 0, 10, 10, 1]	[0, 0, 0, 0, 8, 14]	–	–
PPB	1.81 ± 3.4 (0–11)	12.5 ± 2.0 (10–16)	5.50 ± 3.7 (0–11)	13.1 ± 1.7 (10–16)	13.8 ± 2.3 (8–19)[c]	14.9 ± 2.4 (8–21)[b]

Mean ± SD shown, (round brackets contain range). CMSA shown as the number of participants with each score on the 7-point scale. Abbreviations: arterial ischemic stroke (AIS), periventricular venous infarction (PVI), L (left), R (right), M (mixed), Assisting Hand Assessment (AHA), Melbourne Assessment of Unilateral Upper Limb Function (MA), Behavioural Inattention Test (BIT), Modified Ashworth Scale (MAS), Chedoke-McMaster Stroke Assessment (CMSA), Purdue Pegboard (PPB). Missing data from [a] eight, [b] one, [c] nine, and [d] three participants

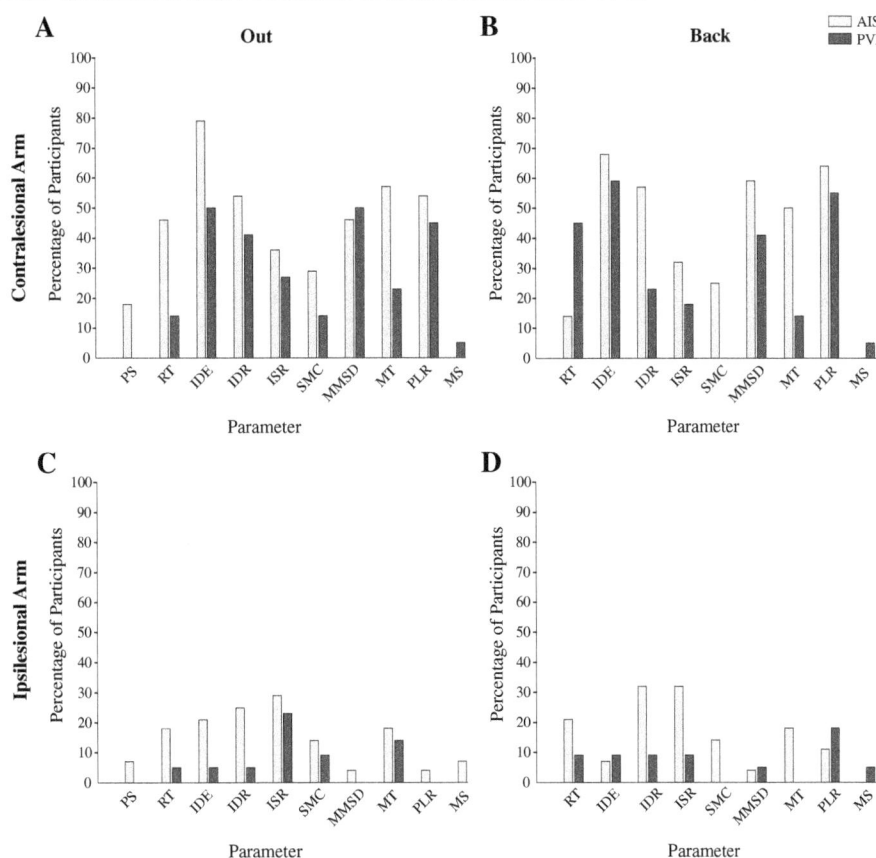

Fig. 2 Failure on reaching parameters. The percentage of individuals within the arterial ischemic stroke (AIS) and periventricular venous infarction (PVI) groups that fell outside 95% range of controls for reaches made out (**a, c**) and back (**b, d**) for each arm. Abbreviations: posture speed (PS), reaction time (RT), initial direction error (IDE), initial distance ratio (IDR), initial speed ratio (ISR), speed maxima count (SMC), minimum-maximum speed difference (MMSD), movement time (MT), path length ratio (PLR), maximum speed (MS)

< 0.001) when reaching out. The AIS group followed a similar trend with shorter (t(26) = − 2.03, $p = 0.05$), and slower movements (Z = 2.11, $p < 0.05$ and t(26) = − 2.30, $p < 0.05$, respectively) in reaching out versus back, while the PVI group had shorter (t(21) = − 2.73, $p = 0.01$) and slower speed (t(21) = − 3.59, $p < 0.01$) movements with more sub-movements (t(21) = 2.70, $p = 0.01$) reaching out versus back.

Ipsilesional / dominant reaching
Reaching out with their ipsilesional arm, the AIS group showed impairments in 7 parameters (Table 2). Compared to controls' dominant arm reaching, the AIS group had slower reaction times (F(2,196) = 16.2, $p < 0.001$), larger initial direction error (F(2,196) = 9.16, $p < 0.001$), shorter (F(2,196) = 7.69, $p = 0.001$) and slower (F(2,196) = 17.1, $p < 0.001$) initial movements, more sub-movements (F(2,196) = 4.07, $p < 0.05$), greater movement time (F(2,196) = 8.89, $p < 0.001$), and slower speed (F92196) = 9.80, $p < 0.001$). PVI participants only showed reduced initial speed ratio (F(2,196) = 17.1, $p < 0.01$) compared to controls. As a group,

AIS participants had greater initial direction error when reaching out compared to PVI ($p < 0.05$).

Reaching back, the AIS group showed impairment in 6 parameters while the PVI group was not different from controls. AIS participants had slower reaction times (F(2,196) = 11.8, $p < 0.001$), greater initial direction error (F(2,196) = 10.0, $p < 0.001$), shorter (F(2,196) = 10.2, $p < 0.001$) and slower (F(2,196) = 13.8, $p < 0.001$) initial movements, greater movement time (F(2,196) = 8.98, $p < 0.001$), and slower overall speed (F(2,196) = 12.0, $p < 0.001$). The AIS group had greater movement time ($p < 0.05$) and slower maximum speed ($p < 0.05$) in their movements compared to the PVI group reaching back with their ipsilesional limb.

Differences in ipsilesional / dominant reaches out and back
Control participants had slower reaction times (Z = − 2.02, $p < 0.05$), greater initial direction error (Z = − 4.92, $p < 0.001$), shorter initial movements (Z = 5.35, $p < 0.001$), slower initial speed (Z = 2.95, $p < 0.001$), more

Table 2 Comparison of mean robotic visually guided reaching performance between the stroke groups and healthy controls

	AIS		PVI		Controls	
	Out	Back	Out	Back	Out	Back
Contralesional/non-dominant upper extremity						
PS (cm/s)	0.29 ± 0.2*		0.20 ± 0.09		0.21 ± 0.1	
RT (s)	0.49 ± 0.2*†	0.46 ± 0.1*†	0.43 ± 0.1‡	0.42 ± 0.1‡	0.37 ± 0.08	0.36 ± 0.09
IDE (°)	10.24 ± 6.2*†	10.70 ± 8.6*†	8.60 ± 4.3‡	8.30 ± 4.1‡	4.16 ± 1.4	3.56 ± 1.4
IDR	0.65 ± 0.2*	0.69 ± 0.1*†	0.69 ± 0.2‡	0.77 ± 0.1‡	0.84 ± 0.1	0.89 ± 0.08
ISR	0.92 ± 0.07*	0.93 ± 0.08*†	0.94 ± 0.06‡	0.97 ± 0.04	0.98 ± 0.03	0.98 ± 0.03
SMC	2.74 ± 0.7*	2.73 ± 0.9*†	2.49 ± 0.5‡	2.24 ± 0.4	2.15 ± 0.4	2.00 ± 0.4
MMSD (cm/s)	2.03 ± 1.6*	2.21 ± 1.2*	2.11 ± 1.4‡	1.95 ± 1.5‡	0.79 ± 0.6	0.80 ± 0.7
MT (s)	1.36 ± 0.3*†	1.33 ± 0.3*†	1.20 ± 0.3‡	1.15 ± 0.2‡	0.97 ± 0.2	0.95 ± 0.2
PLR	1.59 ± 0.5*	1.60 ± 0.4*†	1.51 ± 0.3‡	1.45 ± 0.2‡	1.20 ± 0.1	1.22 ± 0.1
MS (cm/s)	13.21 ± 1.9*†	14.00 ± 1.7*	16.08 ± 3.7	16.12 ± 3.9	16.80 ± 4.0	17.76 ± 4.3
Ipsilesional/dominant upper extremity						
PS (cm/s)	0.23 ± 0.2		0.22 ± 0.1		0.21 ± 0.1	
RT (s)	0.44 ± 0.1*	0.42 ± 0.1*	0.41 ± 0.1	0.40 ± 0.1	0.35 ± 0.08	0.35 ± 0.08
IDE (°)	6.12 ± 3.3*†	5.67 ± 2.1*	5.01 ± 1.8	5.08 ± 2.2	4.52 ± 1.7	3.97 ± 2.0
IDR	0.76 ± 0.1*	0.81 ± 0.1*	0.79 ± 0.1	0.85 ± 0.1	0.84 ± 0.1	0.88 ± 0.08
ISR	0.95 ± 0.04*	0.96 ± 0.05*	0.96 ± 0.04‡	0.97 ± 0.04	0.98 ± 0.03	0.99 ± 0.02
SMC	2.47 ± 0.6*	2.22 ± 0.5	2.21 ± 0.4	2.03 ± 0.4	2.20 ± 0.4	2.03 ± 0.4
MMSD (cm/s)	0.84 ± 0.6	0.74 ± 0.7	0.89 ± 0.4	0.80 ± 0.9	1.03 ± 0.8	1.08 ± 0.9
MT (s)	1.09 ± 0.2*	1.05 ± 0.2*†	1.00 ± 0.2	0.94 ± 0.2	0.94 ± 0.2	0.90 ± 0.2
PLR	1.22 ± 0.1	1.25 ± 0.2	1.21 ± 0.1	1.22 ± 0.1	1.22 ± 0.1	1.23 ± 0.1
MS (cm/s)	13.64 ± 2.6*	14.32 ± 2.1*†	15.91 ± 4.1	17.11 ± 4.6	16.94 ± 3.7	18.09 ± 3.8

Scores are shown as mean ± standard deviation. Statistical significance (p < 0.05) is indicated for differences between AIS and controls (*), PVI and controls (‡), and between AIS and PVI groups (†). Abbreviations: arterial ischemic stroke (AIS), periventricular venous infarction (PVI), posture speed (PS), reaction time (RT), initial direction error (IDE), initial distance ratio (IDR), initial speed ratio (ISR), speed maxima count (SMC), minimum-maximum speed difference (MMSD), movement time (MT), path length ratio (PLR), maximum speed (MS)

sub-movements (t(146) = 5.72, $p < 0.001$), shorter movement time (t(146) = 5.27, $p < 0.001$), and slower maximum hand speed (t(146) = − 9.93, $p < 0.001$) when reaching out compared to back. The AIS group made shorter initial movements (t(27) = − 2.12, $p < 0.05$), more sub-movements (t(27) = 3.06, $p < 0.01$), had greater movement time (Z = − 2.14, $p < 0.05$), and lower maximal speed (t(27) = − 2.31, p < 0.05) when reaching out. Similar to AIS, PVI subjects demonstrated shorter initial movements (t(21) = − 3.04, $p < 0.01$), reduced initial speed (Z = 2.02, p = 0.05), more sub-movements (t(21) = 2.40, p < 0.05), longer movement times (t(21) = 2.94, p < 0.01), and slower overall speed (t(21) = − 2.96, $p < 0.01$) when reaching out versus back.

Inter-limb differences

When reaching out, controls displayed faster reaction times (Z = − 4.46, $p < 0.001$) and larger min-max speed differences (t(146) = − 3.82, $p < 0.001$) with the dominant arm, but all other parameters were similar between limbs. The AIS group displayed slower reaction times (Z = − 3.22, p =

0.001), larger initial direction error (Z = − 3.58, $p < 0.001$), smaller initial movements (Z = 4.13, $p < 0.001$), larger min-max speed difference (Z = − 3.87, $p < 0.001$), slower movement time (t(26) = 4.13, $p < 0.001$) and longer movements (Z = − 4.20, $p < 0.001$) when reaching with the contralesional arm. The PVI group demonstrated larger initial direction errors (Z = − 3.78, $p < 0.001$), min-max speed differences (t(21) = 3.83, $p < 0.001$), slower movement time (t(21) = 3.26, $p < 0.01$) and longer movements (Z = − 4.11, $p < 0.001$) with the contralesional versus the ipsilesional arm.

Reaching back, controls demonstrated slower reaction time (Z = − 3.08, $p < 0.01$), min-max speed difference (Z = 3.59, p < 0.001), and slower movement time (t(146) = 3.72, p < 0.001) with their non-dominant arm. The AIS group displayed greater reaction time (Z = − 3.17, p < 0.01), larger initial direction error (Z = − 3.39, $p < 0.001$), shorter initial movements (t(26) = − 4.36, $p < 0.001$), greater min-max speed difference (t(26) = 5.73, p < 0.001), slower (t(26) = 4.15, p < 0.001) and longer movements (Z = − 4.18, $p < 0.001$) with their contralesional versus their ipsilesional arm. The PVI group showed

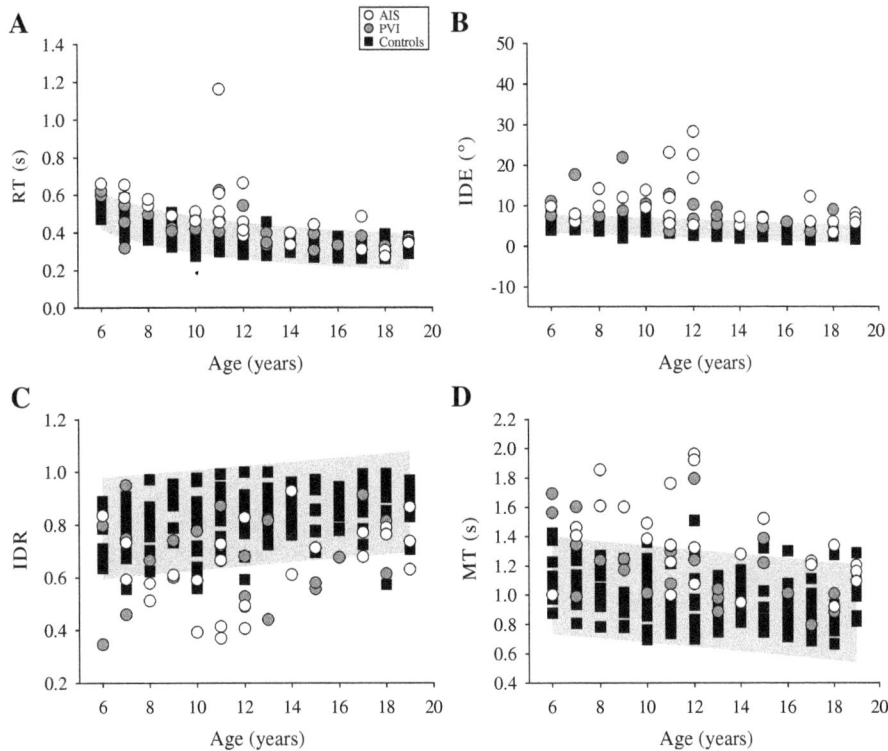

Fig. 3 Contralesional/non-dominant reaching performance. The reaching performance out for (**a**) reaction time (RT), (**b**) initial direction error (IDE), (**c**) initial distance ratio (IDR), and (**d**) movement time (MT) is shown for the arterial ischemic stroke (AIS), periventricular venous infarction (PVI), and control subjects represented by open circles, filled circles and black squares, respectively. The 95% prediction bands of control performance (grey box) with their non-dominant limb in each measure are shown

greater initial direction error (t(21) = 3.60, p < 0.01), larger min-max speed difference (t(21) = 3.35, p < 0.01), slower (t(21) = 4.65, p < 0.001) and longer movements (t(21) = 4.62, p < 0.001) with the contralesional arm.

Hemispheric damage and reaching performance

AIS participants with left ($n = 18$) versus right ($n = 10$) hemispheric damage showed no statistically significant differences in reaching performance out and back with either arm. Further no statistically significant differences were observed in PVI cases with left ($n = 11$) versus right (n = 11) hemispheric damage when reaching out and back with either limb.

Clinical assessments and reaching performance

AHA scores were lower in AIS cases (61.3 ± 20.5) compared to the PVI group (75.2 ± 16.7, t(31) = − 2.04, $p <$ 0.05; Table 1). MA scores were lower in the AIS (69.1 ± 21.8) group compared to PVI (89.4 ± 11.1, U = 67.0, p < 0.05). Ipsilateral deficits determined by the CMSA (score = 6) were found in four AIS and five PVI participants. CMSA scores were lower in AIS than PVI cases in their contralesional arm (U = 171.5, $p <$ 0.01) and hand (U = 82.5, $p <$ 0.001) than the ipsilesional. CMSA scores of the ipsilesional arm (U = 282, $p =$ 0.45) and hand (U =

266, $p =$ 0.30) were comparable between AIS and PVI groups. Several reaching parameters were moderately correlated with our clinical measures in the AIS group (Table 3). While some significant correlations were observed between clinical measures and robotic parameters in the ipsilesional limb of the AIS group, we observed a greater number of significant correlations in the contralesional limb of the AIS group. No statistically significant correlations were observed between clinical and robotic reaching scores out or back with either limb in PVI.

Discussion

Children with perinatal stroke demonstrated significant impairments in reaching with their contralesional limb compared to typically developing subjects. On average, deficits were associated with stroke type and were greater in AIS compared to PVI, similar to our recent studies of sensory function [18, 19]. Our findings in the contralesional limb are more detailed than previous kinematic studies in hemiparetic children, but align with observations of increased reaction times and movement times [31–34]. The AIS group also showed significant deficits when completing the reaching task with their ipsilesional limb compared to the dominant arm of controls. Our

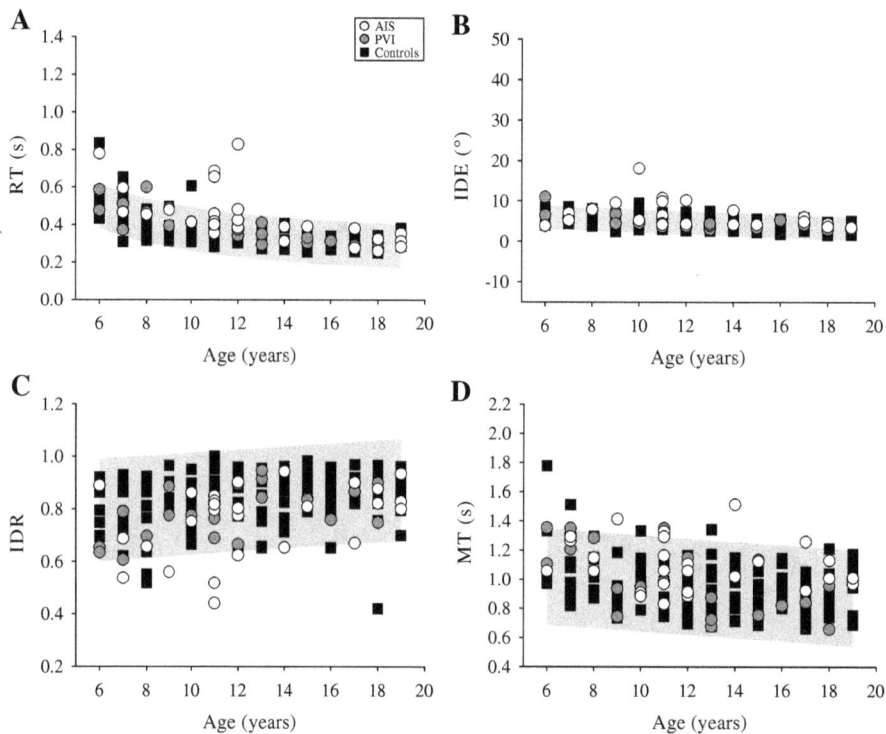

Fig. 4 Ipsilesional/dominant reaching performance. The reaching performance out for (**a**) reaction time (RT), (**b**) initial direction error (IDE), (**c**) initial distance ratio (IDR), and (**d**) movement time (MT) is shown for the arterial ischemic stroke (AIS), periventricular venous infarction (PVI), and control subjects represented by open circles, filled circles and black squares, respectively. The 95% prediction bands of control performance (grey box) with their dominant limb in each measure are shown

findings draw attention to the importance of stroke type in determining upper limb motor impairment, and these results can serve to inform models of developmental plasticity following early unilateral brain injury.

Post-stroke therapies often promote task-specific training to improve motor function and independence [33, 34]. In children, modified constraint and bimanual therapies can improve range of movement of the paretic limb as well as motor connectivity in the lesioned hemisphere [35, 36]. To our knowledge, no therapeutic trial has ever targeted specific kinematic deficits. In the present study we examined specific aspects of movement including postural control (e.g. posture speed), movement initiation (e.g. reaction time, initial direction error), feedback/corrective phases of movement (e.g. speed maxima count), as well as overall movement metrics (e.g. movement time). The precision and detail provided by robotic measures may facilitate more individualized therapy approaches in the future specifically targeting difference aspects of movement, either through traditional therapy approaches or more technologically advanced techniques. Further, robots have the ability to measure both small and large changes in motor function over time. These types of measurements have significant potential to quantify responses to novel interventions and also quantify motor development in

children. In future research, the types of assessments described in this study could be employed to help determine which patients should be included in clinical trials.

Our confirmation that the "unaffected" limb often has abnormal motor function in children with perinatal stroke and HCP has important implications. Early unilateral brain injuries can result in reduced strength, dexterity, speed, and increased clumsiness of the ipsilesional arm [6, 8, 37–39]. Our study adds detailed kinematic data to this body of literature supporting the concept that a unilateral injury can lead to bilateral motor impairments. Developmental plasticity models suggest sensory function almost always remains contralateral while motor control is often divided between both the lesioned and contralesional hemisphere [40], the degree of which is associated with clinical function [14]. Such dissociation of communication between sensory and motor cortices in the contralateral hemisphere may lead to worse functional deficits. The fact that the better arm for which children with HCP are heavily dependent upon for daily function is specifically impaired in many parameters warrants new focus on improved recognition and possible redirection of therapeutic efforts.

Reaching performance was worse in reaches made out versus back in our groups, regardless of the limb being

Table 3 Clinical correlations with robotic reaching performance

| | AIS | | | | PVI | | | |
| | Contralesional | | Ipsilesional | | Contralesional | | Ipsilesional | |
	Out	Back	Out	Back	Out	Back	Out	Back
AHA								
PS (cm/s)	0.070		−0.076		− 0.33		0.00	
RT (s)	−0.32	− 0.19	− 0.39	− 0.41	− 0.36	− 0.23	0.0060	− 0.054
IDE (°)	− 0.58	− 0.57	− 0.20	0.053	− 0.18	− 0.47	− 0.014	− 0.090
IDR	0.51	0.63*	0.14	0.065	0.34	0.29	0.21	0.26
ISR	0.35	0.25	−0.12	0.17	0.22	0.26	0.14	0.091
SMC	−0.67*	− 0.48	− 0.041	0.028	− 0.33	0.26	0.079	0.35
MMSD (cm/s)	−0.55	− 0.75*	− 0.40	− 0.24	− 0.42	0.14	− 0.11	0.43
MT (s)	−0.60*	− 0.72*	0.24	0.066	−0.64*	− 0.55	− 0.19	− 0.062
PLR	− 0.41	− 0.52	− 0.43	− 0.18	− 0.44	− 0.32	0.24	0.36
MS (cm/s)	0.073	0.063	−0.41	− 0.40	0.31	0.47	0.48	0.45
MA								
PS (cm/s)	0.10		0.11		−0.46		−0.16	
RT (s)	− 0.36	−0.37	− 0.31	−0.36	− 0.53	−0.36	− 0.42	−0.32
IDE (°)	−0.47	−0.46	− 0.12	−0.022	− 0.25	−0.49	− 0.20	−0.061
IDR	0.32	0.46	0.12	0.13	0.13	0.22	0.17	0.040
ISR	0.31	0.19	−0.039	0.15	0.0050	0.44	−0.11	−0.14
SMC	−0.53	−0.32	− 0.0050	−0.0040	− 0.23	0.35	0.083	0.52
MMSD (cm/s)	−0.42	−0.63*	− 0.45	−0.45	− 0.39	0.090	− 0.096	0.49
MT (s)	−0.50	−0.56	0.12	−0.047	− 0.34	−0.34	− 0.18	0.0020
PLR	−0.34	−0.50	− 0.47	−0.26	− 0.37	−0.24	0.15	0.27
MS (cm/s)	0.039	0.059	−0.34	−0.31	0.14	0.27	0.44	0.30
CMSA Arm								
PS (cm/s)	0.14		−0.29		−0.18		−0.022	
RT (s)	−0.19	−0.16	− 0.022	−0.070	− 0.38	−0.27	0.19	0.17
IDE (°)	−0.48	−0.52*	0.16	−0.28	− 0.39	−0.19	− 0.37	0.0090
IDR	0.56*	0.69*	−0.062	0.25	0.54	0.22	0.051	−0.32
ISR	0.50	0.35	−0.41	−0.072	0.47	0.34	−0.24	−0.18
SMC	−0.64*	−0.48	0.13	−0.081	− 0.29	0.11	0.18	−0.0010
MMSD (cm/s)	−0.49	−0.55*	− 0.15	−0.0040	− 0.34	0.11	− 0.17	0.017
MT (s)	−0.61*	−0.56*	0.19	0.35	−0.33	−0.13	0.26	−0.071
PLR	−0.45	−0.51*	0.20	−0.061	− 0.36	−0.16	− 0.037	−0.031
MS (cm/s)	−0.061	0.25	0.010	−0.19	0.16	0.29	−0.025	0.067
CMSA Hand, mean (SD)								
PS (cm/s)	−0.11		0.10		0.31		−0.15	
RT (s)	−0.26	−0.37	0.086	0.10	−0.26	−0.47	− 0.039	−0.027
IDE (°)	−0.43	−0.37	0.013	−0.050	− 0.047	0.21	− 0.083	−0.074
IDR	0.36	0.36	0.22	0.14	0.37	−0.010	−0.18	− 0.31
ISR	0.21	0.16	0.045	−0.014	0.23	−0.21	−0.12	− 0.43
SMC	−0.59*	− 0.32	−0.26	− 0.20	−0.15	− 0.14	0.36	0.13
MMSD (cm/s)	−0.56*	−0.55*	−0.33	−0.15	− 0.0050	0.056	− 0.034	−0.22
MT (s)	−0.65*	−0.49	− 0.37	−0.070	− 0.33	−0.48	0.33	0.10

Table 3 Clinical correlations with robotic reaching performance *(Continued)*

	AIS				PVI			
	Contralesional		Ipsilesional		Contralesional		Ipsilesional	
	Out	Back	Out	Back	Out	Back	Out	Back
PLR	−0.53*	−0.57*	−0.034	−0.096	−0.11	−0.25	−0.38	−0.25
MS (cm/s)	−0.13	0.12	0.10	0.0010	0.18	0.15	−0.41	−0.47
PPB								
PS (cm/s)	−0.0020		−0.20		0.23		−0.30	
RT (s)	−0.24	−0.27	−0.51*	−0.56*	−0.27	−0.21	−0.53	−0.52
IDE (°)	−0.37	−0.35	0.061	−0.45	−0.080	−0.21	−0.45	−0.15
IDR	0.55*	0.57*	0.13	0.35	0.52	0.19	0.49	−0.22
ISR	0.30	0.23	−0.075	0.078	0.40	0.12	0.066	−0.026
SMC	−0.56*	−0.41	−0.026	−0.10	−0.30	0.016	−0.19	0.27
MMSD (cm/s)	−0.53*	−0.55*	0.021	−0.45	−0.32	0.055	−0.31	0.28
MT (s)	−0.61*	−0.54*	−0.022	−0.13	−0.56*	−0.50	−0.11	−0.13
PLR	−0.40	−0.44	−0.031	−0.26	−0.32	−0.29	−0.20	0.029
MS (cm/s)	0.069	0.16	0.19	−0.040	0.29	0.36	0.27	0.33

Partial Spearman's correlations controlling for the effects of age were conducted between robotic measures and clinical motor assessments. R values of each correlation are shown. An asterisks (*) denotes significant correlations following Bonferroni correction for multiple comparisons (6 comparisons, α = 0.05, p < 0.008). Abbreviations: arterial ischemic stroke (AIS), periventricular venous infarction (PVI), Assisting Hand Assessment (AHA), Melbourne Assessment of Unilateral Upper Limb Function (MA), Chedoke-McMaster Stroke Assessment (CMSA), Purdue Pegboard (PPB), posture speed (PS), reaction time (RT), initial direction error (IDE), initial distance ratio (IDR), initial speed ratio (ISR), speed maxima count (SMC), minimum-maximum speed difference (MMSD), movement time (MT), path length ratio (PLR), maximum speed (MS)

used. These findings are not surprising and are likely due to the fact that reaches out are to one of four peripheral targets presented pseudo-randomly, but following every peripheral target the reach back was to the same, central target. These findings demonstrate that despite some motor impairment, children with perinatal stroke are almost universally able to use the predictability of a reaching task to optimize their movements.

The two cerebral hemispheres are specialized to facilitate and control different aspects of function. In adults, it has been found that the left hemisphere has greater control over visual integration and initial trajectory features of movement such as movement direction and acceleration, while the right hemisphere is more involved in limb position and posture [41, 42]. Accordingly, left hemispheric damage in adults has been associated with limb apraxia and impaired motor sequencing [43], whereas right hemisphere damage may produce deficits in positional accuracy and target localization [44]. In stark contrast, in our still developing pediatric subjects, we found no differences in reaching performance between stroke cases with left versus right hemisphere damage. An oversimplified, speculative suggestion would be that younger brains harbour "greater" neuroplasticity. More specifically, perinatal stroke studies of language function have shown that side of lesion has little impact on long-term outcome [45]. Our data here supports this and reports new evidence that side of lesion has little

impact on major motor function. This is somewhat surprising as the resistance of language to early injury is often attributed to it not being "installed" at the time of injury, whereas the motor system is clearly already functioning before birth.

We also examined how kinematic parameters aligned with traditional clinical measures of motor function. In prior studies in adults with stroke we have demonstrated strong relationships with a number of clinical measures of impairment and disability using similar kinematic measures in both the contralesional [15–17] and ipsilesional limbs [46]. The reaching performance of the contralesional arm showed moderate correlations for the AIS group with multiple different clinical scores. This was not surprising given the importance of reaching in many of the activities required for the performance of these tasks. However, the same associations were not seen in the PVI stroke group, consistent with some of our other data describing clear differences between stroke groups [18, 19].

Our findings of greater impairments in the AIS group are perhaps not surprising and appear consistent with our previous work [18, 19]. It has been hypothesized that children with AIS experience poorer sensorimotor outcomes due to the larger nature of the arterial stroke in the middle cerebral artery territory, affecting both cortical and subcortical structures crucial for both sensory and motor functions [47]. Conversely, the smaller, subcortical PVI lesions selectively injure only the white matter with sparing of the cortex. Additional evidence suggests that sensory pathways can often re-route around such lesions to maintain connections to the appropriate sensory cortex which itself is often damaged in arterial lesions [48]. The timing of these strokes may also have implications for the development of motor and sensory systems where the timing of PVI earlier in gestation when sensory-motor tracts are less developed may facilitate more adaptive developmental plasticity to achieve closer to normal organization and greater function [2, 49]. These models are increasingly informed by both human and preclinical studies [14, 49–51] but precisely how they dictate clinical function remains incompletely understood.

Limitations

With our large sample of typically developing controls, we were able to assess trends of motor function across childhood. The longitudinal profile of motor control and how it improves across childhood is well described, as are historical reports of gross motor development in children with HCP [52]. However, the kinematics we recorded provide a deeper, more detailed description of how motor control changes with age. Establishing these profiles in healthy controls provides opportunity and context to better interpret dysfunction in children with HCP and perinatal stroke. Despite our large age range, our reported age effects by reaching parameter are cross-sectional rather than developmental. Future longitudinal studies over this age range are required to characterize the developmental effects of perinatal stroke on motor control. Furthermore, additional aspects of upper limb movement, including range of motion or force exertion are not assessed by the current visually guided reaching task and warrant further investigation in future studies.

Conclusions

In this study, we quantified bilateral motor control in children with perinatal stroke. Traditional interventional strategies focus on improving motor function in the contralesional, paretic arm and independence. We found that several hemiparetic children showed significant impairments in reaching movements of both their contralesional and ipsilesional arms. Although ipsilesional motor deficits may occur less severely than those in the contralesional limb, impairment in the ipsilesional limb may be detrimental especially in stroke survivors that rely on that arm as their primary or preferred limb in daily activities. More research is needed to determine whether treating these ipsilesional impairments could, in fact, improve overall function of the children. Future studies using robotic technology must investigate the clinical relevance of robotically measured motor dysfunction in the upper limbs of children with perinatal stroke.

Abbreviations

AHA: Assisting Hand Assessment; AIS: Arterial ischemic stroke; BIT: Behavioural Inattention Test; CMSA: Chedoke-McMaster Stroke Assessment; HCP: Hemiparetic cerebral palsy; IDE: Initial direction error; IDR: Initial distance ratio; ISR: Initial speed ratio; KINARM: Kinesiological Instrument for Normal and Altered Reaching Movements; MA: Melbourne Assessment of Unilateral Upper Limb Function; MAS: Modified Ashworth Scale; MMSD: Minimum-maximum speed difference; MS: Maximum speed; MT: Movement time; PLR: Path length ratio; PPB: Purdue pegboard; PS: Posture speed; PS_{max}: Maximum posture speed; PS_{min}: Minimum posture speed; PVI: Periventricular venous infarction; RT: Reaction time; SMC: Speed maxima count

Acknowledgements

We acknowledge the support of J Yajure, M Metzler, and M Piitz.

Funding

This project was funded through an Alberta Children's Hospital Canadian Institutes of Health Research Trainee Studentship, Alberta Innovates – Health Solutions graduate studentship, Hotchkiss Brain Institute's Robertson Fund, and a Cerebral Palsy International Research Foundation Grant.

Authors' contributions

SPD, AK, and AMK participated in the design of the study. AMK participated in patient recruitment, data collection, data analysis, and the drafting of the manuscript. JAS, AK, and SPD participated in data analysis and drafting of the manuscript. All authors read and approved the final manuscript.

Competing interests

All authors confirm no conflicts of interest.

Author details

[1]University of Calgary, Calgary, AB T2N 2T9, Canada. [2]Section of Neurology, Department of Pediatrics, Alberta Children's Hospital Research Institute, Calgary, AB, Canada. [3]Department of Clinical Neurosciences, Foothills Medical Centre, Hotchkiss Brain Institute, 1403 – 29th St. NW, Calgary, AB, Canada.

References

1. Raju TN, Nelson KB, Ferriero D, Lynch JK. Ischemic perinatal stroke: summary of a workshop sponsored by the National Institute of Child Health and Human Development and the National Institute of Neurological Disorders and Stroke. Pediatrics. 2007;120:609–16.
2. Kirton A, Deveber G, Pontigon AM, Macgregor D, Shroff M. Presumed perinatal ischemic stroke: vascular classification predicts outcomes. Ann Neurol. 2008;63:436–43.
3. Kirton A. Modeling developmental plasticity after perinatal stroke: defining central therapeutic targets in cerebral palsy. Pediatr Neurol. 2013;48:81–94.
4. Tomhave WA, Van Heest AE, Bagley A, James MA. Affected and contralateral

hand strength and dexterity measures in children with hemiplegic cerebral palsy. J Hand Surg. 2015;40:900–7.

5. Gordon AM, Charles J, Duff SV. Fingertip forces during object manipulation in children with hemiplegic cerebral palsy. II: bilateral coordination. Dev Med Child Neurol. 1999;41:176–85.

6. Steenbergen B, Veringa A, de Haan A, Hulstijn W. Manual dexterity and keyboard use in spastic hemiparesis: a comparison between the impaired hand and the "good" hand on a number of performance measures. Clin Rehabil. 1998;12:64–72.

7. Brown JV, Schumacher U, Rohlmann A, Ettlinger G, Schmidt RC, Skreczek W. Aimed movements to visual targets in hemiplegic and normal children: is the "good" hand of children with infantile hemiplegia also normal? Neuropsychologia. 1989;27:283–302.

8. Holmström L, Vollmer B, Tedroff K, Islam M, Persson JKE, Kits A, et al. Hand function in relation to brain lesions and corticomotor-projection pattern in children with unilateral cerebral palsy. Dev Med Child Neurol. 2010;52:145–52.

9. Rich TL, Menk J, Rudser K, Feyma T, Gillick B. Less-affected hand function in children with hemiparetic unilateral cerebral palsy: a comparison study with typically developing peers. Neurorehabil Neural Repair. 2017;31:965–76.

10. Eyre JA. Corticospinal tract development and its plasticity after perinatal injury. Neurosci Biobehav Rev. 2007;31:1136–49.

11. Eyre JA, Taylor JP, Villagra F, Smith M, Miller S. Evidence of activity-dependent withdrawal of corticospinal projections during human development. Neurology. 2001;57:1543–54.

12. Staudt M. Reorganization after pre- and perinatal brain lesions. J Anat. 2010; 217:469–74.

13. van der Aa NE, Verhage CH, Groenendaal F, Vermeulen RJ, de Bode S, van Nieuwenhuizen O, et al. Neonatal neuroimaging predicts recruitment of contralesional corticospinal tracts following perinatal brain injury. Dev Med Child Neurol. 2013;55:707–12.

14. Zewdie E, Damji O, Ciechanski P, Seeger T, Kirton A. Contralesional corticomotor neurophysiology in hemiparetic children with perinatal stroke: developmental plasticity and clinical function. Neurorehabil Neural Repair. 2016;31:261–71.

15. Coderre AM, Zeid AA, Dukelow SP, Demmer MJ, Moore KD, Demers MJ, et al. Assessment of Upper-Limb Sensorimotor Function of Subacute Stroke Patients Using Visually Guided Reaching. Neurorehabil Neural Repair. 2010; 24(6):528–41.

16. Dukelow SP, Herter TM, Bagg SD, Scott SH. The independence of deficits in position sense and visually guided reaching following stroke. J Neuroengineering Rehabil. 2012;9:72.

17. Semrau JA, Herter TM, Scott SH, Dukelow SP. Examining differences in patterns of sensory and motor recovery after stroke with robotics. Stroke J Cereb Circ. 2015;46:3459–69.

18. Kuczynski AM, Dukelow SP, Semrau JA, Kirton A. Robotic quantification of position sense in children with perinatal stroke. Neurorehabil Neural Repair. 2016;30:762–72.

19. Kuczynski AM, Semrau JA, Kirton A, Dukelow SP. Kinesthetic deficits after perinatal stroke: robotic measurement in hemiparetic children. J Neuroengineering Rehabil. 2017;14:13.

20. Cole L, Dewey D, Letourneau N, Kaplan BJ, Chaput K, Gallagher C, et al. Clinical characteristics, risk factors, and outcomes associated with neonatal hemorrhagic stroke: a population-based case-control study. JAMA Pediatr. 2017;171(3):230–38.

21. Kitchen L, Westmacott R, Friefeld S, MacGregor D, Curtis R, Allen A, et al. The pediatric stroke outcome measure: a validation and reliability study. Stroke. 2012;43:1602–8.

22. Eliasson AC, Krumlinde-sundholm L, Rosblad B, Beckung E, Arner M, Ohrvall AM, et al. The manual ability classification system (MACS) for children with cerebral palsy: scale development and evidence of validity and reliability. Dev Med Child Neurol. 2006;48:549–54.

23. Bohannon RW, Smith MB. Interrater reliability of a modified Ashworth scale of muscle spasticity. Phys Ther. 1987;67:206–7.

24. Scott SH. Apparatus for measuring and perturbing shoulder and elbow joint positions and torques during reaching. JNeurosciMethods. 1999;89:119–27.

25. Dukelow SP, Herter TM, Moore KD, Demers MJ, Glasgow JI, Bagg SD, et al. Quantitative assessment of limb position sense following stroke. Neurorehabil Neural Repair. 2010;24:178–87.

26. James MA. Use of the Medical Research Council muscle strength grading system in the upper extremity. J Hand Surg. 2007;32:154–6.

27. Gowland C, Stratford P, Ward M, Moreland J, Torresin W, Van Hullenaar S, et

al. Measuring physical impairment and disability with the Chedoke-McMaster stroke assessment. Stroke. 1993;24:58–63.

28. Krumlinde-sundholm L, Eliasson A-C. Development of the assisting hand assessment: a Rasch-built measure intended for children with unilateral upper limb impairments. Scand J Occup Ther. 2003;10:16–26.

29. Randall M, Johnson LM, Reddihough D. The Melbourne assessment of unilateral upper limb function. Melbourne: Royal Children's Hospital, Melbourne; 1999.

30. Oldfield RC. The assessment and analysis of handedness: the Edinburgh inventory. Neuropsychologia. 1971;9:97–113.

31. Wilson B, Cockburn J, Halligan P. Development of a behavioral test of visuospatial neglect. Arch Phys Med Rehabil. 1998;68:98–102.

32. Chang J-J, Wu T-I, Wu W-L, Su F-C. Kinematical measure for spastic reaching in children with cerebral palsy. Clin Biomech Bristol Avon. 2005;20:381–8.

33. Rönnqvist L, Rösblad B. Kinematic analysis of unimanual reaching and grasping movements in children with hemiplegic cerebral palsy. Clin Biomech Bristol Avon. 2007;22:165–75.

34. Jaspers E, Desloovere K, Bruyninckx H, Klingels K, Molenaers G, Aertbeliën E, et al. Three-dimensional upper limb movement characteristics in children with hemiplegic cerebral palsy and typically developing children. Res Dev Disabil. 2011;32:2283–94.

35. Aboelnasr EA, Hegazy FA, Altalway HA. Kinematic characteristics of reaching in children with hemiplegic cerebral palsy: a comparative study. Brain Inj. 2016:1–7.

36. Valvano J. Activity-focused motor interventions for children with neurological conditions. Phys Occup Ther Pediatr. 2004;24:79–107.

37. Eliasson AC, Krumlinde-sundholm L, Shaw K, Wang C. Effects of constraint-induced movement therapy in young children with hemiplegic cerebral palsy: an adapted model. Dev Med Child Neurol. 2005;47:266–75.

38. Boyd R, Sakzewski L, Ziviani J, Abbott DF, Badawy R, Gilmore R, et al. INCITE: a randomised trial comparing constraint induced movement therapy and bimanual training in children with congenital hemiplegia. BMCNeurol. 2010; 10:4.

39. Haaland KY, Delaney HD. Motor deficits after left or right hemisphere damage due to stroke or tumor. Neuropsychologia. 1981;19:17–27.

40. Chestnut C, Haaland KY. Functional significance of ipsilesional motor deficits after unilateral stroke. Arch Phys Med Rehabil. 2008;89:62–8.

41. Sainburg RL, Schaefer SY. Interlimb differences in control of movement extent. J Neurophysiol. 2004;92:1374–83.

42. Schaefer SY, Haaland KY, Sainburg RL. Ipsilesional motor deficits following stroke reflect hemispheric specializations for movement control. Brain J Neurol. 2007;130:2146–58.

43. Harrington DL, Haaland KY. Hemispheric specialization for motor sequencing: abnormalities in levels of programming. Neuropsychologia. 1991;29:147–63.

44. Haaland KY, Prestopnik JL, Knight RT, Lee RR. Hemispheric asymmetries for kinematic and positional aspects of reaching. Brain J Neurol. 2004;127:1145–58.

45. Kirton A, DeVeber G. Life after perinatal stroke. Stroke J Cereb Circ. 2013;44: 3265–71.

46. Semrau JA, Herter TM, Kenzie JM, Findlater SE, Scott SH, Dukelow SP. Robotic characterization of Ipsilesional motor function in subacute stroke. Neurorehabil Neural Repair. 2017;31:571–82.

47. Kirton A, Armstrong-Wells J, Chang T, Deveber G, Rivkin MJ, Hernandez M, et al. Symptomatic neonatal arterial ischemic stroke: the International Pediatric Stroke Study. Pediatrics. 2011;128:e1402–10.

48. Staudt M. (re-)organization of the developing human brain following periventricular white matter lesions. Neurosci Biobehav Rev. 2007;31:1150–6.

49. Kirton A. Predicting developmental plasticity after perinatal stroke. Dev Med Child Neurol. 2013;

50. Gillick B, Menk J, Mueller B, Meekins G, Krach LE, Feyma T, et al. Synergistic effect of combined transcranial direct current stimulation/constraint-induced movement therapy in children and young adults with hemiparesis: study protocol. BMC Pediatr. 2015;15:178.

51. Kirton A. Advancing non-invasive neuromodulation clinical trials in children: lessons from perinatal stroke. Eur J Paediatr Neurol EJPN Off J Eur Paediatr Neurol Soc. 2016;21(1):75–103.

52. Rosenbaum PL, Walter SD, Hanna SE, Palisano RJ, Russell DJ, Raina P, et al. Prognosis for gross motor function in cerebral palsy: creation of motor development curves. JAMA. 2002;288:1357–63.

7

Technical development of transcutaneous electrical nerve inhibition using medium-frequency alternating current

Yushin Kim[1,2], Hang-Jun Cho[2] and Hyung-Soon Park[2]*

Abstract

Background: Innovative technical approaches to controlling undesired sensory and motor activity, such as hyperalgesia or spasticity, may contribute to rehabilitation techniques for improving neural plasticity in patients with neurologic disorders. To date, transcutaneous electrical stimulation has used low frequency pulsed currents for sensory inhibition and muscle activation. Yet, few studies have attempted to achieve motor nerve inhibition using transcutaneous electrical stimulation. This study aimed to develop a technique for transcutaneous electrical nerve inhibition (TENI) using medium-frequency alternating current (MFAC) to suppress both sensory and motor nerve activity in humans.

Methods: Surface electrodes were affixed to the skin of eight young adults to stimulate the median nerve. Stimulation intensity was increased up to 50% and 100% of the pain threshold. To identify changes in sensory perception by transcutaneous MFAC (tMFAC) stimulation, we examined tactile and pressure pain thresholds in the index and middle fingers before and after stimulation at 10 kHz. To demonstrate the effect of tMFAC stimulation on motor inhibition, stimulation was applied while participants produced flexion forces with the index and middle fingers at target forces (50% and 90% of MVC, maximum voluntary contraction).

Results: tMFAC stimulation intensity significantly increased tactile and pressure pain thresholds, indicating decreased sensory perception. During the force production task, tMFAC stimulation with the maximum intensity immediately reduced finger forces by ~ 40%. Finger forces recovered immediately after stimulation cessation. The effect on motor inhibition was greater with the higher target force (90% MVC) than with the lower target (50% MVC). Also, higher tMFAC stimulation intensity provided a greater inhibition effect on both sensory and motor nerve activity.

Conclusion: We found that tMFAC stimulation immediately inhibits sensory and motor activity. This pre-clinical study demonstrates a novel technique for TENI using MFAC stimulation and showed that it can effectively inhibit both sensory perception and motor activity. The proposed technique can be combined with existing rehabilitation devices (e.g., a robotic exoskeleton) to inhibit undesired sensorimotor activities and to accelerate recovery after neurologic injury.

Keywords: Electrical stimulation, Nerve inhibition, Kilohertz-frequency alternating current, Surface electrode, Force, Sensory, Pain, Motor

* Correspondence: hyungspark@kaist.ac.kr
[2]Department of Mechanical Engineering, Korea Advanced Institute of Science and Technology (KAIST), Daejeon 34141, Republic of Korea
Full list of author information is available at the end of the article

Background

In patients with neurologic disorders, the presence of undesired sensorimotor activity is a major clinical challenge. For example, hypersensitization, spasticity, hypertonia, and/or dystonia causes sensory and motor impairment in patients with brain injuries. To control pathologic neuromuscular conditions, researchers have introduced various therapeutic interventions such as transcutaneous electrical stimulation, oral medications, injections of botulinum neurotoxin, local anesthetics, physical therapy, rehabilitation robotic training, and surgery [1–3].

Compared to analgesic drugs, transcutaneous electrical stimulation has fewer side effects and, thus, has become a popular therapeutic technique for inhibition of undesired sensory activity, such as excessive pain or hyperalgesia [4]. For instance, to suppress excessive pain, surface electrodes are attached at the site of pain and a low frequency pulsed current (1–100 Hz) is applied [5]. Low frequency currents have also been used in functional electrical stimulation (FES) or neuro-muscular electrical stimulation (NMES), in which the current acts an excitatory agent for muscle contraction [6]. Similarly, current techniques for transcutaneous electrical stimulation have been developed using low frequency currents aimed at either inhibiting sensory perception or exciting muscle fibers (i.e., inducing contraction). This technique cannot be used for motor inhibition, which is essential for suppression of undesired motor activities (e.g., spasticity, hypertonia, dystonia).

There is some evidence supporting the feasibility of using transcutaneous electrical nerve inhibition (TENI) to reduce undesired nerve activity [7, 8]. Previous animal studies demonstrated that electrical stimulation with medium-frequency alternating currents (MFAC, 2 kHz – 40 kHz) inhibits motor nerve activity [8–12]. Those studies found that MFAC inhibits peripheral nerve activity and muscle force production when implanted electrodes directly deliver electrical currents to the peripheral nerve [9, 12]. Furthermore, the MFAC stimulus has shown intensity-dependent characteristics (i.e., a higher intensity stimulus induces greater nerve inhibition) and time-dependent characteristics (i.e., suppression occurs immediately after stimulus application) [8–11]. Most literature reporting MFAC techniques has been limited to animal studies because current MFAC techniques require surgical procedures to directly implant or insert electrodes into the target muscle. Development of a technique in which MFAC could be applied using transcutaneous electrical stimulation, with good skin penetration and effective nerve inhibition (e.g., TENI), could allow wider clinical application to suppress undesired sensory and motor activities. In addition, future applications of TENI could include combinations with other rehabilitation engineering techniques, such as with a robotic exoskeleton, to reduce pain and/or spasticity and to enhance functional recovery in neurologic patients.

One potential challenge with TENI is the proper targeting of axon fibers in a particular peripheral nerve. In general, the target of electrical stimulation, a peripheral nerve, is located below a layer of fat and muscle that may act as an electrical insulator [13]. Furthermore, applying MFAC to the muscle belly can induce muscle contraction rather than nerve inhibition. A previous study has proposed that MFAC delivered to the neuromuscular junction acts to release neurotransmitters at the end of the intramuscular axons [11]. This action can be avoided by moving/placing electrodes away from muscle bellies. Fortunately, there are specific regions in which peripheral nerves pass below a thin layer of subcutaneous fat and non-muscular tissue, such as the location of the median nerve proximal to the wrist. Moreover, previous studies have demonstrated that MFAC can penetrate soft tissues approximately 2.5 cm from the surface of the skin [14, 15] and may transmit a stimulating current from the skin to a layer below subcutaneous fat [16]. These results support the technical feasibility of TENI using MFAC.

In this study, we aimed to develop a technique for inhibiting human sensorimotor activities with TENI using MFAC. We hypothesized that transcutaneous MFAC (tMFAC) stimulation of the distal median nerve would 1) reduce sensory perception in the index and middle fingers and 2) inhibit force production by the two fingers. We also expected that a higher stimulus intensity would result in greater inhibition of both sensory and motor nerve activity compared to a lower stimulus intensity.

Methods

Design

We applied tMFAC stimulation to the distal median nerve. To confirm the effect of tMFAC stimulation on sensory perception, we performed the Semmes–Weinstein monofilament examination and pressure algometry to the index and middle fingers. To identify the motor inhibitory effects caused by TENI, we applied tMFAC stimulation for 5 s while participants continuously pressed force sensors with the index and middle fingers and measured the reduction in force during stimulation. We also monitored the safety of using TENI with MFAC.

Participants

Eight healthy young adults (age: 24.8 ± 3.0 y, height: 172.4 ± 7.2 cm, weight: 64.9 ± 7.6 kg, six males, two females) participated in this study. All participants, except one, were right-handed. Potential participants were excluded from the study if they reported musculoskeletal pain, diabetes mellitus, hypertension, autoimmune disease, and any surgical history or neurologic disorder. Written informed consent was obtained from all participants prior to participation. The experimental protocol was approved by Institutional Review Board of the Korea Advanced Institute of Science and Technology.

Apparatus

The participants were seated on a chair and their arms were positioned on a testing table. The height of the chair was adjusted such that participants could put their arms on the table with both shoulders at approximately 35° of abduction and 45° of flexion and elbows at approximately 45° of flexion (Fig. 1a). A rigid Styrofoam™ board was used to support both wrists and forearms.

To measure the forces from the index and middle fingers of each participant's non-dominant hand, two piezoelectric force sensors (CSBA-20LS, Curiotech, Korea) were mounted inside a plastic frame. The position of the sensors could be adjusted in the medial–lateral direction, within a range of 100 mm, such that the sensors were placed at the head of the proximal phalanx of each participant's index and middle fingers, these positions were maintained throughout the experiment.

Analog output signals from the sensors were processed using separate AC/DC conditioners (RW-ST01A, SMOWO, Shanghai China). A cotton cover was attached to the upper surface of each sensor to prevent friction generated by slipping and to limit the influence of finger skin temperature on the piezo-electric signals. A 16-bit A/D board (NI 6211, National Instruments, Austin, TX USA) converted processed analog input into digital signals at 1000 Hz. Data were low-pass filtered with a 3rd order Butterworth filter at 25 Hz. Raw data were acquired using LabVIEW (LabVIEW 2010, National Instruments, Austin, TX USA).

To apply tMFAC stimulation through surface electrodes (Hypoallergenic Electrodes, Roscoe Medical/Compass Health Brands, Middleburg Heights, OH USA), we used an electrotherapy device (InTENSity Select Combo II, Roscoe Medical/Compass Health Brands, Middleburg Heights, OH USA). In order to create a biphasic, steady, unmodulated alternating current of 10 kHz in a square-wave pulse, we selected the manual IF (interferential) program mode provided by the device. Two electrodes (Channel 1) were attached on the skin. The other two electrodes (Channel 2) were not used to avoid any affect due to interference. An oscilloscope (TDS2012C, Tektronix, Beaverton, OR, USA) was used to confirm the pulse (unmodulated square-wave at 10 kHz) and current intensity (mA) created at the Channel 1 electrodes. When electrical stimulation started, the stimulus intensity gradually increased for 0.3 s.

Procedure

Preparation

To identify the location of the median nerve, participants were asked to execute a finger-to-thumb opposition task with wrist flexion (Fig. 2a). Then, the locations of the palmaris longus tendon was confirmed and its radial side was used to identify the location of the median nerve. The skin over the median nerve was cleaned with a 70% isopropyl alcohol pad. Electrode 1 (2 × 1 cm) was placed on the skin overlying the median nerve near the transverse carpal ligament (Fig. 2b). Electrode 2 (5 × 5 cm) was placed over the ipsilateral olecranon process, proximal to Electrode 1 (Fig. 2c). In each test, surface

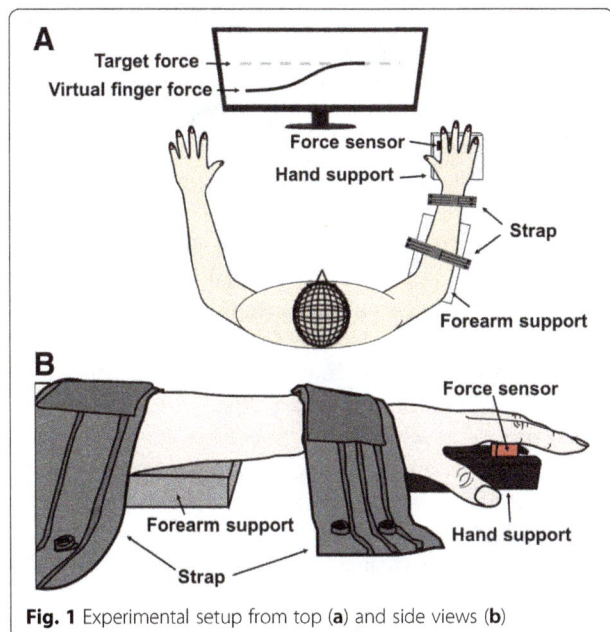
Fig. 1 Experimental setup from top (a) and side views (b)

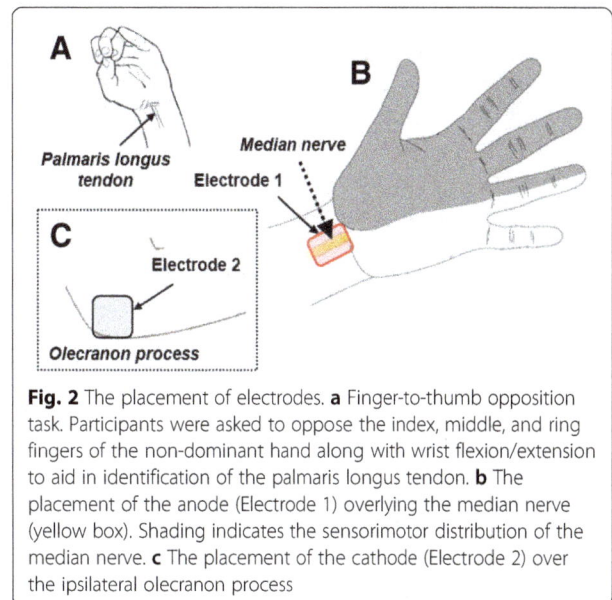
Fig. 2 The placement of electrodes. a Finger-to-thumb opposition task. Participants were asked to oppose the index, middle, and ring fingers of the non-dominant hand along with wrist flexion/extension to aid in identification of the palmaris longus tendon. b The placement of the anode (Electrode 1) overlying the median nerve (yellow box). Shading indicates the sensorimotor distribution of the median nerve. c The placement of the cathode (Electrode 2) over the ipsilateral olecranon process

electrodes were optimally placed where the sensation evoked by electrical stimulation was strongest at the tip of the index and middle fingers. Electrode placement was slightly adjusted if MFAC stimulation induced undesired muscle contraction secondary to direct stimulation of the neuromuscular junction or asynchronous firing of the nerve [11]. For example, if stimulation caused thenar muscle contraction, the location of the electrodes was moved slightly (approximately 0.5 cm) toward the ulnar or the proximal side. Subsequently, we monitored whether subjects perceived sensory changes in the median nerve-innervated areas, primarily the 2nd and the 3rd fingers but not in areas innervated by other nerves such as the 4th and the 5th fingers. To determine the maximum intensity acceptable to a participant, electrical stimulation was gradually increased to individual pain threshold [17, 18], which was found to be 31.4 ± 4.4 mA.

Identification of sensory inhibition

To identify the effect of tMFAC stimulation on sensory perception, we performed the Semmes–Weinstein monofilament examination and pressure algometry that measure tactile and pressure pain thresholds, respectively. Two measurements were performed to the skin at the tip of the index or middle finger. During sensory testing, the non-dominant hand was placed on a desk with the palm up. The sensory test was performed under three conditions: baseline, 100% intensity, and 50% intensity. In the baseline condition, sensory testing was performed without any stimulation. In the 100% and 50% intensity conditions, measurement was performed while applying tMFAC. In each condition, three measurement trials were conducted for each finger. Tactile and pressure pain thresholds were taken as the average of three measurements.

For the Semmes–Weinstein monofilament examination, we used a set of 20 nylon monofilaments (Touch Test Sensory Evaluators, North Coast Medical, Gilroy, CA USA), graded according to monofilament diameter. Measurements were made by pressing each monofilament to the skin. Measurements started with the smallest diameter monofilament (an ascending method of threshold testing) [19]. The monofilament was held in contact with the skin until it bent, and then removed after 1 s. Participants were asked to close their eyes and to indicate whether they could sense the monofilament stimulation [20]. In the 100% and 50% intensity conditions, we applied tMFAC for 5 s and performed monofilament examination within 1 to 3 s after starting the tMFAC stimulation, so that participants could not anticipate the onset of pressure. We recorded tactile threshold in milligram force as directed by the manufacturer and force values were presented using a logarithmic scale [21, 22].

To perform pressure algometry, we used a 1-cm diameter algometer (EFFEGI FPK 20, Facchini SRL, Alfonsine RA Italy). Pressure was applied to the skin in a perpendicular direction using the algometer. Participants were instructed to report when they felt a transition from a touch or pressure sensation to noxious pain, corresponding to each individual's pressure pain threshold. Pressure was increased at a rate of 1 kg/cm^2 and released after the subject reported pain [23]. This method has previously shown high trial-to-trial reliability [24]. In the 100% and 50% intensity conditions, we applied pressure after starting the tMFAC stimulation. When pressure pain threshold was identified, the tMFC stimulation was stopped. All pressure pain threshold values were recorded in kg/cm^2.

Identification of motor inhibition

To measure finger forces, a customized plastic frame (120×110 mm) with an arch was placed underneath the palm to maintain approximately 0° of wrist extension and metacarpophalangeal flexion (Fig. 1b). Two straps fixed the participant's wrist and forearm to a testing platform to limit force transmission from proximal muscles and from the elbow and shoulder joints.

A finger-pressing task was designed, such that subjects pressed a force sensor with the head of the proximal phalanx of each index and middle finger (Fig. 1b). Wrist and hand position was optimized to maximize the contribution of the intrinsic hand muscles (e.g., lumbrical and interosseous muscles) [25, 26]. To determine the target force, participants were asked to press the sensors using maximum voluntary contraction (MVC), such that they produced their maximum finger force. During MVC measurement, a digital monitor provided visual feedback on virtual finger forces, calculated as the sum of the forces produced by the index and middle fingers. MVC measurement were repeated three times and the values were averaged.

After three to five practice trials, the finger-pressing tasks were conducted using electrical stimulation. The finger-pressing tasks were conducted under four conditions with two target forces (90% and 50% MVC) and two tMFAC stimulation intensities (100% and 50% maximum intensity). Each of the four conditions were repeated three times consecutively. In total, 12 experimental trials were conducted with a 60-s rest period between each trial.

In the finger-pressing tasks, participants were asked to match the virtual finger force to the target force. A digital monitor displayed two lines corresponding to the target force and the participant's virtual finger force. The finger-pressing task was performed for 15 s. The two target forces, 90% and 50% of MVC, were selected in random order. Raw force values were recorded and displayed in newtons (N).

During the finger-pressing tasks, we applied tMFAC stimulation within 1 to 5 s after starting the task, such that participants could not anticipate the onset of stimulation. To avoid a startle response associated with the onset of electrical stimulation, the stimulus intensity gradually increased for 0.3 s after the time of onset. The stimulus immediately stopped after 5 s. Participants were asked to continue performing the finger-pressing task whether or not stimulation sensations were felt. Visual feedback on force production was maintained during electrical stimulation.

The participants were also asked to report any paresthesias, dysesthesias, or fatigue. If hypersensitive fear, severe fatigue, discomfort, or any abnormal change was reported during a task trial, the experiment was immediately stopped.

Data analysis
All finger forces were normalized by each participant's virtual finger force at MVC. Data are presented as a percentage of MVC (% MVC). To investigate changes in force production induced by tMFAC stimulation, we divided the time-varying force trajectory measured during the finger-pressing task into three phases, based on virtual finger force values (Fig. 3). Phase 1 was the baseline period in which the participants successfully matched

the virtual finger force with the target force, prior to the stimulation. To determine a reference value for meaningful force changes, we calculated a reduction threshold based on the 68–95–99.7 rule, in which the values are skewed if the values in a normally distributed data set are less than two standard deviations from the mean [27]. A reduction threshold was calculated [Reduction Threshold = Mean Total Finger Force – 2 x (Standard Deviation of the Total Finger Force)] using the virtual finger force for the 1 s prior to the onset of stimulation [27, 28]. Phase 2 was the period that MFAC influenced finger force production. In this period, t1 and t2 were defined as onset and offset times for inhibitory effects on motor neuron signals. Specifically, t1 was defined as the time interval in which finger forces decreased below the reduction threshold, after introduction of tMFAC stimulation and t2 was defined as the time interval between cessation of the stimulation to the time of minimum force production, indicating the time for recovery of finger force production from MFAC effects. Finally, Phase 3 was defined as the period after the stimulation, in which finger forces completely recovered above the reduction threshold.

To examine finger-pressing performance during the task, the mean squared error (MSE) of two-finger forces with respect to the target force was calculated for each phase. MSE values were computed using raw force data (N) to allow comparison of finger-pressing performance

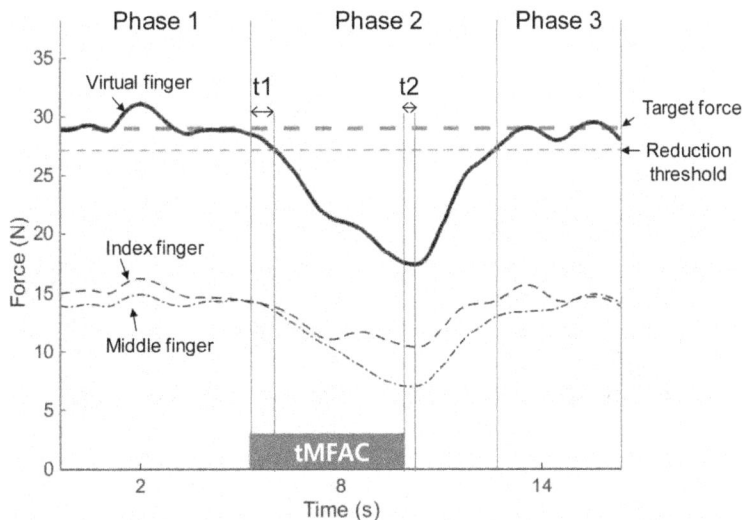

Fig. 3 A sample of a force trajectory in the finger-pressing task using the index and middle fingers. Virtual finger forces represent the sum of the index and middle finger forces. The target force is determined using 90% and 50% of a maximum voluntary contraction in the virtual finger. The reduction threshold is a reference value calculated by subtracting three standard deviations from the mean force during Phase 1. Phase 1 is the baseline period wherein the participants matched the virtual finger force to the target force before transcutaneous medium-frequency alternating current (tMFAC) stimulation was delivered. Phase 2 is the period from onset of tMFAC stimulation to the point that the virtual finger force recovers to reach the reduction threshold. Phase 3 is the period in which virtual finger force has completely recovered. In Phase 2, t1 and t2 were defined as onset and offset times for blockade of motor neuron signals, respectively. For instance, t1 represents the time from tMFAC stimulation onset to the time when virtual finger force falls below the reduction threshold. Also, t2 represents the time from tMFAC stimulation cessation to the time when virtual finger force begins to increase

between different target force conditions (e.g., 90% and 50% MVC). To quantify force reduction induced by tMFAC stimulation, the mean and minimum values of the index, middle, and two-finger forces in each phase were calculated using the normalized force data (% MVC). Data collected from the same experimental conditions were averaged for each participant.

Statistical analysis

Data are presented using mean and standard deviation values. To compare tactile thresholds among baseline, 100%, and 50% intensities of tMFAC stimulation, the Friedman test was used for each of the index and middle fingers, and then as a post-hoc test. One-way repeated measures analysis of variance (ANOVA) was performed for the comparison of pressure pain thresholds among baseline, 100%, and 50% intensities of tMFAC stimulation in the index and middle fingers. If ANOVA results indicated significant interactions, multiple pairwise comparisons were conducted using Duncan's new multiple range test. The Wilcoxon signed-rank test was used with a Bonferroni adjustment (accepted α was 0.0167). One-way repeated measures ANOVA was also conducted to compare finger forces between the three phases using normalized mean and minimum values. To compare MSE values with three factors, the three-way repeated measures ANOVA was conducted (i.e., target forces (90% vs. 50%), stimulation intensities (100% vs. 50%), and phases (Phase 1 vs. 2 vs. 3)). The intraclass correlation coefficient (ICC) was calculated for trial-to-trial reliability of pain threshold and MVC measurements. In the study, the level of significance was set at $p < 0.05$.

Results

In the monofilament test, tMFAC stimulation increased tactile thresholds in both the index and middle fingers (Table 1). Also, higher stimulation intensity provided a greater inhibition of tactile sensation. Stimulation at 100% intensity significantly increased the tactile threshold to approximately twice that of the baseline condition. Stimulation at 50% intensity also significantly increased the tactile threshold to approximately 1.5

times the baseline condition. Stimulation at either 100% or 50% intensity also significantly increased the pain threshold (Table 1). Similar to the tactile threshold, a higher intensity created a greater inhibitory effect on pain. On average, the pain threshold increased 43% and 17% over baseline levels with 100% and 50% stimulation intensities, respectively. The trial-to-trial reliability was good for pressure pain thresholds (ICC ≥ 0.778).

The mean virtual MVC was 28.8 ± 2.9 N, contributed by the index (15.1 ± 1.6 N) and middle (13.7 ± 1.8 N) fingers. The trial-to-trial reliability was good for MVC measurement (ICC = 0.737). The target force in the finger-pressing task was 25.8 ± 2.5 N at a level of 90% MVC and 14.9 ± 2.1 N at 50% MVC.

tMFAC stimulation significantly reduced mean finger forces during Phase 2 when compared to Phases 1 and 3 in most experimental conditions (Fig. 4). Specifically, significant differences in the mean and minimum forces for all fingers (index, middle, and virtual fingers) were seen between the three phases, with the single exception of the experimental condition with 50% MVC and 50% stimulation intensity, in which there was no difference in the mean and minimum forces generated by the middle finger between phases. Changes in the minimum forces in each phase support the finding that tMFAC stimulation reduced the finger forces by almost half, especially in the 90% MVC and 100% stimulation intensity experimental condition (Fig. 5). In the minimum forces, tMFAC stimulation at maximum intensity decreased the virtual finger force by 40% and 14% when the target force was 90% and 50% MVC, respectively. When the intensity was 50% of pain threshold, the virtual finger force was reduced by 25% and 4% at target forces of 90% and 50% MVC, respectively.

Stimulation with the tMFAC technique altered motor performance when the participants performed a finger-pressing task (Fig. 6). A significant difference between MSE values was shown between target forces (90% vs. 50%, F = 6.987, $p = 0.033$), stimulation intensities (100% vs. 50%, F = 7.035, $p = 0.033$), and phases (Phase 1 vs. 2 vs. 3, F = 8.291, $p = 0.004$). Significant interactions were found between factors ($p < 0.05$). Three groups were identified by posthoc testing: (1) The

Table 1 Changes in tactile [log10 (10 × force in mg)] and pain threshold (kg/cm²) after tMFAC stimulation

	Baseline	100% intensity	50% intensity	Significance
Index finger				
Tactile threshold[a]	2.3 (2.3–2.6)	4.7 (4.3–6.0)	3.6 (3.1–3.6)	χ^2: 16.00, p: < 0.001
Pain threshold[b]	3.2 ± 0.4	4.4 ± 0.5	3.7 ± 0.2	F: 20.042, p: < 0.001
Middle finger				
Tactile threshold[a]	2.5 (2.3–2.6)	5.0 (4.7–6.0)	3.9 (3.4–4.3)	χ^2: 16.00, p: < 0.001
Pain threshold[b]	3.0 ± 0.3	4.5 ± 0.5	3.6 ± 0.3	F: 28.230, p: < 0.001

Values are expressed as median values (inter-quartile range)[a] and means ± standard deviations[b]

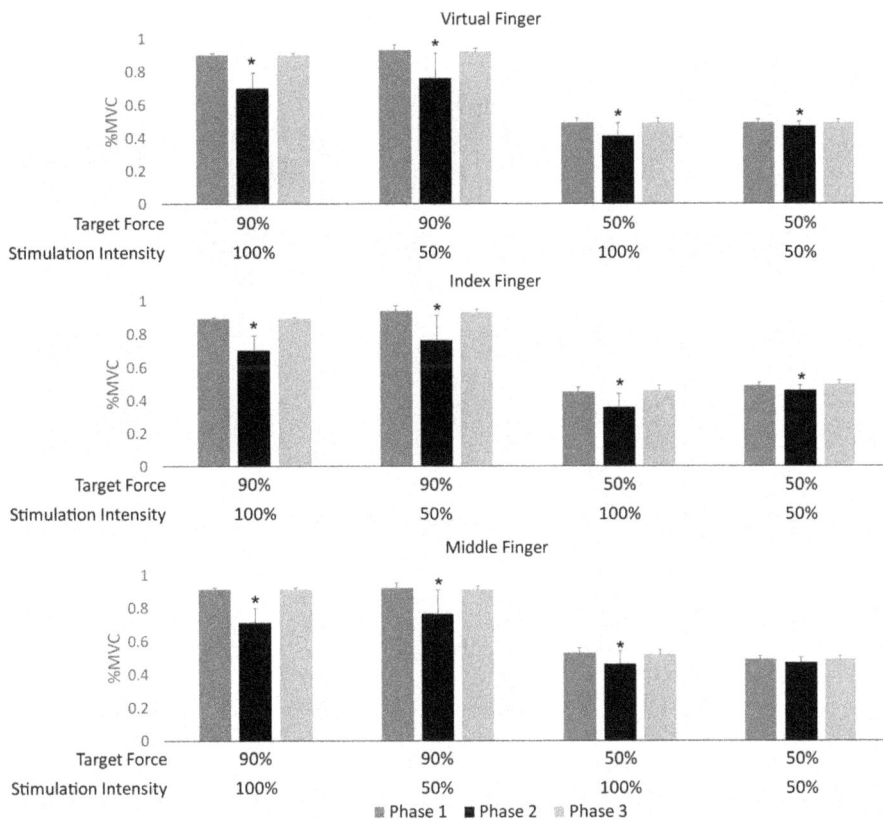

Fig. 4 Mean finger force by phase in each experimental condition. Data are presented as mean ± standard deviation of force, normalized by the maximal voluntary contraction (%MVC) of corresponding fingers for each participant. Virtual finger force indicates the sum of the index and middle finger forces. *: significantly lower force in Phase 2 than that of Phases 1 or 3 ($p < 0.05$, Duncan's new multiple range test)

experimental condition with 90% MVC and 100% stimulation intensity demonstrated the highest MSE during Phase 2 ($p < 0.05$; noted ** in Fig. 6), with respect to the other experimental conditions. (2) Two other experimental conditions, 50% MVC with 100% stimulation intensity and 90% MVC with 50% stimulation intensity, demonstrated elevated MSE during Phase 2, compared to the other experimental conditions ($p < 0.05$; noted * in Fig. 6). (3) MSE values during all other experimental conditions were not significantly different.

The time intervals t1 and t2, were tested to determine onset and offset times of inhibition and recovery of motor responses by tMFAC stimulation. In general, t1 values showed that motor inhibition occurred within one second of stimulation onset. Inhibition and recovery responses under sub-maximal stimulation intensity were usually faster when compared to those at maximum stimulation intensity. When the target force was 90% MVC, the inhibition period (t1) was 0.61 ± 0.19 s for 100% stimulation intensity and 0.38 ± 0.31 s for that of 50% intensity and the recovery period (t2) was 0.34 ± 0.25 s at 100% intensity and 0.19 ± 0.16 s at 50% intensity. When the target force was 50% MVC, t1 was 0.58 ± 0.25 s for 100% intensity and 0.42 ± 0.24 s for 50%

intensity, while t2 was 0.17 ± 0.14 s and 0.21 ± 0.18 s for 100% and 50% stimulation intensity, respectively.

No participants dropped out of the experiment and no adverse effects were reported by the participants during or after the stimulation.

Discussion

The current study demonstrates that tMFAC inhibits both sensory and motor nerve activity. To immediately suppress human sensory perception, various technical approaches for transcutaneous electrical stimulation have been suggested in both low- and medium-frequency ranges [5, 8]. However, the transcutaneous electrical stimulation that immediately depresses human motor activities has not been investigated. Only earlier animal studies using implanted electrodes have demonstrated that delivering MFAC to the peripheral nerve can immediately depress motor nerve conduction, resulting in muscle force reduction [10–12]. Thus, it remained unclear whether tMFAC applied through surface electrodes can inhibit both sensory and motor nerve activity. To our knowledge, this is the first human behavior study to describe a TENI technique that reduces both

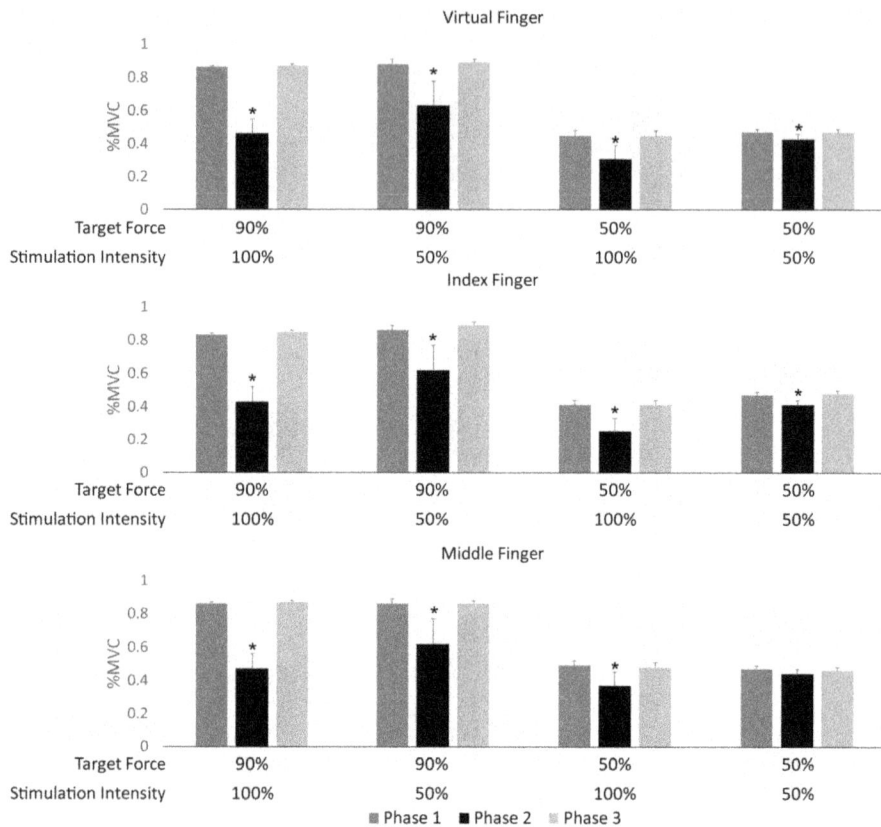

Fig. 5 Minimum finger force by phase in each experimental condition. Data are presented as mean ± standard deviation of force, normalized by the maximal voluntary contraction (%MVC) of corresponding fingers for each participant. Virtual finger force indicates the sum of the index and middle finger forces. *: significantly lower force in Phase 2 than that of Phases 1 or 3 (p < 0.05, Duncan's new multiple range test)

sensory perception and muscle force production by applying tMFAC. We found that tMFAC stimulation immediately reduced finger force production and demonstrated recovery from the inhibition effect after cessation of stimulation. We have also shown that

inhibition effects by tMFAC were safe in our healthy participants.

The inhibition effect of tMFAC differed with the level of stimulation intensity. Our results showed that tMFAC stimulation with a higher intensity created a stronger

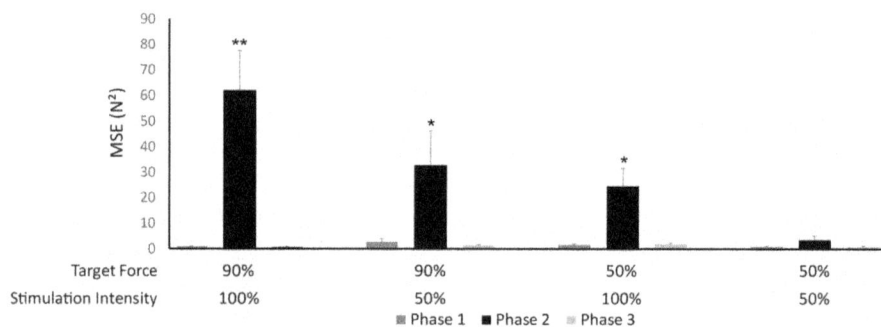

Fig. 6 Comparison of mean squared error (MSE) between experimental conditions. MSE was compared with three factors, i.e., target forces (90% vs. 50%), stimulation intensities (100% vs. 50%), and phases (Phase 1 vs. 2 vs. 3). Phases 1, 2, and 3 indicate pre-stimulation, stimulation, and post-stimulation periods, respectively. Here, a higher MSE value represents performance error that finger forces are produced apart from a target during a finger-pressing task. **: The condition presenting the highest MSE value compared to the other conditions (p < 0.05, Duncan's new multiple range test). *: The condition presenting the second highest MSE value in experimental conditions (p < 0.05, Duncan's new multiple range test)

inhibition effect in nerve responses. Similar results were also found in earlier animal studies that applied MFAC to the peripheral nerve through implanted electrodes [9–12]. In human subjects, one study demonstrated that MFAC delivered at fixed stimulation intensity using implanted electrodes reduced pain in amputees [29]. Most previous studies using non-invasive methods applied electrical stimulation above the muscle belly [14, 16, 30] and used modulated tMFAC, e.g., interferential current [14, 16]. Those studies focused on delivering interferential current below the muscle belly for sensory inhibition only. Also, kilohertz carrier frequency was used to deliver interferential currents (50–100 Hz) deeper under the tissue. In a very relevant study, Avedano-Coy et al. compared the sensory inhibition effect between tMFAC and TENS applied to the radial nerve in the forearm [7]. They showed that pressure pain thresholds increased about 20% with tMFAC, whereas TENS increased the thresholds by 30%. Although TENS was superior to tMFAC in [7], our result showed a greater increase in pressure pain threshold with tMFAC (43% increase). The major reason would be that we applied greater current intensity. Given that the stimulus intensity of tMFAC (18.0 ± 3.5 mA) used in [7] was a motor threshold that was about 57% of the pain threshold (31.4 ± 4.4 mA) used in the present study, our result (43% increase) is consistent with the result in [7]. Furthermore, it should be noted that the greater current intensity (31.4 ± 4.4 mA) used for tMFAC in our study compared to that used with TENS (16.6 ± 4.0 mA) in [7] does not mean that greater electrical energy was delivered to the subjects, because the magnitude of voltage decreases as frequency increases due to the frequency-dependent characteristics of skin impedance [31]. However, as applying MFAC at low intensity is insufficient to show nerve inhibition effects [11], further studies are necessary to demonstrate the efficacy of MFAC and TENS at various intensities.

In this study, we identified finger force reduction caused by tMFAC, although the intensity of the current was above the motor threshold. Low-frequency currents (1–100 Hz) used for FES or NMES increase muscle force when the intensity of the current is increased above the motor threshold. However, this is not the case with the MFAC. It has been demonstrated that the application of MFAC causes a change in membrane potential that is localized to the area just under the electrodes [32, 33] and is not transmitted to the neuromuscular junction [34]. However, a few cases reported in the literature describe MFAC-induced muscle contraction [11]. The first case is that of transient firing of a nerve at the onset of MFAC stimulation resulting in a reflexive muscle response. This response is inevitable, but does not last longer than 2 s. Thus, we applied electrical stimulation for 5 s and measured steady state responses. The second case is that of MFAC directly delivered to the neuromuscular junction where it acts to release neurotransmitters at the end of the intramuscular axons. Therefore, we positioned surface electrodes away from the muscle belly. The third case is that of asynchronous firing observed when nerve responses are not synchronized with the stimulating pulses. In a previous study [11], asynchronous firing was observed if electrical intensity was not adequate to completely stimulate the nerve, and an increase in stimulation intensity could eliminate asynchronous firing. Thus, we increased stimulation intensities up to the pain threshold. The median nerve consists of both sensory and motor fibers. Thus, it is reasonable to infer that tMFAC stimulation depolarizes the membrane potential in both the sensory and the motor fibers, resulting in the inhibition of sensory perception and finger force production.

We also found that higher intensity resulted in a stronger inhibition effect in finger force production. In the finger-pressing task, tMFAC stimulation at maximum intensity resulted in 40% and 14% virtual finger force reduction when the target force was 90% and 50% MVC, respectively. Since previous animal studies that used implanted electrodes showed 100% blockade of muscle force production [9–12], force reduction in this study may be attributed to a partial blockade effect. Applying higher intensity would increase the amount of force reduction but this is inapplicable in humans due to pain perception. The magnitude of decreased force output is comparable to that in a previous study in which the administration of local anesthetic agents to the distal median nerve decreased pinch grip force by 60% [35].

In this study, it is likely that tMFAC stimulation results in decreased force production through a combination of both disturbed sensory perception and suppressed peripheral nerve activity. In previous studies, digital anesthesia (that only blocks sensory feedback) reduced finger force production by 26–30% [36, 37]. Given that sensory feedback provides a net facilitatory effect on motor output in the central nervous system [38, 39], a disturbance in sensory perception produced by tMFAC stimulation may suppress motor neuron excitability [40]. In addition, we postulate that tMFAC stimulation directly inhibits motor nerve activity by inducing nerve signal propagation failure and/or neurotransmitter depletion at the neuromuscular junction [8]. In the current study, participants were instructed to press force sensors using the head of proximal phalanx with simultaneous extension of the interphalangeal joints, because this position emphasizes the contribution of intrinsic hand muscles (85%) [25]. If tMFAC stimulation affects the activity of the median nerve, the actions of lumbrical muscles innervated by the median nerve would be inhibited, resulting in a decrease in MCP flexion forces. A previous cadaver study demonstrated that during free movement of the fingers, the first lumbrical muscle acting alone can produce MCP flexion forces as low as 5 N [26]. Another study also demonstrated that the first lumbrical muscle can contribute 19% of finger flexion force, when participants pressed force sensors with the proximal phalanx in that study [41]. These studies support the idea that tMFAC stimulation inhibited MCP flexion forces contributed by the lumbrical muscles.

Our finger-pressing task demonstrated that the level of nerve inhibition differed with the magnitude of force production. Our findings indicate that a higher target force results in a greater force reduction by tMFAC stimulation. We propose that compensations within the motor system result in a smaller inhibition effect with a target force of 50% MVC, compared to a target force of 90% MVC. In the human motor system, there are abundant degrees of freedom between motor elements (e.g., body segments, muscle forces, and joints). This complex system makes it possible to obtain the same motor performance using different motor elements [42, 43]. Given that human fingers contain two types of muscles based on the origin of insertion, i.e., the intrinsic and extrinsic hand muscles, compensations between these muscles might influence motor performance during a finger-pressing task, especially when a target force is low.

Both motor and sensory nerve inhibition by tMFAC stimulation may deserve consideration as a clinical approach for reducing spasticity or pain. Spastic paralysis is defined as a motor disorder that shows increased muscle tone in a static posture and/or dynamic motor behaviors due to hyperexcitability of the stretch reflex or exaggerated cutaneous reflexes. Some earlier studies demonstrated that electrical stimulation was effective for the management of spasticity [44, 45]. In addition to spasticity, another study provided preliminary evidence on the efficacy and safety of MFAC for post-amputation pain [29]. Given that tMFAC stimulation can inhibit both motor and sensory responses, this intervention might effectively suppress spasticity and pain. However, since the current study was conducted in healthy subjects, the efficiency of tMFAC in neurologic disorders needs further investigation through clinical trials.

There are some limitations in this study. First, this is an uncontrolled study involving a small number of young healthy subjects. Although significant sensory and motor inhibition were observed in this study, the inclusion of a broader age range and/or patient population with a control group would be needed in future studies to strengthen our findings. Second, small maximum current intensity (31 mA) was used which is much smaller than the max-

imum current in commercial devices (100 mA [46]) and previous studies (120 mA [47–49]). Considering the intensity-dependent characteristics of tMFAC stimulation, the comfort of any tMFAC-induced sensations can be critical to achieving the desired inhibitory effects. Hence, for clinical applications, we suggest a pre-adaptation period of over 10 min of tMFAC stimulation to rapidly reduce MFAC-induced sensation and increase comfort [29]. This may result in enhanced tolerance of higher stimulation intensities, and, therefore, increased inhibition effects. Although no pre-adaptation period was used in the present experimental protocol, this period is recommended for future studies. We applied electrical simulation for a short period (5 s) because this pre-clinical study aimed to identify the technical feasibility of TENI using tMFAC and we intended to minimize the task period to reduce fatigue effects. A longer application period would be required to observe force trajectories for when a steady minimum force was reached after tMFAC stimulation. Finally, we applied MFAC at 10 kHz based on data from a previous study that used interferential current stimulation and demonstrated that, for a range of 1 Hz to 35 kHz, 10 kHz was optimal for stimulating subcutaneous tissues with minimal discomfort [30]. However, since interferential current stimulation was designed for a different technical purpose, in which low-frequency burst currents are generated for neuromuscular stimulation beneath the subcutaneous layer, further studies are required to find the optimal frequency for TENI.

Conclusions

In this study, we developed a technique for TENI using tMFAC stimulation. We found that tMFAC stimulation significantly reduced both sensory perception and finger force production. Higher tMFAC stimulation intensities resulted in greater inhibitory effects. Motor activity was reduced immediately after stimulation. Additionally, the inhibition effect was greater when higher forces were produced. We expect that tMFAC stimulation will provide a convenient and versatile modality to inhibit undesired nerve activity, with minimal side effects. For instance, the tMFAC stimulation technique may be combined with currently used rehabilitation devices (e.g., a continuous passive motion machine, exoskeleton, or orthosis). However, the effect of tMFAC on spasticity or pain remains unknown. Further clinical studies are needed to clarify the feasibility and efficacy of TENI using tMFAC in patients with neurologic disorders.

Acknowledgements
The authors would like to thank K.S. Lee for help with an experimental setup.

Funding
This research was supported by the Ministry of Education through the National Research Foundation of Korea (NRF-2017R1A6A3A01011909). Also, this work was supported by the ICT R&D program of MSIP/IITP. [2017-0-01724, Development of A soft wearable suit using intelligent information and meta-material/structure technology for fall prediction and prevention].

Authors' contributions
YK contributed in conceiving study concept, analyzing data, and drafting manuscript. HSC helped in conceiving the study concept, data collection, and interpretation. HSP conceived the study and supervised the whole project. All authors read and approved the final manuscript.

Competing interests
No benefits in any form have been or will be received from a commercial party related directly or indirectly to the participant of this manuscript. The authors declare that they have no competing interests.

Author details
[1]Major in Sport, Health & Rehabilitation, Department of Health Administration and Healthcare, Cheongju University, Cheongju 28503, Republic of Korea. [2]Department of Mechanical Engineering, Korea Advanced Institute of Science and Technology (KAIST), Daejeon 34141, Republic of Korea.

References
1. Bhakta BB. Management of spasticity in stroke. Br Med Bull. 2000;56:476–85.
2. Gallichio JE. Pharmacologic management of spasticity following stroke. Phys Ther. 2004;84:973–81.
3. Lagalla G, Danni M, Reiter F, Ceravolo MG, Provinciali L. Post-stroke spasticity management with repeated botulinum toxin injections in the upper limb. Am J Phys Med Rehabil. 2000;79:377–84. quiz 91-4
4. Wang B, Tang J, White PF, Naruse R, Sloninsky A, Kariger R, Gold J, Wender RH. Effect of the intensity of transcutaneous acupoint electrical stimulation on the postoperative analgesic requirement. Anesth Analg. 1997;85:406–13.
5. Rennie S. Electrophysical agents - contraindications and precautions: an evidence-based approach to clinical decision making in physical therapy foreword. Physiother Can. 2010;62:1–3.
6. Damiano DL, Prosser LA, Curatalo LA, Alter KE. Muscle plasticity and ankle control after repetitive use of a functional electrical stimulation device for foot drop in cerebral palsy. Neurorehabil Neural Repair. 2013;27:200–7.
7. Avendano-Coy J, Gomez-Soriano J, Goicoechea-Garcia C, Basco-Lopez JA, Taylor J. Effect of Unmodulated 5-kHz alternating currents versus transcutaneous electrical nerve stimulation on mechanical and thermal pain, tactile threshold, and peripheral nerve conduction: a double-blind, placebo-controlled crossover trial. Arch Phys Med Rehabil. 2017;98:888–95.
8. Ward AR. Electrical stimulation using kilohertz-frequency alternating current. Phys Ther. 2009;89:181–90.
9. Tanner JA. Reversible blocking of nerve conduction by alternating-current excitation. Nature. 1962;195:712–3.
10. Bhadra N, Kilgore KL. High-frequency electrical conduction block of mammalian peripheral motor nerve. Muscle Nerve. 2005;32:782–90.
11. Bowman BR, McNeal DR. Response of single alpha motoneurons to high-frequency pulse trains. Firing behavior and conduction block phenomenon. Appl Neurophysiol. 1986;49:121–38.
12. Ackermann DM Jr, Ethier C, Foldes EL, Oby ER, Tyler D, Bauman M, Bhadra N, Miller L, Kilgore KL. Electrical conduction block in large nerves: high-frequency current delivery in the nonhuman primate. Muscle Nerve. 2011; 43:897–9.
13. Doheny EP, Caulfield BM, Minogue CM, Lowery MM. Effect of subcutaneous fat thickness and surface electrode configuration during neuromuscular electrical stimulation. Med Eng Phys. 2010;32:468–74.
14. Petrofsky J. The effect of the subcutaneous fat on the transfer of current through skin and into muscle. Med Eng Phys. 2008;30:1168–76.
15. Beatti A, Rayner A, Chipchase L, Souvlis T. Penetration and spread of interferential current in cutaneous, subcutaneous and muscle tissues. Physiotherapy. 2011;97:319–26.
16. Petrofsky J, Laymon M, Prowse M, Gunda S, Batt J. The transfer of current through skin and muscle during electrical stimulation with sine, square, Russian and interferential waveforms. J Med Eng Technol. 2009;33:170–81.
17. Aarskog R, Johnson MI, Demmink JH, Lofthus A, Iversen V, Lopes-Martins R, Joensen J, Bjordal JM. Is mechanical pain threshold after transcutaneous electrical nerve stimulation (TENS) increased locally and unilaterally? A randomized placebo-controlled trial in healthy subjects. Physiother Res Int. 2007;12:251–63.
18. Lee J, Napadow V, Park K. Pain and sensory detection threshold response to acupuncture is modulated by coping strategy and acupuncture sensation. BMC Complement Altern Med. 2014;14:324.
19. Velstra IM, Bolliger M, Baumberger M, Rietman JS, Curt A. Epicritic sensation in cervical spinal cord injury: diagnostic gains beyond testing light touch. J Neurotrauma. 2013;30:1342–8.
20. Cuypers K, Levin O, Thijs H, Swinnen SP, Meesen RL. Long-term TENS treatment improves tactile sensitivity in MS patients. Neurorehabil Neural Repair. 2010;24:420–7.
21. Ellaway PH, Catley M. Reliability of the electrical perceptual threshold and Semmes-Weinstein monofilament tests of cutaneous sensibility. Spinal Cord. 2013;51:120–5.
22. Birke JA, Brandsma JW, Schreuders TA, Piefer A. Sensory testing with monofilaments in Hansen's disease and normal control subjects. Int J Lepr Other Mycobact Dis. 2000;68:291–8.
23. Fischer AA. Pressure algometry over normal muscles. Standard values, validity and reproducibility of pressure threshold. Pain. 1987;30:115–26.
24. Nussbaum EL, Downes L. Reliability of clinical pressure-pain algometric measurements obtained on consecutive days. Phys Ther. 1998;78:160–9.
25. Li ZM, Zatsiorsky VM, Latash ML. Contribution of the extrinsic and intrinsic hand muscles to the moments in finger joints. Clin Biomech (Bristol, Avon). 2000;15:203–11.
26. Ranney DA, Wells RP, Dowling J. Lumbrical function: interaction of lumbrical contraction with the elasticity of the extrinsic finger muscles and its effect on metacarpophalangeal equilibrium. J Hand Surg Am. 1987;12:566–75.
27. Altman DG, Bland JM. Detecting skewness from summary information. BMJ. 1996;313:1200.
28. Hodges PW, Bui BH. A comparison of computer-based methods for the determination of onset of muscle contraction using electromyography. Electroencephalogr Clin Neurophysiol. 1996;101:511–9.
29. Soin A, Shah NS, Fang ZP. High-frequency electrical nerve block for postamputation pain: a pilot study. Neuromodulation. 2015;18:197–205. discussion –6
30. Ward AR, Robertson VJ. Sensory, motor, and pain thresholds for stimulation with medium frequency alternating current. Arch Phys Med Rehabil. 1998; 79:273–8.
31. Spach MS, Barr RC, Havstad JW, Long EC. Skin-electrode impedance and its effect on recording cardiac potentials. Circulation. 1966;34:649–56.
32. Tai C, de Groat WC, Roppolo JR. Simulation of nerve block by high-frequency sinusoidal electrical current based on the Hodgkin-Huxley model. IEEE Trans Neural Syst Rehabil Eng. 2005;13:415–22.
33. Zhang X, Roppolo JR, de Groat WC, Tai C. Mechanism of nerve conduction block induced by high-frequency biphasic electrical currents. IEEE Trans Biomed Eng. 2006;53:2445–54.
34. Bhadra N, Bhadra N, Kilgore K, Gustafson KJ. High frequency electrical conduction block of the pudendal nerve. J Neural Eng. 2006;3:180–7.
35. Kozin SH, Porter S, Clark P, Thoder JJ. The contribution of the intrinsic muscles to grip and pinch strength. J Hand Surg Am. 1999;24:64–72.
36. Augurelle AS, Smith AM, Lejeune T, Thonnard JL. Importance of cutaneous feedback in maintaining a secure grip during manipulation of hand-held objects. J Neurophysiol. 2003;89:665–71.

37. Duque J, Vandermeeren Y, Lejeune TM, Thonnard JL, Smith AM, Olivier E. Paradoxical effect of digital anaesthesia on force and corticospinal excitability. Neuroreport. 2005;16:259–62.

38. Cash RF, Isayama R, Gunraj CA, Ni Z, Chen R. The influence of sensory afferent input on local motor cortical excitatory circuitry in humans. J Physiol. 2015;593:1667–84.

39. Rocco-Donovan M, Ramos RL, Giraldo S, Brumberg JC. Characteristics of synaptic connections between rodent primary somatosensory and motor cortices. Somatosens Mot Res. 2011;28:63–72.

40. Tokimura H, Di Lazzaro V, Tokimura Y, Oliviero A, Profice P, Insola A, Mazzone P, Tonali P, Rothwell JC. Short latency inhibition of human hand motor cortex by somatosensory input from the hand. J Physiol. 2000;523(Pt 2):503–13.

41. Ketchum LD, Thompson D, Pocock G, Wallingford D. A clinical study of forces generated by the intrinsic muscles of the index finger and the extrinsic flexor and extensor muscles of the hand. J Hand Surg Am. 1978;3:571–8.

42. Gottlieb GL. Muscle activation patterns during two types of voluntary single-joint movement. J Neurophysiol. 1998;80:1860–7.

43. Kim Y, Koh K, Yoon B, Kim WS, Shin JH, Park HS, Shim JK. Examining impairment of adaptive compensation for stabilizing motor repetitions in stroke survivors. Exp Brain Res. 2017;235:3543–52.

44. Levin MF, Huichan CWY. Relief of Hemiparetic spasticity by Tens is associated with improvement in reflex and voluntary motor functions. Electroencephalogr Clin Neurophysiol. 1992;85:131–42.

45. Sahin N, Ugurlu H, Albayrak I. The efficacy of electrical stimulation in reducing the post-stroke spasticity: a randomized controlled study. Disabil Rehabil. 2012;34:151–6.

46. Tyler WJ, Boasso AM, Mortimore HM, Silva RS, Charlesworth JD, Marlin MA, Aebersold K, Aven L, Wetmore DZ, Pal SK. Transdermal neuromodulation of noradrenergic activity suppresses psychophysiological and biochemical stress responses in humans. Sci Rep. 2015;5:13865.

47. Roig M, Reid WD. Electrical stimulation and peripheral muscle function in COPD: a systematic review. Respir Med. 2009;103:485–95.

48. Durmus D, Alayli G, Canturk F. Effects of quadriceps electrical stimulation program on clinical parameters in the patients with knee osteoarthritis. Clin Rheumatol. 2007;26:674–8.

49. O'Keeffe DT, Lyons GM. A versatile drop foot stimulator for research applications. Med Eng Phys. 2002;24:237–42.

8

Myocontrol is closed-loop control: incidental feedback is sufficient for scaling the prosthesis force in routine grasping

Marko Markovic[1†], Meike A. Schweisfurth[1,2*†] (iD), Leonard F. Engels[3], Dario Farina[1,4] and Strahinja Dosen[1,5]

Abstract

Background: Sensory feedback is critical for grasping in able-bodied subjects. Consequently, closing the loop in upper-limb prosthetics by providing artificial sensory feedback to the amputee is expected to improve the prosthesis utility. Nevertheless, even though amputees rate the prospect of sensory feedback high, its benefits in daily life are still very much debated. We argue that in order to measure the potential functional benefit of artificial sensory feedback, the baseline open-loop performance needs to be established.

Methods: The myoelectric control of naïve able-bodied subjects was evaluated during modulation of electromyographic signals (*EMG task*), and grasping with a prosthesis (*Prosthesis task*). The subjects needed to activate the wrist flexor muscles and close the prosthesis to reach a randomly selected target level (routine grasping). To assess the baseline performance, the tasks were performed with a different extent of implicit feedback (proprioception, prosthesis motion and sound). Finally, the prosthesis task was repeated with explicit visual force feedback. The subjects' ability to scale the prosthesis command/force was assessed by testing for a statistically significant increase in the median of the generated commands/ forces between neighboring levels. The quality of control was evaluated by computing the median absolute error (MAE) with respect to the target.

Results: The subjects could successfully scale their motor commands and generated prosthesis forces across target levels in all tasks, even with the least amount of implicit feedback (only muscle proprioception, EMG task). In addition, the deviation of the generated commands/forces from the target levels decreased with additional feedback. However, the increase in implicit feedback, from proprioception to prosthesis motion and sound, seemed to have a more substantial effect than the final introduction of explicit feedback. Explicit feedback improved the performance mainly at the higher target-force levels.

Conclusions: The study establishes the baseline performance of myoelectric control and prosthesis grasping force. The results demonstrate that even without additional feedback, naïve subjects can effectively modulate force with good accuracy with respect to that achieved when increasing the amount of feedback information.

Keywords: Myoelectric prosthesis, Baseline, Routine grasping, Grasping force, Sensory feedback, Closed-loop control

---

* Correspondence: MeikeAnnika.Schweisfurth@haw-hamburg.de
†Marko Markovic and Meike A. Schweisfurth contributed equally to this work.
[1]Applied Rehabilitation Technology Lab (ART-Lab), Department of Trauma Surgery, Orthopedics and Plastic Surgery, University Medical Center Göttingen, Georg-August-University, 37075 Göttingen, Germany
[2]Faculty of Life Sciences, Hochschule für Angewandte Wissenschaften Hamburg, Ulmenliet 20, 21033 Hamburg, Germany
Full list of author information is available at the end of the article

Background

The hands are an essential part of our body and our most important tool to interact with the world. Not only do we grasp, move, and explore objects using the hands, but they also contribute to our interaction and communication with other living beings through the language of gestures. This refined control of the hands is due to a seamless integration of feedforward motor commands and an elaborate network of sensory feedback (i.e., touch, temperature, nociception, proprioception, kinesthetic feedback) we receive [1].

The loss of a hand in people with transradial amputation can have a pronounced effect on the performance of daily-life activities and the general quality of life. The state-of-the-art in recovering hand function in persons with transradial amputation is to equip them with myoelectric prostheses. These systems are controlled through the activity of the hand and wrist flexor and extensor muscles in the residual limb, recorded by surface electromyography (sEMG). This is a robust and intuitive control scheme for simple, single degree of freedom grippers, since the muscles that were originally used to control the hand and wrist are now employed to open (extensors) and close (flexors) the prosthesis. However, the restoration of lost functions is only partial, as commercially available myoelectric prostheses do not provide explicit sensory feedback about the prosthesis state. The only exception is a recently presented system [2] providing a simple feedback of touch onset using a single vibration motor embedded in the distal part of the prosthesis.

Sensory integration is crucial for motor execution, adaptation and learning [3]. Therefore, as long as no sensory feedback is provided, prosthetic hands are believed to remain suboptimal assistive devices, rather than full bionic hand replacements [4]. Researchers have implemented different methods to provide reliable, intuitive feedback to the user [5]. Most solutions follow the general approach known as sensory substitution [6], in which an alternative sensory modality is used to compensate for the lost sense. In this, the prosthesis is equipped with sensors measuring the system state (joint angles) and interaction with the environment (grasping force), and the sensor data are transmitted to the user through electrical or mechanical stimulation eliciting tactile sensations [7]. The feedback information is coded by changing stimulation parameters, intensity and/or frequency (parameter modulation) and/or location (spatial modulation). In electrical stimulation, low-intensity electrical current pulses are delivered to the skin through surface electrodes, activating superficial skin afferents [8], or directly to the peripheral nerves [9] and/or brain [10] using implantable interfaces. The most common method to deliver direct mechanical stimulation, on the other hand, is to use vibration motors [7]. These can be simple pager vibrators [11–13] with a single input

controlling both intensity and frequency, or more advanced voice-coil devices [14], which can modulate the stimulation parameters independently (two control inputs). The prosthesis grasping force was considered most often as the variable to feed back [5], as it cannot be easily assessed visually (contrary to joint angles, for example).

However, even in the absence of explicit force feedback from the prosthesis, the control is not completely "open-loop" since the users can still rely on incidental information sources. First, the prosthesis responds proportionally, that is, the stronger the contraction of the user muscles, the faster the velocity of closing and hence the higher the resulting contact force when grasping. Therefore, the user can rely on the proprioceptive feedback from the remaining muscles (sense of contraction) to control the force. In addition, the user can exploit visual feedback to estimate and adjust the velocity of closing, and thereby indirectly and predictively the resulting grasping force [15]. This strategy can be facilitated by additional cues, such as the sound from the motor and the perception of vibrations transmitted through the socket. Finally, humans are capable of internalizing the dynamics of the system they are controlling [16, 17]. They can use these internal models to operate the system predictively through precomputed feedforward commands. This process translates, at least partly, to the control of prosthetics [18]. For example, it was shown that prosthesis users are able to scale the applied grasping forces in an anticipatory manner depending on the perceived state of the target object (fragile vs. rigid) [19].

Prosthesis users can exploit implicit feedback sources in their daily use of the prosthetic device [20, 21]. However, the quality of control achievable by using incidental feedback has never been systematically investigated. This assessment is important because it represents the baseline performance of "open-loop" control. Such baseline can then be used as a reference to evaluate explicit feedback strategies. This could contribute to clarifying the role of feedback and to quantifying the benefits of closing the loop in upper-limb prosthetics, especially because there is no unanimous agreement whether and to what extent explicit feedback is functionally useful for prosthesis control. Studies on the topic are indeed often contradictive [14, 22–24] and/or inconclusive [25].

In most studies, a specific solution was presented, and the prosthesis performance with feedback was compared to that without the feedback. These are important developments that can demonstrate the effectiveness of a particular feedback interface. However, such studies do not explicitly reveal the reasons why the presented feedback improved or failed to improve the performance. To address the latter, basic studies in controlled conditions should be performed to investigate the general nature of the mechanisms governing closed-loop control in prosthetics. The present study aims at closing that gap in the literature by investigating the role of incidental and explicit feedback sources in prosthesis control. We first determined the "open-loop" baseline and then compared it to the performance achieved using ideal explicit feedback. The subjects' task was to control the magnitude of muscle activation and prosthesis grasping force. In the baseline condition, the subjects relied on natural proprioception from their muscles plus visual and audio cues related to prosthesis movement, whereas in the explicit feedback condition, the information on the generated grasping force was shown on a computer screen. The aim was to assess the impact of different amounts of implicit feedback on prosthesis force control and to investigate if and how much the performance can be improved by supplementing the implicit sources with explicit force information.

Materials and methods
Ethics and consent
Ten able-bodied subjects (22 ± 3 yrs., 6 men, 4 women) participated in the experiment. Subjects were informed about the experiment both in writing and orally. The study was approved by the Ethics committee of the University of Göttingen (04/2016). All experiments were conducted in accordance with the declaration of Helsinki, and all participants provided written informed consent prior to participation in the experiments.

Experimental setup
The experimental setup consisted of: 1) a Michelangelo hand controlled proportionally using a single dry EMG electrode with embedded amplification, filtering and rectification circuit (13E200, Otto Bock Healthcare GmbH, Vienna, AT); 2) a wooden block to be grasped by the prosthesis; and 3) a standard desktop computer with a 22″ screen. The control-loop was implemented in Matlab Simulink 2015b (MathWorks, US) using a flexible test bench for the assessment of the closed-loop human manual control [26] and executed on the host PC in real time at 100 Hz. Since it has an integrated rectification and filtering circuit, the EMG electrode outputs the envelope of the acquired EMG (smoothed signal). The provided EMG envelope was sampled at 100 Hz by the embedded prosthesis controller and sent to the host PC via a Bluetooth link, where it was additionally filtered using a 2nd order Butterworth low-pass filter with a cut-off frequency of 2 Hz. Visual feedback for the subject was displayed on the computer screen. The average Bluetooth communication latency was around 80 ms.

The subjects sat comfortably in front of a desk with the computer screen positioned approximately 75 cm away from them (Fig. 1). The prosthesis was securely fixed to

the surface of the table, between the subject and the computer monitor. Therefore, the subjects had a clear view of the prosthesis and could also hear the motor sound, with the peak frequencies in the range from 170 Hz to 500 Hz corresponding to different prosthesis closing speeds (20–100% of maximum speed). A rigid object was fixed to the prosthesis' thumb, so that when the prosthesis closed, it grasped the object. Prior to the experiment, the optimal placement for the EMG electrodes was determined by palpating the ventral aspect of the forearm during wrist/hand flexion movement. The skin was prepared with a small amount of abrasive gel (everi, SpesMedica, IT), and an elastic band was used to strap the electrode firmly to the forearm. The subjects kept their arm in a comfortable semi-upright position, resting their elbow on a cushion placed on the desk and maintained the same position throughout the experiment. Importantly, the subjects' wrist was left free and unimpaired during the experiment. The analog electrode gain was adjusted so that the signal fluctuated around 85% of the amplifier saturation level when the subjects performed maximum muscle activation, exploiting thereby the full range of the analog amplifier.

Experimental tasks
The experiment comprised three parts in which the subjects controlled two output variables, namely, the level of muscle contraction (*EMG task*) or the level of grasping force when controlling the prosthesis (*Prosthesis task*). The grasping force was controlled in two tasks, first without (*Prosthesis task without feedback*) and then with an explicit visual force feedback shown on the computer screen (*Prosthesis task with feedback*). The generated and reference muscle activations and prosthesis forces were all normalized to the interval [0%, 100%], as explained below.

In the *EMG task* (Fig. 1a), the prosthesis was turned off, and no feedback was provided during the task. The subjects were asked to contract their hand/wrist flexor muscles (the hand was not) to reach a given target level and to maintain the contraction until the trial counter expired (2 s, Fig. 2a1). After each contraction, the subjects had to relax the muscles to initiate a new trial. The filtered myoelectric command was used as the momentary estimate of the muscle activation level. To normalize the signal, the maximum activation was measured as the strongest contraction that the subjects could maintain for 2 s without fatiguing. The muscle signal maximum was defined as the average of five measurements. Finally, the muscle activation signal was normalized by linearly mapping the range between 10 and 100% of the obtained maximum to the interval [0%, 100%]. A myoelectric prosthesis generally operates proportionally, and the level of muscle activation is therefore translated into the magnitude of grasping force. Therefore, the role of the EMG task was to assess how well the subjects could generate the commands to

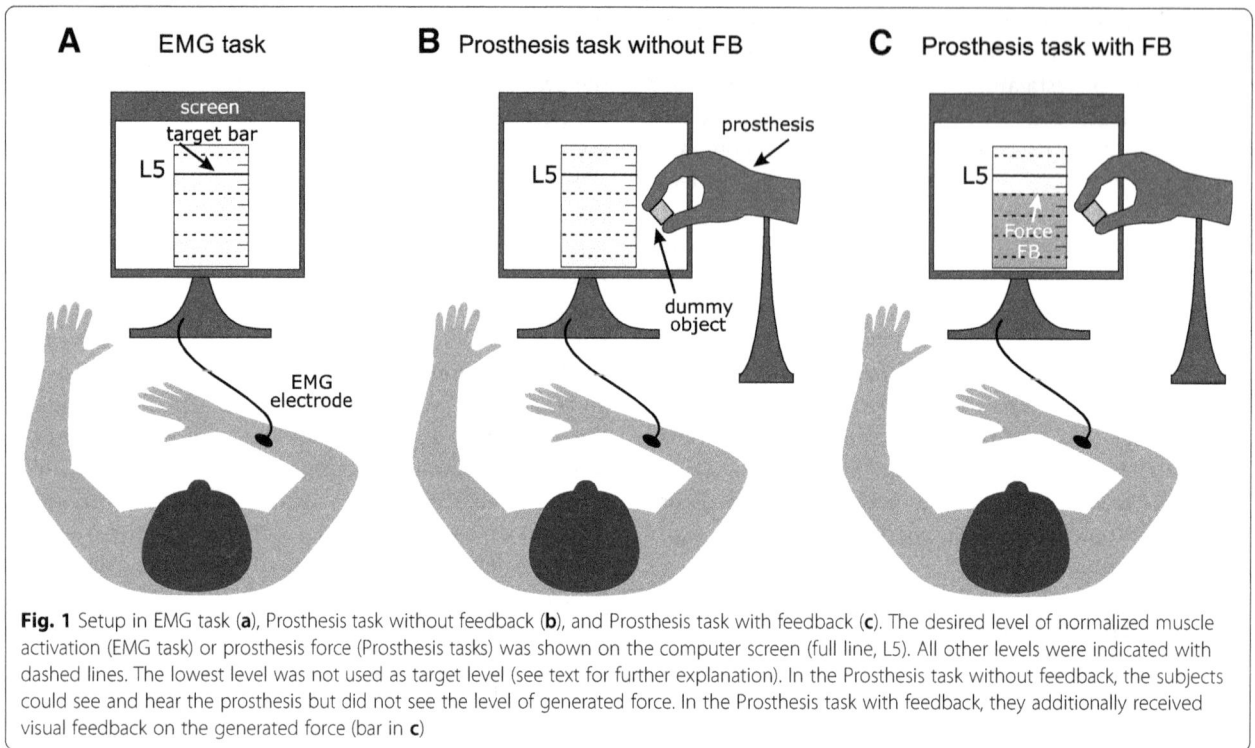

Fig. 1 Setup in EMG task (**a**), Prosthesis task without feedback (**b**), and Prosthesis task with feedback (**c**). The desired level of normalized muscle activation (EMG task) or prosthesis force (Prosthesis tasks) was shown on the computer screen (full line, L5). All other levels were indicated with dashed lines. The lowest level was not used as target level (see text for further explanation). In the Prosthesis task without feedback, the subjects could see and hear the prosthesis but did not see the level of generated force. In the Prosthesis task with feedback, they additionally received visual feedback on the generated force (bar in **c**)

the prosthesis (i.e., muscle-activation levels) by relying only on the natural proprioception from their own muscles (sense of contraction).

In both prosthesis tasks (Fig. 1b-c), the subjects were asked to close the prosthesis using the power grip (all

fingers) so that a given target level of force was generated upon contacting the object. The task was performed by contracting the hand/wrist flexor muscles to close the prosthesis from the fully opened position. While the EMG calibration remained the same as in the *EMG task*, the

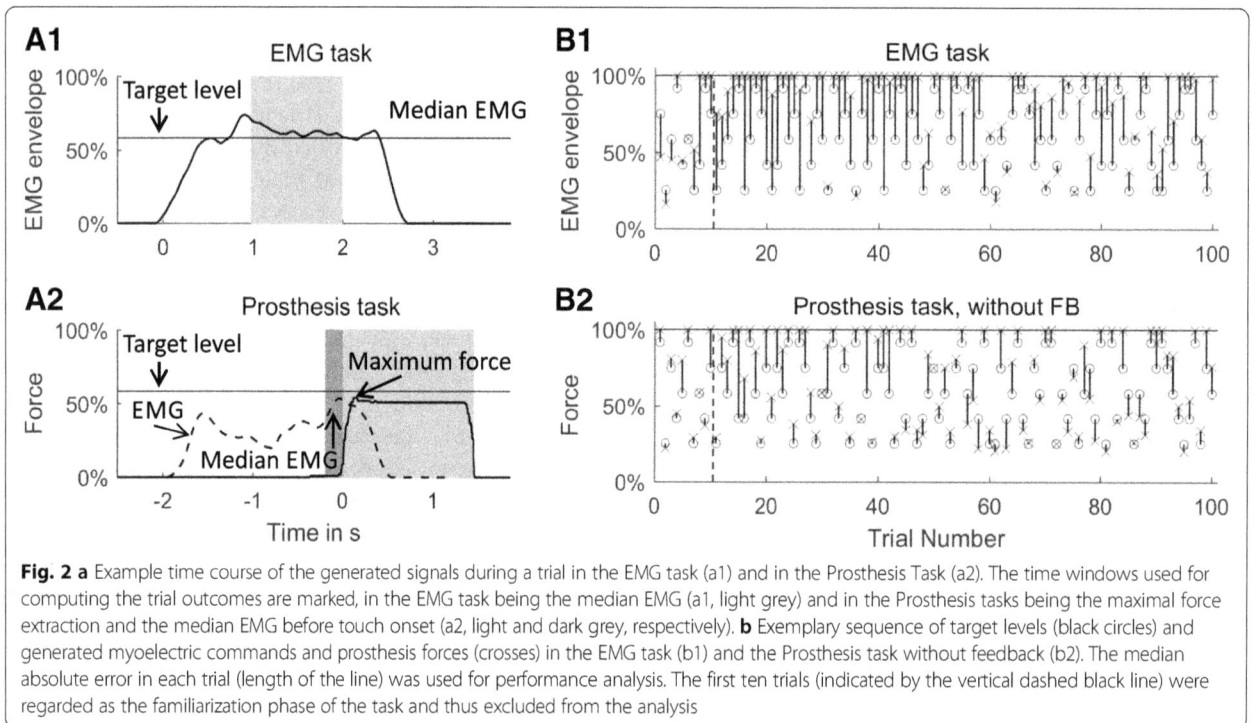

Fig. 2 a Example time course of the generated signals during a trial in the EMG task (a1) and in the Prosthesis Task (a2). The time windows used for computing the trial outcomes are marked, in the EMG task being the median EMG (a1, light grey) and in the Prosthesis tasks being the maximal force extraction and the median EMG before touch onset (a2, light and dark grey, respectively). **b** Exemplary sequence of target levels (black circles) and generated myoelectric commands and prosthesis forces (crosses) in the EMG task (b1) and the Prosthesis task without feedback (b2). The median absolute error in each trial (length of the line) was used for performance analysis. The first ten trials (indicated by the vertical dashed black line) were regarded as the familiarization phase of the task and thus excluded from the analysis

force was normalized with respect to the maximum prosthesis force (~ 100 N). The myoelectric signal proportionally controlled the velocity of closing and the resulting grasping force. The prosthesis input-output function was rather linear, so that the normalized myoelectric input produced approximately the same magnitude of the normalized grasping force (i.e., X % of EMG led to X % of force). The subjects were instructed to activate the flexor muscles to the level that they estimate would lead to the desired grasping force and then maintain the contraction until the prosthesis closed (Fig. 2a2). Therefore, the subjects performed virtually the same protocol as in the EMG task, but this time they could observe the prosthesis response, that is, closing motion as well as motor sound. Since the prosthesis was non-backdrivable and the subjects controlled only the prosthesis closing (using a single EMG channel), the force could not be decreased after contact. When the prosthesis closed around the object, the subject could relax his/her muscles and the prosthesis opened automatically 1.75 s after touch onset.

In the *Prosthesis task without feedback* no explicit force feedback was given (Fig. 1b). The aim was to assess if the subjects would generate better myoelectric commands than in the *EMG task*, by activating the muscles more consistently and accurately, if they received additional incidental feedback (prosthesis motion and sound plus muscle proprioception). Here, the subjects were instructed to focus and rely on all the feedback cues available. In addition, the forces generated in this test established the baseline of force control with no explicit force feedback.

In the *Prosthesis task with feedback* the measured maximum force was shown on the computer screen, revealing to the subject the force that they were generating in that trial (Fig. 1c). The aim was to assess if the subjects would further improve the generation of myoelectric commands and/or the quality of force control, if they were provided with explicit feedback on the generated forces. The subjects were instructed to follow the same strategy as in the two previous tasks, that is, to close the hand using one continuous contraction so that the generated force was produced directly upon contacting the object, without the need to steer the force once the hand was closed. Therefore, the visual feedback was not used to modulate the muscle activation (prosthesis force) during an ongoing trial. Instead, the feedback provided the outcome of the present trial (generated grasping force) and the subject used this information to adjust the muscle activation in the next grasp. Again, the subjects were instructed to focus and rely on all available feedback cues.

Experimental protocol

The tasks were ordered according to the increasing amount of feedback information, that is, the subjects first performed the *EMG task* (proprioception), followed by the *Prosthesis task without feedback* (proprioception, prosthesis), and finally the *Prosthesis task with feedback* (proprioception, prosthesis, force). This sequence was chosen so that, in each new task, the subjects were provided with additional feedback sources, thereby preventing unwanted across-task learning effects [18], which could potentially mask the impact of less feedback on performance. In each trial, the aim was to produce the indicated level of muscle activation (*EMG task*) or force (*Prosthesis tasks*), as explained in the previous section. The full signal range [0%, 100%] was divided into six equal intervals, and the middle points of the intervals, from the second to the sixth, were adopted as the five target levels (upper five dashed lines, Fig. 1). It should be noted that, due to the inherent coupling mechanism in the prosthesis, generating a command to close the prosthesis at the minimum velocity consistently produced forces within the 2nd interval (see [27] for a comparable discussion). This is the reason why the first interval was not considered as target. The subjects were informed about that coupling, and as will be discussed in the following paragraph, they knew how to exploit it. The trials were organized into 20 sequences of 5 trials, and within each sequence, all target levels appeared once in a randomized order (Fig. 2b1 and b2). Therefore, there were 100 trials per task, with 20 trials per target level (out of which the last 18 were used for analysis, see section Data Analysis). To prevent fatigue, the subjects took a 2-min break after 50 trials. In each trial, the target level was indicated on the computer screen, textually (L2 to L6) and as a horizontal line on the vertical bar (Fig. 1a).

Before starting the *EMG task*, the subjects were trained on how to produce the maximum (100%) and minimum value (just above zero) of the myoelectric command. To this aim, they were provided with visual feedback of the myoelectric command and asked to generate the respective values for several consecutive trials. Once they were sufficiently accurate in reaching them, they repeated the same task with eyes closed. The training was finished when they could generate the maximum/minimum myoelectric command five times in a row without relying on the visual feedback. At this point, it was assumed that the subjects had calibrated their control of muscle activation (*EMG task*). The subjects then performed the sequence of grasping trials. They were instructed to use the learned minimum/maximum values as a reference to scale their motor commands to the target level indicated in the trials. Importantly, before starting the *Prosthesis task* the subjects were introduced in detail to the basics of the prosthesis operation, including proportional control, the linear relation between closing velocity and generated force, and the non-backdrivability. The prosthesis closing and force control was demonstrated by closing it, via artificially-generated signals, at the maximum and minimum velocity for several times. The subjects were also allowed to close the prosthesis five times without receiving explicit force feedback, in order to get familiar with its control.

Data analysis

The trial outcome in the *EMG task* (generated myoelectric command) was the median of the generated muscle activation, computed over the last 1-s window of the 2-s trial duration (Fig. 2a1). In the *Prosthesis tasks*, the maximum of the generated grasping force (generated force) and the median EMG in the last 200 ms before touch onset (generated myoelectric command) were used as trial outcomes (Fig. 2a2). The time offset of 200 ms was introduced because of the prosthesis' mechanical inertia; that is, the time delay for building up the grasping force in response to a given EMG command. To account for the subjects' familiarization with the experimental condition, the first ten trials of each task were excluded from the analysis. The Kolmogorov-Smirnov tests showed that the data were not normally distributed; consequently, we used non-parametric tests for statistical analysis and median and interquartile range to report the results. The significance level was set to a Type-I error level of 0.05 ($p < 0.05$) in all tests described below.

Scaling across target levels

The goal of this analysis was to evaluate, separately for each of the three tasks, if the subjects could successfully scale their myoelectric commands and generated prosthesis forces according to the indicated target levels. To this aim, the medians of the generated muscle activations and prosthesis forces were determined for each target level and subject and statistically compared across target levels within the same task. A Friedman test was applied to evaluate statistically significant differences between levels 2 to 6. If present, Bonferroni-Holmes-corrected Wilcoxon signed-ranks tests were used to assess statistically significant differences between the neighboring levels (four tests per Friedman test). The analysis revealed how many statistically different levels of myoelectric commands and prosthesis forces the subjects could generate. In the ideal case, this would be equal to the number of target levels (five).

Performance between tasks

Myoelectric command generation was analyzed separately from force generation. The goal of this analysis was to assess if and how the amount of feedback altered the reproducibility of myoelectric commands and consequently the quality of force generation. To gain a more detailed insight into the impact of feedback in prosthesis force control, a level-wise force analysis was performed between the two *Prosthesis tasks (with* vs. *without explicit feedback)*. The exact procedures for these two analyses are described in the

remainder of this paragraph. Levels 2 and 6 were excluded as the prosthesis control was very different from the other levels. Namely, when aiming at level 6, the subjects often saturated both EMG command as well as the prosthesis force (normalized myoelectric commands and forces were close to 100%). Therefore, the true distribution of the generated myoelectric commands and prosthesis forces at level 6 could not be captured. For the target level 2, the subjects exploited the coupling inherent in the prosthesis, as explained in the section Experimental Protocol. They realized that to reach the 2nd level, they simply needed to produce the minimal myoelectric command to close the prosthesis at the minimum velocity, as the prosthesis could not generate lower forces. Therefore, they consistently undershot in the produced EMG (see Fig. 3a2 and a3). For the remaining levels 3 to 5, the median absolute error (MAE), defined as the absolute difference between the generated and desired muscle activation/prosthesis force, was calculated to assess the performance. The MAE was determined separately for each task (also for myoelectric command and force in the *Prosthesis task*), target level, and subject. To perform an overall analysis, the mean MAE across target levels was calculated for each subject and task. A Friedman test was applied to compare the overall performance in myoelectric command generation between the three tasks. If the test indicated significant differences, the tasks were compared pairwise using Bonferroni-Holmes-corrected Wilcoxon signed-rank tests. This analysis was performed to evaluate how the amount of feedback contributed to the control performance. Similarly, for the *Prosthesis tasks* the quality of force control (average MAE across levels 3 to 5) with and without explicit feedback was statistically compared using a Wilcoxon signed-rank test. To assess the force-control impact on individual levels, the same analysis was additionally performed separately for target levels 3 to 5.

Results
Scaling across target levels

Figure 3 depicts the distribution of the per-subject medians of the generated muscle activations and grasping forces across target levels in each task. For level 2 in the *Prosthesis task*, the subjects generated forces close to the target level while undershooting substantially with the myoelectric commands (compare Fig. 3a2, a3, b2 and b3), exploiting the coupling mechanism described in the section Experimental protocol. For level 6, the subjects often saturated the commands as well as the forces, as discussed above, resulting in (artificially) dense distributions and medians close to 100%. Generally, the results demonstrated that the subjects could successfully scale their generated muscle activations and/or forces according to the indicated target levels, even without any direct feedback on the controlled variable. In each task consistently ($p < 0.05$ in each Friedman test), the overall medians of the generated muscle

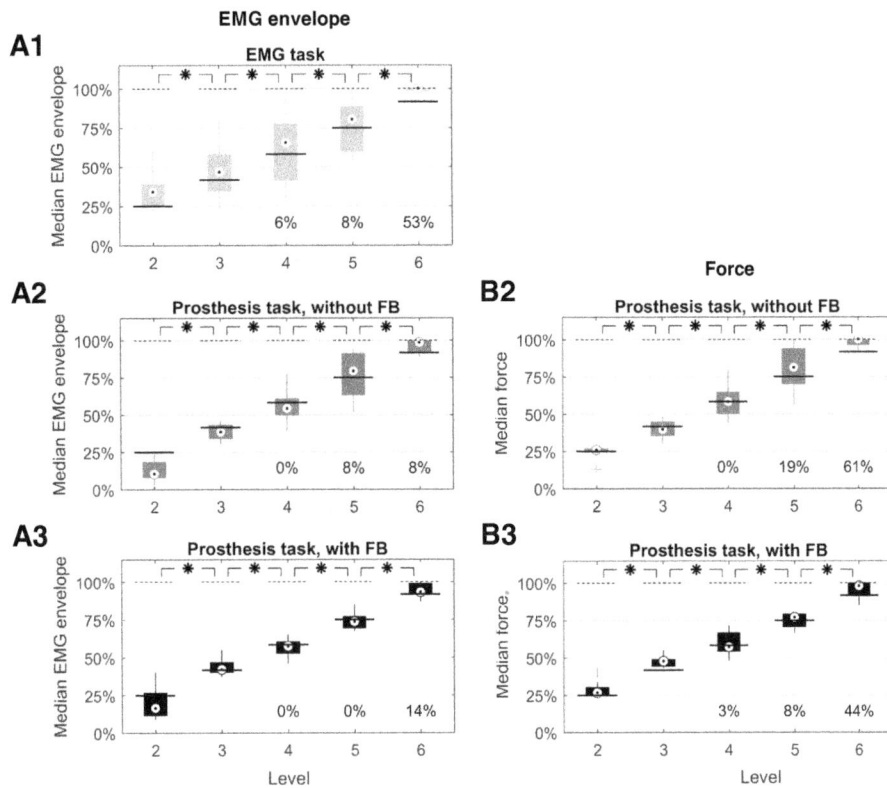

Fig. 3 Distribution of generated muscle activations (a1 to a3) and prosthesis forces (b2 to b3) for each target level. For the *EMG task* (a1, light grey) and the *Prosthesis task without* (a2, b2, dark grey) and *with* (a3, b3, black) *feedback*, the distribution of the (per-subject) median of muscle activations (**a**) / forces (**b**) is visualized using boxplots, depicting the overall median (circle), interquartile range (box), maximal/minimal values (lines) and outliers (pluses). Black continuous lines denote the target levels, black dashed lines the level of saturation. For each task, significant differences between the muscle activations / forces generated while aiming at the neighboring target levels are marked with an asterisk ($p < 0.05$, Bonferroni-Holmes corrected). For levels 4 to 6, the median percentage of saturations per subject is given

activations and grasping forces significantly increased ($p <$ 0.05 after Bonferroni-Holmes correction) from one target level to the next, for all the neighboring levels, clearly showing the subjects' scaling ability. The range between the overall medians in the extreme levels was 66% for the *EMG task*, 88% in the EMG envelope and 74% in force for the *Prosthesis task without feedback*, and 76% in the EMG envelope and 71% in force for the *Prosthesis task with feedback*. The addition of the feedback sources seemed to have a beneficial effect on the scaling, as the dispersion of the subject-specific medians became lower, observable by comparing the interquartile ranges (the length of the boxplots), from Fig. 3a1 over a2 to a3 and from b2 to b3.

Performance between tasks

Figure 4 shows the overall MAE (across levels 3 to 5, as described in the Methods) for the generated muscle activations and grasping forces for each task, assessing the quality of myoelectric-command generation and prosthesis-force control between the tasks. The overall median MAE of the generated muscle activations was largest for the *EMG task* (22%), lower in the *Prosthesis task without feedback* (15%)

and lowest in the *Prosthesis task with feedback* (12%). The pairwise differences were all statistically significant, as revealed by a Friedman test ($p < 0.001$) and significant post-hoc comparisons. Adding prosthesis motion and sound to proprioception significantly improved the command generation performance (*EMG task* vs. *Prosthesis task without feedback*), and providing explicit visual feedback improved the myoelectric control even further (*Prosthesis task without feedback* vs. *with feedback*). In the *Prosthesis task*, the improved myoelectric control also resulted in more accurate force generation, as the MAE of the generated forces decreased slightly but significantly when the explicit force feedback was introduced (Fig. 4, forces, 13% vs. 14% in the *Prosthesis task* with vs. without feedback). The quality of force control for each individual target level is presented in Fig. 5. The explicit feedback was not beneficial for level 3 but significantly improved force control at the higher levels (4 and 5, median improvement of 4% and 6%, respectively).

Discussion

There have been no systematic studies so far assessing the baseline ability of human subjects to generate

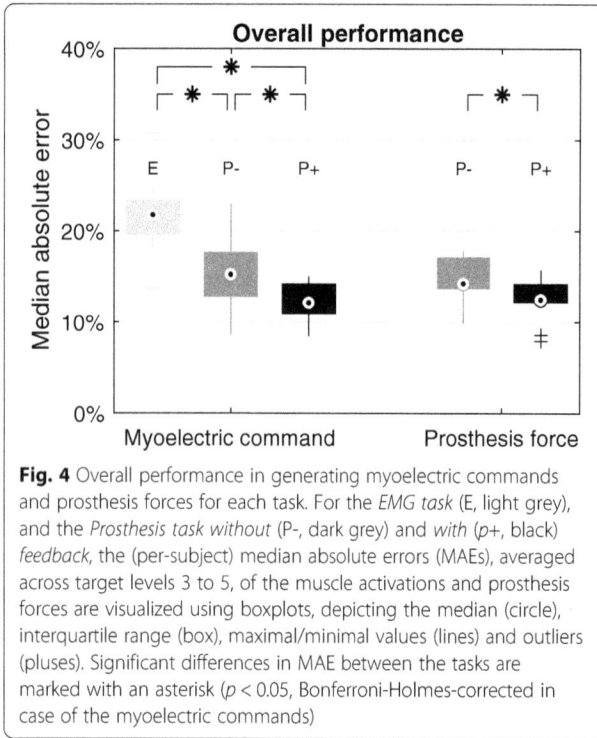

Fig. 4 Overall performance in generating myoelectric commands and prosthesis forces for each task. For the *EMG task* (E, light grey), and the *Prosthesis task without* (P-, dark grey) and *with* (p+, black) *feedback*, the (per-subject) median absolute errors (MAEs), averaged across target levels 3 to 5, of the muscle activations and prosthesis forces are visualized using boxplots, depicting the median (circle), interquartile range (box), maximal/minimal values (lines) and outliers (pluses). Significant differences in MAE between the tasks are marked with an asterisk ($p < 0.05$, Bonferroni-Holmes-corrected in case of the myoelectric commands)

myoelectric commands and control a prosthesis force at a range of levels in "open-loop", that is, with no explicit feedback on the grasp outcome. We have investigated incidental and explicit feedback in the context of prosthesis grasping. However, it is likely that the insights could be generalized to controlling other prosthesis functions. For example, the subjects might be able to control the wrist rotation speed (e.g., rotate slowly or

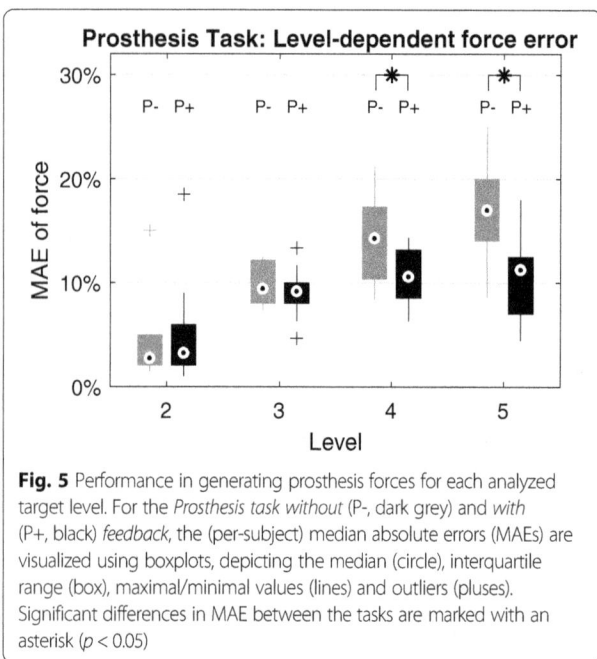

Fig. 5 Performance in generating prosthesis forces for each analyzed target level. For the *Prosthesis task without* (P-, dark grey) and *with* (P+, black) *feedback*, the (per-subject) median absolute errors (MAEs) are visualized using boxplots, depicting the median (circle), interquartile range (box), maximal/minimal values (lines) and outliers (pluses). Significant differences in MAE between the tasks are marked with an asterisk ($p < 0.05$)

quickly) using muscle proprioception and motor sound, without even looking at the hand. Finally, it should be emphasized that implicit and explicit feedback are components of the larger human motor control scheme that needs to be considered in its totality in order to properly model and understand closed-loop prosthesis control. This includes, among others, the ability of the subject to learn, predict, and adapt [19, 28–30], which is likely to have a substantial effect on the use and relevance of the feedback in general (either explicit or implicit).

Our results demonstrated that even in naïve users, the control without explicit feedback is not completely blind (open loop) but, on the contrary, surprisingly good. This could explain the unexpected outcome in some studies [13, 14, 25], where artificial feedback failed to provide any benefit. In other studies, the task was to produce few force levels (e.g., low, medium and high) [9, 12, 31] and the present experiment demonstrated that the subjects can already do more than that even with only minimal implicit feedback (muscle proprioception). Nevertheless, we argue that this type of feedback is useful for gross control tasks (force control during routine grasping); more delicate tasks, such as individual finger control in a dexterous prosthesis [32] or the use of prosthesis for haptic exploration [33], would still require artificial tactile feedback.

Looking at the *EMG task* only, this study shows that the feedback obtained through muscle proprioception is an important feature inherently available in myocontrol, essentially making myocontrol closed-loop control. This feedback source would not be present with other types of interfacing, such as nerve interfacing for motor commands without a target muscle. Using muscles for control is therefore very beneficial not just because they provide good control signals, but also because they provide very intuitive feedback.

The subjects could indeed generate five distinct levels, but they would not necessarily match the actual target levels, as the mean absolute error was between 10 and 20%. The quality of myoelectric control consistently improved with the addition of more feedback sources. Increasing the amount of implicit information, from proprioception only to proprioception and prosthesis motion and sound, and finally providing explicit feedback, steadily decreased the error in generating myoelectric commands. Interestingly, the improvement was more substantial when introducing the prosthesis (*EMG task* to *Prosthesis task without feedback*) compared to when adding explicit feedback on top of prosthesis motion and sound (*Prosthesis task without feedback* to *Prosthesis task with feedback*). The improvement in myoelectric control due to explicit feedback translated into better force control, but this benefit was modest overall.

The explicit force feedback significantly improved the performance when the uncertainty of myocontrol was high, since the EMG signals become more variable as the contraction level increases [34]. Overall, these results point to the importance of considering the implicit feedback when designing a closed-loop prosthetic system. In the present study, for example, the impact of increasing the implicit feedback on performance was more substantial than that of introducing the explicit information. It should also be considered that the provided explicit sensory feedback was ideal, being provided as continuous visual feedback. In reality, no feedback modality could provide such an accurate feedback on EMG or force in a real-life application. Therefore, the improvement observed here should be the very best that feedback can provide; yet, its benefit was rather small.

However, it should be noted that the controllability in the *Prosthesis task* was somewhat limited due to the inherent characteristics of a myoelectric prosthesis. The non-back-drivability, high impedance, and non-linear effects due to friction, especially while the prosthesis is closed around the object, might be a reason why the improvement in performance with the explicit feedback was limited. Effectively, this has prevented the subjects from exploiting the force feedback in real-time (i.e., within a single trial). Instead, the explicit feedback was used intermediately, on a trial-to-trial basis. The subjects used the feedback to assess the task outcome, and based on the discrepancy between the intended and generated force level, they adjusted their motor command in the next trial. Finally, although the two tasks in the present study have been performed using a Michelangelo hand prosthesis, the general mechanisms of prosthesis operation (proportionality, non-backdrivability) are common to most commercial systems and, therefore, allow us to interpret the study conclusions in a more general and broader relevance. Likewise, the first condition (*EMG task*), demonstrating the vital role of muscle proprioception during myocontrol, is fully device independent.

Generally, the good baseline performance (*Prosthesis task without feedback*) suggests that force-feedback interfaces require a reasonably good resolution (< 15%) in order to have a chance to provide a benefit (increased performance with respect to the baseline), especially at the higher force levels. This is valuable information and should be considered in the future design of feedback interfaces.

Study limitations

In the present study, the forearm muscles have been used, since they are relevant for controlling hand prostheses. However, we believe that the subjects would be able to exploit the incidental feedback in a similar manner when using other muscles, e.g., upper arm (transhumeral prosthesis). Nevertheless, this needs to be confirmed experimentally, as the controllability (fine vs. gross movements) and proprioception might be somewhat different.

We only tested a homogenous group of naïve able-bodied subjects. Proprioceptive feedback from the muscles is also available to people with amputation, albeit somewhat different depending on the extent of amputation, shortening of muscles, and changes of attachment points. General skills as well as the interpretation and exploitation of the visual and auditory cues should be similar, and in addition, a person with amputation could exploit the incidental cues available through the prosthesis socket. Therefore, we expect that the results would not be significantly different in naïve persons with amputation, and even more so, the general conclusions regarding the importance of incidental feedback in prosthesis control. In experienced people with amputation, the baseline performance is likely to be even better than suggested here, due to extensive prosthesis use [35].

It would certainly be interesting to further compare performance with prosthesis users, considering also their age and level of physical activity, as these factors might influence muscle proprioception [36, 37] but also vision and audition, which deteriorate with age.

Next, the present study has been purposefully conducted in well controlled laboratory conditions to obtain isolated insights into different feedback components, as explained in *Introduction*. Therefore, there was no background noise that could mask the prosthesis sounds, the hand was always clearly visible, and the task consisted of repeatable grasping of the same object. These conditions might facilitate the reliance on implicit feedback. In daily life, however, users will most likely encounter more challenging circumstances, which could make explicit feedback more important. For example, in our recent study, we have demonstrated that explicit feedback becomes relevant when the task complexity increases [38]. Hence, it is all the more important to validate our findings in amputees.

Conclusion

This study provides a first systematic investigation of how implicit (proprioception, prosthesis sound, vision of the prosthesis) and explicit feedback (visual force information) interact to influence the performance of grasping force control. We showed that muscle proprioception alone already allows to scale the grasping forces. Adding the incidental feedback from the prosthesis improved the accuracy of this scaling by decreasing the deviations from the target levels. Importantly, the improvement was more substantial when increasing the amount of incidental feedback than when the explicit force feedback was introduced. These insights emphasize that a myoelectric interface already provides closed-loop control with good performance. Therefore, artificial feedback needs to be carefully designed to outperform this baseline and become truly effective.

Funding
We acknowledge the financial support by the German Ministry for Education and Research (BMBF) under the project INOPRO and the European Commission under the MYOSENS (FP7-PEOPLE-2011-IAPP-286208) project.

Authors' contributions
MM, MAS, DF, and SD conceived the study and designed the experiment. MAS and MM programmed the setup and analyzed the data. MM, MAS, and LFE conducted the experiments. MM, MAS, DF, and SD interpreted the results. MM, MAS, and SD wrote the manuscript. All authors read and approved the final manuscript.

Competing interests
The authors declare that they have no competing interests.

Author details
[1]Applied Rehabilitation Technology Lab (ART-Lab), Department of Trauma Surgery, Orthopedics and Plastic Surgery, University Medical Center Göttingen, Georg-August-University, 37075 Göttingen, Germany. [2]Faculty of Life Sciences, Hochschule für Angewandte Wissenschaften Hamburg, Ulmenliet 20, 21033 Hamburg, Germany. [3]Biorobotics Institute, Scuola Superiore Sant'Anna, Viale R. Piaggio, 34, 56025 Pontedera, PI, Italy. [4]Neurorehabilitation Engineering Department of Bioengineering Imperial College London, London SW7 2AZ, UK. [5]Faculty of Medicine, Department of Health Science and Technology, Center for Sensory-Motor Interaction, Aalborg University, DE-9220 Aalborg, Denmark.

References
1. MacKenzie C, Iberall T. The grasping hand. Amsterdam: Elsevier; 2010.
2. "Vincent Systems GmbH, VINCENTevolution 2." [Online]. Available: http://vincentsystems.de/en/prosthetics/vincent-evolution-2/. [Accessed: 20 May 2018].
3. Rothwell JC, Traub MM, Day BL, Obeso JA, Thomas PK, Marsden CD. Manual motor performance in a deafferented man. Brain. 1982;105(Pt 3):515–42.
4. Scott RN, Parker PA. Myoelectric prostheses : state of the art. J Med Eng Technol. 1988;12(4):143–51.
5. Antfolk C, D'Alonzo M, Rosén B, Lundborg G, Sebelius F, Cipriani C. Sensory feedback in upper limb prosthetics. Expert Rev Med Devices. 2013;10(1):45–54.
6. Bach-y-Rita P, Kercel SW. Sensory substitution and the human–machine interface. Trends Cogn Sci. 2015;7(12):541–6.
7. Kaczmarek K, Webster JG, Bach-y-Rita P, Tompkins WJ. Electrotactile and vibrotactile displays for sensory substitution systems. IEEE Trans Biomed Eng. 1991;38(1. Ieee):1–16.
8. Szeto AY, Saunders FA. Electrocutaneous stimulation for sensory communication in rehabilitation engineering. IEEE Trans Biomed Eng. 1982; 29(4):300–8.
9. Raspopovic S, Capogrosso M, Petrini FM, Bonizzato M, Rigosa J, Di Pino G, Carpaneto J, Controzzi M, Boretius T, Fernandez E, Granata G, Oddo CM, Citi L, Ciancio AL, Cipriani C, Carrozza MC, Jensen W, Guglielmelli E, Stieglitz T, Rossini PM, Micera S. Restoring natural sensory feedback in real-time bidirectional hand prostheses. Sci Transl Med. 2014;6(222):222ra19.
10. Tabot GA, Dammann JF, Berg JA, Tenore FV, Boback JL, Vogelstein RJ, Bensmaia SJ. Restoring the sense of touch with a prosthetic hand through a brain interface. Proc Natl Acad Sci U S A. 2013;110(45):18279–84.
11. Witteveen HJB, Droog EA, Rietman JS, Veltink PH. Vibro- and electrotactile user feedback on hand opening for myoelectric forearm prostheses. IEEE Trans Biomed Eng. 2012;59(8):2219–26.
12. Saunders I, Vijayakumar S. The role of feed-forward and feedback processes for closed-loop prosthesis control. J Neuroeng Rehabil. 2011;8(1):60.
13. Cipriani C, Zaccone F, Micera S, Carrozza MC. On the shared control of an EMG-controlled prosthetic hand: analysis of user-prosthesis interaction. IEEE Trans Robot. 2008;24(1):170–84.
14. Witteveen HJB, Rietman HS, Veltink PH. Vibrotactile grasping force and hand aperture feedback for myoelectric forearm prosthesis users. Prosthetics Orthot Int. 2015;39(3):204–12.
15. Ninu A, Dosen S, Muceli S, Rattay F, Dietl H, Farina D. Closed-loop control of grasping with a myoelectric hand prosthesis: which are the relevant feedback variables for force control? IEEE Trans Neural Syst Rehabil Eng. 2014;22(5):1041–52.
16. Kawato M, Wolpert DM. Internal models for motor control. Novartis Found Symp. 1998;218:291–304.
17. Todorov E. Optimality principles in sensorimotor control. Nat Neurosci. 2004; 7(9):907–15.
18. Dosen S, Markovic M, Wille N, Henkel M, Koppe M, Ninu A, Frömmel C, Farina D. Building an internal model of a myoelectric prosthesis via closed-loop control for consistent and routine grasping. Exp Brain Res. 2015;233(6): 1855–65.
19. Lum PS, Black I, Holley RJ, Barth J, Dromerick AW. Internal models of upper limb prosthesis users when grasping and lifting a fragile object with their prosthetic limb. Exp Brain Res. 2014;232(12):3785–95.
20. Zafar M, Van Doren CL. Effectiveness of supplemental grasp-force feedback in the presence of vision. Med Biol Eng Comput. 2000;38(3):267–74.
21. Pistohl T, Joshi D, Ganesh G, Jackson A, Nazarpour K. Artificial proprioceptive feedback for myoelectric control. IEEE Trans Neural Syst Rehabil Eng. 2015; 23(3):498–507.
22. Xu H, Zhang D, Huegel J, Xu W, Zhu X. Effects of different tactile feedback on myoelectric closed-loop control for grasping based on Electrotactile stimulation. IEEE Trans Neural Syst Rehabil Eng. 2015;24(8):827–36.
23. Pylatiuk C, Kargov A, Schulz S. Design and evaluation of a low-cost force feedback system for myoelectric prosthetic hands. JPO J Prosthetics Orthot. 2006;18(2):57–61.
24. Hasson CJ, Manczurowsky J. Effects of kinematic vibrotactile feedback on learning to control a virtual prosthetic arm. J Neuroeng Rehabil. 2015;12(1):1–16.
25. Brown JD, Paek A, Syed M, O'Malley MK, Shewokis PA, Contreras-Vidal JL, Davis AJ, Gillespie RB. An exploration of grip force regulation with a low-impedance myoelectric prosthesis featuring referred haptic feedback. J Neuroeng Rehabil. 2015;12(1):104.
26. Dosen S, Markovic M, Hartmann C, Farina D. Sensory feedback in prosthetics: a standardized test bench for closed-loop control. IEEE Trans Neural Syst Rehabil Eng. 2015;23(2):267–76.
27. Schweisfurth MA, Markovic M, Dosen S, Teich F, Graimann B, Farina D. Electrotactile EMG feedback improves the control of prosthesis grasping force. J Neural Eng. 2016;13(5):056010.
28. Dosen S, Markovic M, Somer K, Graimann B, Farina D. EMG biofeedback for online predictive control of grasping force in a myoelectric prosthesis. J Neuroeng Rehabil. 2015;12(1):55.
29. Štrbac M, Isaković M, Belić M, Popović I, Simanić I, Farina D, Keller T, Došen S. Short-and long-term learning of feedforward control of a myoelectric prosthesis with sensory feedback by amputees. IEEE Trans. Neural Syst Rehabil Eng. 2017;25(11):2133–45.
30. Johnson RE, Kording KP, Hargrove LJ, Sensinger JW. Does EMG control lead to distinct motor adaptation? Front Neurosci. 2014;8:302.
31. Chatterjee A, Chaubey P, Martin J, Thakor N. Testing a prosthetic haptic feedback simulator with an interactive force matching task. JPO J Prosthetics Orthot. 2008;20(2):27–34.
32. Vallbo AB, Johansson RS. Properties of cutaneous mechanoreceptors in the human hand related to touch sensation. Hum Neurobiol. 1984;3(1):3–14.
33. Franceschi M, Seminara L, Dosen S, Valle M, Farina D, Member S. A system for electrotactile feedback using electronic skin and flexible matrix electrodes: experimental evaluation. IEEE Trans Haptics. 2016;1412(c):1–14.
34. Parker P, Englehart K, Hudgins B. Myoelectric signal processing for control of powered limb prostheses. J Electromyogr Kinesiol. 2006;16(6):541–8.
35. Amsuess S, Gobel P, Graimann B, Farina D. A multi-class proportional Myocontrol algorithm for upper limb prosthesis control: validation in

real-life scenarios on amputees. IEEE Trans Neural Syst Rehabil Eng. 2014;23(5):827–36.

36. Lee NK, Kwon YH, Son SM, Nam SH, Kim JS. The effects of aging on visuomotor coordination and proprioceptive function in the upper limb. J Phys Ther Sci. 2013;25:627–9.

37. Ribeiro F, Oliveira J. Aging effects on joint proprioception: the role of physical activity in proprioception preservation. Eur Rev Aging Phys Act. 2007;4(2):71–6.

38. Markovic M, Schweisfurth MA, Engels LF, Bentz T, Wüstefeld D, Farina D, Dosen S. The clinical relevance of advanced artificial feedback in the control of a multi-functional myoelectric prosthesis. J Neuroeng Rehabil. 2018;15(1): 1–15.

Sensor-based postural feedback is more effective than conventional feedback to improve lumbopelvic movement control in patients with chronic low back pain

Thomas Matheve[1]* , Simon Brumagne[2], Christophe Demoulin[3] and Annick Timmermans[1]

Abstract

Background: Improving movement control can be an important treatment goal for patients with chronic low back pain (CLBP). Although external feedback is essential when learning new movement skills, many aspects of feedback provision in patients with CLBP remain currently unexplored. New rehabilitation technologies, such as movement sensors, are able to provide reliable and accurate feedback. As such, they might be more effective than conventional feedback for improving movement control. The aims of this study were (1) to assess whether sensor-based feedback is more effective to improve lumbopelvic movement control compared to feedback from a mirror or no feedback in patients with chronic low back pain (CLBP), and (2) to evaluate whether patients with CLBP are equally capable of improving lumbopelvic movement control compared to healthy persons.

Methods: Fifty-four healthy participants and 54 patients with chronic non-specific LBP were recruited. Both participant groups were randomised into three subgroups. During a single exercise session, subgroups practised a lumbopelvic movement control task while receiving a different type of feedback, i.e. feedback from movement sensors, from a mirror or no feedback (=control group). Kinematic measurements of the lumbar spine and hip were obtained at baseline, during and immediately after the intervention to evaluate the improvements in movement control on the practised task (assessment of performance) and on a transfer task (assessment of motor learning).

Results: Sensor-based feedback was more effective than feedback from a mirror ($p < 0.0001$) and no feedback ($p < 0.0001$) to improve lumbopelvic movement control performance (Sensor vs. Mirror estimated difference 9.9° (95% CI 6.1°-13.7°), Sensor vs. Control estimated difference 10.6° (95% CI 6.8°-14.3°)) and motor learning (Sensor vs. Mirror estimated difference 7.2° (95% CI 3.8°-10.6°), Sensor vs. Control estimated difference 6.9° (95% CI 3.5°-10.2°)). Patients with CLBP were equally capable of improving lumbopelvic movement control compared to healthy persons.

Conclusions: Sensor-based feedback is an effective means to improve lumbopelvic movement control in patients with CLBP. Future research should focus on the long-term retention effects of sensor-based feedback.

Keywords: Low back pain, Feedback, Movement control, Motor learning, Sensors, Technology

* Correspondence: Thomas.Matheve@uhasselt.be
[1]Rehabilitation Research Center - Biomed, Faculty of Medicine and Life Sciences, Hasselt University, Hasselt, Belgium
Full list of author information is available at the end of the article

Background

The lifetime prevalence of low back pain (LBP) is reported to be as high as 84%, whereas the estimated prevalence of chronic LBP (CLBP) is approximately 23% [1]. Globally, it is the leading cause of disability [2] and one of the most important reasons for work absenteeism, resulting in a high socioeconomic burden [3].

Patients with CLBP form a heterogeneous group, which is exemplified by the differences in movement patterns within this population. While some patients with CLBP stiffen their spine and avoid spinal movements, others show the opposite pattern and adopt end range postures or move excessively into their painful direction [4]. For the latter type of patients, movement control exercises are often prescribed [5]. The aim of these exercises is to learn how to control movements into the painful direction, thereby reducing the mechanical load on the painful structures and decreasing peripheral nociceptive input [6].

Changing movement patterns requires motor learning. The importance of external feedback (i.e. feedback coming from a source external to the person performing the task [7]) in motor learning has been well established, and optimizing the way feedback is provided is therefore essential [8, 9]. While there is an abundance of literature on the role of extrinsic feedback to improve motor learning in a healthy population, many aspects of feedback provision in patients with LBP remain currently unexplored [9]. When patients with LBP perform lumbar movement control exercises in the absence of a therapist, they typically have to rely on visual feedback (e.g. from a mirror) or palpation [10]. However, the reliability and accuracy of these types of feedback can be questioned [11, 12], which may lead to a suboptimal learning process [7]. With the development of rehabilitation technologies, new opportunities for providing external feedback have emerged [13]. For example, wireless inertial motion sensors can be used to provide easy to understand and accurate feedback to the patient (e.g. via an avatar) [13, 14]. As such, sensor-based postural feedback might be more effective than conventional feedback for improving movement control, which in turn may enhance treatment effects.

Although movement control exercises are widely used in a variety of chronic pain populations, little is known about the influence of chronic pain on the capacity to learn new movement skills. From a theoretical perspective, it has been suggested that patients with CLBP might have a reduced motor learning capacity [15]. One of the reasons for this hypothesis is that LBP can negatively influence proprioceptive acuity, leading to impaired intrinsic feedback from the lumbar spine [16]. As a consequence, patients with LBP might have to rely more on external feedback and become more dependent on it [7]. In addition, pain demands attention and can distract patients from the

movement task [17], which might in turn interfere with the learning process [15]. However, empirical evidence for a reduced motor learning capacity in patients with CLBP is currently lacking and the scantly available research in other chronic pain populations shows equivocal results [18, 19].

Therefore, the aims of this study were (1) to assess whether sensor-based feedback is more effective to improve lumbopelvic movement control compared to feedback from a mirror or no feedback in patients with chronic low back pain (CLBP), and (2) to evaluate whether patients with CLBP are equally capable of improving lumbopelvic movement control compared to healthy persons.

Methods
Design

A randomised controlled trial including healthy persons and patients with CLBP was conducted. Both groups of participants were randomised into three subgroups, each receiving a different type of feedback during the intervention, i.e. feedback from sensors, a mirror or no feedback (= control group). Randomisation was done with a computerised random sequence generator and allocation concealment was obtained by using sequentially numbered, sealed, opaque envelopes prepared by a person not further involved in the study.

The intervention consisted of a single exercise session during which participants practised a movement control task while receiving their assigned type of feedback. Movement control was assessed with lumbopelvic kinematics, which were obtained at baseline, during and immediately after the intervention.

Participants

Participants were recruited at private physiotherapy and GP practices and via social media. To be included, all participants needed to be between 18 and 65 years old and patients had to be diagnosed with chronic non-specific LBP (> 3 months, ≥3 days/week). Exclusion criteria for all participants were: spinal surgery in the past, an underlying serious disease or a physical problem interfering with daily life activities (e.g. severe knee pain), signs or symptoms of nerve root involvement, performance of lumbopelvic movement control exercises in the past year and pregnancy. Healthy subjects were also excluded if they experienced LBP in the past year.

To ensure that participants were able to achieve an improvement in movement control, the performance on the baseline movement control tasks was an additional inclusion criterion. To be included, the maximal lumbar range of motion during the baseline movement control tasks had to exceed 10° (0° would be a perfect performance). Participants with less range of motion on either of the baseline movement control tasks were excluded. Although this threshold of 10° was set a priori, the lumbar range of motion could only be calculated after completion of the full protocol. Therefore, all of the included participants completed the protocol, but only those fulfilling the abovementioned criterion were included in the final analysis.

Assessments
Baseline assessments
Sociodemographic data were obtained from all participants. Patients with CLBP also completed the Numeric pain rating scale (NPRS) [20] to assess current pain and the average pain during the past 7 days, the Roland Morris Disability questionnaire (RMDQ) [21] to assess disability and the Tampa scale for kinesiophobia (Miller RP, Kori SH, Todd DD: The Tampa Scale, unpublished) to assess the fear of movement/re-injury due to physical activity. After completing the questionnaires, participants performed two movement control tasks, i.e. a lifting task followed by a waiter's bow (Fig. 1). Both tasks were standardised for the participants' height and assessed with lumbopelvic kinematic measurements in the sagittal plane. Before the baseline kinematic measurements, the tasks were explained and demonstrated in a standardised way. For the lifting task, participants started from a relaxed standing position and were asked to lift a box with handles from a platform on the floor and to put it back down, while maintaining their lumbar curvature (i.e. not to flex or extend the lumbar spine). Participants were allowed to flex their knees as far as they wanted to. The distance from the box to the hallux was 15 cm. The dimensions of the box were 40 × 30 × 23.5 cm, and it weighed 4 kg. The top of the box was positioned 10 cm below the apex of the subjects' patella. For the waiter's bow, participants started with slightly flexed knees (±20°). Participants were instructed to keep their knees in the same position and to

bend forward in the hips while maintaining their lumbar curvature. Participants had to touch the middle of a stool, marked with a piece of tape, which was positioned 15 cm in front of the hallux, and to return to their starting position. No familiarisation was allowed, and each task was performed five times at a self-selected speed.

Assessments during and after the intervention
Kinematics were also obtained during and three minutes after the intervention. For the post-intervention kinematic assessment, participants first performed the waiter's bow and then the lifting task as described above. Immediately after the post-intervention kinematic assessment, all participants were asked to complete the Borg-scale for perceived exertion [22], and to answer two questions on a 0 to 10 numeric rating scale: 'what was your average LBP intensity during the experiment?' (0 = no pain at all, 10 = worst imaginable pain), 'how fearful were you to damage your back?' (0 = not fearful at all, 10 = extremely fearful). If significant between group differences would be present on the post-intervention questionnaires, these would be controlled for in the data analysis, as they might influence movement patterns [23–25].

Equipment
The Valedo®motion research tool (Hocoma, Switzerland) was used to assess the lumbopelvic kinematics and to provide feedback in the sensor groups. This system consists of a laptop and three wireless inertial measurement sensors, which contain a magnetometer, 3D-accelerometer and a 3D-gyroscope. The sensors were placed on the spinous process of L1 and S1, and 20 cm above the lateral femoral condyle (Fig. 1). All three sensors were used for the kinematic assessment, while only the L1 and S1 sensors were used to provide feedback in the sensor groups. Details

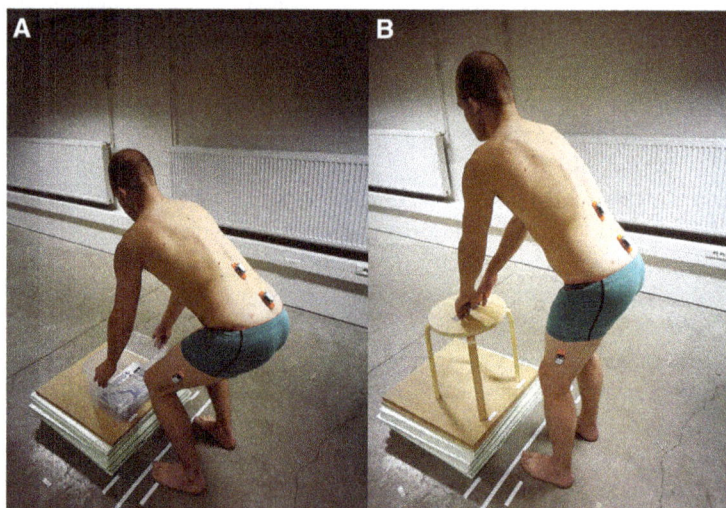

Fig. 1 Movement control tasks. **a** Lifting task. **b** Waiter's bow

on the kinematic data acquisition have been previously described [26].

Intervention

During the intervention, participants practised the waiter's bow during three sets of six repetitions while they received their assigned form of feedback. Each set of exercises was separated by one minute of rest. The lifting task was not practised. The feedback in the different groups was provided as follows:

Sensor group

The sensor-feedback was given via an avatar on a computer screen in front of the participants. The avatar was controlled by two movement sensors that were placed on the spinous process of L1 and S1. The upper body of the avatar corresponded with the S1-sensor and the green rectangle with the L1-sensor (Fig. 2). First, the system was calibrated when the participants assumed the starting position so that the green rectangle was placed in the middle of the avatar's upper body. Participants were instructed to keep the green rectangle on the avatar during the exercises, as this meant that the lumbar curvature was

maintained (Fig. 2a). If the rectangle moved anteriorly of the avatar, this corresponded with a lumbar flexion (Fig. 2b), while a posterior displacement indicated a lumbar extension.

Mirror group

A large mirror was placed laterally to the participants so they could see the stool and their whole body, and observe their spinal curvature during the exercises.

Control group

No feedback was provided.

Before the exercise trials, participants were explained how to use pelvic tilts to adjust the lumbar curvature. Hereafter, they were allowed to perform up to five pelvic tilts, during which participants in the sensor group could see how pelvic movements affected the position of the green rectangle relative to the avatar, participants in the mirror group could observe in the mirror how the pelvic tilts changed their lumbar curvature, while the control group received no feedback.

Outcome measures for addressing the primary and secondary aims of the study
Primary aim - effectiveness of feedback

The influence of the different types of feedback on movement control performance and motor learning was of primary interest. Performance can be measured during or shortly after training, whereas motor learning can be assessed with a transfer test [27]. As the participants only practised the waiter's bow, we used the differences between baseline and post-intervention kinematics of the waiter's bow as a measure of performance, while differences in the lifting task kinematics were used as a measure for motor learning. For each repetition, the maximal range of motion in the lumbar spine and hip joint was calculated and expressed in absolute values. Lumbar spine angles were calculated from the L1 and S1 sensors, while hip joint angles were calculated from the S1 and femoral sensors. This method is highly reliable for both tasks in this study (ICCs = 0.89–0.93) [26]. The minimal detectable change between two measurements for the lifting task is 5.3° for the lumbar spine and 8.8° for the hip, while for the waiter's bow this is 6.5° and 11.8°, respectively [26]. An improvement in movement control was defined as a decrease in the lumbar range of motion and an increase in the hip range of motion between baseline and post-intervention assessment. In addition to statistical significance, the abovementioned minimal detectable changes were used to interpret the results.

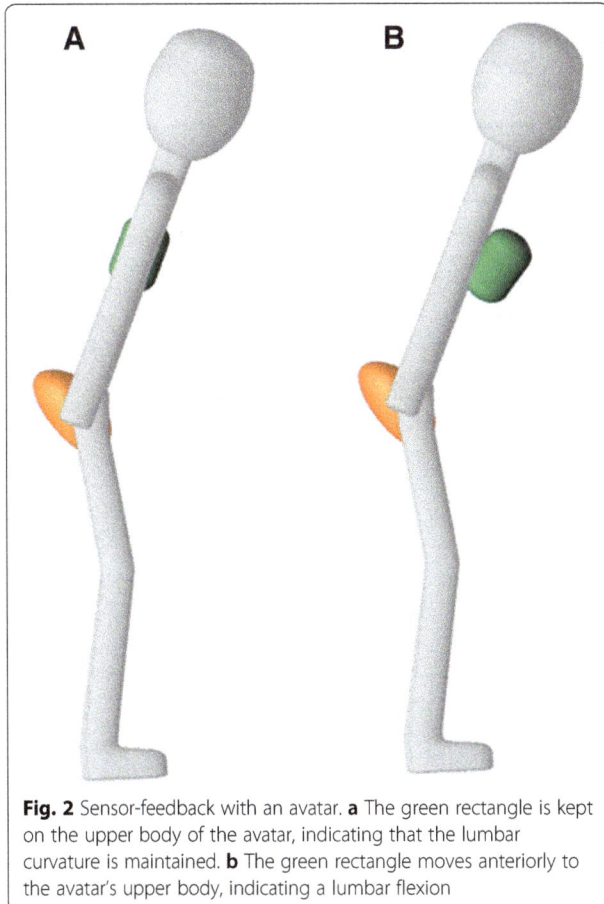

Fig. 2 Sensor-feedback with an avatar. **a** The green rectangle is kept on the upper body of the avatar, indicating that the lumbar curvature is maintained. **b** The green rectangle moves anteriorly to the avatar's upper body, indicating a lumbar flexion

Secondary aim – Comparison between healthy persons and patients with CLBP

The differences between healthy subjects and patients with CLBP in movement control performance improvement and motor learning was evaluated. This was done by comparing the change in lumbopelvic kinematics between baseline and post-intervention between both participant groups. In addition, the evolution of the performance on

the waiter's bow task during the intervention was compared. In this way, it could be determined whether healthy participants and patients with CLBP needed the same number of repetitions to achieve an improvement on the waiter's bow.

To investigate whether participants became dependent on the external feedback, the performance on the last exercise trial (with feedback) was compared with the

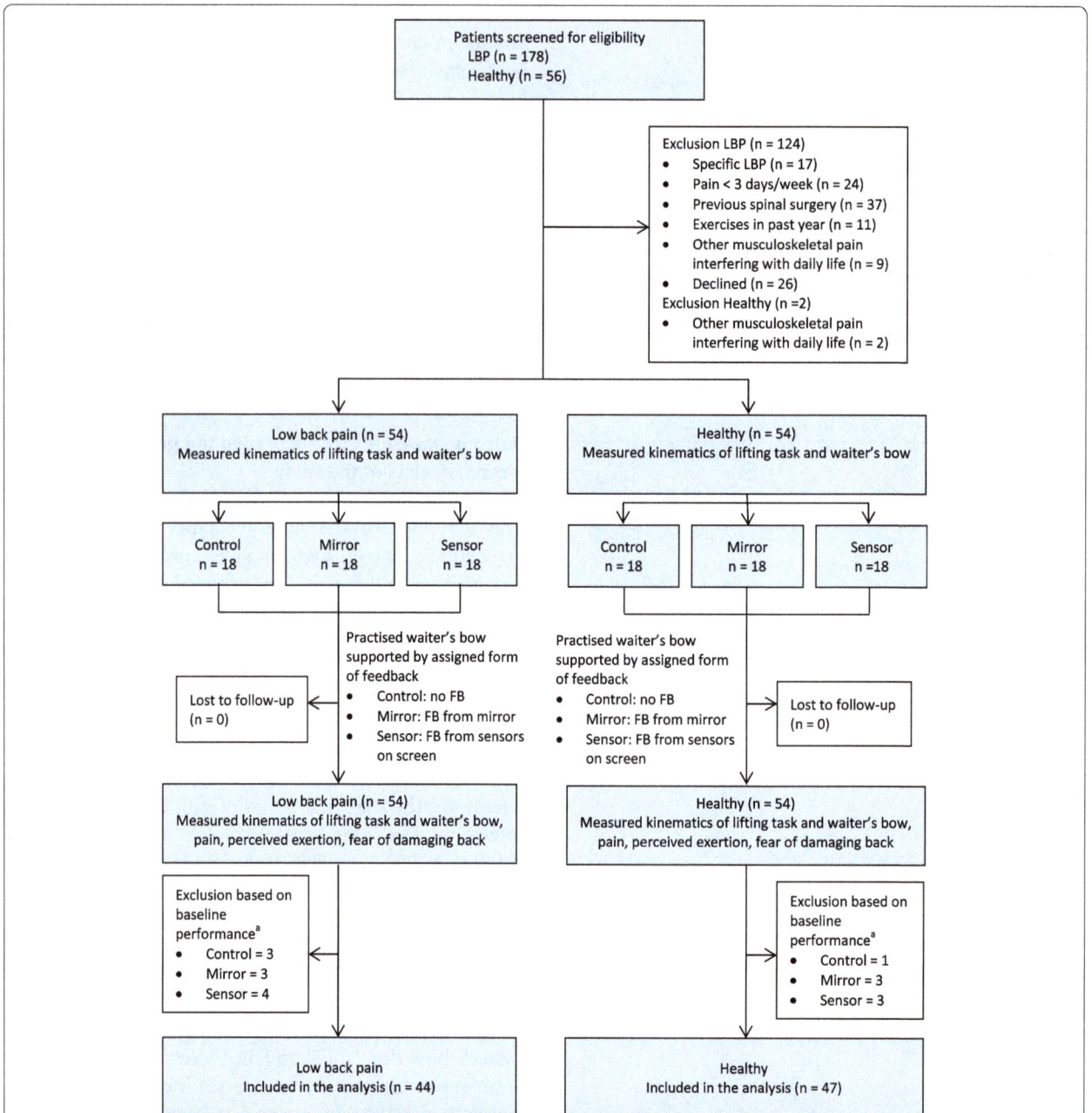

Fig. 3 Design and flow of participants through the trial. FB = feedback. [a] Participants were excluded after the trial, based on their performance on the baseline movement control tasks (exclusion criterion set a priori). Because the performance on the baseline kinematic measurements was calculated after trial completion, all participants were measured post-intervention, but only 44 participants in the low back pain group and 47 participants in the healthy group were included in the final analysis

post-intervention performance (without feedback) on the waiter's bow. A significant decline on the post-intervention performance would indicate such dependence [7].

Data analysis

The statistical analysis was performed with SAS JMP Pro (Version 12.2). To examine the effectiveness of the feedback and the difference in movement control improvement between healthy participants and patients with CLBP, a multiple linear regression was performed. The following variables were entered in the initial model to predict the differences between baseline and post-intervention kinematics: type of feedback (i.e. control, mirror or sensor), health status (i.e. healthy or CLBP), joint (i.e. lumbar spine or hip) and all their pairwise interactions. To control for the baseline values of the lumbar spine and hip angles, this variable was also put in the initial model. The variable 'joint' was included in the model because the movements of the spine and hip were considered to be related to each other. The final model was obtained by stepwise backward regression. The variable with the least significant p-value was left out first, and this was repeated until all the variables reached significance ($p < 0.05$). A Tukey all pairwise comparison was used as a post-hoc test.

A mixed model was used to assess the difference between healthy participants and patients with CLBP in the evolution of the performance on the waiter's bow task. This model was also used to examine the difference between the last repetition of the intervention and the post-intervention performance on the waiter's bow. The same variables from the linear regression were included in the mixed model, but 'repetition number' (i.e. baseline, repetitions during the intervention and post-intervention

measurements were numbered) and its pairwise interactions with other variables were added as fixed factors. 'Participant' was used as a random factor to account for multiple measurements for the same participant.

Sample size calculation was based on an effect size (f^2) of 0.2, power of 0.80 and α-level of 0.05. With these parameters, a total sample size of 80 participants was needed. Taking into account an attrition rate of 30% because of baseline performance on the movement control tests, 54 healthy persons and 54 patients with CLBP had to be recruited.

Results

The flow of participants through the study is shown in Fig. 3. Ten (19%) patients with CLBP and seven (13%) healthy participants were excluded based on their baseline performance on the movement control tasks. No significant differences in demographics (Table 1) and baseline scores on kinematic outcome measures (Table 2, first column) were observed between groups.

Effectiveness of feedback

The results of the linear regression and post-hoc tests are presented in Table 3 (see Additional file 1 for a detailed sum of squares table). In both the healthy participants and patients with CLBP, the sensor group improved significantly more than the mirror and control group (post-hoc tests, $p < 0.0001$), while no differences were observed between the mirror and control group (post-hoc tests, $p > 0.91$). These results were obtained for both the waiter's bow and the lifting task, as well as for the lumbar spine and hip. The improvements in the sensor groups were also larger than the measurement error (i.e.

Table 1 Baseline characteristics of the participants

Characteristic	Patients with chronic low back pain			Healthy persons			p-value
	Control (n = 15)	Mirror (n = 15)	Sensor (n = 14)	Control (n = 17)	Mirror (n = 15)	Sensor (n = 15)	
Sociodemographic data							
Age (years)	43 (12)	36 (13)	40 (17)	37 (10)	40 (14)	33 (14)	0.31
Gender, n female (%)	5 (33)	7 (47)	6 (43)	10 (59)	6 (40)	8 (53)	0.31
Height (cm)	176 (11)	175 (7)	171 (8)	174 (5)	170 (9)	172 (9)	0.38
Weight (kg)	78 (14)	69 (12)	70 (11)	70 (11)	63 (11)	71 (13)	0.05
LBP Questionnaires							
Onset LBP (years)[a]	3 (7)	4 (6)	6 (10)				0.56
NPRS 7 days (0–10)	4.9 (1.5)	4.5 (1.9)	4.5 (1.4)				0.72
NPRS current (0–10)	3.1 (2.0)	2.9 (1.9)	3.2 (2.2)				0.93
RMDQ (0–24)	7.7 (3.5)	7.5 (4.9)	6.6 (3.3)				0.69
TSK (17–68)	37.9 (5.5)	37.1 (6.9)	37.1 (8.6)				0.94

Data are mean (SD), unless mentioned otherwise

LBP low back pain, *NPRS* Numeric pain rating scale, *NPRS 7 days* average pain during the past 7 days measured with a NPRS, *NPRS current* current pain measured with a NPRS, *RMDQ* Roland-Morris Disability Questionnaire, *TSK* Tampa scale for kinesiophobia

[a]Median (IQR)

Table 2 Baseline and post-intervention maximal range of motion in the lumbar spine and hip joint

			Baseline	Post-intervention	Mean difference (95%CI)
Chronic low back pain					
Waiter's bow					
Lumbar spine		Control	17.9 (5.9)	17.5 (6.6)	−0.4 (−2.9 to 2.0)
		Mirror	18.5 (4.3)	15.8 (2.7)	−2.7 (−0.5 to −0.2)
		Sensor	16.2 (6.2)	6.5 (4.7)	−9.7 (−13.9 to −5.5)[a]
Hip		Control	27.8 (16.3)	28.3 (15.8)	0.5 (−4.7 to 5.8)
		Mirror	36.0 (13.7)	38.5 (14.2)	2.5 (−3.4 to 8.4)
		Sensor	31.4 (9.8)	46.1 (11.8)	14.7 (6.4 to 23.0)[a]
Lifting task					
Lumbar spine		Control	23.7 (7.2)	22.0 (10.6)	−1.7 (−5.1 to 1.8)
		Mirror	20.5 (7.2)	18.9 (4.7)	−1.6 (−4.1 to 1.0)
		Sensor	21.0 (7.5)	13.9 (7.8)	−7.2 (−3.7 to −10.7)[a]
Hip		Control	89.2 (13.6)	87.3 (14.7)	−1.9 (−7.9 to 4.1)
		Mirror	91.1 (13.6)	86.3 (19.2)	−4.9 (−11.5 to 1.8)
		Sensor	89.7 (12.8)	95.4 (9.8)	5.7 (−0.1 to 11.5)
Healthy subjects					
Waiter's bow					
Lumbar spine		Control	20.5 (7.3)	18.7 (9.7)	−1.8 (−6.3 to 2.8)
		Mirror	22.2 (7.7)	20.6 (9.8)	−1.6 (−5.1 to 1.8)
		Sensor	21.5 (6.1)	8.2 (4.4)	−13.3 (−17.9 to −9.4)[a]
Hip		Control	26.1 (10.5)	33.4 (13.8)	7.2 (−1.6 to 12.9)
		Mirror	27.7 (12.7)	33.5 (15.1)	5.8 (1.1 to 10.4)
		Sensor	30.7 (10.1)	45.1 (7.4)	14.5 (9.2 to 19.7)[a]
Lifting task					
Lumbar spine		Control	24.1 (10.7)	22.4 (11.0)	−1.8 (−3.0 to −0.7)
		Mirror	27.8 (7.0)	26.9 (7.3)	−0.9 (−3.7 to 1.8)
		Sensor	27.0 (8.3)	19.8 (7.0)	−7.1 (−2.6 to −11.7)[a]
Hip		Control	88.0 (13.1)	86.7 (12.7)	−1.3 (−8.8 to 2.1)
		Mirror	92.4 (13.3)	92.6 (7.8)	0.2 (−4.2 to 4.6)
		Sensor	83.9 (14.1)	92.1 (10.7)	8.2 (3.1 to 13.3)

All data are expressed as angles in degrees (°). Data for baseline and post-intervention are mean (SD). Mean difference = post-intervention minus baseline
[a]Mean difference > measurement error

minimal detectable change), except for the hip during the lifting task (Table 2). There were no between groups differences in the post-intervention questionnaires (see Additional file 2).

Based on the type III sum of squares tables (see Additional file 1), it is clear that the type of feedback is the most important factor contributing to the variance that is explained by the final regression models of the waiter's bow and lifting task, while the factor joint only explains a small proportion. A significant part of the variance that is explained by the final model of the lifting task can be attributed to the baseline scores on the kinematic assessments. Participants who had a worse performance on the baseline lifting task had a larger improvement.

Comparison between healthy persons and patients with CLBP

The variable health status (i.e. healthy or CLBP) and its interaction with repetition number were not retained in the final mixed model (Table 4). This indicates that patients with CLBP were equally capable of improving lumbopelvic movement control, and that the evolution of the performance on the waiter's bow task was similar between both participant groups (see Fig. 4 for an example of the sensor groups). These results are further supported by the fact that only a small proportion of the variance that is explained by the final model can be attributed to each of the variables pertaining to our second research question (see Additional file 3 for a detailed

Table 3 Results of the linear regression analysis and post-hoc tests for type of feedback

Linear regression		Post-hoc multiple comparisons for type of FB		
Fixed effects	p-value	Comparison	Estimated differences between groups (95% CI)	p-value
Waiter's bow				
Initial model				
Health status	0.09			
Type of FB	< 0.0001			
Joint	0.01			
Baseline score kinematics	0.06			
Health status*type of FB	0.61			
Health status*Joint	0.71			
Type of FB*Joint	0.94			
Final model				
Type of FB	< 0.0001	Mirror minus Control	0.6 (− 3.1 to 4.4)	0.91
Joint	0.04	Sensor minus Control	10.6 (6.8 to 14.3)	< 0.0001[a]
		Sensor minus Mirror	9.9 (6.1 to 13.7)	< 0.0001[a]
Lifting task				
Initial model				
Health status	0.20			
Type of FB	< 0.0001			
Joint	0.029			
Baseline score kinematics	0.003			
Health status*type of FB	0.65			
Health status*Joint	0.44			
Type of FB*Joint	0.57			
Final model				
Type of FB	< 0.0001	Mirror minus Control	−0.3 (− 3.7 to 3.0)	0.97
Joint	0.02	Sensor minus Control	6.9 (3.5 to 10.2)	< 0.0001[a]
Baseline score kinematics	0.002	Sensor minus Mirror	7.2 (3.8 to 10.6)	< 0.0001[a]

FB Feedback, *Health status* healthy of CLBP, *Joint* lumbar spine or hip, *Type of FB* sensor, mirror or control

[a]in favour of the sensor group

sum of squares table). Post-hoc tests also showed that there were no differences between the performance on the last exercise trial and the post-intervention assessment of the waiter's bow. This demonstrates that participants in the mirror and sensor groups did not become dependent on the feedback.

Discussion

The primary aim of this study was to compare the effectiveness of different types of external feedback to improve lumbopelvic movement control in healthy persons and patients with CLBP. Our results show that sensor-based postural feedback was more effective to improve lumbopelvic movement control than feedback from a mirror or no feedback. Furthermore, being provided with feedback from a mirror did not lead to better results than receiving no feedback at all.

We hypothesize that the lack of improvement in the mirror group could be explained by the difficulty for unexperienced persons to visually detect changes in the lumbar curvature during the waiter's bow. Although physiotherapists can reliably assess the waiter's bow by observation, observer training may play an important role in this assessment [28]. Possibly, a longer teaching and familiarization period before the intervention could have enhanced the effectiveness of the mirror-feedback.

In contrast, the very short introduction to the sensor-feedback was sufficient to improve lumbopelvic movement control. We believe that the avatar provided more accurate and easy-to-understand feedback, which required no advanced training in order to interpret it correctly. It has been shown that abstract visualisations can be more effective than very realistic feedback (e.g. via a video or mirror) because they can provide information about key features of the task only, without overwhelming the

Table 4 Results for the mixed model

Fixed effects	p-value
Initial model	
Health status	0.40
Type of FB	< 0.0001
Joint	< 0.0001
Baseline score kinematics	< 0.0001
Repetition number	< 0.0001
Health status*type of FB	0.83
Health status*Joint	0.01
Type of FB*Joint	0.08
Repetition number*type of FB	< 0.0001
Repetition number*Health status	0.28
Repetition number*Joint	0.09
Final model	
Health status	0.38
Type of FB	< 0.0001
Baseline score kinematics	< 0.0001
Joint	< 0.0001
Repetition number	< 0.0001
Health status*Joint	0.01
Repetition number*Type of FB	< 0.0001

FB Feedback, *Health status* healthy of CLBP, *Joint* lumbar spine or hip, *Type of FB* sensor, mirror or control

participants with irrelevant information [8]. Participants in the sensor group only had to look at the green dot relative to the avatar's upper body, while participants in the mirror group could also see movements in other body regions that were irrelevant to the task.

In addition, the screen displaying the avatar could be placed in front of the participants, whereas the mirror had to be positioned laterally to visualise the movements in the sagittal plane. Although this difference in position could be interpreted as a confounding factor because participants in the mirror group had to turn their heads in order to view their spinal curvature, the possibility to place the computer screen in the most convenient position should rather be considered as an inherent advantage of the sensor-feedback.

Finally, the improvements on the lifting task were partially explained by the baseline kinematic scores. Participants who performed worse on the lifting task at baseline assessment had a significantly larger improvement, which indicates that the motor learning effect was more pronounced in these participants. This might be explained by the fact that persons who performed worse at the baseline lifting task also had a larger potential for improvement.

Besides a mirror, various other types of conventional feedback, including tape or palpation [10], can be used to support patients during lumbopelvic movement exercises. The rationale for comparing the sensor-based feedback to feedback from a mirror was twofold: First, a mirror is frequently being used or recommended to provide postural feedback during lumbopelvic movement

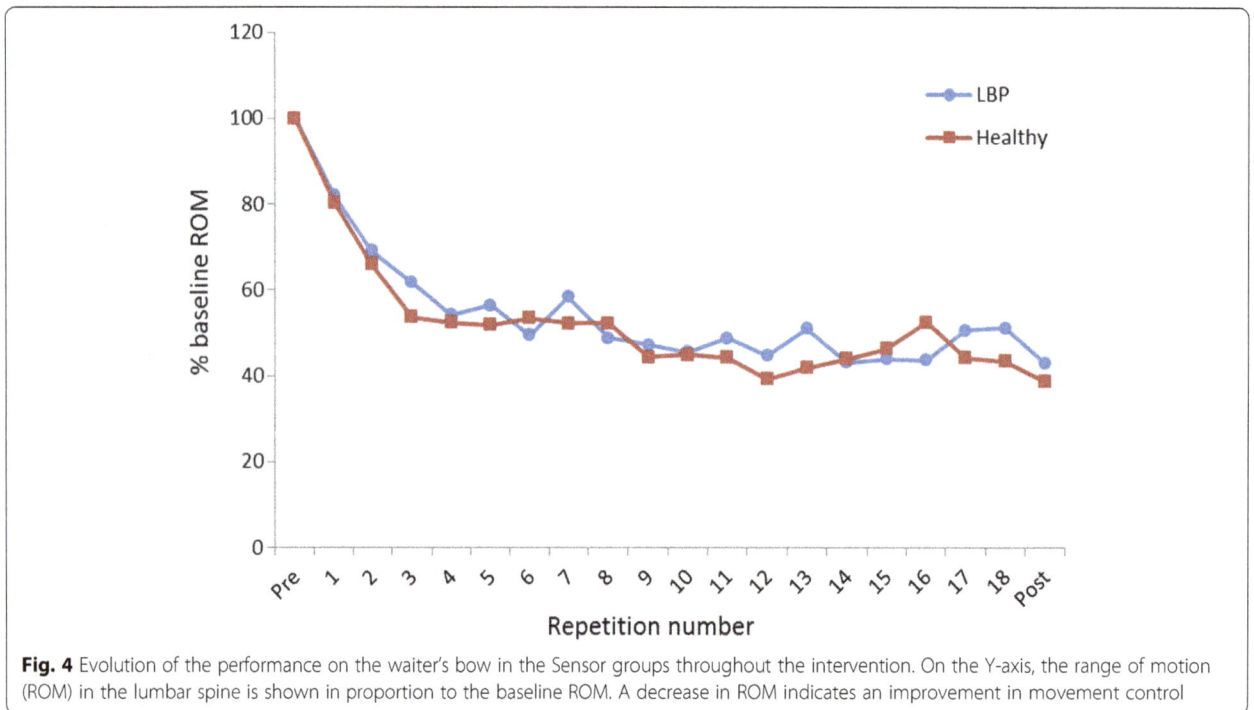

Fig. 4 Evolution of the performance on the waiter's bow in the Sensor groups throughout the intervention. On the Y-axis, the range of motion (ROM) in the lumbar spine is shown in proportion to the baseline ROM. A decrease in ROM indicates an improvement in movement control

control exercises [10, 29–31]. Second, and more importantly, both the mirror and sensors provided visual feedback, whereas palpation and a tape provide tactile feedback. Because visual motion detection is processed differently than tactile motion detection [32], we chose to compare the sensor feedback to feedback from a mirror.

Healthy subjects and patients with CLBP were equally capable of improving lumbopelvic movement control. It has been suggested that pain could negatively influence skill acquisition and motor learning by distracting people from the task they are performing [15]. However, this distraction mainly occurs when the pain is more intense, unfamiliar or unexpected [17]. The patients with CLBP in our study did not report an increase in pain during the exercise trials and there is no reason to assume that the pain they felt was unexpected or unfamiliar. Therefore, it is unlikely that patients with CLBP were distracted from the movement task.

Pain can also affect proprioceptive acuity and impair the intrinsic feedback system [33]. When less reliable intrinsic feedback is available, the dependency on the extrinsic feedback may increase [7]. Overall, patients with CLBP have decreased lumbosacral proprioception compared to healthy persons [16, 34], so it can be argued that removing the external feedback could influence the performance on the waiter's bow more in patients with CLBP than in healthy participants. On the other hand, these proprioceptive impairments may be position specific (e.g. sit versus stance) [34] and little is known about proprioception during dynamic tasks [16], such as the ones in the present study. Our results show that omitting the external feedback had no influence on the performance on the waiter's bow in both participant groups. This suggests that patients with CLBP also used information from the sensorimotor system to adjust their spinal curvature during the exercise trials [8], and that they did not rely more on the external feedback than healthy subjects. The improvements on the lifting task in the sensor groups further support this notion, as it indicates that both participant groups were able to transfer their newly learned skills to a different task. Therefore, it seems appropriate to use concurrent sensor-based feedback during the initial learning phase of movement control tasks in patients with CLBP.

Several limitations apply to this study. First, motor learning was only assessed with a transfer test, and not with a retention test. Both the transferability of practised skills and the long-term retention effects are important aspects of motor learning [27]. Because it is impossible to provide movement control training during every single activity an individual needs to perform, persons should be able to implement their newly acquired skills during activities that were not practised. In addition, the movement control improvements should be retained in the long term. However, because a retention test was not included in this study, we cannot make any statements regarding the longstanding effects of the sensor-based feedback.

Second, the mobility of the lower limb joints was not evaluated at baseline assessment. According to the concept of relative flexibility, a restriction in one joint could influence the movements in an adjacent joint [6]. Especially during the lifting task, more end range movements were necessary in the hip joint. As such, a restriction in hip joint mobility could have influenced the lumbar movements. On the other hand, participants with any physical problems other than LBP (e.g. hip or knee pain) that interfered with daily life activities were excluded from this study. Therefore, we believe it is unlikely that a (pathological) restriction of lower limb joint mobility would have significantly influenced the movement patterns in the lumbar spine.

Finally, our measurement and feedback system only contained three sensors. Due to these technical limitations, we could only measure the movements in the lumbar spine and hip joint. Consequently, we cannot exclude that some patients might have used compensatory movements in the thoracic spine while performing the movement control tasks. On the other hand, the reduction in lumbar ROM in the sensor group was accompanied by an increase in hip joint motion, indicating movements in the hip joint and lumbar spine were coupled.

Conclusions

The recent development of rehabilitation technologies creates new possibilities for therapists and patients to support the rehabilitation process. As such, evaluating the effectiveness of these rapidly evolving technological systems poses an important challenge. The present study shows that sensor-based postural feedback is more effective than feedback from a mirror or no feedback to improve lumbopelvic movement control in the short term. Patients with CLBP were equally capable of improving lumbopelvic movement control as compared to healthy participants. Future research should focus on the long-term retention effects and evaluate whether supporting exercises with sensor-based feedback leads to larger improvements in pain and disability compared to conventional exercise therapy.

Acknowledgements
We would like to thank Dr. Robin Bruyndonckx and Dr. Francesca Solmi for their advice on the statistical analysis.

Authors' contributions
TM conceptualised the study, and SB and AT refined the design. TM and CD collected the data. TM drafted the manuscript, and SB, CD and AT revised it for important intellectual content and helped interpret the data. All authors read and approved the final manuscript.

Competing interests
The authors declare that they have no competing interests.

Author details
[1]Rehabilitation Research Center - Biomed, Faculty of Medicine and Life Sciences, Hasselt University, Hasselt, Belgium. [2]Department of Rehabilitation Sciences, KU Leuven – University of Leuven, Leuven, Belgium. [3]Department of Sport and Rehabilitation Sciences, University of Liege, Liege, Belgium.

References
1. Airaksinen O, Brox JI, Cedraschi C, Hildebrandt J, Klaber-Moffett J, Kovacs F, Mannion AF, Reis S, Staal JB, Ursin H, Zanoli G. Chapter 4. European guidelines for the management of chronic nonspecific low back pain. Eur Spine J. 2006;15(Suppl 2):S192–300.
2. Hurwitz EL, Randhawa K, Yu H, Cote P, Haldeman S. The global spine care initiative: a summary of the global burden of low back and neck pain studies. Eur Spine J. 2018. https://doi.org/10.1007/s00586-017-5432-9 .
3. Dagenais S, Caro J, Haldeman S. A systematic review of low back pain cost of illness studies in the United States and internationally. Spine J. 2008;8:8–20.
4. O'Sullivan P. Diagnosis and classification of chronic low back pain disorders: maladaptive movement and motor control impairments as underlying mechanism. Man Ther. 2005;10:242–55.
5. Luomajoki HA, Bonet Beltran MB, Careddu S, Bauer CM. Effectiveness of movement control exercise on patients with non-specific low back pain and movement control impairment: a systematic review and meta-analysis. Musculoskeletal Science Practice. 2018;36:1–11.
6. Sahrmann SA. Movement System Impairment Syndromes of the Extremities, Cervical and Thoracic Spines. 1st ed. St. Louis: Mosby; 2010.
7. Magill RA. Motor Learning and Control. Concepts and applications. 8th ed. Boston: McGraw-Hill; 2007.
8. Sigrist R, Rauter G, Riener R, Wolf P. Augmented visual, auditory, haptic, and multimodal feedback in motor learning: a review. Psychon Bull Rev. 2013;20:21–53.
9. Ribeiro DC, Sole G, Abbott JH, Milosavljevic S. Extrinsic feedback and management of low back pain: a critical review of the literature. Man Ther. 2011;16:231–9.
10. Hodges PW, Van Dillen LR, McGill SM, Brumagne S, Hides JA, Moseley GL. Integrated clinical approach to motor control interventions in low back and pelvic pain. In: Hodges PW, Cholewicki J, Van Dieen JH, editors. Spinal Control: The rehabilitation of back pain State of the art and science. 1st ed. London: Churchill Livingstone; 2013. p. 243–309.
11. Elgueta-Cancino E, Schabrun S, Danneels L, Hodges P. A clinical test of lumbopelvic control: development and reliability of a clinical test of dissociation of lumbopelvic and thoracolumbar motion. Man Ther. 2014;19:418–24.
12. Haneline MT, Cooperstein R, Young M, Birkeland K. Spinal motion palpation: a comparison of studies that assessed intersegmental end feel vs excursion. J Manip Physiol Ther. 2008;31:616–26.
13. Wang Q, Markopoulos P, Yu B, Chen W, Timmermans A. Interactive wearable systems for upper body rehabilitation: a systematic review. J Neuroeng Rehabil. 2017;14:20.
14. Matheve T, Claes G, Olivieri E, Timmermans A. Serious gaming to support exercise therapy for patients with chronic nonspecific low back pain: a feasibility study. Games Health J. 2018;7:262–270.
15. Boudreau SA, Farina D, Falla D. The role of motor learning and neuroplasticity in designing rehabilitation approaches for musculoskeletal pain disorders. Man Ther. 2010;15:410–4.
16. Brumagne S, Janssens L, Claeys K, Pijnenburg M. Altered variability in proprioceptive control strategy in people with recurrent low back pain. In: Hodges P, Cholewicki J, Van Dieën JH, editors. Spinal control: The rehabilitation of back pain. 1st ed. London: Churchill Livingstone; 2013. p. 135–44.
17. Eccleston C, Crombez G. Pain demands attention: a cognitive-affective model of the interruptive function of pain. Psychol Bull. 1999;125:356–66.
18. Vallence AM, Smith A, Tabor A, Rolan PE, Ridding MC. Chronic tension-type headache is associated with impaired motor learning. Cephalalgia. 2013;33: 1048–54.
19. Parker RS, Lewis GN, Rice DA, McNair PJ. The association between Corticomotor excitability and motor skill learning in people with painful hand arthritis. Clin J Pain. 2017;33:222–30.
20. Chapman JR, Norvell DC, Hermsmeyer JT, Bransford RJ, DeVine J, McGirt MJ, Lee MJ. Evaluating common outcomes for measuring treatment success for chronic low back pain. Spine (Phila Pa 1976). 2011;36:S54–68.
21. Roland M, Morris R. A study of the natural history of back pain. Part I: development of a reliable and sensitive measure of disability in low-back pain. Spine (Phila Pa 1976). 1983;8:141–4.
22. Borg GA. Psychophysical bases of perceived exertion. Med Sci Sports Exerc. 1982;14:377–81.
23. Vaisy M, Gizzi L, Petzke F, Consmuller T, Pfingsten M, Falla D. Measurement of lumbar spine functional movement in low back pain. Clin J Pain. 2015;31:876–85.
24. Trost Z, France CR, Thomas JS. Examination of the photograph series of daily activities (PHODA) scale in chronic low back pain patients with high and low kinesiophobia. Pain. 2009;141:276–82.
25. van Dieen JH, van der Burg P, Raaijmakers TA, Toussaint HM. Effects of repetitive lifting on kinematics: inadequate anticipatory control or adaptive changes? J Mot Behav. 1998;30:20–32.
26. Matheve T, De Baets L, Rast F, Bauer C, Timmermans A. Within/between-session reliability and agreement of lumbopelvic kinematics in the sagittal plane during functional movement control tasks in healthy persons. Musculoskelet Sci Pract. 2018;33:90–8.
27. Soderstrom NC, Bjork RA. Learning versus performance: an integrative review. Perspect Psychol Sci. 2015;10:176–99.
28. Carlsson H, Rasmussen-Barr E. Clinical screening tests for assessing movement control in non-specific low-back pain. A systematic review of intra- and inter-observer reliability studies. Man Ther. 2013;18:103–10.
29. Vibe Fersum K, O'Sullivan P, Skouen JS, Smith A, Kvale A. Efficacy of classification-based cognitive functional therapy in patients with non-specific chronic low back pain: a randomized controlled trial. Eur J Pain. 2013;17:916–28.
30. O'Sullivan PB, Caneiro JP, O'Keeffe M, Smith A, Dankaerts W, Fersum K, O'Sullivan K. Cognitive functional therapy: an integrated behavioral approach for the targeted Management of Disabling low Back Pain. Phys Ther. 2018;98:408–23.
31. Sheeran L, van Deursen R, Caterson B, Sparkes V. Classification-guided versus generalized postural intervention in subgroups of nonspecific chronic low back pain: a pragmatic randomized controlled study. Spine (Phila Pa 1976). 2013;38:1613–25.
32. Nakashita S, Saito DN, Kochiyama T, Honda M, Tanabe HC, Sadato N. Tactile-visual integration in the posterior parietal cortex: a functional magnetic resonance imaging study. Brain Res Bull. 2008;75:513–25.

33. Roijezon U, Clark NC, Treleaven J. Proprioception in musculoskeletal rehabilitation. Part 1: basic science and principles of assessment and clinical interventions. Man Ther. 2015;20:368–77.
34. Tong MH, Mousavi SJ, Kiers H, Ferreira P, Refshauge K, van Dieen J. Is there a relationship between lumbar proprioception and low back pain? A systematic review with meta-analysis. Arch Phys Med Rehabil. 2017;98: 120–36. e122

10

Dissociating motor learning from recovery in exoskeleton training post-stroke

Nicolas Schweighofer[1][*] , Chunji Wang[2], Denis Mottet[3], Isabelle Laffont[4], Karima Bakthi[4], David J. Reinkensmeyer[5] and Olivier Rémy-Néris[6]

Abstract

Background: A large number of robotic or gravity-supporting devices have been developed for rehabilitation of upper extremity post-stroke. Because these devices continuously monitor performance data during training, they could potentially help to develop predictive models of the effects of motor training on recovery. However, during training with such devices, patients must become adept at using the new "tool" of the exoskeleton, including learning the new forces and visuomotor transformations associated with the device. We thus hypothesized that the changes in performance during extensive training with a passive, gravity-supporting, exoskeleton device (the Armeo Spring) will follow an initial fast phase, due to learning to use the device, and a slower phase that corresponds to reduction in overall arm impairment. Of interest was whether these fast and slow processes were related.

Methods: To test the two-process hypothesis, we used mixed-effect exponential models to identify putative fast and slow changes in smoothness of arm movements during 80 arm reaching tests performed during 20 days of exoskeleton training in 53 individuals with post-acute stroke.

Results: In line with our hypothesis, we found that double exponential models better fit the changes in smoothness of arm movements than single exponential models. In contrast, single exponential models better fit the data for a group of young healthy control subjects. In addition, in the stroke group, we showed that smoothness correlated with a measure of impairment (the upper extremity Fugl Meyer score - UEFM) at the end, but not at the beginning, of training. Furthermore, the improvement in movement smoothness due to the slow component, but not to the fast component, strongly correlated with the improvement in the UEFM between the beginning and end of training. There was no correlation between the change of peaks due to the fast process and the changes due to the slow process. Finally, the improvement in smoothness due to the slow, but not the fast, component correlated with the number of days since stroke at the onset of training – i.e. participants who started exoskeleton training sooner after stroke improved their smoothness more.

Conclusions: Our results therefore demonstrate that at least two processes are involved in in performance improvements measured during mechanized training post-stroke. The fast process is consistent with learning to use the exoskeleton, while the slow process independently reflects the reduction in upper extremity impairment.

Keywords: Motor learning, Motor adaptation, Motor recovery, Stroke, Neurorehabilitation, Exoskeleton, Rehabilitation robotics, Movement analysis

* Correspondence: schweigh@usc.edu
[1]Biokinesiology and Physical Therapy, University of Southern California, Los Angeles, USA
Full list of author information is available at the end of the article

Background

Initial behavioral changes post-stroke largely result from "spontaneous recovery", which is greatest in the first month and continues for ~ 6 months [1]. Spontaneous recovery involves reduction in lesion edema, ischemic penumbra, and brain reorganization [2, 3]. However, motor training consisting of thousands of movements over weeks has been shown to influence the speed and the level of recovery via slow re-organization of surviving neural networks in animals, and is thought to have a similar effect in humans [4–8]. Thus, "recovery" can be thought of as a process of spontaneous recovery modulated by use-dependent plasticity; this recovery is often characterized as a reduction of impairment, measured using clinical scales such as the UEFM scale, which tests the ability to perform a variety of arm and hand movements.

Because therapists can only deliver a fraction of such large doses of training, a number of robotic or mechanized devices have been developed to retrain arm movements post-stroke in a semi-automated manner, see for reviews [9–13]. Upper extremity training with such devices, or even reach training without any mechanical support, has been shown to improve reaching movements' speed, smoothness, and range (e.g., [14–16]).

During robotic or gravity-supported mechanized training, novel sensorimotor interactions must be learned. For instance, the passive Armeo Spring exoskeleton (Hocoma Inc.), which was used in the present study, applies novel forces to the participant's arm, because adjustable springs compensate for the impact of gravity on the upper and lower arm. In addition, novel visuo-motor transformations must be learned, because the movements' goals and hand movements are presented visually on a monitor in front of the participants. To perform fast and accurate movements, participants thus need to learn to compensate for these new forces and visuo-motor transformations. Even after learning to compensate for these perturbations, further performance improvements would be expected with ongoing practice [16, 17].

As a result, the causes of the observed improvements in motor performance shown by individuals post-stroke during exoskeleton training are unclear: Are the improvements due to learning to move the new "tool" of the exoskeleton, or to a reduction of impairment, or both? And, are the two putative processes related? Answering these questions could provide insights into the more general problem of learning new motor tasks after stroke, and even perhaps into the problem of relearning to control the arm with the residual neural hardware that the stroke presumably has re-configured.

Here, our objective was to identify if performance improvements followed two processes during exoskeleton training post-stroke. 53 individuals with moderate impairments due to a stroke between 20 and 90 days prior to enrollment received Armeo Spring training twice a day, every weekday, for four consecutive weeks. Vertical arm reaching tests, performed on the Armeo Spring, were given before and after each session. A group of 11 young healthy control subjects received training for 1 week for comparison of putative motor learning effects.

We used double exponential mixed-effects models to decompose test performance data into faster and slower improvements of performance. Our measure of performance was movement smoothness during pointing tests, given by the average number of peaks in the hand trajectory velocity profiles, a measure that has been previously shown to be sensitive to stroke impairment [14, 15]. The use of an exponential term to model performance gains was motivated by the well-known negatively accelerated gains in performance as a function of training in most motor learning tasks [18], and by recent studies showing that changes in performance in arm reach training in non-disabled and post-stroke individuals can be well modeled with exponentials [19, 20]. The use of the mixed-effects in the nonlinear model was motivated by the high variability in impairment, spontaneous recovery, motor learning, and responsiveness to therapy post-stroke [19, 21, 22]. We compared the fit of double exponentials to single exponentials in the stroke group and in a group of young healthy control subjects. We then tested whether the slow component could assess recovery by comparing changes in smoothness due to the slow component to changes in the Upper Extremity Fugl Meyer (UEFM) pre- and post-training. We also tested whether the fast and slow components correlated with each other, as well as with the start time of the exoskeleton training, relative to the onset of the stroke.

Methods
Participants
We analyzed arm kinematic data from a sub-cohort of participants included in the experimental group of the REM-AVC clinical trial (NCT01383512), a multi-center RCT of mechanized arm therapy post-stroke. This RCT aimed at evaluating the medico-economic benefits in post-acute stroke of 4 weeks of standard care and motor arm therapy with Armeo Spring vs. standard care and self-rehabilitation. Kinematic and clinical data of 53 participants with a single stroke in the territory of the middle cerebral artery (MCA) were available for the present study (30 males, 19 females, 4 gender not available; 59.3 ± 13.9 years old; UEFM at baseline 24.7 ± 9.1, days since stroke 56 ± 21 days - all reported values are mean ± standard deviation; see Table 1). The participants were scheduled to receive 4 weeks of Armeo Spring training, 5 days/week, twice/day, for a total of 40 sessions. A performance test was given before and

after each training session (thus, for a total of $2 \times 2 \times 5 \times 4 = 80$ tests). For each test, we recorded upper limb kinematics during fast and accurate pointing movements (performed with the Armeo Spring) between targets in the vertical plane. Baseline UEFM was measured in the week before training and again in the week following training by physical or occupational therapists who were all trained to administer the UEFM. To quantify normative performance, 11 non-disabled individuals (4 females, 23.5 ± 2.0 years) performed 10 training sessions for 5 days. A performance test was given before and after each training session (thus, for a total of $2 \times 2 \times 5 = 20$ tests).

The Armeo spring device

The Armeo Spring exoskeleton is based on the T-WREX device [23]. It has six degrees of freedom, summarized in Fig. 1b. It has two adjustable gravity-compensating springs, at the upper arm and the forearm respectively.

Lengths of the segments are adjustable to adapt to the user's arm length. There are no motors at any joints; users must move their arms actively to control the exoskeleton. The arm is attached to the exoskeleton via Velcro straps; movement of the user's trunk is mildly constrained by a Velcro strap at the upper arm.

The device records all joint angles and calculates in real time the end effector location through a forward kinematics model of the exoskeleton (developed by Hocoma, Inc.). The end effector location is used to control a cursor on a screen, displayed in the vertical plane in front of the user.

Exoskeleton training and testing

A training session lasted between 20 and 30 min, and consisted of a performance test (the "Ladybug Test" Fig. 1a) that required moving the cursor to acquire targets shown on the screen, a number of different video games (selected by the therapists and patients in each session), and a

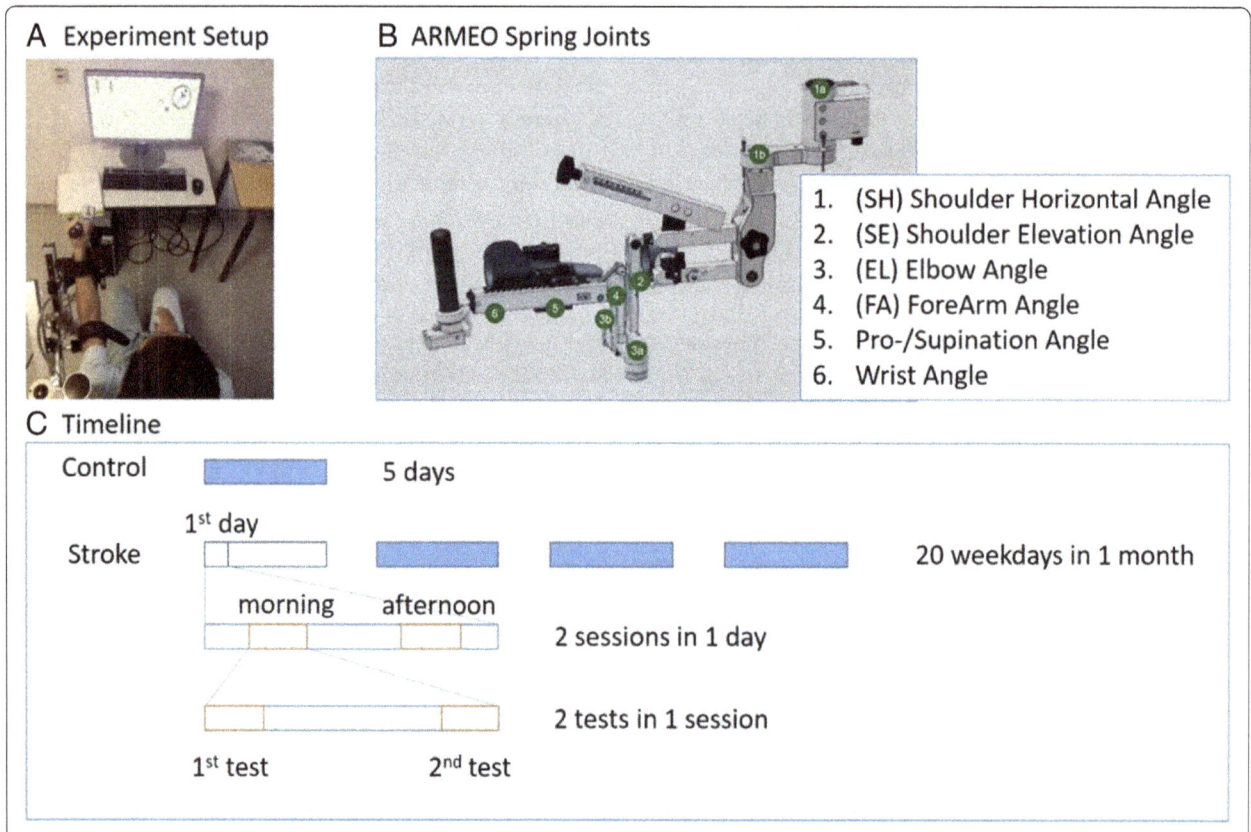

Fig. 1 Methods. **a**. Experiment setup: Participants sat in front of a vertical screen on which the video games were displayed. In the "Ladybug Test" given at the beginning and end of each training session, the cursor on the screen represented movements of the end-effector (hand) in the frontal plane as the participant attempted to acquire targets. **b**. The exoskeleton used in this study, the Armeo Spring device. Summation of joints 1a and 1b gives the Shoulder Horizontal (SH) angle, joint 2 the Shoulder Elevation (SE) angle, joint 3a (for the right arm) and 3b (for the left arm) the elbow (EL) angle, joint 4 the ForeArm (FA) angle, joint 5 the pronation and supination angle, and joint 6 the wrist angle. **c**. Training and testing schedule: each day, a session was administered in the morning and a second in the afternoon. The Ladybug test was administered at the beginning and end of each training session. The stroke group received 20 consecutive weekdays of training, whereas the control group received 5 consecutive days of training

Table 1 Participants information

Group	No.	Age	Affected Side	Gender	UEFM pre to post	Post Stroke Days	Prescribed No. of Tests
Stroke	53	59 ± 14	29 L, 24R,	30 M, 19F, 4 Missing	25 ± 9 to 39 ± 14 4 Missing	56 ± 21 4 Missing	80 in 4 weeks
Control	11	23 ± 2	–	7 M, 4F	–	–	20 in 1 week

second Ladybug test (thus, there were two Ladybug tests/session, and four tests per day). All games and tests, including the Ladybug test, were developed by Hocoma as part of the Armeo Spring software.

The Ladybug test was a two-dimensional pointing task in the frontal plane. In this test, the user was instructed to catch ladybug targets that appeared sequentially on the screen by moving the cursor to the target locations. The movement along the dimension perpendicular to the frontal (coronal) plane was ignored in the control of the cursor. The sequence of target locations appeared random to the subject, but was fixed in each test. The user had limited time to catch the ladybug (< 10 s). After a ladybug was caught, or the time limit was reached, the ladybug disappeared and the next ladybug appeared at a new location. There were four possible difficulty levels for the test; difficulty was modulated both by the number of targets and by the workspace size; from easy to difficult: 12 targets, 24 × 16 cm (horizontal × vertical); 20 targets, 36 × 27 cm; 32 targets, 45 × 36 cm and 48 targets, 63 × 45 cm. In the stroke group, test difficulty was adjusted by the therapist based on the patient's performance and motivation. In the control group, difficulty was set to the highest level. Here, we only analyzed end-effector trajectory data from these tests, that is, not from the video games in between the tests.

Data analysis
Preprocessing
We filtered the end effector trajectory with a second order Butterworth filter [24] with a cutoff frequency of 5 Hz. We defined a trial as the movement between two consecutive targets. A trial was considered successful if it started from a previously caught target and led to the catching of the next target. Only successful trials, that is, trials in which the participant caught the next ladybug within the pre-specified time of 10 s (control 99.8%, stroke 78.2%) were included in the analysis. We excluded tests in which participants caught less than 25% of the ladybugs (0.7% of all tests in stroke group, 0% in control group).

Task space performance
We characterized performance in a test via the average number of peaks in the velocity profile of each successful movements. To calculate the number of peaks in each test, we computed the derivative of velocity (tangential

acceleration) and counted the number of times it went from positive to negative. We then took the average of number of peaks (p) of all successful trials in the test. Note that the best possible performance is 1 velocity peak per movement.

Mixed effect models of learning and recovery
We modeled the dynamics of average number of peaks p in the velocity profiles in each test as exponential functions of time t represented by test number, with mixed effects [25]. For participants in the control group, visual observation seemed to indicate that changes in the average number of peaks decreased according to a single exponential-like decay. We therefore considered a model with a single exponential formulation, which gives performance for each test as:

$$p_{i,j} = A_i \exp(-B_i t_j) + 1 + \epsilon_{i,j}, \tag{1}$$

where t_j is the test number j, A_i is the mixed-effect coefficient representing the amplitude of the exponential for participant i, B_i is the mixed-effect coefficient representing the learning rate, and $\epsilon_{i,j}$ is the residual. We chose an asymptote of 1 because it is the theoretical lower limit of number of peaks in velocity profiles.

For the participants in the stroke group, visual observation seemed to indicate that changes in number of peaks over four weeks of training was initially fast and then slower. We therefore considered a model with two exponential components

$$p_{i,j} = A_i^f \exp\left(-B_i^f t_j\right) + A_i^s \exp\left(-B_i^s t_j\right) + 1 + \epsilon_{i,j}, \tag{2}$$

where, for all participants, the A^f, A^s, B^f and B^s were constraint to be positive; in addition, $B^f > B^s$; thus, the first term represents a fast component and the second a slow component. Note that the model of Eq. (1) comprises 5 parameters (the mean and standard deviations of the amplitude and the learning rate, and the residual standard deviation) and the model of Eq. (2) comprises 9 parameters. The mean parameters are the fixed effects and the standard deviation capture the random effects, which model the large variability in lesion, impairment, spontaneous recovery, motor learning, and responsiveness to therapy post-stroke [19, 21, 22].

In model development, it is possible to increase the fit by adding parameters, but doing so may result in overfitting. The Bayesian Information Criterion (BIC) attempts to resolve this problem by introducing a penalty term for the number of parameters in the model. For the control group, the BIC showed that a model with a single exponential better fit the data than a model with two exponentials. We also verified that a model with random effects on both the amplitude and the learning rate better fit the data than a model with only fixed effects. In contrast, for the stroke group, a model with two exponentials better fit the data than a model with a single exponential for this group. We also verified that a model with random effects on the amplitudes and the learning rates for both components better fit the data than a model with only fixed effects. The models were all fit with the function *nlmefit()* in Matlab 2016a. Our predefined threshold for statistical significance was 0.05. All analyses were performed in Matlab.

Results

Participants in the stroke group performed an average of 74 ± 13 performance tests, with a range of 33 to 86 tests. 36% of the participants performed 80 tests or more.[1] All participants in the control group performed the 20 tests. Participants typically showed large changes in performance during the duration of training. Figure 2 shows representative trajectories in both task space and joint space for a participant in the stroke group (UEFM pre = 39, post = 63) and a comparison for a participant in the control group. After training, the trajectories in task space were straighter, and the joint trajectories appeared smoother, but still less so than for the individual in the control group.

Figure 3 shows the average number of velocity peaks in each trial as well as the models plotted with the fixed effects. The participants in the stroke group exhibited large improvements in the number of peaks, with a decrease of approximately three peaks per movement on average over the course of training (Fig. 3b). Control subjects also showed an improvement in performance, but exhibited fewer number of peaks on average before training, and as a result a smaller overall improvement was possible (Fig. 3a).

Figure 3c shows examples of data and model fits for four individuals post-stroke. The slow component, due to a small learning rate, was approximately linear; thus, the average number of peaks continued to decrease until

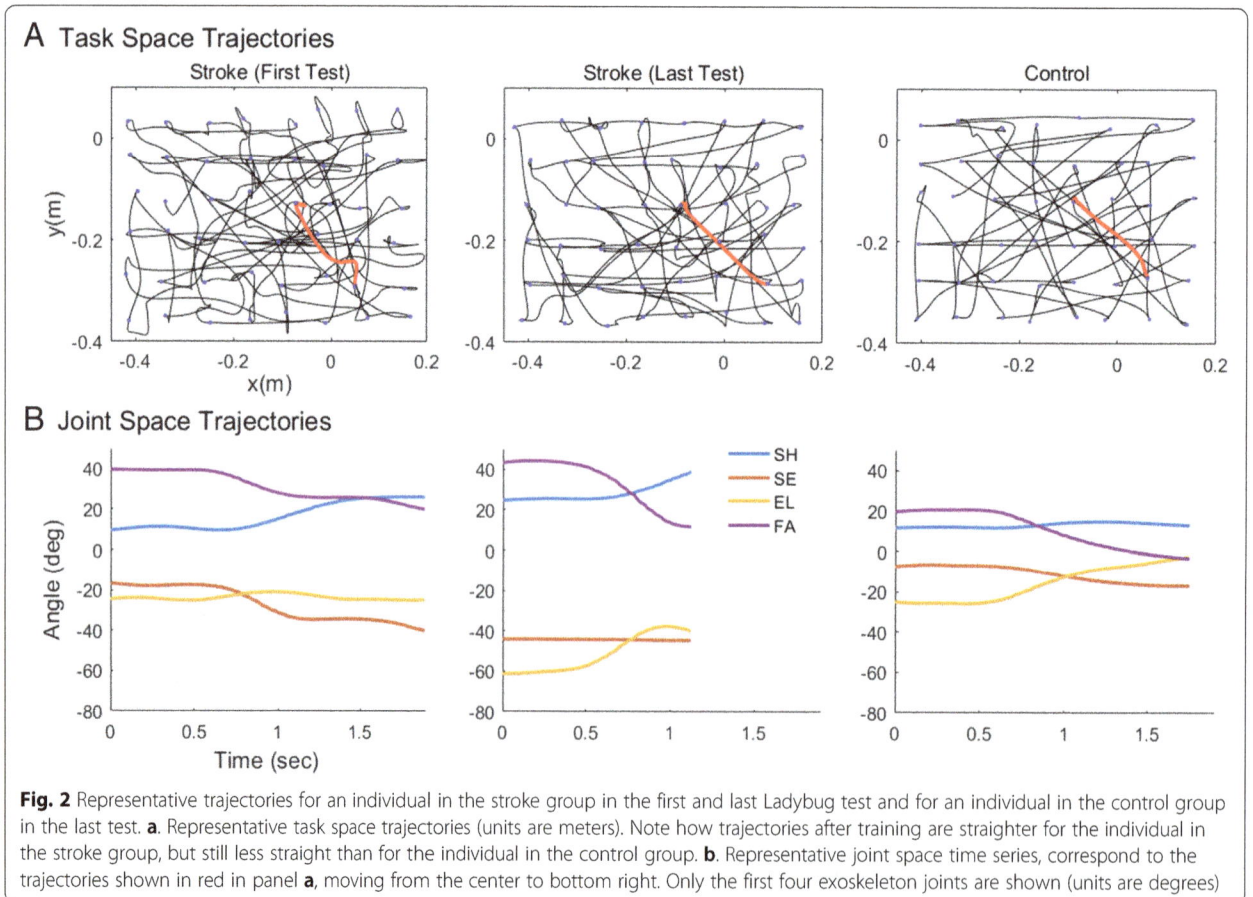

Fig. 2 Representative trajectories for an individual in the stroke group in the first and last Ladybug test and for an individual in the control group in the last test. **a**. Representative task space trajectories (units are meters). Note how trajectories after training are straighter for the individual in the stroke group, but still less straight than for the individual in the control group. **b**. Representative joint space time series, correspond to the trajectories shown in red in panel **a**, moving from the center to bottom right. Only the first four exoskeleton joints are shown (units are degrees)

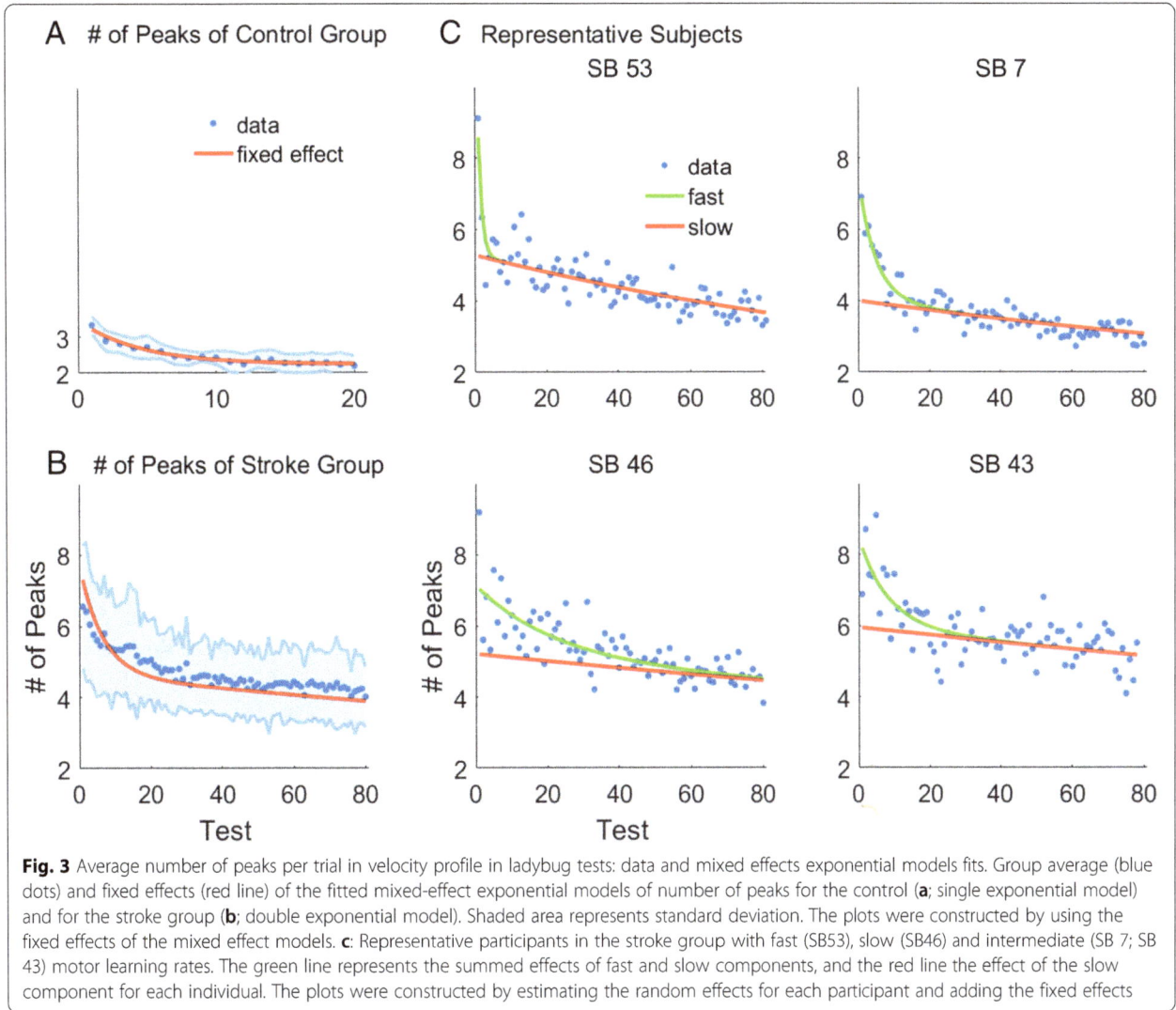

Fig. 3 Average number of peaks per trial in velocity profile in ladybug tests: data and mixed effects exponential models fits. Group average (blue dots) and fixed effects (red line) of the fitted mixed-effect exponential models of number of peaks for the control (a; single exponential model) and for the stroke group (b; double exponential model). Shaded area represents standard deviation. The plots were constructed by using the fixed effects of the mixed effect models. c: Representative participants in the stroke group with fast (SB53), slow (SB46) and intermediate (SB 7; SB 43) motor learning rates. The green line represents the summed effects of fast and slow components, and the red line the effect of the slow component for each individual. The plots were constructed by estimating the random effects for each participant and adding the fixed effects

the end of training. In contrast, the fast component decayed much faster, and usually reached an asymptote during training. For the stroke group, the slow learning rate corresponded to a time constant of 352 ± 123 tests, and the fast learning rate corresponded to a time constant of 13 ± 19 tests. For the control group, the time constant was 4.4 ± 1.6 tests (Note: there were 4 tests per day for both the stroke and control groups, but training and testing was only performed on weekdays, thus we cannot estimate the time constants in days).

For the stroke group, the average number of peaks estimated by the mixed effect model at the last test (test 80) for each participant was significantly correlated with the UEFM post-training (least square regression: $p = 0.0003$; $r = -0.52$; Fig. 4a). In contrast, the UEFM pre-training did not correlate with the number of peaks at test 1, as estimated by the model ($p = 0.10$). This indicates that the average number of peaks in the velocity

profiles as measured by the exoskeleton is only a good indicator of impairment after sufficient practice.

Because we hypothesized that the slow component will measure recovery, we correlated the changes in number of peaks from start to end of training due to the slow component with the changes in UEFM from pre- to post-training. We found that the changes in number of peaks from test 1 to test 80 due to the slow component was significantly correlated with the change of UEFM (both least square and robust regression: $p < 0.0001$; $r = -0.64$; Fig. 4b). In contrast, the changes in number of peaks from before to after training due to the fast component did not correlate with the change of UEFM ($p = 0.33$). In addition, there was no correlation between the change of peaks due to the fast process and the changes due to the slow process ($p = 0.37$).

Finally, we investigated whether the time at which the subjects began the exoskeleton training, relative to the

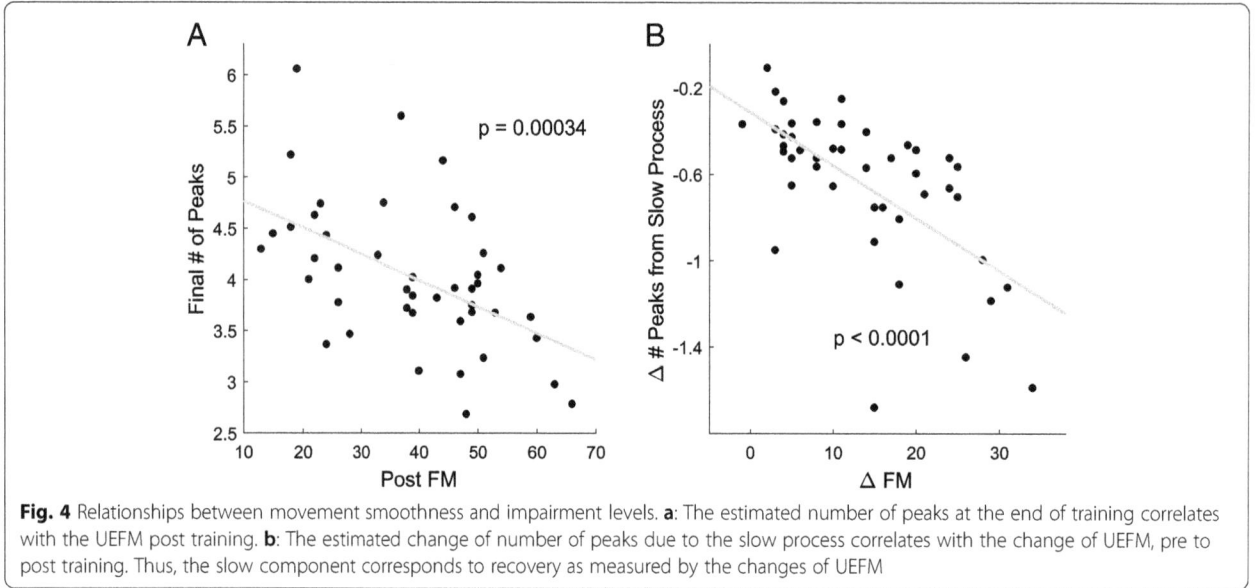

Fig. 4 Relationships between movement smoothness and impairment levels. **a**: The estimated number of peaks at the end of training correlates with the UEFM post training. **b**: The estimated change of number of peaks due to the slow process correlates with the change of UEFM, pre to post training. Thus, the slow component corresponds to recovery as measured by the changes of UEFM

onset stroke, correlated with either motor learning, as estimated via the fast component, or motor recovery, as estimated via the slow component. We found that days since stroke to start of training correlated with the changes in number of peaks from test 1 to test 80 due to the slow component ($p = 0.0063$; Fig. 5): subjects who began training earlier had a greater reduction in peaks. There was no correlation between days since stroke and the changes in number of peaks due to the fast process ($p = 0.26$). Note that we also assessed possible effects of gender, hand

affected, and age but found no correlation with changes in the number of peaks due to either fast or slow processes.

Discussion

We characterized changes in sensorimotor performance in 53 post-stroke individuals during 4 weeks of mechanized motor training with double exponential mixed-effect models. Sensorimotor performance was quantified with the average number of peaks in velocity profiles, an indicator of movement smoothness, in frontal plane reaching tests given before and after each training session. A model that estimated a fast improvement in smoothness via a fast decreasing exponential component, and a slow improvement in smoothness via a slow decreasing exponential component provided a better fit to the data than a model with a single exponential for individual post-stroke. For individuals post-stroke, our results show that the slow, but not the fast component, assessed reduction in upper extremity impairment (i.e. recovery, as we have defined it), because 1) the final average number of peaks as estimated by the model correlated with the post-training UEFM, 2) the changes in number of peaks due to the slow component, but not the overall changes in number of peaks, correlated with the changes in UEFM from pre- to post-training, and 3) the changes in number of peaks due to the slow component, but not the fast component, correlated with the number of days since stroke at the onset of training. The fast component therefore presumably tracked performance improvement due to learning to perform arm movements with the Armeo Spring exoskeleton. Evidence for such motor learning was additionally supported by the fact that non-disabled subjects also showed fast improvements in average number of peaks albeit with a single time constant about three times

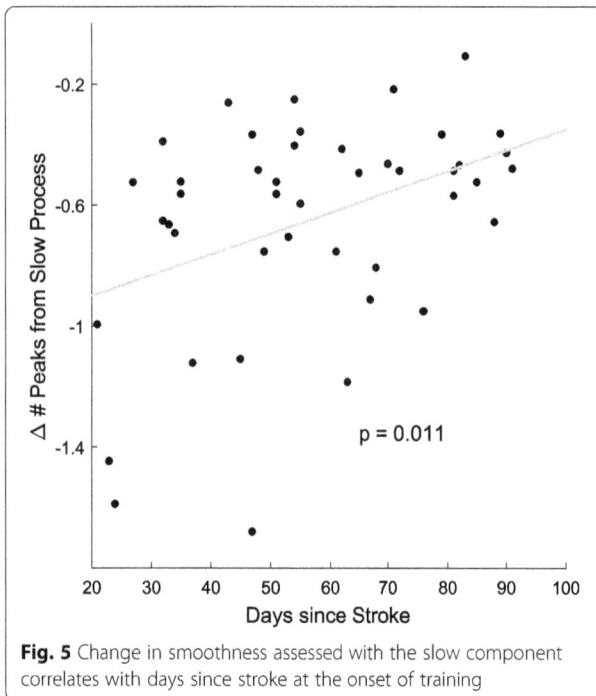

Fig. 5 Change in smoothness assessed with the slow component correlates with days since stroke at the onset of training

shorter than that for the fast component of the stroke group. This difference in time constants could be due to age (e.g., [26]) or the effects of stroke, but the single time constant presumably reflects the process of learning to move the exoskeleton, a task the individuals with stroke also had to learn.

There was no correlation between the change of peaks due to the fast process and the changes due to the slow process. This suggests that learning to use the tool of the exoskeleton progresses relatively independently of the ongoing the reduction in upper extremity impairment (c.f., [27]). In other words, there appears to be limited transfer between learning the task of pointing with the exoskeleton, and learning the various movement tasks associated with scoring well on the UEFM.

Early in training in the stroke group, the velocity profiles have multiple peaks and the appearance of a sequence of pulses, suggesting that the pointing task is being executed as a sequence of sub-movements [28]. As previously found in individuals post-stroke [14, 15, 28], these disconnected sub-movements blend to form a trajectory profile with fewer peaks as recovery proceeds. Previous work on a 2D rehabilitation robot showed that such sub-movements exhibited a remarkably invariant speed-vs.-time profile; this was proposed as evidence for dynamic movement primitives, which would constitute fundamental building blocks of complex motion [28]. It is therefore possible that during training, individuals post-stroke relearn incrementally how to (re-)combine multiple primitives for smooth and accurate motor control [29–31].

Our results also show that the rate of motor recovery, but not the rate of motor learning, was higher when subjects started exoskeleton training sooner after their stroke. Animal research has shown that motor training effectiveness depends on time post-stroke, suggesting a critical window of plasticity [3]. In humans, earlier training has been associated with better outcomes [32, 33] although too early intensive training may lead to subpar outcomes [2, 34]. The critical window has been hypothesized to be due to enhanced level of plasticity in the neural milieu near the infarct [3]. Plastic processes involved in force field adaptation or visuo-motor adaptation, as experienced when performing movements with the Armeo Spring, are thought to occur in the cerebellum [35–38]. The participants included did not have cerebellar strokes (since a stroke in the MCA was an inclusion criterion in REM-AVC). Our results thus suggest that the initial cerebellar-dependent motor learning phase does not follow a critical window of plasticity for lesions occurring in the territory of the MCA. In contrast, our findings are overall consistent with a larger rate of spontaneous recovery early after stroke, e.g. [1].

Stroke is characterized by high variability in impairment, spontaneous recovery, and responsiveness to therapy [21].

We have previously shown that including mixed-effects in non-linear models can account for between-individual differences in performance and changes of performances during motor training post-stroke [19]. Here, similarly, we therefore used non-linear mixed effects to precisely account for differences in baseline performance, as well as learning and recovery for each participant. The double exponential model with only nine free fixed parameters (4 means, 4 variances and a noise parameter) fit all data from 53 participants post-stroke simultaneously. Thus, a single mixed-effects model can account for the large between-individual variability in initial and final performance, in learning-related performance changes, and in recovery performance changes. However, although our modeling method identified two time-dependent processes, additional processes are presumably involved, as we have shown with motor adaptation in non-disabled individuals [38]. More sensitive tests that use fewer targets and repeated movements would be needed to identify faster components.

A limitation of our study is the use of arm reaching tests with different difficulty levels set by the therapists for each individual depending on performance. As a results, the number and position of targets varied across and within participants in the stroke group. For this reason, typical metrics used in motor adaptation studies such as maximum deviation from the straight line between the start and target positions could not be used. Hence, our choice to use the average number of peaks in velocity profiles, which does not directly depend on movement amplitudes and is dimensionless. The number of peaks in velocity profiles has long been used to quantify movement smoothness in non-disabled subjects, e.g. [39], and has been previously shown to decrease following robotic training post-stroke [14, 15]). Furthermore, previous studies of arm reaching post-stroke have linked number of peaks in velocity profiles to clinical scores such as the UEFM [40, 41]. Finally, in the present study, the average number of peaks in velocity profiles in each Ladybug test appeared little sensitive to changes in test difficulty, as we verified that that test difficulty was not significant when included as a covariate in the regression analyses. Note however that a robust metric has recently been proposed to measure smoothness in arm movements, the spectral arc-length metric [42]. Nonetheless, these authors concluded that the number of peaks "performs fairly well on the movements made by stroke subjects", but not on those by non-disabled individuals, presumably because, as we found, the number of peaks are much larger in individuals post-stroke.

Predicting the chances of a patient responding to a specific intervention would be highly useful to clinicians. Because "classical" neurorehabilitation studies generate few repeated measures, typically not during training, the ability to predict recovery based on such data is limited, e.g., [43]. In contrast, studies investigating robotic or mechanized training, such as in the current study, generate large amount of kinematic data that provide a solution to this paucity of repeated data – see [44]. For instance, addition of kinematic measures of arm movements recorded with MIT-Manus after stroke improved prediction of clinical scales of recovery [45]. However, our data show that care must be taken in using initial performance data (extracted from hand trajectories performed with an exoskeleton) as a marker of recovery, because initial performance is not only degraded by the lesioned motor system, but depends on learning to move the exoskeleton.

Conclusion

Rehabilitation after brain damage is based on the premise that motor learning determines activity-dependent motor recovery after stroke [46]. In this study, kinematic analysis of pointing movements performed during four weeks of motor training with an exoskeleton post-stroke allowed us to identify a fast and a slow process of performance improvement. Because of the fast learning process, changes in kinematic performance early in training were poor predictors of impairment reduction. The current work could not assess, however, whether long-term training with the exoskeleton benefits the patients, as our analyses cannot show a causal effect of motor training on recovery. Such causal effects need to be assessed via clinical trials like REM-AVC or via longitudinal studies in which the dose of training is manipulated as the variable of interest.

Endnote

[1]Some participants did not perform all the sessions for reasons such as fatigue (the session was terminated before the 2nd test was given) or omission by the therapists to include the test in the session. In addition, some therapists did not include the test in the first sessions when patients were instructed on the functioning of the ARMEO.

Acknowledgements
We thank the REM-AVC team for help with data collections for the stroke group, Julien Couadic and Valentine Guiton for extractions of the clinical data from the database. We thank Jim Gordon, Jun Izawa, Carolee Winstein, and members of the CNRL for comments on a previous draft.

Funding
This study was in part supported by the National Institute of Neurological Disorders And Stroke of the National Institutes of Health under Award Numbers R01 HD065438 and R56 NS100528 to NS. The content is solely the responsibility of the authors and does not necessarily represent the official views of the National Institutes of Health. The REM AVC study was funded by the French ministry of health (STIC program).

Authors' contributions
NS designed the study, analyzed the data and wrote the manuscript. CW analyzed the data, performed the study with non-disabled participants, and wrote the manuscript. DM helped with overall design and with data collection and analysis. IL and KB designed and performed the study with the non-disabled participants. DR provided technical assistance with the Armeo Spring and with the design, and wrote the manuscript. ORN designed the REM-AVC trial and organized the collection of kinematics data for the stroke participants. All authors read and approved the final manuscript.

Competing interests
David Reinkensmeyer receives royalties from UC Irvine for a patent licensed to Hocoma related to Armeo Spring and has an equity interest in Hocoma. The terms of this arrangement have been reviewed and approved by the University of California, Irvine in accordance with its conflict of interest policies.

Author details
[1]Biokinesiology and Physical Therapy, University of Southern California, Los Angeles, USA. [2]Neuroscience graduate Program, University of Southern California, Los Angeles, USA. [3]STAPS, Université de Montpellier, Euromov, Montpellier, France. [4]Montpellier University Hospital, Euromov, IFRH, Montpellier University, Montpellier, France. [5]Departments of Mechanical and Aerospace Engineering, Anatomy and Neurobiology, University of California, Irvine, USA. [6]Université de Bretagne Occidentale, Centre hospitalier universitaire, LaTIM-INSERM UMR1101, Brest, France.

References
1. Duncan PW, Lai SM, Keighley J. Defining post-stroke recovery: implications for design and interpretation of drug trials. Neuropharmacology. 2000;39(5): 835–41.
2. Bains AS, Schweighofer N. Time-sensitive reorganization of the somatosensory cortex post-stroke depends on interaction between Hebbian plasticity and homeoplasticity: a simulation study. *Journal of neurophysiology* 2014:jn. 00433:02013.
3. Murphy TH, Corbett D. Plasticity during stroke recovery: from synapse to behaviour. Nat Rev Neurosci. 2009;10(12):861–72.
4. Nudo RJ, Wise BM, SiFuentes F, Milliken GW. Neural substrates for the effects of rehabilitative training on motor recovery after ischemic infarct. Science. 1996;272(5269):1791–4.
5. Pavlides C, Miyashita E, Asanuma H. Projection from the sensory to the motor cortex is important in learning motor skills in the monkey. J Neurophysiol. 1993;70(2):733–41.
6. Wolf SL, Winstein CJ, Miller JP, Taub E, Uswatte G, Morris D, Giuliani C, Light KE, Nichols-Larsen D. Effect of constraint-induced movement therapy on upper extremity function 3 to 9 months after stroke: the EXCITE randomized clinical trial. JAMA. 2006;296(17):2095–104.
7. Lincoln NB, Willis D, Philips SA, Juby LC, Berman P. Comparison of rehabilitation practice on hospital wards for stroke patients. Stroke. 1996; 27(1):18–23.
8. Jeffers MS, Karthikeyan S, Gomez-Smith M, Gasinzigwa S, Achenbach J, Feiten A, Corbett D. Does stroke rehabilitation really matter? Part B: an algorithm for prescribing an effective intensity of rehabilitation. Neurorehabil Neural Repair. 2018;32(1):73–83.
9. Krebs HI, Volpe BT, Ferraro M, Fasoli S, Palazzolo J, Rohrer B, Edelstein L, Hogan N. Robot-aided neurorehabilitation: from evidence-based to science-based rehabilitation. Top Stroke Rehabil. 2002;8(4):54–70.

10. Kwakkel G, Kollen BJ, Krebs HI. Effects of robot-assisted therapy on upper limb recovery after stroke: a systematic review. Neurorehabil Neural Repair. 2008;22(2):111–21.

11. Marchal-Crespo L, Reinkensmeyer DJ. Review of control strategies for robotic movement training after neurologic injury. J Neuroeng Rehabil. 2009;6:20.

12. Laffont I, Bakhti K, Coroian F, van Dokkum L, Mottet D, Schweighofer N, Froger J: Innovative technologies applied to sensorimotor rehabilitation after stroke. Ann Phys Rehabil Med 2014, 57(8):543–551.

13. Mehrholz J, Platz T, Kugler J, Pohl M. Electromechanical and robot-assisted arm training for improving arm function and activities of daily living after stroke. Cochrane Database Syst Rev. 2008;(4):CD006876.

14. Rohrer B, Fasoli S, Krebs HI, Volpe B, Frontera WR, Stein J, Hogan N. Submovements grow larger, fewer, and more blended during stroke recovery. Mot Control. 2004;8(4):472–83.

15. Rohrer B, Fasoli S, Krebs HI, Hughes R, Volpe B, Frontera WR, Stein J, Hogan N. Movement smoothness changes during stroke recovery. J Neurosci. 2002; 22(18):8297–304.

16. Park H, Kim S, Winstein CJ, Gordon J, Schweighofer N. Short-duration and intensive training improves long-term reaching performance in individuals with chronic stroke. Neurorehabil Neural Repair. 2016;30(6):551–61.

17. Gottlieb GL, Corcos DM, Jaric S, Agarwal GC. Practice improves even the simplest movements. Exp Brain Res. 1988;73(2):436–40.

18. Schmidt RA, Lee T, Winstein C, Wulf G, Zelaznik H: Motor control and learning, 6E. Human kinetics.; 2018.

19. Park H, Schweighofer N. Nonlinear mixed-effects model reveals a distinction between learning and performance in intensive reach training post-stroke. J Neuroeng Rehabil. 2017;14(1):21.

20. Schaefer SY, Duff K. Rapid responsiveness to practice predicts longer-term retention of upper extremity motor skill in non-demented older adults. Front Aging Neurosci. 2015;7:214.

21. Cramer SC. Repairing the human brain after stroke: I. mechanisms of spontaneous recovery. Ann Neurol. 2008;63(3):272–87.

22. Cramer SC. Repairing the human brain after stroke. II Restorative therapies. Ann Neurol. 2008;63(5):549–60.

23. Sanchez RJ, Liu J, Rao S, Shah P, Smith R, Rahman T, Cramer SC, Bobrow JE, Reinkensmeyer DJ. Automating arm movement training following severe stroke: functional exercises with quantitative feedback in a gravity-reduced environment. IEEE Trans Neural Syst Rehabil Eng. 2006;14(3):378–89.

24. Butterworth S: On the theory of filter amplifiers. 1930.

25. Lindstrom MJ, Bates DM. Nonlinear Mixed Effects Models for Repeated Measures Data. Biometrics. 1990;46(3):673–87.

26. Buch ER, Young S, Contreras-Vidal JL. Visuomotor adaptation in normal aging. Learn Mem. 2003;10(1):55–63.

27. Hardwick RM, Rajan VA, Bastian AJ, Krakauer JW, Celnik PA. Motor learning in stroke: trained patients are not equal to untrained patients with less impairment. Neurorehabil Neural Repair. 2017;31(2):178–89.

28. Krebs HI, Aisen ML, Volpe BT, Hogan N. Quantization of continuous arm movements in humans with brain injury. Proc Natl Acad Sci U S A. 1999; 96(8):4645–9.

29. Schaal S. Dynamic movement primitives-a framework for motor control in humans and humanoid robotics. Tokyo: Adaptive motion of animals and machines; 2006. p. 261–80.

30. Huang R, Cheng H, Guo H, Lin X, Zhang J. Hierarchical learning control with physical human-exoskeleton interaction. Inf Sci. 2018;432:584–95.

31. Schaal S, Schweighofer N. Computational motor control in humans and robots. Curr Opin Neurobiol. 2005;15(6):675–82.

32. Horn SD, DeJong G, Smout RJ, Gassaway J, James R, Conroy B. Stroke rehabilitation patients, practice, and outcomes: is earlier and more aggressive therapy better? Arch Phys Med Rehabil. 2005;86(12 Suppl 2): S101–14.

33. Wolf SL, Thompson PA, Winstein CJ, Miller JP, Blanton SR, Nichols-Larsen DS, Morris DM, Uswatte G, Taub E, Light KE, et al. The EXCITE stroke trial: comparing early and delayed constraint-induced movement therapy. Stroke. 2010;41(10):2309–15.

34. Dromerick AW, Lang CE, Birkenmeier RL, Wagner JM, Miller JP, Videen TO, Powers WJ, Wolf SL, Edwards DF. Very early constraint-induced movement during stroke rehabilitation (VECTORS): a single-center RCT. Neurology. 2009; 73(3):195–201.

35. Schweighofer N, Spoelstra J, Arbib MA, Kawato M. Role of the cerebellum in reaching movements in humans. II. A neural model of the intermediate cerebellum. Eur J Neurosci. 1998;10(1):95–105.

36. Bastian AJ. Learning to predict the future: the cerebellum adapts feedforward movement control. Curr Opin Neurobiol. 2006;16(6):645–9.

37. Thach WT, Bastian AJ. Role of the cerebellum in the control and adaptation of gait in health and disease. Prog Brain Res. 2004;143:353–66.

38. Kim S, Ogawa K, Lv J, Schweighofer N, Imamizu H. Neural substrates related to motor memory with multiple timescales in sensorimotor adaptation. PLoS Biol. 2015;13(12):e1002312.

39. Brooks VB, Cooke JD, Thomas JS. The continuity of movements. In: Stein RB, Pearson KG, Smith RS, Redford JB, editors. Control of posture and locomotion. Boston, MA: Springer US; 1973. p. 257–72.

40. Bosecker C, Dipietro L, Volpe B, Krebs HI. Kinematic robot-based evaluation scales and clinical counterparts to measure upper limb motor performance in patients with chronic stroke. Neurorehabil Neural Repair. 2010;24(1):62–9.

41. van Dokkum L, Hauret I, Mottet D, Froger J, Metrot J, Laffont I: The contribution of kinematics in the assessment of upper limb motor recovery early after stroke. Neurorehabil Neural Repair 2014, 28(1):4–12.

42. Balasubramanian S, Melendez-Calderon A, Burdet E. A robust and sensitive metric for quantifying movement smoothness. IEEE Trans Biomed Eng. 2012;59(8):2126–36.

43. Hidaka Y, Han CE, Wolf SL, Winstein CJ, Schweighofer N. Use it and improve it or lose it: interactions between arm function and use in humans post-stroke. PLoS Comput Biol. 2012;8(2):e1002343.

44. Reinkensmeyer DJ, Burdet E, Casadio M, Krakauer JW, Kwakkel G, Lang CE, Swinnen SP, Ward NS, Schweighofer N. Computational neurorehabilitation: modeling plasticity and learning to predict recovery. J Neuroeng Rehabil. 2016;13(1):42.

45. Krebs HI, Krams M, Agrafiotis DK, DiBernardo A, Chavez JC, Littman GS, Yang E, Byttebier G, Dipietro L, Rykman A, et al. Robotic measurement of arm movements after stroke establishes biomarkers of motor recovery. Stroke. 2014;45(1):200–4.

46. Krakauer JW. Motor learning: its relevance to stroke recovery and neurorehabilitation. Curr Opin Neurol. 2006;19(1):84–90.

11

Development of a 3D, networked multi-user virtual reality environment for home therapy after stroke

Kristen M Triandafilou[1*], Daria Tsoupikova[2], Alexander J Barry[1], Kelly N Thielbar[1], Nikolay Stoykov[1] and Derek G Kamper[3,4]

Abstract

Background: Impairment of upper extremity function is a common outcome following stroke, to the detriment of lifestyle and employment opportunities. Yet, access to treatment may be limited due to geographical and transportation constraints, especially for those living in rural areas. While stroke rates are higher in these areas, stroke survivors in these regions of the country have substantially less access to clinical therapy. Home therapy could offer an important alternative to clinical treatment, but the inherent isolation and the monotony of self-directed training can greatly reduce compliance.

Methods: We developed a 3D, networked multi-user Virtual Environment for Rehabilitative Gaming Exercises (VERGE) system for home therapy. Within this environment, stroke survivors can interact with therapists and/or fellow stroke survivors in the same virtual space even though they may be physically remote. Each user's own movement controls an avatar through kinematic measurements made with a low-cost, Kinect™ device. The system was explicitly designed to train movements important to rehabilitation and to provide real-time feedback of performance to users and clinicians. To obtain user feedback about the system, 15 stroke survivors with chronic upper extremity hemiparesis participated in a multisession pilot evaluation study, consisting of a three-week intervention in a laboratory setting. For each week, the participant performed three one-hour training sessions with one of three modalities: 1) VERGE system, 2) an existing virtual reality environment based on Alice in Wonderland (AWVR), or 3) a home exercise program (HEP).

Results: Over 85% of the subjects found the VERGE system to be an effective means of promoting repetitive practice of arm movement. Arm displacement averaged 350 m for each VERGE training session. Arm displacement was not significantly less when using VERGE than when using AWVR or HEP. Participants were split on preference for VERGE, AWVR or HEP. Importantly, almost all subjects indicated a willingness to perform the training for at least 2–3 days per week at home.

Conclusions: Multi-user VR environments hold promise for home therapy, although the importance of reducing complexity of operation for the user in the VR system must be emphasized. A modified version of the VERGE system is currently being used in a home therapy study.

Keywords: Stroke, Rehabilitation, Virtual reality, Serious games, Upper extremity

* Correspondence: ktriandafi@sralab.org
[1]Shirley Ryan AbilityLab, Arms + Hands Lab, Chicago, IL, USA
Full list of author information is available at the end of the article

Background

Chronic upper extremity impairment is all too common among the more than 7 million stroke survivors in the U.S. [1]. These impairments have disabling effects on all facets of life, including self-care, employment, and leisure activities. Repetitive practice of movement, such as arm movement, is thought to improve outcomes for stroke survivors [2–4], but access to the clinic for therapy is often limited by geography or lack of transportation. While almost 50 million Americans live in rural areas, 90% of physical and occupational therapists live in major urban areas [5]. Per capita ratios of therapists to overall population are 50% larger in urban as compared to rural regions of the country [6]. Rates of stroke in these rural areas, however, exceed those of major urban areas [7–9]. Thus, a large number of stroke survivors have limited access to skilled treatment. Data from 21 states found that only 30% of stroke survivors received outpatient rehabilitation, a much lower percentage than that recommended by clinical practice guidelines [10]. Declines seen following discharge from inpatient rehabilitation are undoubtedly exacerbated by limited access to clinical therapy [11].

Disparity in quality of care has been recognized in the acute treatment of stroke for a number of years. This situation has led to the development of telemedicine to extend expert care to individuals during the initial hours and days following the stroke, advance site-independent treatment, and create models of care in rural areas [12–14]. Therapy options after this acute period, however, generally remain limited for stroke survivors in rural areas. Akin to the telemedicine efforts, telerehabilitation treatments have been proposed. However, telerehabilitation interactions are typically limited to off-line monitoring by the therapist [8, 9, 15], phone calls between a therapist and client [16, 17], or videoconferencing [18–20]. While systems allowing more direct interaction have been proposed, the hardware cost and complexity limit applicability for home-based therapy [21–23]. Hence, the therapist is relegated to the role of observer and the intimacy of a clinical therapy session is lost. Therapy options are substantially restricted, as is the available feedback.

Recently, multiple investigators have been exploring means of improving home-based therapy through the development of systems or serious games which permit multiple, simultaneous users [24–30]. These efforts have proposed the inclusion of multiple users as a means to overcome resistance to home-based therapy that may result due to isolation or lack of engagement. Indeed, studies have observed a preference for multi-user vs, single-user therapy when utilizing these systems [26, 29]. However, these systems have largely been limited to control of a one-dimensional or two-dimensional space and both users remain in the same physical location (e.g., side by side). One team of researchers did develop a framework for supporting distant users (such as a therapist in the hospital and a stroke survivor in their home), but game control was limited to one or two dimensions [31, 32].

Here, we describe the development of a fully three-dimensional (3D) virtual reality environment (VRE) for home-based therapy in which multiple, remote users can interact in real time. In this Virtual Environment for Rehabilitative Gaming Exercises (VERGE) system [33], movement of the user is mapped to corresponding movement of an avatar to foster a sense of presence in and engagement with the VRE. The 3D environment encompasses aspects of clinical therapy, such as transport of objects or movement of the hand into specified regions of the upper extremity workspace. Although the importance of 3D movements in VR environments is a topic of debate [34, 35], movements tested in environments with lesser degrees-of-freedom (DOF) are often very limited and dictated by a one DOF robot. These movements differ substantially from the types of movements normally seen in 3D reaching movements [4, 36]. The network architecture of the system allows users to be located remotely from each other, such as a stroke survivor in their home, a therapist in a clinic, or a stroke survivor's friend or relative living in another city or state. The virtual nature of the environment allows even very limited movements in the physical world to have successful functional outcomes in the virtual world, thereby offering a sense of accomplishment and motivation for successive attempts. Additionally, task difficulty can easily be modified in order to maintain the proper level of challenge, which is important for motor learning in general [37] and rehabilitation in particular [38].

We developed and performed preliminary testing of the VERGE system to gauge user response in comparison to two other therapy modalities that could be used for home therapy: an existing virtual reality system based on the Alice in Wonderland story (AWVR) [39] and a home exercise program (HEP). Fifteen stroke survivors completed three, one-hour therapy sessions per week with each of the three therapy modalities (9 sessions total). We hypothesized that the use of the VERGE system would not decrease the amount of arm movement promoted, in comparison with the AWVR and HEP modalities. We further expected that users' self-described engagement would be greatest for the VERGE system due to the presence of a partner.

Methods
VERGE System
Architecture

At its core, VERGE consists of a 3D VRE in which avatars interact with virtual objects. To date, we have created two such VREs, one depicting a dining room and the other a kitchen. The scenes were created in Maya (Autodesk Inc., San Rafael, CA) and imported into Unity 3D (Unity 4.5, Unity Technologies, San Francisco, CA), the software platform controlling VERGE. The VREs are rich in detail in order to provide depth cues [40]. Thus, depth can be conveyed without the need for stereovision, such as that provided by head mounted displays (HMDs). We have found that HMDs can be difficult for stroke survivors to use due to the limited field-of-view and, especially, involuntary coupling between neck and arm motion [41, 42]. The latter may lead to complications with moving the arm while keeping the head steady.

The avatars were created from a custom skeleton in Maya (Autodesk Inc., San Rafael, CA), which was rigged to an existing mesh of the "casual young man" 3D model, purchased and modified for our project (Fig. 1). We created the custom skeleton to match the topology of the existing character while corresponding to the skeletal joint naming convention in Unity 3D. The skeleton (and thus avatar) is animated according to joint angle data captured with a Kinect™ I optical tracker (Microsoft Corp., Redmont, WA). The 3D motion data from the Kinect™ are transmitted to the Unity code through UDP to drive the movement of the avatar in the virtual environment.

The VERGE system employs a central server interacting with peripheral client computers, one for each user. The server receives information from the client computers and controls updating of the scene so that the appropriate view of the scene is shown on each client computer through TCP/IP network architecture. We implemented communication between the client computers through custom libraries in C# (Microsoft Visual Studio). We used two multi-user network models: an authoritative server (server performs all physics calculations) for when more than one user could interact with virtual objects simultaneously and a non-authoritative server (local computation of physics) for when only one user at a time could interact with the virtual environment.

Exercises

We have created three exercises (*Ball Bump, Food Fight, and Trajectory Trace*) employing Unity 3D and C#. These exercise were designed to encourage upper extremity movement, particularly to areas of the workspace that are often difficult to reach, such as those requiring raising the arm and reaching away from the body [43]. For each exercise, VERGE provides a first-person view of the virtual scene, as through the eyes of the avatar, to each user in accordance with previous studies [44]. This helps to establish a sense of presence for the user in the scene. The server displays a third-person view of the VRE.

Ball Bump is played on the table of the dining room VRE created in Maya (Fig. 2a). The goal is to hit a ball back and forth across the table, while avoiding the objects on the table. Contact between the ball and the avatar hand produces a collision that redirects the ball according to the Unity physics engine. Similarly, collisions between the ball and other objects redirect the ball. The ball will fall off the table if a fellow participant misses making contact with it and /or if the user hits the ball in the wrong direction. Pressing a red napkin, located to the side, produces a new ball. Thus, participants are encouraged to reach away from their bodies, especially to contact the napkin or to free the ball when it becomes stuck behind an object. This can be a collaborative exercise, in which the participants try to make as many successful passes as possible before the ball falls

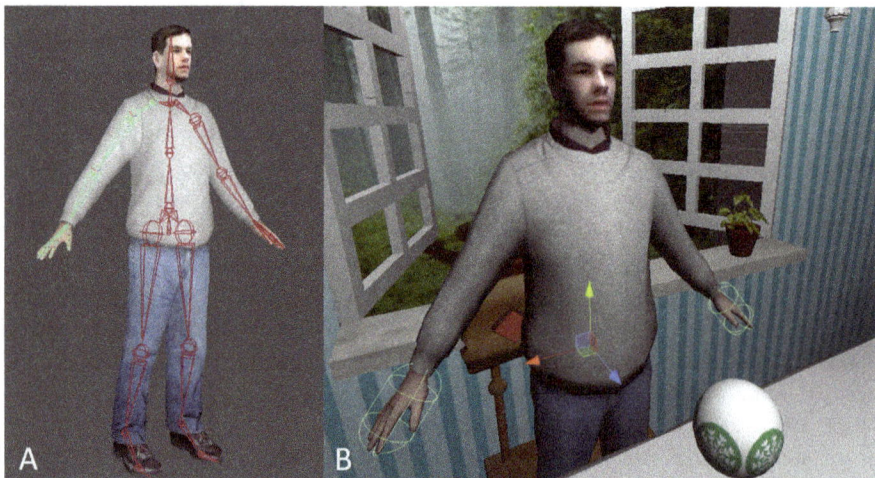

Fig. 1 Avatar kinematics. **a** 3D model of the avatar with underlying custom skeleton as displayed in Maya. **b** Avatar imported into custom scene in Unity. Visible coordinate frame indicates location of right hip joint. Ellipsoid encompassing hands represents the contact regions for the hand colliders

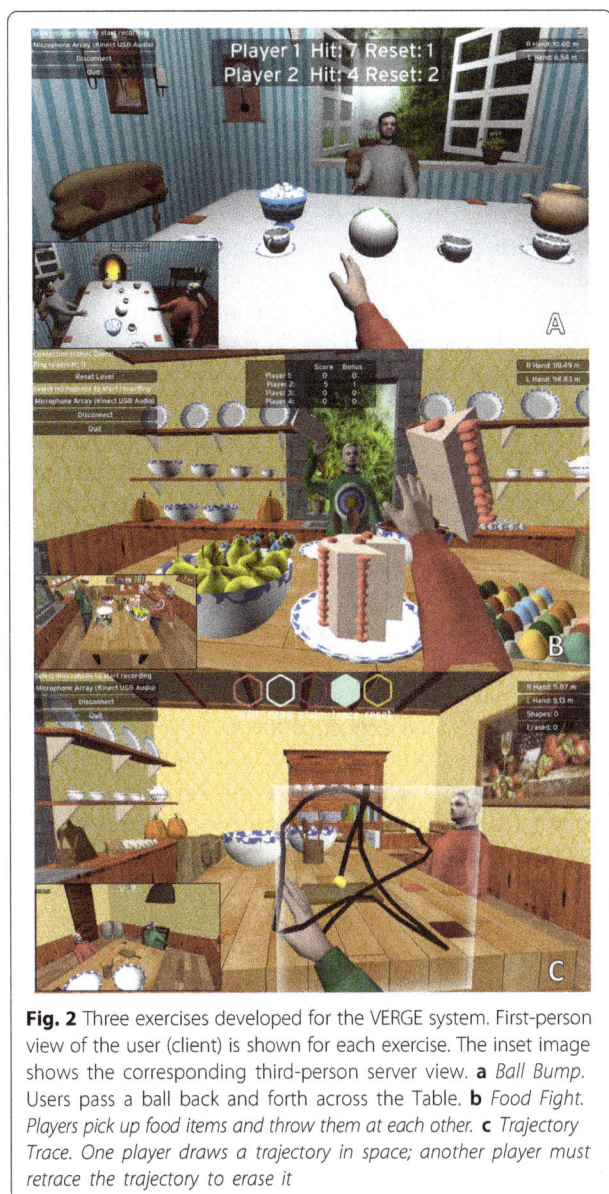

Fig. 2 Three exercises developed for the VERGE system. First-person view of the user (client) is shown for each exercise. The inset image shows the corresponding third-person server view. **a** *Ball Bump.* Users pass a ball back and forth across the Table. **b** *Food Fight.* Players pick up food items and throw them at each other. **c** *Trajectory Trace.* One player draws a trajectory in space; another player must retrace the trajectory to erase it

off the table, or a competitive game in which each player tries to hit the ball past the other player. Prior studies have shown that different users will have different preferences for competitive or collaborative exercises [30].

The *Food Fight* game takes place in the custom kitchen VRE created in Maya. Participants grab different food items and throw them at other avatars (Fig. 2b). The user "grasps" an object by placing the avatar's hand in close proximity and clicking a button on a wireless optical pen mouse (2.4GHz Wireless Optical Pen Mouse Adjustable 500/1000DPI, Docooler) with either hand (stroke survivors typically operate the pen mouse with the ipsilesional hand). The user releases the object by operating another button on the pen mouse; the object's trajectory is determined by the object's velocity vector at

the time of release. Once all of the food items have been thrown (e.g., cake, eggs, and fruit), the user can reset the food items by clicking on the reset button to continue play. We integrated mesh deformations and special effects for food items colliding with other objects. Eggs splatter and appear as yolks, the cake morphs into a pile of crumbs, and the pears and apples deform into broken fruit. Scenes are updated by the central server in authoritative mode.

In the *Trajectory Trace* exercise (Fig. 2c) one participant draws a 3D trajectory in the air. This trajectory is then passed to another participant who attempts to erase it by retracing. The state of the game (Draw, Claim, Trace, or Reset), as well as the initiation and termination of drawing the curve, is controlled by touching a button (located on the avatar's chest) with the less affected hand. The trajectory is anchored to the avatar, such that the user must reach with the arm rather than using the trunk to move the hand to the trajectory, similar to a previous study [45]. The partner (such as a therapist) can specify to which part of the workspace the other player (e.g., a stroke survivor) should practice reaching, by drawing the trajectory in that region. To help with depth perception, a translucent 3D cube outlines the boundaries of the drawn 3D shape. Since the trajectory must be retraced in the same direction in which it was created, we display a yellow sphere to indicate the current starting point. As the user successfully traces the trajectory and it disappears, the 3D depth cube adjusts to match the volume of the remaining trajectory in real time.

Pilot Study

A pilot study was performed to examine the feasibility of the system for use by stroke survivors. Especially, we wanted to test the amount of movement of the impaired arm, particularly to certain regions of the upper extremity workspace. Specifically, we wanted to determine whether employment of the VERGE system reduced arm movement in comparison with other potential home treatment options, namely the AWVR and HEP. We also wanted to compare user engagement across the three modalities.

Participants

Fifteen stroke survivors (10 male/ 5 female) in the chronic stage of recovery participated in this study. Subjects were at least 2 years post-stroke (mean of 17.4 years) and ranged in age from 33 to 81 years. Subjects had upper extremity hemiparesis, rated as Stage 3 - Stage 5 on the Stage of Arm subsection of the Chedoke-McMaster Stroke Assessment Scale [46] by a trained therapist. Subjects had no known orthopedic disease, significant visual deficits, contracture or pain (self-reported pain less than 6 on a 10-point scale) in the arm that would have hampered performing the experiments. Northwestern University's Institutional Review Board (Chicago, IL) approved the study design and each participant signed an informed consent before study enrollment.

Intervention

Each participant took part in a three-week intervention study consisting of 9 one-hour training sessions in a laboratory setting over 3 weeks. During each week, the participant was involved in one of three therapy modalities 1) VERGE, 2) HEP or 3) AWVR. The order of the therapy was randomized for each participant, and all participants took part in all three therapies.

The VERGE therapy utilized the three different exercises previously described. *Ball Bump* was always the first exercise introduced to the participant as it was deemed the simplest to understand, and thus provided a straightforward means for learning to control the avatar in the VRE. *Trajectory Trace* and *Food Fight* were then played, in that order. All exercises for the VERGE therapy were performed with the arm unsupported. Participants performed each exercise for 15 min, with a 5 min resting period between games. For the purposes of this study, the other user was always a member of the study team with experience performing the virtual exercises, in a situation akin to the expert user employed in an aforementioned study [29]. This individual was located in a different room within the same building to simulate home use.

The HEP therapy consisted of pre-defined sets of seated, self-paced arm-hand exercises derived from standard care. These 16 exercises were presented to the participant in the form of a printed handout (see Additional file 1). The HEP consisted of a generalized list of tasks for the specific purposes of this research study, and not one individualized to the needs of a particular patient. In accordance with the other modalities, we instructed participants to work through the handout in three blocks of 15 min of activity followed by 5 min of rest for each training session. Participants performed all tasks while seated at a table. Roughly 30% of the exercises involved arm support (provided by the tabletop) while 70% were unsupported. To limit the potential for participants to perform extra HEP at home, no copies of the HEP protocol were permitted to leave the research facility.

The AWVR is a rich VRE on which we have trained stroke survivors in the past [39]. The environment draws the user into the March Hare's tea party where the participant is guided to perform a number of tasks to spur repetitive practice of movements. We chose three of the available exercises, based on their appropriateness for encouraging arm movement. One exercise, *Tea Stir*, entailed picking up a spoon from a jar and then reaching forward to stir tea in a teacup; the arm remained suspended, unsupported until the spoon "melted" and disappeared (Fig. 3a). This exercise involved crossing the midline of the body and extending the arm laterally. For the *Crabby Cookies* exercise, the participant reached out to a plate of virtual cookies. Once a cookie was touched, it transformed into a crab that scurried across the table and had to be "caught" by touching it (Fig. 3b). Thus, the *Crabby Cookies* exercise required multiple reaches away from the body. The third exercise, *Bottomless Sherry*, required the participant to reach for a glass of sherry, raise it to take a sip, and then set it back on the table to be refilled (Fig. 3c). We instructed participants to place the glass in different locations on the surface of the table to encourage reaching to her range of motion limits. All exercises were performed with the arm unsupported. Participants performed each exercise for 15 min, followed by a 5 min break, over the one-hour session. As the complexity was similar across exercises, order of play was random and often chosen by the participant.

During the first therapy session for each therapy modality, study staff explained the exercises and demonstrated performance. After that, study staff were available throughout each session to answer questions and monitor for safety, but each participant was encouraged to work independently, as if at home. As noted for VERGE, the participant worked together with another member of the study staff, but that individual was located in a separate room.

Outcome measures

As we were especially interested in user response to VERGE, we administered a questionnaire (*VERGE Survey*) employing a 5-point Likert scale [47, 48] at the end of the VERGE training week (see Additional file 2). This questionnaire addressed the different exercises and issues specific to VERGE. Participants completed a different questionnaire (*Weekly Survey*) at the end of each therapy week (including VERGE) to measure the level of engagement in and the perceived potential for the therapy (*See* Additional file 3). We administered a final questionnaire (*Final Survey*), directly comparing the three therapies, at the end of the study (*See* Additional file 4). Additionally, we captured participant kinematics throughout the third session for each therapy modality with the Xsens 3D motion tracker system (MVN, Xsens, Culver City, CA), (Fig. 4). Participants donned the Xsens vest, containing eight inertial measurement units (IMUs) and a headband containing one IMU (per upper extremity configuration). The Xsens system continuously recorded upper extremity movement from the IMU data during all of the exercises.

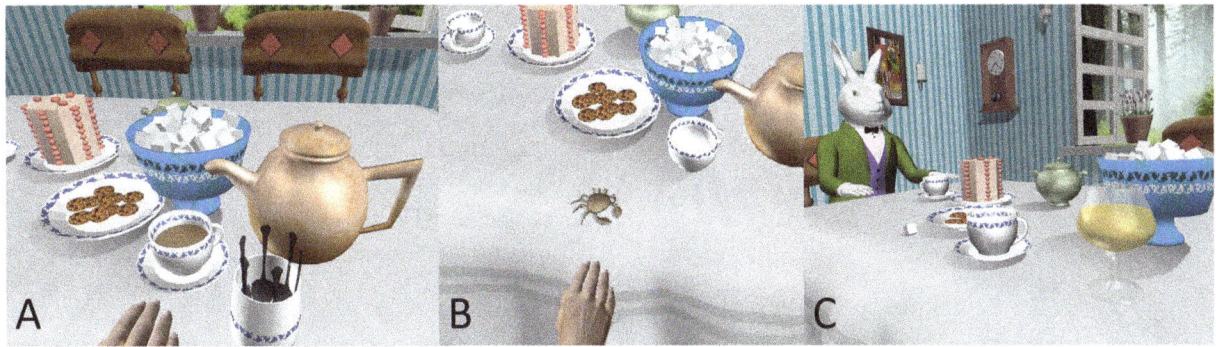

Fig. 3 Three AWVR exercises used for this study. First-person user view is shown. **a** *Tea Stir*. Spoons (foreground) melt when used to stir the hot tea. **b** *Crabby Cookies*. Cookies morph into crabs that run around the table and must be "captured". **c** *Bottomless Sherry*. Sherry glass must be repeatedly lifted to "drink" and set down on the table to refill

Analysis

Descriptive statistics were utilized to compare responses from the *VERGE* Survey. For the *Weekly Surveys*, we used the nonparametric Friedman test to compare participant responses, as measured by the Likert scores, across the treatment modalities. Hand and shoulder displacements were computed from the Xsens data by using the biomechanical toolkit Mokka [49]. Total shoulder movement was subtracted from total hand movement to account for arm displacement resulting purely from trunk translation. We performed non-inferiority tests to examine whether total arm displacement during VERGE was inferior to arm displacement during the other two modalities. The δ was set equal to 10% of the larger of the hand displacement means for AWVR and HEP. Furthermore, we examined which parts of the workspace were accessed. For example, Reach Distance was calculated as the relative distance, normalized by arm length, of the hand away from the shoulder. Thus, a Reach Distance = 0 indicated that the hand was coincident with the shoulder, while a Reach Distance = 1 indicated full arm extension. We defined Hand Elevation as the vertical location of the hand with respect to the shoulder. A value of 0 represented the hand at shoulder height, while a value of 1 indicated that the hand was located at its lowest possible position with respect to the shoulder (i.e., hand at the side with elbow fully extended). We performed non-inferiority tests to examine whether time spent with a Reach Distance ≥ 0.7 and whether the time spent with Hand Elevation ≤ 0.4 were inferior for VERGE than for the other two modalities. The δ was set to 4.5 min, equal to 10% of the total training time. We also created histograms to show the amount of time the hand was positioned at different bins of Reach Distance and Hand Elevation.

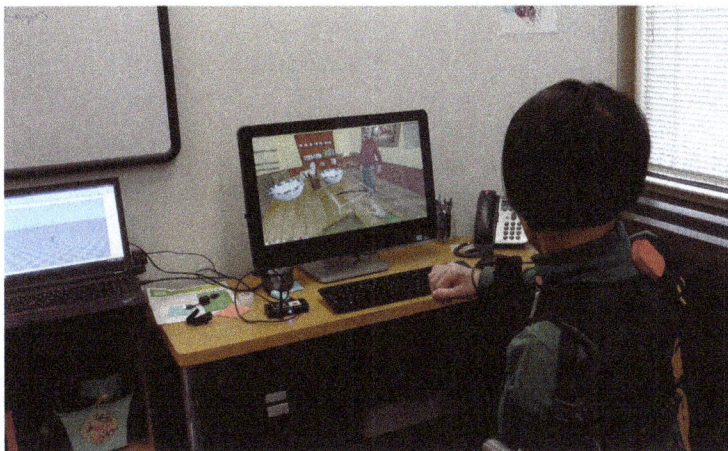

Fig. 4 Stroke survivor training while wearing Xsens. Participant is trying to erase the displayed trajectory in the *Trajectory Trace* exercise in VERGE. While control of the avatar is provided through the Kinect™, the subject is wearing an Xsens 3D motion tracker system vest (MVN, Xsens, Culver City, CA) to provide continuous measurement of the hand and shoulder displacement for experimental analysis

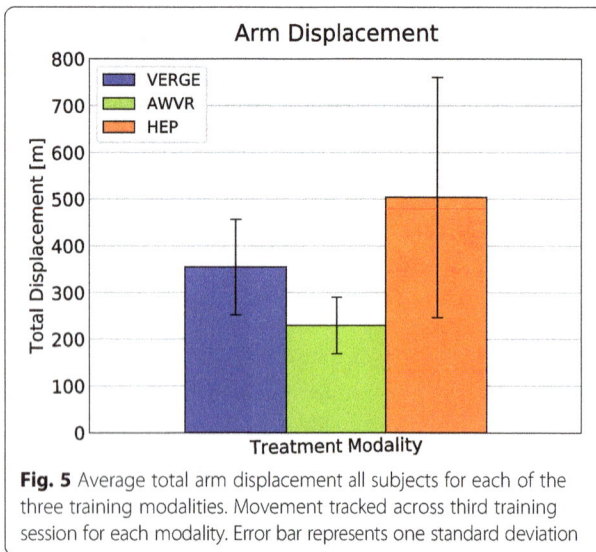

Fig. 5 Average total arm displacement all subjects for each of the three training modalities. Movement tracked across third training session for each modality. Error bar represents one standard deviation

Results

Questionnaires

User feedback gathered for the *VERGE Survey* was generally positive, with 13 of 15 participants indicating that the therapy was *Very* (*n* = 8) or *Extremely* (*n* = 5) productive and 14 of 15 participants indicating that they were *Satisfied* (*n* = 2) or *Very Satisfied* (*n* = 12) with the amount of arm use during the therapy session. Additionally, participants largely enjoyed having a partner as 13 of the 15 participants *Very Much* (*n* = 7) or *Extremely* (*n* = 6) enjoyed playing with a virtual partner and 14 of 15 participants *Agreed* (7) or *Strongly agreed* (7) that training with another virtual partner in the environment increased motivation. Response to the look of the exercises was generally positive as 11 of 15 participants *Very Much* (*n* = 6) or *Extremely* (*n* = 5) liked the 3D graphics of the system. Importantly, 12 of 15 participants *Agreed* (*n* = 5) or *Strongly Agreed* (*n* = 7) that the VERGE system had great potential as home-based rehabilitation.

Results of the *Weekly Survey*, administered at the end of each training modality, are shown in Table 1. Few statistically significant differences were apparent among the three treatment modalities for any of the responses. *Satisfaction with time spent in training* was significantly less for VERGE than for the other modalities; however, all three modalities showed a mean response above 4, which represented *Satisfied* on the survey. Responses were generally quite positive, with the vast majority of responses having a mean value of 4.0 or greater (5-point Likert scale with 3 indicating a neutral response). Importantly, the majority of subjects indicated that if the equipment were available they would *Definitely* (*n* = 10) or *Probably* (*n* = 4) continue at least one of the therapy modalities at home. Overall, they indicated a willingness

to perform the therapy for 2–3 or more days per week (*n* = 15).

The questionnaire directly comparing the training modalities (*Final Survey*) revealed a variety of opinions (Table 2). Participants were fairly split about which of the modalities they found the most engaging (each modality received 5 selections) and which they preferred (5 each selected HEP and AWVR and 4 selected VERGE). However, we observed strong trends favoring HEP regarding ease of understanding (two-thirds of participants selected HEP) and which therapy users would most likely continue in the home (9 of 15 participants selected HEP).

Kinematics

Each therapy modality promoted considerable arm movement. Total arm displacement averaged: 354 m for VERGE, 503 m for HEP, and 229 m for AWVR (Fig. 5). Non-inferiority testing showed that arm displacement produced by participants during the VERGE training was not significantly inferior to HEP or AWVR (Fig. 6a). All three modalities also encouraged extended arm postures and elevated hand positions. Time spent with Reach Distance ≥ 0.7 for VERGE was not inferior to that for the other two modalities (Fig. 6b). Additionally, the largest histogram values occurred for postures at which the hand was extended 70% or more of full-arm length away from the shoulder (Fig. 7a). The VERGE system also promoted elevating the hand at least as much as other modalities. Time spent with Hand Elevation ≤ 0.4 was not inferior for VERGE as compared to AWVR and HEP (Fig. 6c). The histograms revealed that during the VERGE session, subjects spent 18.2% ($\pm$ 14.3%) of the time with the hand at or within 40% of arm length below shoulder height (Fig. 7b), while they spent 10.6% ($\pm$ 0.9%,) with the AWVR and 16.5% ($\pm$ 12.3%) during the HEP.

Discussion

VERGE implementation

We developed a 3D, networked VR system allowing users, physically remote from each other, to interact within a virtual environment. Each user controls an avatar in real time by movement of corresponding body segments. These avatars can manipulate virtual objects located within the environment; multiple avatars can even manipulate the same object, such as a ball hit back and forth. Each user needs only have a computer, wireless mouse, and a Kinect™ device. No special software is required for the user, only an executable version of our code and the Kinect SDK.

This VERGE system was successfully tested by 15 stroke survivors with chronic hemiparesis in the upper extremity. User response was generally positive,

Table 1 Results for *Weekly Survey* administered at the end of week for each modality

Survey Question	VERGE	AWVR	HEP	Friedman
Importance of exercise speed	4.6 (0.6)	4.3 (1.1)	4.6 (0.7)	0.733
Importance of personal progress	4.9 (0.3)	4.5 (0.7)*	4.9 (0.4)	0.038
Importance of performance of activities of daily living	4.6 (0.6)	4.6 (0.8)	4.9 (0.4)	0.522
Importance of ability to perform new tasks	4.5 (1.0)	4.6 (0.7)	4.9 (0.3)	0.264
Importance of greater arm/hand movement	4.8 (0.4)	4.9 (0.5)	4.9 (0.4)	0.717
Level of interest/stimulation from therapy	4.0 (1.0)	4.2 (0.7)	4.1 (1.0)	0.889
Effectiveness/helpfulness for arm/hand	4.2 (0.8)	4.4 (0.6)	4.2 (1.0)	0.368
Satisfaction with ease of use	4.3 (1.0)	4.5 (0.8)	4.4 (1.0)	0.661
Satisfaction with your attention to exercises	4.6 (0.8)	4.3 (0.8)	4.7 (0.6)	0.206
Satisfaction with your desire to complete training	4.8 (0.8)	4.9 (0.4)	4.7 (0.5)	0.311
Satisfaction with progress	4.2 (0.8)	4.3 (0.7)	4.6 (0.6)	0.061
Satisfaction with amount of arm use	4.7 (0.8)	4.7 (0.5)	4.7 (0.5)	1.0
Satisfaction with time spent in training	4.1 (0.8)*	4.6 (0.5)	4.6 (0.5)	0.032
Progress experienced in training	3.7 (1.1)	3.9 (0.9)	3.5 (1.1)	0.565
Amount of arm movement compared to prior treatment	4.1 (0.8)	4.5 (0.6)	4.3 (0.8)	0.439
Continued home use	3.9 (1.4)	4.3 (0.8)	4.0 (1.4)	0.304
Expected frequency of home exercises	3.2 (1.0)	3.3 (0.7)	3.2 (1.2)	0.595
Rehabilitation potential	4.1 (1.1)	4.1 (0.9)	4.4 (0.7)	0.206

Likert scale from 1 to 5 employed. Higher numbers denote more positive responses. Mean (SD)
* indicates significance at the level indicated by the Friedman test statistic

with 85% of the participants expressing satisfaction with the utility of the therapy and 93% indicating satisfaction with the amount of arm movement induced. Indeed, participants moved their hands an average of 350 m (after subtracting shoulder translation) during each session. This far exceeds the amount of hand displacement produced by the 54 movements observed during a typical occupational therapy session [50]. In accordance with previous multi-user training studies [26, 29, 30], the vast majority (14 of 15) participants indicated that they liked having a partner for therapy, despite not being in visual contact with this person.

Table 2 Results of Final Survey comparing the three training paradigms

Characteristic	VERGE	AWVR	HEP
Most engaging	5	5	5
Greatest desire to complete sessions	3	6	6
Moved arm the most	4	4	7
Easiest to understand	1	3	10
Most effective	1	5	8
Preferred form of therapy	4	5	5
Most likely to continue at home	3	3	9

Values listed reflect number of subjects choosing each modality

Comparison with other potential training modalities

Overall, all three therapy options encouraged considerable movement of the hand in space. Non-inferiority testing confirmed that use of the VERGE system did not result in significantly less displacement of the hand than that recorded using the more established AWVR or HEP modalities. As relatively few studies have quantified arm movement during therapy outside of a robotic device, these values provide an important target for therapy. Importantly, all three training modalities encouraged movement away from the body. Arm movements to areas of the workspace which require elbow extension can be challenging for stroke survivors, especially when the arm is unsupported [51, 52], as was the case for VERGE, AWVR, and the majority of HEP. The differences observed in the amount of arm movement between modalities could be a result of confounding factors in exercise design. Specifically, exercises in VERGE were designed to include movements out of synergy and in a large free 3-D space. Although the importance of 3D movements in therapy is a topic of debate [34, 35], many tasks require non-planar movements. VERGE allows practice of such task-based motions. AWVR also included movements out of synergy but the workspace was much more limited in size. HEP included many exercises with proximal arm stabilization, these movements were simpler in that they did not require multiple joint coordination or trunk stabilization.

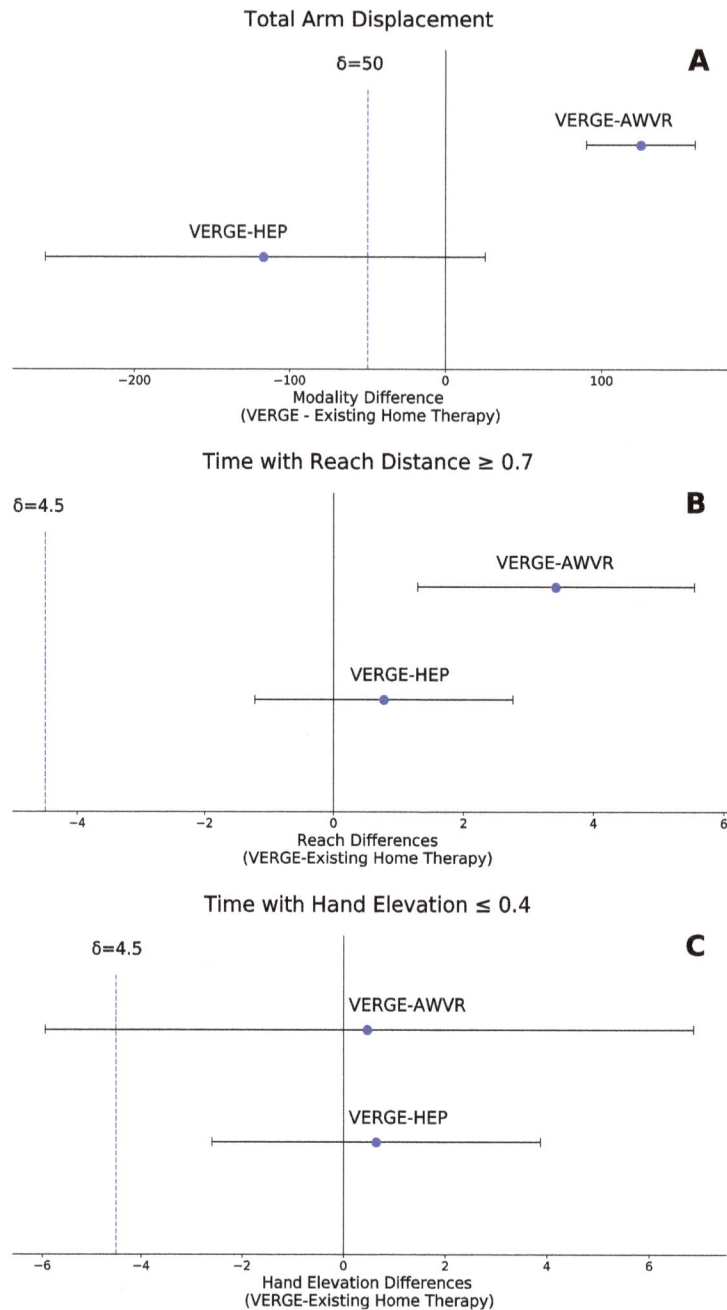

Fig. 6 Non-inferiority tests. **a** Total arm displacement. The δ was set equal to 10% of HEP mean. **b** Time spent (in minutes) with Reach Distance greater than or equal to 70% of arm length. **c** Time spent (in minutes) with Hand Elevation within 40% of arm length with respect to the shoulder. The δ was set equal to 10% of full training time (45 min) for **b** and **c**. VERGE not inferior to HEP or AWVR for any of these measures

During the training sessions, participants spent the most time with their arms extended at least 70% of full range. Participants also spent a considerable portion of time with the hand raised in an upper level of the workspace (within 40% of arm length of the shoulder elevation). With VERGE, for example, participants spent almost 20% of the session with their hand in this region of the workspace despite not having arm support.

Users, however, indicated differences in experience across the treatment modalities. While participants rated the modalities similarly in the weekly questionnaires, they expressed a preference for the HEP in certain areas in the comparative questionnaire, including as the most effective therapy and the treatment they would most likely continue in the home. Some of the appeal is undoubtedly attributable to the ease of use. Two-

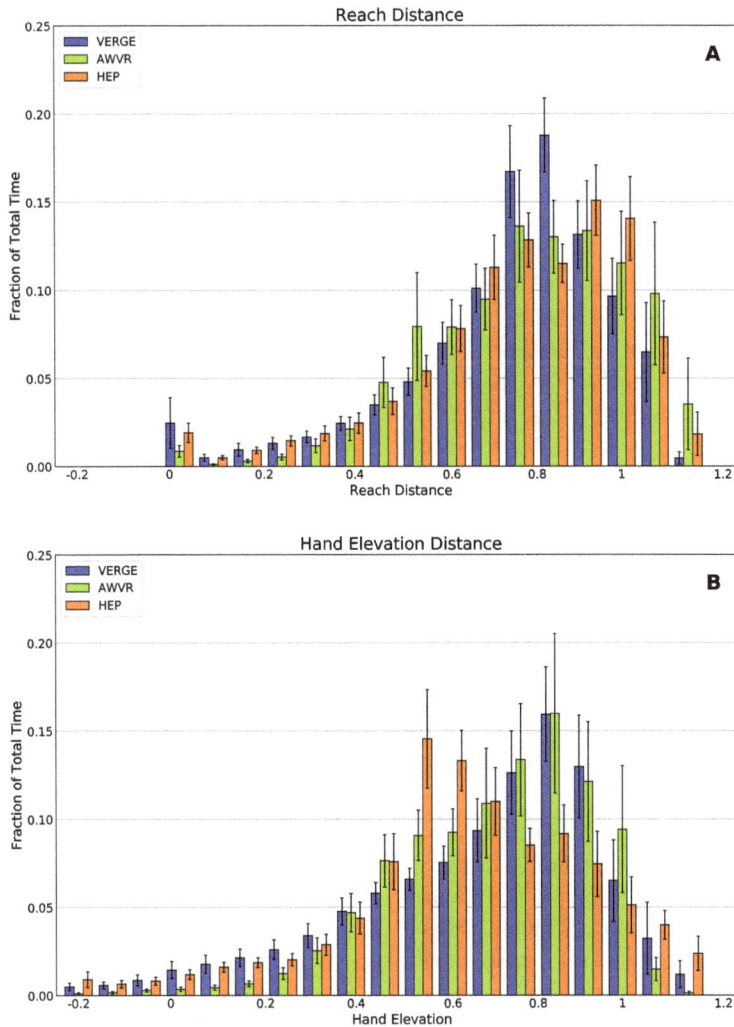

Fig. 7 Histograms, averaged across all subjects, depicting time the hand of the impaired limb spent in different regions of the workspace. **a** Reach Distance. Distance of the hand from the shoulder, represented as a fraction of arm length (0: hand coincident with shoulder; 1: arm fully extended). **b** Hand Elevation Distance. Vertical location of the hand with respect to the shoulder, represented as a fraction of arm length (0, hand elevation equal to shoulder elevation; 1: hand elevation full arm length below shoulder elevation; negative values indicate hand elevation above shoulder elevation). Blue: VERGE, green: AWVR, orange: HEP

thirds of participants chose HEP as the easiest to use. This needs to be addressed in VERGE, as we describe in the following section.

Limitations and lessons learned

The study identified limitations with VERGE that need to be addressed for improved acceptance and utility. For example, the *Trajectory Trace* exercise placed a significant cognitive demand on users. They were required to actively cycle through a sequence of discrete states for each round (Draw, Claim, Trace, Reset) while coordinating with another player (i.e., one player would draw a trajectory while another would claim and trace it). It was sometimes difficult to determine the current state and to remember which came next. Thus, while almost equal

numbers of subjects listed *Ball Bump* or *Food Fight* as their favorite VERGE exercise, none listed *Trajectory Trace*. Despite similar amounts of time spent on each VERGE exercise, hand displacement during *Trajectory Trace* was less than 50% of the amount seen during the *Ball Bump* exercise. Partially attributable to this, over 70% of participants chose HEP as the easiest to understand (only one subject picked VERGE). Clearly, reducing complexity of operation for the user of a therapy paradigm is of paramount importance. We have subsequently modified *Trajectory Trace* to include a visual display indicating the state flow and current state.

Due to the largely collaborative nature of the tasks in VERGE, they included limited quantitative performance measures for the users. Participants stressed the need for objective feedback. As noticeable functional changes may evolve slowly, quantitative assessment of game performance, which can show gains on a much shorter timescale, may provide the motivation needed in the short-term to enable reaching functional milestones. We have subsequently added scoring for each of the exercises. In some cases, both competitive and collaborative scoring is available.

There were limitations with the pilot study as well. While one of the potential benefits of the VERGE system is the inclusion of other players, we did not directly examine preferences for individual vs. partnered training, as previous studies have done [26, 27, 29, 30]. In our study, the three training modalities were quite different from each other. The HEP and AWVR represented existing modalities with potential for use in the home. Factors such as ease of use, the engaging nature of the virtual task, or scoring undoubtedly influenced preferences for the chosen training modality. It should be noted that a large majority of participants expressed enthusiasm for playing with a partner when using VERGE and indicated that they felt that the presence of another user increased motivation. Enthusiasm for multiple players may have been even greater if a friend or relative had served as the playing partner, as was the case in a previous study [26].

Our relatively small sample of participants displayed considerable motivation in repeatedly coming to the laboratory in the hospital for the study and maintaining study adherence. The enthusiasm for therapy may not be as great in the general population. Additionally, only three training sessions were performed with each modality. User responses may have been different after more sessions.

User response may also have been impacted by the fact that this pilot study was performed in the laboratory rather than the home. Coming to the hospital, interacting with people, and receiving compensation may have elevated interest, particularly for the HEP. Compliance rates for conventional home therapy exercise programs have been mixed [53–56].

Conclusions

This represents one of the first tests of stroke survivors interacting with a remote user in a 3D virtual environment for therapy. The VERGE system can be directly utilized for home-based therapy with a family member or friend in their home or a therapist in the clinic. The low cost and minimal requirements make it practical for the clinic or home. Most participants expressed satisfaction with the system and enthusiasm for the virtual partner. However, they did stress the importance of ease of use and feedback of performance. Their responses highlighted the need for technology to be sufficiently flexible to accommodate the different goals and preferences of individual users.

Importantly, participants indicated a strong interest in home therapy. Over 66% responded that they would *Definitely* be willing to continue therapy in the home and 100% responded that they would perform the training at least 2–3 times per week. Two-thirds of participants indicated that they would be willing to perform home-based training 6–7 times per week. While limitations must be addressed, multi-user virtual reality environments hold promise for maintaining engagement in therapy and providing feedback of performance for home users. We are currently undertaking a home therapy study with the VERGE system.

Additional files

Additional file 1: Home Exercise Program (HEP) handout. The HEP consisted of pre-defined sets of seated, self-paced arm-hand exercises derived from the standard of care. These 16 exercises were presented to the participant in the form of a printed handout. (PDF 261 kb)

Additional file 2: VERGE Survey. Questionnaire administered following the VERGE therapy addressing system specific details. (PDF 28 kb)

Additional file 3: Weekly Survey. Questionnaire administered weekly following each therapy modality (including VERGE). (PDF 311 kb)

Additional file 4: Final Survey. Questionnaire administered at the end of the study to compare the three treatment modalities. (PDF 30 kb)

Acknowledgements
The authors would like to thank Jessica Nguyen for her valuable assistance with data analysis and Ning Yuan for his appreciated role with data collection.

Funding
Funded by the US Department of Health and Human Services, National Institute on Disability, Independent Living, and Rehabilitation Research (NIDILRR), Grant #H133E070013.

Authors' contributions
KMT: Research project organization and execution, data acquisition, interpretation, statistical analysis and manuscript writing, review and critique. DT and NS: Design and implementation of the MUVR environment, manuscript review and critique. AJB: Research project execution, data acquisition and analysis, manuscript review and critique. KNT: Design and initial training of the HEP, manuscript review and critique. DGK: Research project conception, design, data review and critique, manuscript writing review and critique. All authors approved the final manuscript.

Competing interests
The authors declare that they have no competing interests.

Author details

[1]Shirley Ryan AbilityLab, Arms + Hands Lab, Chicago, IL, USA. [2]School of Design, University of Illinois at Chicago (UIC), Chicago, IL, USA. [3]UNC/NC State Joint Department of Biomedical Engineering, University of North Carolina at Chapel Hill, Chapel Hill, NC, USA. [4]Closed-Loop Engineering for Advanced Rehabilitation Research Core, University of North Carolina at Chapel Hill, Chapel Hill, NC, USA.

References

1. Benjamin EJ, Blaha MJ, Chiuve SE, Cushman M, Das SR, Deo R, de Ferranti SD, Floyd J, Fornage M, Gillespie C, et al. Heart Disease and Stroke Statistics-2017 Update: A Report From the American Heart Association. Circulation. 2017;135:e146–603.

2. Kwakkel G. Impact of intensity of practice after stroke: issues for consideration. Disabil Rehabil. 2006;28:823–30.

3. Kleim JA, Jones TA. Principles of experience-dependent neural plasticity: implications for rehabilitation after brain damage. J Speech Lang Hear Res. 2008;51:S225–39.

4. Winstein CJ, Stein J, Arena R, Bates B, Cherney LR, Cramer SC, Deruyter F, Eng JJ, Fisher B, Harvey RL, et al. Guidelines for Adult Stroke Rehabilitation and Recovery: A Guideline for Healthcare Professionals From the American Heart Association/American Stroke Association. Stroke. 2016;47:e98–e169.

5. Professions BoH: Rural health profession facts: supply and distribution of health professions in rural america. (Administration HRaS ed. Rockville, MD; 1992.

6. Analysis NCfHW: Distribution of U.S. health care providers residing in rural and urban areas. US Department of Health and Human Services.

7. Liao Y, Greenlund KJ, Croft JB, Keenan NL, Giles WH. Factors explaining excess stroke prevalence in the US Stroke Belt. Stroke. 2009;40:3336–41.

8. Kairy D, Veras M, Archambault P, Hernandez A, Higgins J, Levin MF, Poissant L, Raz A, Kaizer F. Maximizing post-stroke upper limb rehabilitation using a novel telerehabilitation interactive virtual reality system in the patient's home: study protocol of a randomized clinical trial. Contemp Clin Trials. 2016;47:49–53.

9. Wolf SL, Sahu K, Bay RC, Buchanan S, Reiss A, Linder S, Rosenfeldt A, Alberts J. The HAAPI (Home Arm Assistance Progression Initiative) Trial: A Novel Robotics Delivery Approach in Stroke Rehabilitation. Neurorehabil Neural Repair. 2015;29:958–68.

10. CfDCa P. Outpatient rehabilitation among stroke survivors: 21 states and the District of Columbia, 2005. Morb Mortal Wkly Rep. 2007;56:504–7.

11. Hopman WM, Verner J. Quality of life during and after inpatient stroke rehabilitation. Stroke. 2003;34:801–5.

12. Meyer BC, Raman R, Hemmen T, Obler R, Zivin JA, Rao R, Thomas RG, Lyden PD. Efficacy of site-independent telemedicine in the STRokE DOC trial: a randomised, blinded, prospective study. Lancet Neurol. 2008;7:787–95.

13. Morales-Vidal S, Ruland S. Telemedicine in stroke care and rehabilitation. Top Stroke Rehabil. 2013;20:101–7.

14. Muller-Barna P, Hubert GJ, Boy S, Bogdahn U, Wiedmann S, Heuschmann PU, Audebert HJ. TeleStroke units serving as a model of care in rural areas: 10-year experience of the TeleMedical project for integrative stroke care. Stroke. 2014;45:2739–44.

15. Housley SN, Garlow AR, Ducote K, Howard A, Thomas T, Wu D, Richards K, Butler AJ. Increasing Access to Cost Effective Home-Based Rehabilitation for Rural Veteran Stroke Survivors. Austin J Cerebrovasc Dis Stroke. 2016;3:1–11.

16. Hutchison AJ, Breckon JD. A review of telephone coaching services for people with long-term conditions. J Telemed Telecare. 2011;17:451–8.

17. Chumbler NR, Quigley P, Li X, Morey M, Rose D, Sanford J, Griffiths P, Hoenig H. Effects of telerehabilitation on physical function and disability for stroke patients: a randomized, controlled trial. Stroke. 2012;43:2168–74.

18. Staszuk A, Wiatrak B, Tadeusiewicz R, Karuga-Kuzniewska E, Rybak Z. Telerehabilitation approach for patients with hand impairment. Acta Bioeng Biomech. 2016;18:55–62.

19. Levy CE, Silverman E, Jia H, Geiss M, Omura D. Effects of physical therapy delivery via home video telerehabilitation on functional and health-related quality of life outcomes. J Rehabil Res Dev. 2015;52:361–70.

20. Koh GC, Yen SC, Tay A, Cheong A, Ng YS, De Silva DA, Png C, Caves K, Koh K, Kumar Y, et al: Singapore Tele-technology Aided Rehabilitation in Stroke (STARS) trial: protocol of a randomized clinical trial on tele-rehabilitation for stroke patients. BMC Neurol 2015, 15:161.

21. Johnson MJ, Loureiro RCV, Harwin WS. Collaborative tele-rehabilitation and robot-mediated therapy for stroke rehabilitation at home or clinic. Intell Serv Robot. 2008;1:109–21.

22. Lanini J, Tsuji T, Wolf P, Riener R, Novak D. Teleoperation of two six-degree-of-freedom arm rehabilitation exoskeletons. In: IEEE International Conference on Rehabilitation Robotics (ICORR). Singapore: Singapore. IEEE. p. 2015.

23. Song A, Wu C, Ni D, Li H, Qin H. One-Therapist to Three-Patient Telerehabilitation Robot System for the Upper Limb after Stroke. Int J Soc Robot. 2016;8:319–29.

24. Andrade KO, Martins J, Caurin GA, Joaquim RC, Fernandes G. Relative performance analysis for robot rehabilitation procedure with two simultaneous users. In: IEEE RAS & EMBS International Conference on Biomedical Robotics and Biomechatronics; Rome, Italy. IEEE; 2012.

25. Caurin GA, Siqueira AA, Andrade KO, Joaquim RC, Krebs HI. Adaptive strategy for multi-user robotic rehabilitation games. Conf Proc IEEE Eng Med Biol Soc. 2011;2011:1395–8.

26. Gorsic M, Cikajlo I, Goljar N, Novak D. A multisession evaluation of an adaptive competitive arm rehabilitation game. J Neuroeng Rehabil. 2017;14:128.

27. Gorsic M, Cikajlo I, Novak D. Competitive and cooperative arm rehabilitation games played by a patient and unimpaired person: effects on motivation and exercise intensity. J Neuroeng Rehabil. 2017;14:23.

28. Le HH, Loureiro RCV, Dussopt F, Phillips N, Zivanovic A, Loomes MJ: Soundscape and Haptic Cues in an Interactive Painting: a Study with Autistic Children. In IEEE RAS & EMBS International Conference on Biomedical Robotics and Biomechatronics; Rome, Italy. IEEE; 2014.

29. Mace M, Kinany N, Rinne P, Rayner A, Bentley P, Burdet E. Balancing the playing field: collaborative gaming for physical training. J Neuroeng Rehabil. 2017;14:116.

30. Novak D, Nagle A, Keller U, Riener R. Increasing motivation in robot-aided arm rehabilitation with competitive and cooperative gameplay. J Neuroeng Rehabil. 2014;11:64.

31. Andrade KO, Fernandes G, Martins J, Roma V, Joaquim RC, Caurin GA. Rehabilitation robotics and serious games: An initial architecture for simultaneous players. In: Biosignals and Biorobotics Conference (BRC). Rio de Janerio, Brazil: IEEE; 2013.

32. Pires FA, Santos WM, Andrade KO, Caurin GA, Siqueira AA. Robotic platform for telerehabilitation studies based on unity game engine. In: IEEE 3nd International Conference on Serious Games and Applications for Health. Rio de Janeiro, Brazil: IEEE. p. 2014.

33. Tsoupikova D, Stoykov N, Kamper D, Vick R. Virtual reality environment assisting recovery from stroke. Yokohama, Japan: SIGGRAPH ASIA; 2009.

34. Conroy SS, Whitall J, Dipietro L, Jones-Lush LM, Zhan M, Finley MA, Wittenberg GF, Krebs HI, Bever CT. Effect of gravity on robot-assisted motor training after chronic stroke: a randomized trial. Arch Phys Med Rehabil. 2011;92:1754–61.

35. Ellis MD, Sukal-Moulton T, Dewald JP. Progressive shoulder abduction loading is a crucial element of arm rehabilitation in chronic stroke. Neurorehabil Neural Repair. 2009;23:862–9.

36. Reinkensmeyer DJ, McKenna Cole A, Kahn LE, Kamper DG. Directional control of reaching is preserved following mild/moderate stroke and stochastically constrained following severe stroke. Exp Brain Res. 2002; 143:525–30.

37. Guadagnoli MA, Lee TD. Challenge point: a framework for conceptualizing the effects of various practice conditions in motor learning. J Mot Behav. 2004;36:212–24.

38. Onla-or S, Winstein CJ. Determining the optimal challenge point for motor skill learning in adults with moderately severe Parkinson's disease. Neurorehabil Neural Repair. 2008;22:385–95.

39. Tsoupikova D, Stoykov NS, Corrigan M, Thielbar K, Vick R, Li Y, Triandafilou K, Preuss F, Kamper D. Virtual immersion for post-stroke hand rehabilitation therapy. Ann Biomed Eng. 2015;43:467–77.

40. Luo X, Kenyon RV, Kamper D, DeFanti TA. On the Determinants of Size-Constancy in a Virtual Environment. The International Journal of Virtual Reality. 2009;8:43–51.

41. Fischer HC, Stubblefield K, Kline T, Luo X, Kenyon RV, Kamper DG. Hand rehabilitation following stroke: a pilot study of assisted finger extension training in a virtual environment. Top Stroke Rehabil. 2007;14:1–12.

42. Ellis MD, Drogos J, Carmona C, Keller T, Dewald JP. Neck rotation modulates flexion synergy torques, indicating an ipsilateral reticulospinal source for impairment in stroke. J Neurophysiol. 2012;108:3096–104.

43. Tsoupikova D, Triandafilou K, Solanki S, Barry A, Presuss F, Kamper D. Real-

time diagnostic data in multi-user virtual reality post-stroke therapy. Macau. ACM: SIGGRAPH Asia; 2016.

44. Cameirao MS, Badia SB, Duarte E, Frisoli A, Verschure PF. The combined impact of virtual reality neurorehabilitation and its interfaces on upper extremity functional recovery in patients with chronic stroke. Stroke. 2012;43:2720–8.

45. Wittmann F, Lambercy O, Gonzenbach RR, van Raai MA, Hover R, Held J, Starkey ML, Curt A, Luft A, Gassert R. Assessment-driven arm therapy at home using an IMU-based virtual reality system. In: Rehabilitation Robotics (ICORR), 2015 IEEE International Conference on. Singapore: Singapore. IEEE. p. 2015.

46. Gowland C, Stratford P, Ward M, Moreland J, Torresin W, Van Hullenaar S, Sanford J, Barreca S, Vanspall B, Plews N. Measuring physical impairment and disability with the Chedoke-McMaster Stroke Assessment. Stroke. 1993; 24:58–63.

47. Likert R. A technique for the measurement of attitudes. Archives of Psychology. 1932;22:140–55.

48. Norman G. Likert scales, levels of measurement and the "laws" of statistics. Adv Health Sci Educ. 2010;15:625–32.

49. Barre A, Armand S. Biomechanical ToolKit: Open-source framework to visualize and process biomechanical data. Comput Methods Prog Biomed. 2014;114:80–7.

50. Lang CE, Macdonald JR, Reisman DS, Boyd L, Jacobson Kimberley T, Schindler-Ivens SM, Hornby TG, Ross SA, Scheets PL. Observation of amounts of movement practice provided during stroke rehabilitation. Arch Phys Med Rehabil. 2009;90:1692–8.

51. Iwamuro BT, Cruz EG, Connelly LL, Fischer HC, Kamper DG. Effect of a gravity-compensating orthosis on reaching after stroke: evaluation of the Therapy Assistant WREX. Arch Phys Med Rehabil. 2008;89:2121–8.

52. Sukal TM, Ellis MD, Dewald JP. Shoulder abduction-induced reductions in reaching work area following hemiparetic stroke: neuroscientific implications. Exp Brain Res. 2007;183:215–23.

53. Duncan P, Richards L, Wallace D, Stoker-Yates J, Pohl P, Luchies C, Ogle A, Studenski S. A randomized, controlled pilot study of a home-based exercise program for individuals with mild and moderate stroke. Stroke. 1998;29: 2055–60.

54. Jurkiewicz MT, Marzolini S, Oh P. Adherence to a home-based exercise program for individuals after stroke. Top Stroke Rehabil. 2011;18:277–84.

55. Sluijs EM, Kok GJ, van der Zee J: Correlates of exercise compliance in physical therapy. Phys Ther 1993, 73:771–782; discussion 783-776.

56. Chen CY, Neufeld PS, Feely CA, Skinner CS. Factors influencing compliance with home exercise programs among patients with upper-extremity impairment. Am J Occup Ther. 1999;53:171–80.

12

Automated functional upper limb evaluation of patients with Friedreich ataxia using serious games rehabilitation exercises

Bruno Bonnechère[1,2,3*] (iD), Bart Jansen[2,3], Inès Haack[1], Lubos Omelina[2,3], Véronique Feipel[4], Serge Van Sint Jan[1] and Massimo Pandolfo[5]

Abstract

Background: Friedreich ataxia (FRDA) is a disease with neurological and systemic involvement. Clinical assessment tools commonly used for FRDA become less effective in evaluating decay in patients with advanced FRDA, particularly when they are in a wheelchair. Further motor worsening mainly impairs upper limb function. In this study, we tested if serious games (SG) developed for rehabilitation can be used as an assessment tool for upper limb function even in patients with advanced FRDA.

Methods: A specific SG has been developed for physical rehabilitation of patients suffering from neurologic diseases. The use of this SG, coupled with Kinect sensor, has been validated to perform functional evaluation of the upper limbs with healthy subjects across lifespan. Twenty-seven FRDA patients were included in the study. Patients were invited to perform upper limb rehabilitation exercises embedded in SG. Motions were recorded by the Kinect and clinically relevant parameters were extracted from the collected motions. We tested if the existence of correlations between the scores from the serious games and the severity of the disease using clinical assessment tools commonly used for FRDA. Results of patients were compared with a group a healthy subjects of similar age.

Results: Very highly significant differences were found for time required to perform the exercise (increase of 76%, $t(68) = 7.22$, $P < 0.001$) and for accuracy (decrease of 6%, $t(68) = -3.69$, $P < 0.001$) between patients and healthy subjects. Concerning the patients significant correlations were found between age and time ($R = 0.65$, $p = 0.015$), accuracy ($R = -0.75$, $p = 0.004$) and the total displacement of upper limbs. ($R = 0.55$, $p = 0.031$). Statistically significant correlations were found between the age of diagnosis and speed related parameters.

Conclusions: The results of this study indicate that SG reliably captures motor impairment of FRDA patients due to cerebellar and pyramidal involvement. Results also show that functional evaluation of FRDA patients can be performed during rehabilitation therapy embedded in games with the patient seated in a wheelchair.

Keywords: Serious games, Assessment, Evaluation, Friedreich Ataxia, Kinect sensor

* Correspondence: bbonnech@ulb.ac.be
[1]Laboratory of Anatomy, Biomechanics and Organogenesis (LABO) [CP 619], Université Libre de Bruxelles, Lennik Street 808, 1070 Brussels, Belgium
[2]Department of Electronics and Informatics – ETRO, Vrije Universiteit Brussel, Brussels, Belgium
Full list of author information is available at the end of the article

Background

Friedreich ataxia (FRDA) is an autosomal recessive disease with neurological and systemic involvement. Most commonly, loss of balance in a child or adolescent is the first symptom. Within a few years, trunk and limb ataxia become prominent, accompanied by dysarthria, oculomotor abnormalities and weakness. At the onset of disease, ataxia is mostly due to loss of large proprioceptive primary sensory neurons in the dorsal root ganglia (DRGs), with associated atrophy of the posterior columns and spinocerebellar tracts. With progression, cerebellar ataxia, due to atrophy of the dentate nucleus, becomes prevalent. Also with progression, distal axonal loss in the pyramidal tracts that cause further motor impairment [1, 2]. Most affected individuals become unable to walk within 10–15 years since disease onset, but then continue to deteriorate because of worsening upper limb ataxia, weakness, dysarthria, and eventually dysphagia. Clinical assessment tools commonly used for FRDA, such as the Scale for Assessment and Rating of Ataxia (SARA) [3], the Friedreich Ataxia Rating Scale (FARS) [4], and the International Cooperative Ataxia Rating Scale (ICARS) [5], become less effective in evaluating progression in patients with advanced FRDA, particularly when they are in a wheelchair and when upper limb function is impaired. This is partly due to a ceiling effect in these scales, in which gait and balance item have a major weight, but also to the characteristics of the disease [6, 7]. In FRDA, pyramidal symptoms like slowing and impairment of rapid alternating movements and difficulties in raising arms to point a target, eventually greatly affect performance in upper limb coordination tests, making their scoring more erratic. Hence the need for a more integrated tool to assess upper limb motor function in FRDA, particularly in wheelchair-bound patients with advanced disease.

Commercial video games have significantly evolved over the last decade. Today computer performance and play experience allow new perspectives for rehabilitation. Thanks to new gaming controllers (Nintendo Wii FitTM, Microsoft Xbox KinectTM, etc.) video game playing has changed from a passive (e.g., the player is seated on a sofa using a very simple controller) to an active experience: players have to move in order to interact with games (e.g., the player is truly active with a game controller requesting full body movements). Clinicians are now prospecting the new potential use of these games in rehabilitation mainly through testing available commercial games with patients suffering from various neurological pathologies (e.g. Cerebral Palsy [8], stroke [9], Parkinson disease [10]). Although encouraging results have been observed, especially in terms of motivation, there are several problems related to the use of commercial video games in rehabilitation. The player motion accuracy requested from the player during the games is low while most therapists will aim to improve patient joint control and coordination and the motion that

must be performed to control the games do not correspond to rehabilitation exercises. Furthermore, there is currently no possibility to record the motion performed by the patients during those kind of exercises. However, collecting this information could be important to: (i) allow to provide direct feedback to patient and eventually correct the motion if they are not performed in the right way and (ii) to provide information to therapists in case of telerehabilitation exercises when the patient is performing exercises at home without the clinicians' supervision [11].

In order to tackle the above-mentioned limitations, specific games must be developed for rehabilitation purposes [12]. Such kind of games, called serious games (SG) (i.e. games designed with a primary purpose other than pure entertainment), must be designed taking into account real clinical needs and constraints (e.g. simple visual background, based on relevant clinical schemes, range of motion and speed required to perform the exercises must be adaptable, etc.) [13] and allow to record motions performed by the patients [14, 15].

Depending on the joints and the kind of motions performed, results obtained with the Kinect sensor must be analyzed carefully. However, it was shown that using the displacement of wrist relative to trunk appears to be a good approach to evaluate upper limb function during rehabilitation exercises using serious games [15]. Furthermore, results obtained from Kinect and gold-standard optoelectronic device to assess upper limb functions are significantly correlated [16].

In this study, we tested if SG can be used as an assessment tool for upper limb function in patients with advanced FRDA. First, we determined if the scores obtained in the SG are able to differentiate patients and healthy participants. Then, we correlated SG results with genetic and clinical parameters of disease severity. To the authors best knowledge, there is currently no study about the use of SG to perform functional evaluation of patients with FRDA simultaneously with physical rehabilitation exercises.

Methods

Patients

Twenty-seven patients were included in the study, characteristics of the patients are presented in Table 1. They were all enrolled in the European Friedreich Ataxia Consortium for Translational Studies (EFACTS, Clinicaltrials.gov identifier NCT02069509) natural history study, the first prospective pan-European FRDA registry designed to define clinical rating scales and quality of life measures, which can be used in clinical trials. Since its inception in 2010, EFACTS has enrolled more than 800 genetically confirmed FRDA patients in nine European countries. SG was added to the EFACTS follow-up protocol at the Brussels site as an additional functional assessment. Data presented here are cross-sectional, for each patient they have been obtained at

Table 1 Characteristics of the patients included in the study

Variables	N	Mean (std)
Age (years)	27	26,0 (12.2)
Duration of the disease (years)	27	15.0 (7,44)
SARA score	27	22,5 (9,2)
ADL score	27	16,9 (6.7)
GAA-1 number of repeats	15	608.2 (306.4)
9 R 1 (s)	25	72.01 (42.3)
9 R 2 (s)	25	68.1(41.6)
9 L 1 (s)	25	87.2 (57.1)
9 L 2 (s)	25	79.3 (47.0)
CCFS F score (with writing)	25	1.33 (0.37)
CCFS H score (without writing)	25	1.31 (0.37)

time of a single annual EFACTS visit. The study was approved by the local institutional Ethics Committee (ref. P2010/132) and patients gave written informed consent.

A database of healthy subjects ranging from 5 to 90 years was created in a previous study with the aim of using these data for comparison with patients by selecting the appropriate age range [15]. Exclusion criteria for the healthy subjects were neurological conditions, balance deficits or orthopedic disorders in the last six months. Forty-three healthy subjects have been used as an age-matched control group (26 (11) years old, 20 women).

Clinical evaluation

The clinical assessment of EFACTS patients includes structured interviews, questionnaires, performance-based coordination tests, clinical disease rating scales and neuropsychological functional measures. Sampling of biomaterials and genetic analysis complement the examination. GAA repeat lengths for both alleles (GAA-1 and GAA-2) are determined at the ULB Laboratory of Experimental Neurology [17] Table 1.

Details of the clinical assessment have been previously reported [6]. Briefly, clinical tests whose scores have been correlated with those obtained from the SG include the Scale for the Assessment and Rating of Ataxia (SARA) [3], which quantifies ataxia symptoms based on eight items with a maximum score of 40; the Inventory of Non-Ataxia Symptoms (INAS) [18], which provides a checklist of non-ataxia symptoms such as changes in reflexes, other motor and sensory symptoms, ophthalmological findings, urinary dysfunction, and cognitive impairment; the Spinocerebellar Ataxia Functional Index (SCAFI), consisting of timed performance measures including an 8 m walk at maximum speed, the nine-hole peg test, and the rate of repeating the syllables "PATA" within 10s; the Cerebellar Composite Functional Score (CCFS) [19], a computerized set of timed tests of upper limb coordination performed

with the dominant hand that includes a rapidly alternating click test, the 9-hole peg test and an optional writing test, which generates a composite score (higher values correspond to more impairment) including (F) or excluding (H) the optional writing test; the functional staging for ataxia part of the Friedreich Ataxia Rating Scale (FARS) [4]; the basic activities of daily living (ADL) part of the FARS was used to assess impairment in the ability to perform daily life activities.

The serious game

Participants played one mini-game specially developed for physical rehabilitation as part of a previous project (called ICT4Rehab), the Wipe Out game [13]. The player has to clean the screen virtually covered by some virtual fog using a tissue controlled by medio-lateral and inferior-superior displacements of the upper limb (wrist) relative to the trunk (Fig. 1). Spatial displacements of the players were recorded by a Kinect sensor [14]. Motion data were stored in standard format (i.e., C3D) for further analysis. Participants were invited to stand in front of the screen and the sensor. Patients were asked to play the games three times. The mean of the three repetitions was used for statistical analysis. This was similar to previously published functional evaluation protocols using SG [15].

Data processing

The use of this SG has been validated to perform functional evaluation of the upper limbs with healthy subjects across lifespan [15]. Two parameters were processed from the games: the time required to clean 90% of the screen and the accuracy. The accuracy of the motion was assessed by computing the number of times that the subject is placing the cloth in the same position on the screen (Eq.1). The number of frames where the cloth was in a position that had already been cleaned were computed ("cleaned" frames). The result was finally expressed in percentage. The higher the accuracy score, the better the results in term of performance.

$$\text{accuracy} = 100 - \left(\left(\frac{\text{Number of "cleaned" frames}}{\text{Total number of frames}} \right) \times 100 \right)$$

(1)

Several parameters were then processed from the motion performed by the patients and recorded by the Kinect, those parameters are adapted from previous studies on the validation of scores to assess dynamic balance during rehabilitation exercises [20]: the total displacement of the wrist related to the trunk (DOT) based on medio-lateral (ML) and top-down (TD) displacements (Eq. 2), the area of 95% confidence prediction ellipse (Area) (Eq. 3), the dispersion of the trajectory from the mean position in ML and TD directions (RMS_{ML} and RMS_{TD}) (Eqs. 4 and 5), the

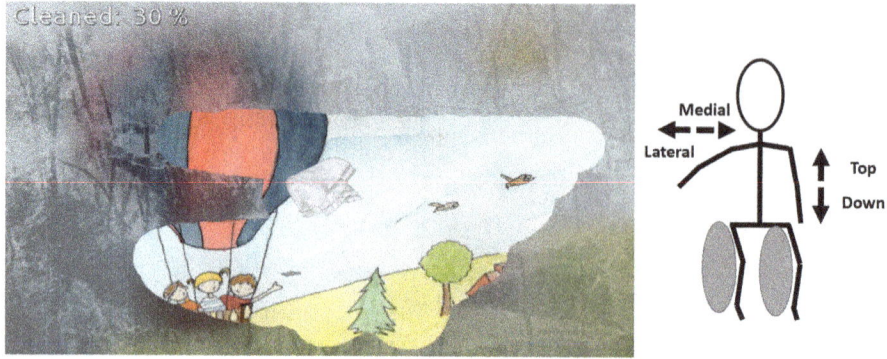

Fig. 1 Screenshot of the game

range of displacement (R_{ML} and R_{TD} (Eqs. 6 and 7), the mean velocity displacement (MV_{ML} and MV_{TD}) (Eqs. 8 and 9) and the total mean velocity (TMV) (Eq. 10).

$$DOT = \sum_{i=1}^{N} \sqrt{ML(i)^2 + TD(i)^2} \qquad (2)$$

$$Area = \pi \times prod\left(2.4478 \times \sqrt{svd(eig(\ cov(ML, TD)))}\right) \qquad (3)$$

$$RMS_{ML} = \frac{1}{N}\sqrt{\sum_{i=1}^{N} ML(i)^2} \qquad (4)$$

$$RMS_{TD} = \frac{1}{N}\sqrt{\sum_{i=1}^{N} TD(i)^2} \qquad (5)$$

$$R_{ML} = \max(ML) - \min(ML) \qquad (6)$$

$$R_{TD} = \max(TD) - \min(TD) \qquad (7)$$

$$MV_{ML} = \frac{f}{N}\sum_{i=1}^{N-1}|ML(i+1) - ML(i)| \qquad (8)$$

$$MV_{TD} = \frac{f}{N}\sum_{i=1}^{N-1}|TD(i+1) - TD(i)| \qquad (9)$$

$$TMV = \frac{f}{N}\sum_{i=1}^{N-1}\sqrt{(ML(i+1) - ML(i))^2 + (TD(i+1) - TD(i))^2} \qquad (10)$$

Data were processed and plotted using a customized software routine developed in Matlab 2017.

Statistics

To detect a difference of 40% of the time required to perform the exercise between patients and control with 80% power and a two-sided type I error of 5%, we calculated that we need to include 24 patients.

Normality of each parameter was checked using the Shapiro-Wilk tests and by graphical analysis (histogram, boxplot and normal Q-Q plot). Pearson's correlation coefficients were used to determine if the scores from the SG were correlated with the clinical evaluation. Independent sample T-test were applied to compare patients

and healthy subjects. Statistics were performed with SPSS 20 and RStudio (version 1.1.442) with R version 3.4.4, significance level was set at 0.05.

Results

Age is an important factor for both gross and fine motor control [21, 22] and since the range of age is important in our group of patients (from 6 to 48 years old) results for time and accuracy were plotted according to the age of the participants and compared to results of the healthy control group in Figs. 2 and 3 respectively. Quadratic fitting with 95% CI were plotted since it has been previously demonstrated that this fitting was the most adapted for this kind of data [15]. Very highly significant differences were found for time (increased of 76%, $t(68) = 7.22$, $P < 0.001$) and for accuracy (decreased of 6%, $t(68) = -3.69$, $P < 0.001$) between healthy subjects and patients. Results of all the studied parameters are presented in Table 2. Since no significant differences were found between right and left side for any of the parameters mean values were presented.

Pearson's correlation coefficients are presented in Table 3. Statistically significant correlations were found between age and Time ($R = 0.65$, $p = 0.015$), accuracy ($R = -0.75$, $p = 0.004$) and the total displacement of upper limbs (DOT) ($R = 0.55$, $p = 0.031$). Statistically significant correlations were found between the age of diagnosis and the speed related parameters ($R = -0.53$, $p = 0.021$ and $R = -0.49$, $p = 0.029$ for MV_{ML} and MV_{IS} respectively).

Statistically significant correlations were found for TD displacements ($R = 0.48$ and 0.47 for ranges and RMS) and the basic activities of daily living.

Correlations were found between the nine-hole peg tests and the DOT ($R = 0.60$, $p = 0.012$), the area ($R = 0.59$, $p = 0.025$), the amplitudes ($R = 0.45$, $p = 0.041$ and $R = 0.49$, $p = 0.033$ for ML and TD displacements respectively). For the speed correlations were found only for the TD direction ($R = 0.43$, $p = 0.030$) not for ML.

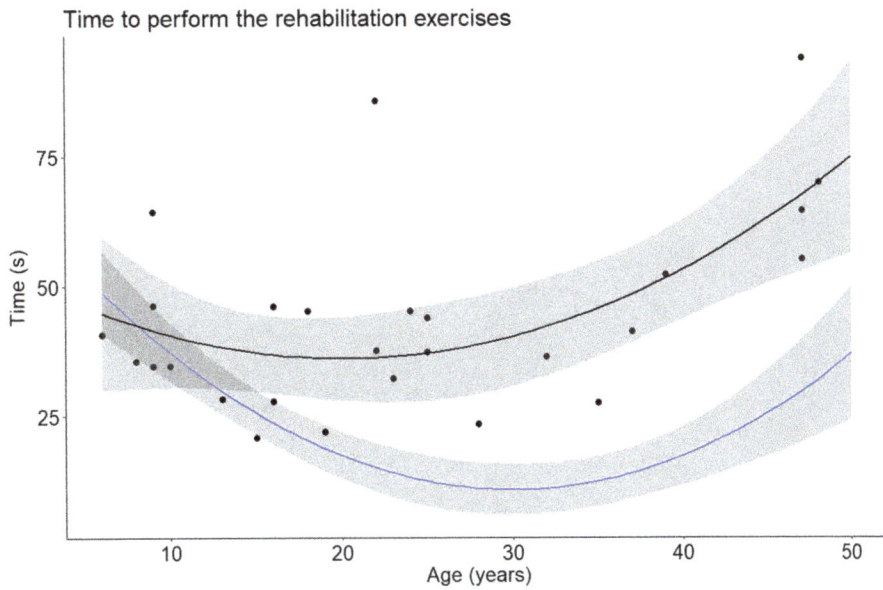

Fig. 2 Mean and 95% confidence interval (CI) of the time for healthy subjects (blue) and patient results (black). Black dots represent individual results of the patients

Concerning the comparison with the genetic analysis statistically significant correlations were found between the parameters extracted from the SG (DOT, RMS_{ML}, RMS_{TD} and R_{ML}) and GAA-1.

Discussion

During the course of FRDA, patients gradually become unable to stand and walk. Therefore, it is essential that an upper limb coordination test like SG can be performed with the patient seated in a wheelchair. Although previous studies reported some limitations of the Kinect sensor to measure upper limb joint angles of patients in wheelchairs [23], this study demonstrates it is feasible to combine rehabilitation exercises and functional evaluation of FRDA patients, even the more disabled ones.

The first aim of this study was to determine if functional analysis performed with the SG can be used to differentiate

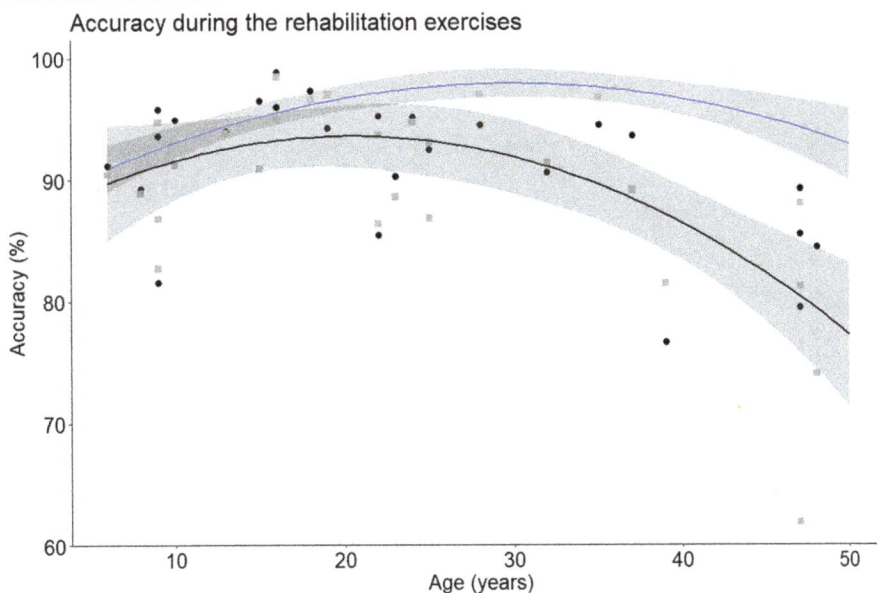

Fig. 3 Mean and 95% CI of the accuracy for healthy subjects (blue) and patient results (black). Black dots (right side) and grey squares (left side) represent individual results of the patients. Since no statistically significant difference were found between right and left side mean of the two sides was used for the fitting

Table 2 Mean (std) results for patients and control

Variables	Patients ($n = 27$)	Control ($n = 43$)	T-test	Difference [95% CI]
Time (s)	44 (18)	25 (15)	$t(68) = 7.22$, $P < 0.001$	19 [12; 29]
Accuracy (%)	88 (7)	94 (6)	$t(68) = 3.69$, $P < 0.001$	6 [3; 9]
DOT (cm)	1462 (664)	1150 (350)	$t(68) = 2.24$, $P = 0.026$	312 [40; 583]
Area (cm^2)	1421 (913)	1278 (576)	$t(68) = 0.74$, $P = 0.458$	143 [− 242; 528]
RMS$_{ML}$ (cm)	10 (3)	8 (4)	$t(68) = 2.38$, $P = 0.018$	2 [0.3; 3.7]
RMS$_{TD}$ (cm)	7 (3)	5 (2)	$t(68) = 3.06$, $P = 0.003$	2 [0.7; 3.3]
R$_{ML}$ (cm)	55 (11)	48 (8)	$t(68) = 2.86$, $P = 0.005$	7 [2.2; 11.8]
R$_{TD}$ (cm)	44 (10)	39 (7)	$t(68) = 2.27$, $P = 0.024$	5 [0.7; 9.3]
MV$_{ML}$ (cm/s)	38 (16)	56 (10)	$t(68) = 5.23$, $P < 0.001$	18 [13; 24]
MV$_{TD}$ (cm/s)	33 (14)	53 (9)	$t(68) = 6.61$, $P < 0.001$	20 [14; 26]
TMV (cm/s)	57 (20)	81 (10)	$t(68) = 5.19$, $P < 0.001$	26 [16; 32]

P-value is the results of T-tests

patient and healthy subjects. Statistically significant differences were obtained for most of the studied parameters except for the area ($p = 0.37$) indicating that the patients stay within an acceptable range in the limits of the screen. By separately analyzing the two components (medio-lateral and top-down) of motion we observed that the difference is due to a too large amplitude in the ML direction whereas there is no difference at the TD level.

Figures 2 and 3 show that until the age of 20 patients seem to remain in the confidence interval of the control group, differences only appeared later in the course of the disease. Similar trends were found for all parameters. In order to better visualize this phenomenon, results were normalized and expressed as a percentage of control group values. In Fig. 4 results are plotted according to disease duration. There was a statistically significant correlation between disease duration and decreased speed ($R = 0.64$, $p = 0.002$). Interestingly, the decrease in speed was associated with a significant reduction of accuracy ($R = − 0.67$, $p = 0.001$). We also analyzed the relation between speed and accuracy. For FRDA there is a higher correlation ($R = − 0.87$, $p < 0.001$) than for healthy subjects ($R = − 0.72$, $p < 0.001$). We divided the subjects according to age (bellow or above 20 years old) and plotted the results in Fig. 5. For participants aged less than 20 years the slope of the regression line was $\beta = − 1.8$, $p = 0.022$, $R^2 = 0.42$ for FRDA and $\beta = − 3.5$, $p < 0.001$, $R^2 = 0.54$ for healthy subjects. For participants older than 20 years the slope of the regression line is: $\beta = − 2.3$, $p < 0.001$, $R^2 = 0.68$ for FRDA and $\beta = − 1.4$, $p < 0.001$, $R^2 = 0.46$ for healthy subjects.

These results indicate that SG reliably captures motor impairment of FRDA patients due to cerebellar and pyramidal involvement. Results also show that functional

Table 3 Pearson's correlation coefficients (R) between scores obtained from the SG and the clinical evaluation

Variables	Time	Accuracy	DOT	Area	RMS$_{ML}$	RMS$_{TD}$	R$_{ML}$	R$_{TD}$	MV$_{ML}$	MV$_{TD}$	TMV
Age (year)	**.63****	**−.73****	**.57***	−.16	−0.04	−.20	−.06	−.20	−.16	−.20	−.41
Age of diagnosis (year)	.44	**−.64****	.28	−.10	−.23	−.12	−.18	−.36	**−.53***	**−.49***	−.19
Duration of the disease (year)	**.64****	**−.67****	**.48****	−.25	.26	.26	.32	.06	−.16	−.25	−.25
SARA score	.27	−.21	**.46***	.32	.35	.24	.32	.29	.25	.21	.21
ADL score	.13	.15	**.38**	.37	**.50***	**.59***	**.39***	**.50***	.36	.28	.28
GAA-1 number of repeats	−.18	.28	**.61***	.39	**.47***	**.58***	**.64****	.39	.26	.01	.11
9 R 1 (s)	.14	.22	**.61***	**.64***	.01	**.59***	**.50***	**.49***	**.38***	**.46***	**.41***
9 R 2 (s)	.15	.0.20	**.61***	**.63***	−.02	**.55***	**.48***	**.50***	.37	**.46***	**.41***
9 L 1 (s)	.18	**.65****	**.61***	**.51***	.36	**.59***	.41	**.48***	.30	**.40***	.32
9 L 2 (s)	−.16	0.11	**.63***	**.60***	.12	**.54***	**.43***	**.49***	.32	**.41***	.24
CCFS F score (with writing)	−.13	.29	.16	.36	−.13	.15	**−.43***	.18	**.47***	.37	**.44***
CCFS H score (without writing)	−.18	.37	.11	.33	.23	.26	.31	.19	.30	.27	.30

*Significant correlation ($P < .05$)
**Significant correlation ($P < .01$)

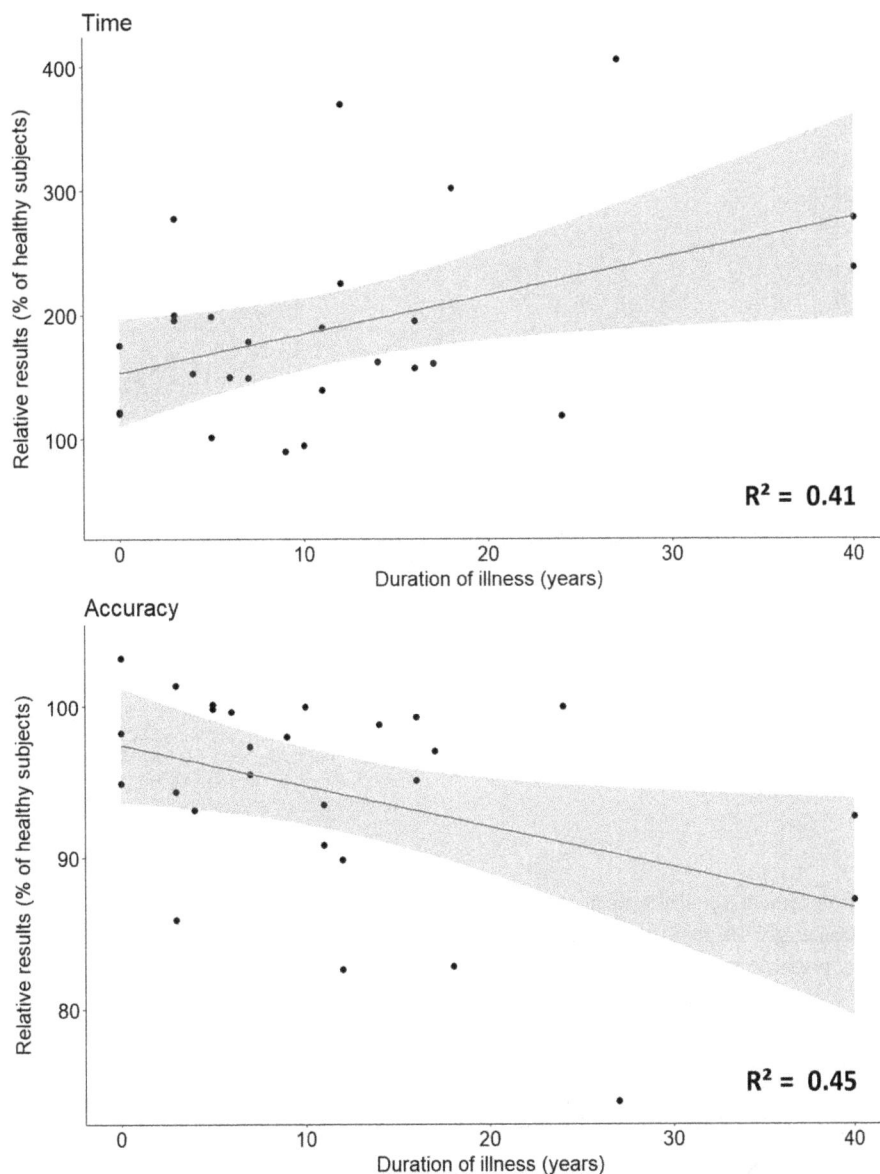

Fig. 4 Results of the time and accuracy expressed in percentage of the values of healthy subjects according to the duration of the disease. Linear fitting with 95% CI is presented with R^2

evaluation of FRDA patients can be performed during rehabilitation therapy embedded in games. Younger patients who still perform within the confidence interval of the control group are likely to have a mainly afferent ataxia due to DRG pathology, so that it is probable that their motor performance under visual control is not degraded. The fact that GAA-1 correlates with several SG parameters is in agreement with other observations that the severity of the genetic mutation not only affects the age of symptom onset, but also the subsequent rate of progression and severity of symptoms [7]. Analysis of a larger sample and prospective follow-up of patients will assess the value of SG as a potential outcome

measure for clinical trials, particularly in more advanced patients for which current evaluation tools becomes less effective with the evolution of the disease.

One limitation of this study is that only one session of measurement has been done, because patients only come once a year to the hospital for the EFACTS follow-up. Therefore, longitudinal studies are needed to determine the reproducibility of measurements and the influence of training, habituation or fatigue on the results.

Finally, the last point is to integrate these solutions into patients' home to motivate them to perform the rehabilitation exercises. In addition to this aspect of

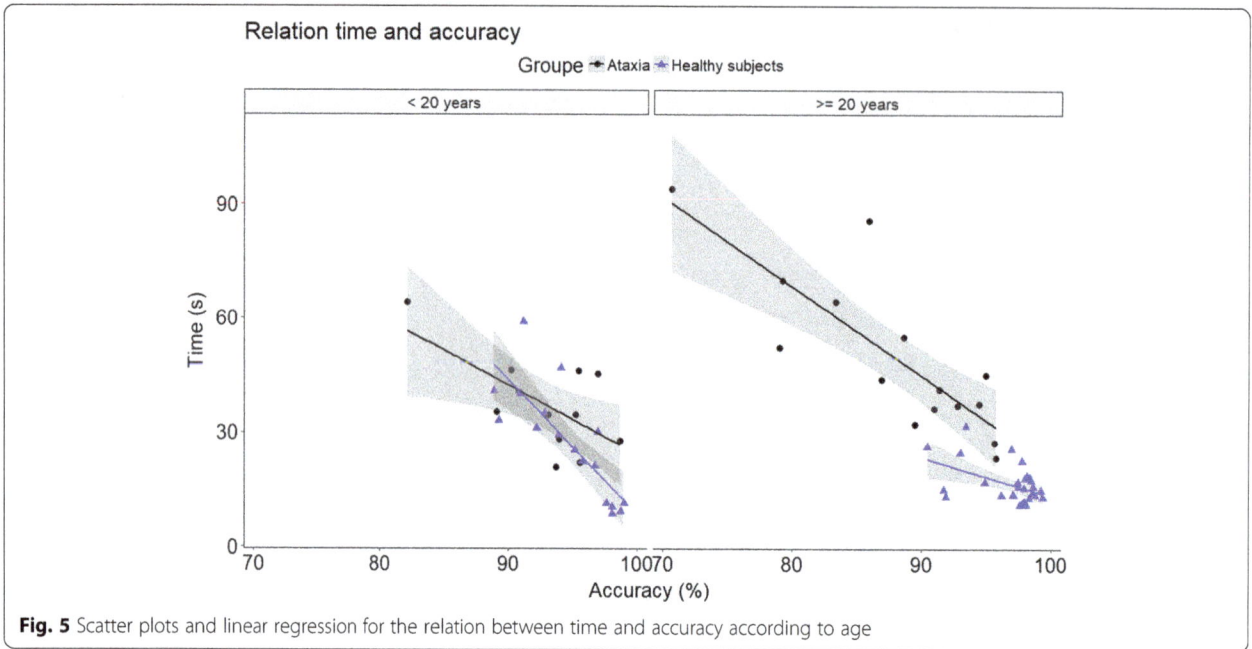

Fig. 5 Scatter plots and linear regression for the relation between time and accuracy according to age

motivation these kinds of solutions allow and evaluation of the quality of the rehabilitation exercise and thus a longitudinal follow-up for both patients and clinicians.

Conclusion

The use of new technologies in rehabilitation, including SG, is becoming increasingly important. In this study demonstrated that it is possible to combine rehabilitation exercises using SG and automated upper limb functional assessment in FRDA patients in wheelchairs. Future works are needed to determine if such kind of solution can be successfully integrated in the rehabilitation program and whether the kind of data presented in this paper can be used to predict disease progression.

Acknowledgements
We extend our deepest thanks to all the participants who participated in this study. Thanks to Mrs. Alaerts and Fadel for their technical assistance.

Funding
This study is a part of the ICT4Rehab and RehabGoesHome projects (www.ict4rehab.org). Those projects were funded by Innoviris (Brussels Capital Region).

Authors' contributions
BB, BJ and SVSJ were responsible for the conception and design of the study. MP performed clinical investigations and acquired clinical data. BB and IH performed rehabilitation exercises using SG. The data were analyzed by BB and VF. BB drafted the report and MP, LO, BJ, VF and SVSJ provided substantial input to the first draft. BB created the figures. All authors reviewed the manuscript and give final approval of the version to be submitted. The study was supervised by MP.

Competing interest
The authors declares that they have no competing interest.

Author details
[1]Laboratory of Anatomy, Biomechanics and Organogenesis (LABO) [CP 619], Université Libre de Bruxelles, Lennik Street 808, 1070 Brussels, Belgium. [2]Department of Electronics and Informatics – ETRO, Vrije Universiteit Brussel, Brussels, Belgium. [3]imec, Leuven, Belgium. [4]Laboratory of Functional Anatomy (LAF), Université Libre de Bruxelles, Brussels, Belgium. [5]Department of Neurology, Erasme Hospital, Brussels, Belgium.

References
1. Harding AE. Friedreich's ataxia: a clinical and genetic study of 90 families with an analysis of early diagnostic criteria and intrafamilial clustering of clinical features. Brain. 1981;104:589–620.
2. Koeppen AH. Friedreich's ataxia: pathology, pathogenesis, and molecular genetics. J Neurol Sci. 2011;303:1–12.
3. Schmitz-Hübsch T, Montcel du ST, Baliko L, Berciano J, Boesch S, Depondt C, et al. Scale for the assessment and rating of ataxia: development of a new clinical scale. Neurology. 2006;66:1717–20.
4. Subramony SH, May W, Lynch D, Gomez C, Fischbeck K, Hallett M, et al. Measuring Friedreich ataxia: interrater reliability of a neurologic rating scale. Neurology. 2005;64:1261–2.
5. Metz G, Coppard N, Cooper JM, Delatycki MB, Dürr A, Di Prospero NA, et al. Rating disease progression of Friedreich's ataxia by the international cooperative Ataxia rating scale: analysis of a 603-patient database. Brain. 2013;136:259–68.

6. Reetz K, Dogan I, Costa AS, Dafotakis M, Fedosov K, Giunti P, et al. Biological and clinical characteristics of the European Friedreich's Ataxia consortium for translational studies (EFACTS) cohort: a cross-sectional analysis of baseline data. Lancet Neurol. 2015;14:174–82.

7. Reetz K, Dogan I, Hilgers R-D, Giunti P, Mariotti C, Dürr A, et al. Progression characteristics of the European Friedreich's Ataxia consortium for translational studies (EFACTS): a 2 year cohort study. Lancet Neurol. 2016;15:1346–54.

8. Bonnechère B, Jansen B, Omelina L, Degelaen M, Wermenbol V, Rooze M, et al. Can serious games be incorporated with conventional treatment of children with cerebral palsy? A review. Res Dev Disabil. 2014;35:1899–913.

9. Putrino D. Telerehabilitation and emerging virtual reality approaches to stroke rehabilitation. Curr Opin Neurol. 2014;27:631–6.

10. Arias P, Robles-García V, Sanmartín G, Flores J, Cudeiro J Virtual reality as a tool for evaluation of repetitive rhythmic movements in the elderly and Parkinson's disease patients Ross O, editor PLoS ONE 2012;7:e30021.

11. Antón D, Goñi A, Illarramendi A. Exercise recognition for Kinect-based telerehabilitation. Methods Inf Med Schattauer GmbH. 2015;54:145–55.

12. van Dooren M, Visch V, Spijkerman R, Goossens R, Hendriks V. Personalization in game Design for Healthcare: a literature review on its definitions and effects. IJSG. 2016;3:3–25.

13. Omelina L, Jansen B, Bonnechère B, Van Sint Jan S, Cornelis J. Serious games for physical rehabilitation: Designing highly configurable and adaptable games. Proceedings. Ninth international conference on disability, virtual reality and associated technologies. Laval. 2012. pp. 195–201.

14. van Diest M, Stegenga J, Wörtche HJ, Postema K, Verkerke GJ, Lamoth CJC. Suitability of Kinect for measuring whole body movement patterns during exergaming. J Biomech. 2014;47:2925–32.

15. Bonnechère B, Sholukha V, Omelina L, Van Vooren M, Jansen B, Van Sint Jan S. Suitability of functional evaluation embedded in serious game rehabilitation exercises to assess motor development across lifespan. Gait Posture. 2017;57:35–9.

16. Bonnechère B, Sholukha V, Omelina L, Van Sint Jan S, Jansen B. 3D analysis of upper limbs motion during rehabilitation exercises using the Kinect™ sensor: development, laboratory validation and clinical application. Sensors. 2018;18:2216.

17. Pandolfo M. Friedreich ataxia: detection of GAA repeat expansions and frataxin point mutations. Methods Mol Med. 2006;126:197–216.

18. Schmitz-Hübsch T, Coudert M, Bauer P, Giunti P, Globas C, Baliko L, et al. Spinocerebellar ataxia types 1, 2, 3, and 6: disease severity and nonataxia symptoms. Neurology. 2008;71:982–9.

19. Tanguy Melac A, Mariotti C, Filipovic Pierucci A, Giunti P, Arpa J, Boesch S, et al. Friedreich and dominant ataxias: quantitative differences in cerebellar dysfunction measurements. J. Neurol. Neurosurg. Psychiatr. 2017;:jnnp–2017-316964.

20. Bonnechère B, Jansen B, Omelina L, Sholukha V, Van Sint Jan S. Validation of the balance Board for Clinical Evaluation Balance during serious gaming rehabilitation exercices. J E Health. 2016;22(9):709–17.

21. Trewartha KM, Garcia A, Wolpert DM, Flanagan JR. Fast but fleeting: adaptive motor learning processes associated with aging and cognitive decline. J Neurosci. 2014;34:13411–21.

22. Teulier C, Lee DK, Ulrich BD. Early gait development in human infants: plasticity and clinical applications. Brumley MR, editor Dev Psychobiol Wiley-Blackwell; 2015;57:447–458.

23. Hwang S, Tsai C-Y, Koontz AM. Feasibility study of using a Microsoft Kinect for virtual coaching of wheelchair transfer techniques. Biomed Tech (Berl). 2017;62:307–13.

13

Exploiting the heightened phase synchrony in patients with neuromuscular disease for the establishment of efficient motor imagery BCIs

Kostas Georgiadis[1,2]* ⓘ, Nikos Laskaris[1,3], Spiros Nikolopoulos[2] and Ioannis Kompatsiaris[2]

Abstract

Background: Phase synchrony has extensively been studied for understanding neural coordination in health and disease. There are a few studies concerning the implications in the context of BCIs, but its potential for establishing a communication channel in patients suffering from neuromuscular disorders remains totally unexplored. We investigate, here, this possibility by estimating the time-resolved phase connectivity patterns induced during a motor imagery (MI) task and adopting a supervised learning scheme to recover the subject's intention from the streaming data.

Methods: Electroencephalographic activity from six patients suffering from neuromuscular disease (NMD) and six healthy individuals was recorded during two randomly alternating, externally cued, MI tasks (clenching either left or right fist) and a rest condition. The metric of Phase locking value (PLV) was used to describe the functional coupling between all recording sites. The functional connectivity patterns and the associate network organization was first compared between the two cohorts. Next, working at the level of individual patients, we trained support vector machines (SVMs) to discriminate between "left" and "right" based on different instantiations of connectivity patterns (depending on the encountered brain rhythm and the temporal interval). Finally, we designed and realized a novel brain decoding scheme that could interpret the intention from streaming connectivity patterns, based on an ensemble of SVMs.

Results: The group-level analysis revealed increased phase synchrony and richer network organization in patients. This trend was also seen in the performance of the employed classifiers. Time-resolved connectivity led to superior performance, with distinct SVMs acting as local experts, specialized in the patterning emerged within specific temporal windows (defined with respect to the external trigger). This empirical finding was further exploited in implementing a decoding scheme that can be activated without the need of the precise timing of a trigger.

Conclusion: The increased phase synchrony in NMD patients can turn to a valuable tool for MI decoding. Considering the fast implementation for the PLV pattern computation in multichannel signals, we can envision the development of efficient personalized BCI systems in assistance of these patients.

Keywords: Phase synchrony, Chronnectomic patterns, BCI, Classifier-ensembles

* Correspondence: georgiaki@csd.auth.gr
[1]AIIA lab, Informatics Department, AUTH, Thessaloniki, Greece
[2]Information Technologies Institute (ITI), Centre for Research & Technology Hellas, Thessaloniki-Thermi, Greece
Full list of author information is available at the end of the article

Background

According to World Health Organization (WHO) approximately 15% of the global population experiences some kind of disability with a 2–4% being reported as severe.[1] Brain Computer Interfaces (BCIs) receive continuous attention as an emerging technology for rehabilitation and restoration of communication in people with disabilities. BCIs create a communication channel between the brain and machines, such as computers, as they "translate" brain signals into machine commands without requiring any muscle or peripheral nerve activity [1, 2]. The idea of "mind reading" was first conceived by Berger [3], but only in the past few years BCI implementations were made plausible. BCIs can be implemented with various approaches, but electroencephalography (EEG) has been proven to be the most popular choice due to its non-invasiveness, low cost and advantage of being employed with minimal effort even in home environments.

EEG-based BCIs can be categorized as exogenous or endogenous depending on whether external stimulation is provided to the user. Event-related (evoked) potential, ERP(EP), BCIs belong to the exogenous BCIs as the brain activation is measured after a specific event (or delivered stimulus). Most often visual stimuli are encountered, since they are more naturally perceived, with the most notable examples being transient [4], code-modulated [5] and steady-state [6, 7] visual responses to flickering patterns. While exogenous BCIs achieve high performance, their design inherently contradicts with the perspective of asynchronous (i.e. self-paced) BCIs, and this is the main reason why endogenous BCIs currently receive significant attention, even though a considerable training period, that can last from a couple of days to several months, is required for the user before harnessing such a system. The most prominent paradigm of endogenous BCIs is the one that requires the user to perform a mental task, including movement imagination of limb(s) or even tongue [8–12], speech imagination [13, 14] and mental arithmetic [15, 16]. In the case of movement imagination, called hereafter motor imagery (MI), particularly, brain decoding usually relies on the sensorimotor rhythm (SMR) detected in the EEG signal from the electrodes located over the sensory-motor cortex, the part of the brain that is associated with planning, control and execution of voluntary movements [17].

MI related modulations in brain activity, associated with both μ and β rhythms over the sensorimotor areas are often reported in EEG studies and the approach of event-related desynchronization/synchronization (ERD/ERS) that estimates the power increase/decrease during the MI task or once it is completed, has been developed to capture them [18–20]. A second popular approach is the technique of common spatial patterns (CSPs) [21]

and its alternatives [22–25], where spatial filtering is combined with classification so as to decode the intended movement. Signal-amplitude characteristics, derived in the time domain, are exploited in all these approaches. Phase synchrony has recently entered into the picture and led to novel alternative ways in decoding an indented movement by describing the functional inter-areal interactions during MI [26, 27]. The metric of phase locking value (PLV) is usually employed and features from either the static or dynamic connectivity patterns, as they emerge over the sensor space, have been demonstrated to facilitate the effective decoding of user's intentions [28, 29].

In the related literature of MI-BCIs, there are only a few studies that deal with the option of a self-initiated motion. In two of them, Scherer et al. [30] and Chae et al. [31], a two-stage classification scheme is adopted. The first stage takes over the detection of (the onset of) an MI-event, while the second stage performs the final read out (i.e. the direction of the movement). Additionally, a "brain switch" has been implemented based on the β rhythm rebound (i.e. ERS) that appears at the end of a particular MI event. Either a simple thresholding scheme [32] or linear discriminant analysis [33] is employed to flag a significant departure from the ongoing activity that corresponds to an "idling" (baseline) state. Once an MI event is detected, the associated command is given to the actuator.

The above mentioned MI-BCI approaches have been investigated in several studies with participants suffering from motor disabilities, including amyotrophic lateral sclerosis (ALS) [34, 35], spinal cord injury (SCI) [36, 37], multiple sclerosis (MS) [38, 39] and chronic strokes (CS) [40, 41]. However, only a limited number of studies have been done on people suffering from neuromuscular disease (NMD) [42]. In contrast with SCI and CS, NMD is a progressive condition that often initiates with the affection of specific group of muscles and finally spreads to many other groups, resulting in gradual loss of a patient's fine motor skills. Therefore, significant mental effort is required by the patients to make a move or even attempt to move their limbs in their everyday life for several years, prior to the complete loss of their movement control. In this direction, the initial motivation of this study was to examine how NMD-patients, as novice BCI users, would perform in simple MI tasks (imagination of left/right hand movement) without any training and/or feedback. We hypothesized that, due to long-lasting self-organization, phase synchrony would govern their re-configured brain networks and could be detected in the sensor space when they were cued to imagine a limb movement (which for them is almost equivalent to try to realize the same movement).

The contribution of this paper is threefold. We first show that NMD patients are characterized by increased level of both phase-synchrony and network organization with respect to healthy controls. Next, we demonstrate a nearly optimal performance for a decoding scheme that exploits, in a personalized fashion, the connectivity patterns emerging during cued imaginary movement. Finally, we describe a novel algorithmic procedure that could adapt the proposed decoding scheme for a self-paced BCI scenario and provide a "proof-of-concept" using the available data. Besides the documented effectiveness, our proposal is supported by the computational efficiency of the adopted PLV implementation (see Appendix).

Methods

Participants

A total of twelve individuals (7 males and 5 females, aged 36.08 ± 6.45) participated in this study, separated into two groups. More specifically, the first group consists of six people suffering from NMD and the second of six able-bodied with a matching socio-demographic profile. Table 1 provides information about each participant, while a more detailed description (e.g. inclusion criteria, clinical characteristics) can be found in [43]. All subjects had normal or corrected-to-normal vision and none of them had taken any psycho-active or psycho-tropic substance. Participants had no prior experience with SMR protocols, or any other BCI protocol. Prior to the experimental session, subjects and their caretakers were informed about the experimental procedure. A consent form, thoroughly read, was signed by the participants or in cases of inability by their caretakers. The experimental protocol was approved by the Ethical Committee of MDA HELLAS.

Experimental environment

During the experimental procedure, participants were seated in a comfortable armchair placed 50 cm from a 22-in. Liquid Crystal Display with the EEG cap attached on their scalp. In cases where subjects used a wheelchair, appropriate modifications were made to make them feel as comfortable as possible. Throughout the entire process, subjects were instructed to place both hands in the armrests and to minimize any kind of upper limb movement in order to minimize the artifactual activity.

Experimental design

The experimental procedure required the subjects to imagine the movement of their left or right hand. Prior to the MI task, a 3 min recording of resting state was realized. The cue for the initiation of movement imagination was given by a red arrow (onset), appearing either on the left or right side of the screen, pointing in the same direction and indicating the corresponding imagery movement. The arrow remained on the screen for approximately 5 s, indicating the continuation of movement imagination to the subject. Once the arrow disappeared from the screen, subjects could rest and prepare themselves for the next arrow appearance. Prior to the arrow presentation, a fixation cross was displayed on the screen for 3 s, indicating the beginning of a new trial. Figure 1 illustrates the sequence of events during a single trial. The experimental session was divided in two sub-sessions performed during the same day, each one consisting of 20 random arrow appearances, equally distributed among the two classes, resulting in 40 trials (20 for each imagery movement class). Between the two sessions subjects had the opportunity to rest for five to 10 min. *OpenVibe*,[2] a free and open-source platform was used to design the experimental protocol and to synchronize the EEG recording with the timestamps from the visual triggers.

EEG recording

The brain activity was recorded, with a sampling frequency of 256 Hz, using the BePlusLTM Bioelectric Signal Amplifier,[3] an EEG scanner with $61 + 2$ (ground and reference) electrodes placed according to the 10–10 International System. Using an electro-conductive cream, the impedance for all electrodes was set bellow $10K\Omega$ before beginning the recording in every session.

Table 1 Subject Demographics

Able-bodied subjects			NMD patients			
Participant ID	Gender	Age	Participant ID	Gender	Age	Condition
S1	F	46	P1	M	35	SMA III
S2	F	31	P2	M	44	Muscular Dystrophy
S3	M	40	P3	M	32	Muscular Dystrophy Type II
S4	M	43	P4	F	36	Tunesian Muscular Dystrophy
S5	F	39	P5	M	25	Duchene Muscular Dystrophy
S6	M	29	P6	F	33	Tunesian Muscular Dystrophy

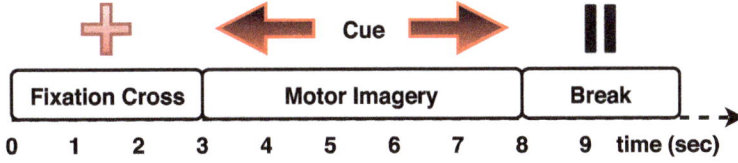

Fig. 1 The timeline of the experimental procedure (depicted for a single-trial)

Pre-processing

During the offline processing, the EEG signals were band-pass filtered within (0.5–45 Hz) with a third-order Butterworth filter (applied in zero-phase filtering mode), prior to the trial segmentation so as to avoid edge effects. The segmentation process resulted in 20 trials for each MI task (left and right) and 20 trials for the resting state. Using a procedure based on spectral analysis and working for each subject independently "bad" sensors were identified visually and excluded from further analysis. It is important to stress out here than on average no more than 5 sensors were rejected and the remaining ("good") ones, denoted hereby as N_{sensor} ($56 \leq N_{sensor} \leq 61$), were employed in the subsequent average re-reference procedure. Independent component analysis (ICA) [44] was then used as a means to reduce artifacts that usually arise from eyes, muscles or cardiac pulse. Using a semi-supervised procedure that employed the ranking of independent components (ICs), based on kurtosis /skewness and the visual inspection of their spectra and topographies, artifactual components were identified and removed before reconstructing the multichannel single-trial data. For the purposes of this work, seven commonly used EEG frequency bands were defined: δ (1–4) Hz; θ (4–8) Hz; $\alpha1$ (8–10) Hz; $\alpha2$ (10–13) Hz; $\beta1$ (13–20) Hz; $\beta2$ (20–30) Hz; γ (30–45) Hz and the neural activity of each brain rhythm was examined independently. Once again, band-pass filtering was implemented via third-order Butterworth filters, applied in zero-phase mode.

PLV-measurements and functional connectivity patterns

Phase synchronization is a well-established concept for describing the coordinated function of distinct neural assemblies based on the recorded signals. When studied at the level of sensor space, the brain signals recorded at distinct sites are used (by one of the available estimators) to detect whether the relative phases of the underlying oscillatory processes bear any systematic relation across time. The Phase Locking Value (PLV) measurement, introduced by Lachaux et al. [45], is a very popular estimator of phase synchrony, with the great advantage of computational simplicity that motivated its use in the context of MI-BCIs. Considered as a function, PLV gets as input two signal traces and outputs a scalar ranging between 0 and 1, with 1 indicating the functionally

coupling between the brain areas associated with the signals and 0 indicating functional independence. Given a pair of single-trial signals $x_k(t)$ $x_r(t)$, with $k,r = 1...N_{sensor}$ and $t = t_1... t_2$, from distinct recording sites, PLV is estimated as follows:

$$PLV(x_k, x_r) = \frac{1}{t_2-t_1} \left| \sum_{t_1}^{t_2} \exp(i \, \Delta\phi(t)) \right| \quad (1)$$

with $\Delta\phi(t) = \phi_k(t)-\phi_r(t)$ denoting the difference between the instantaneous phases of the two processes and discrete time parameter t running along the latencies of interest (for instance the 5 s interval during the presentation of an arrow on the screen). Each phase signal $\phi_k(t)$ is derived by applying the Hilbert transform to the corresponding band-limited brain activity $x_k(t)$. In our implementation, the PLV computations extend to every pair of sensors, by efficiently parallelizing the computations implied by eq.(1), as shown in Appendix. In this way, for each frequency band, an $[N_{sensor} \times N_{sensor}]$ matrix is formed with entries $W_{kr} = PLV(x_k,x_r)$. Adopting the popular perspective of complex networks, this matrix is treated as a weighted adjacency matrix $\mathbf{W}$ encapsulating the connectivity pattern of a graph that spans the sensor space and reflects the brain's functional organization. Considering the symmetry in PLV measurements, $PLV(x_k,x_r) = PLV(x_r,x_k)$ and the fact that all diagonal elements W_{kk} equal 1, it is easy to realize that a more economical description of a connectivity pattern can be obtained by vectorizing the upper triangular part of W, i.e. gathering all $\frac{N_{sensor} \times (N_{sensor}-1)}{2}$ elements W_{kr} with $r < k$ in a single vector, denoted as vec($\mathbf{W}$).

Network metrics

The functional connectivity graph defined by $\mathbf{W}$ matrix, with nodes the recording sites and edges the links between the sites weighed by the associated pairwise PLV values, can be characterized based on network topology metrics [46, 47]. In our study, the network characterization was based on weighted graphs and aimed at revealing the self-organization tendencies of the underlying cortical network and contrasting them between healthy and NMD condition. Towards this end, the following three well-known metrics were estimated and compared between recording conditions (rest vs MI), as well as, physiological states (health vs NMD).

Strength equals to the sum of connectivity weights attached to a given node. It may serve, approximately, as a centrality measure, indicating the importance of the associated brain region within the observed network organization:

$$S_k = \sum_{r \neq k} w_{kr} \quad (2)$$

Global/Local Efficiency is a metric which expresses how efficiently information is transferred via the network, at a global/local level. Network's efficiency is directly linked with the concept of *shortest paths*, which in our case were estimated after turning the functional coupling strengths w_{kr} to pairwise distances $d_{kr} = 1 - w_{kr}$ and applying the Dijkstra's algorithm. Adopting the formulation of global efficiency (GE) as defined in (Latora and Marchiori [48]):

$$GE = \frac{1}{N_{sensors}(N_{sensors}-1)} \sum_{k,r \neq k} \frac{1}{l_{rk}} \quad (3)$$

with l_{rk} denoting the length of shortest path between nodes (i.e. sensors) r and k.

Local efficiency (LE) is estimated by first restricting the above computations to each subgraph G_k, containing the neighbors of a node k, and then integrating across nodes:

$$
\begin{aligned}
LE &= \frac{1}{N_{sensors}} \sum_{r \neq k} LE(k) \\
&= \frac{1}{N_{sensors}} \sum_{r \neq k} \frac{1}{N_{G_k}(N_{G_k}-1)} \sum_{i,j \in G_k} \frac{1}{l_{ij}} \quad (4)
\end{aligned}
$$

Time-indexed patterns of functional connectivity

In an attempt to track more precisely the dynamics of cortical self-organization during MI, we derived multiple instantiations of the connectivity pattern for each single-trial, by means of a stepping window that confined the integration in eq. (1) within successive (overlapping) temporal segments. The width of window, T_{window}, was defined according to the "cycle-criterion" (CC) [49, 50], that adapts the temporal resolution so as 3 cycles from the lowest frequency of the band-limited brain signal to be included at each step along the time-axis.[4] In this way, a sequence vec($\mathbf{W}[\tau]$), $\tau = 1,2...N_\tau$ was derived that encapsulated the evolving functional connectivity during a single event of hand movement imagination. This sequence is indexed via discrete variable τ, differing from the original time variable t of the signals, to indicate that a lower temporal resolution may be utilized for reducing computational burden and memory storage. The motivation for analyzing the dynamics of connectivity patterns stemmed from previous studies, which had demonstrated that transiently formed couplings during MI [34, 35], may be useful for brain decoding.

Feature screening

The number N_{pairs} of features corresponding to the derived PLV measurements was high. This number was ranging from 1596 to 1830, depending on the number of "bad"

sensors, in the case of "static" connectivity patterns, where one vector vec([$\mathbf{W}$]) was assigned to each single trial. This number had to be multiplied by the number of employed steps when we were dealing with time-indexed connectivity patterns (vec($\mathbf{W}[\tau]$)). This was an extremely high number of features, relatively to the small number of available trials. Apart from the theoretical issues raised by the "curse of dimensionality", it was clear that not all possible couplings would carry highly discriminative information useful for the task of decoding left from right MI [51]. For this reason, we resorted to a "filter" approach for selecting features. Specifically, we utilized the Matlab's *rankfeatures*[5] command (with the option of "Wilcoxon" criterion), so as to rank the features (coupling strengths or time-resolved coupling strengths between pair of recording sites) and select the most reliable ones to participate in the subsequent design of a classifier.

More specifically, in the case of static connectivity patterns the operation of this command, denoted as follows

$$
\begin{aligned}
Score(r) = rankfeatures\ (\ &\left\{ vec\left({}^{left}\mathbf{W}^i \right) \right\}_{i=1:N_{trials}}, \\
&\left\{ vec\left({}^{right}\mathbf{W}^j \right) \right\}_{j=1:N_{trials}}), \\
&r = 1, 2...N_{pairs} \quad (5)
\end{aligned}
$$

resulted in a vector of scores reflecting the relative discriminative power of each coupling. Feature selection was accomplished by identifying the set of 10 most discriminative couplings.

For the case of time-indexed connectivity, we adopted a distinct procedure that elaborated on the temporal patterning of the functional connectivity as this was unfolding during MI. The previous command was applied repeatedly at every latency τ of the stepping window resulting in a time-indexed score

$$
\begin{aligned}
Score(r,\tau) = rankfeatures\ (\ &\left\{ vec\left({}^{left}\mathbf{W}^i[\tau] \right) \right\}_{i=1:N_{trials}}, \\
&\left\{ vec\left({}^{right}\mathbf{W}^j[\tau] \right) \right\}_{j=1:N_{trials}}), \quad (6) \\
&\tau = 1, 2..., N_\tau
\end{aligned}
$$

To identify the most important features among the ($N_{pairs} \cdot N_\tau$) available ones, a permutation test was applied. The available connectivity patterns from "left" and "right" trials were randomly partitioned, several times, into two groups and the computations implied by eq.(7) were repeated for every random splitting. The computed $\{{}^{rand}Score(r,\tau)\}_{1:Nrand}$ measurements were used to form a "baseline" distribution of scores associated with the random case, where no differences between imagination of a left and right hand movement would be detectable. From the formed distribution, the value of

Score-index corresponding to the margin of 99.9% was identified and utilized as a threshold, **thr$_{99.9\%}$**, that was applied to the actual Score(r,τ) measurements so as to keep only the statistical significant couplings (*p*-value < 0.001). After this trimming step that zeroed most of the measurements, a sparse matrix appeared that contained some spurious entries (associated with couplings that occasionally become significant for short lasting intervals). An additional data-sieving step (based on simple rowwise median filtering) was applied that eliminated most of them. The rationale behind this last step was the detection of couplings that could be considered as both "useful" and "stable" regarding their discriminatory power. Such a reinforcement of consistency in time was motivated by the need for an economical decoding procedure and the possibility of making it functional without knowing the absolute timing (as it will be explained later). A pair-dependent profile was derived by the sequence of these operation as shown below, where the operator H(·) denotes Heaviside step function operator and $\mathbf{1^N}$ is column-vector of N ones.

$$I(r,t) = H(\ Score(r,\tau) - \mathbf{thr_{99.9\%}}),$$
$$r = 1, 2, ... Npairs\ , t = 1, 2, ... N\tau$$

$$\hat{I}_{[\,N_{pairs} \times N_\tau\,]} = runningMedian_{rowwise}(I)$$

$$Profile(r) = \hat{I}.\mathbf{1}^{N_\tau} \qquad (7)$$

Finally, feature selection was accomplished by detecting the non-zero entries in this profile. A demonstration of this sequence of algorithmic steps can be seen in Fig. 2.

SVM-classifiers as MI-direction decoders

Support Vector Machines (SVMs) constitute a family of well-established classification algorithms [52], that is very popular among BCI practitioners [53, 54]. In the basic binary formulation, the training algorithm of SVM is designed to determine the optimal hyper-plane that separates two classes, while maximizing the margin between them. It selects the single hyperplane that guarantees optimal generalization, meaning that it can cope better with new (unseen) data. The class of an unseen pattern is determined based on its relative position with respect to the learned hyperplane, while a confidence level for this decision can be estimated by considering its distance to the hyperplane [55]. For the purposes of this study, a linear hyper-plane was selected for the MI-direction decoding as it provided satisfactory results at low computational load (a combination of high importance for online implementations). In all cases

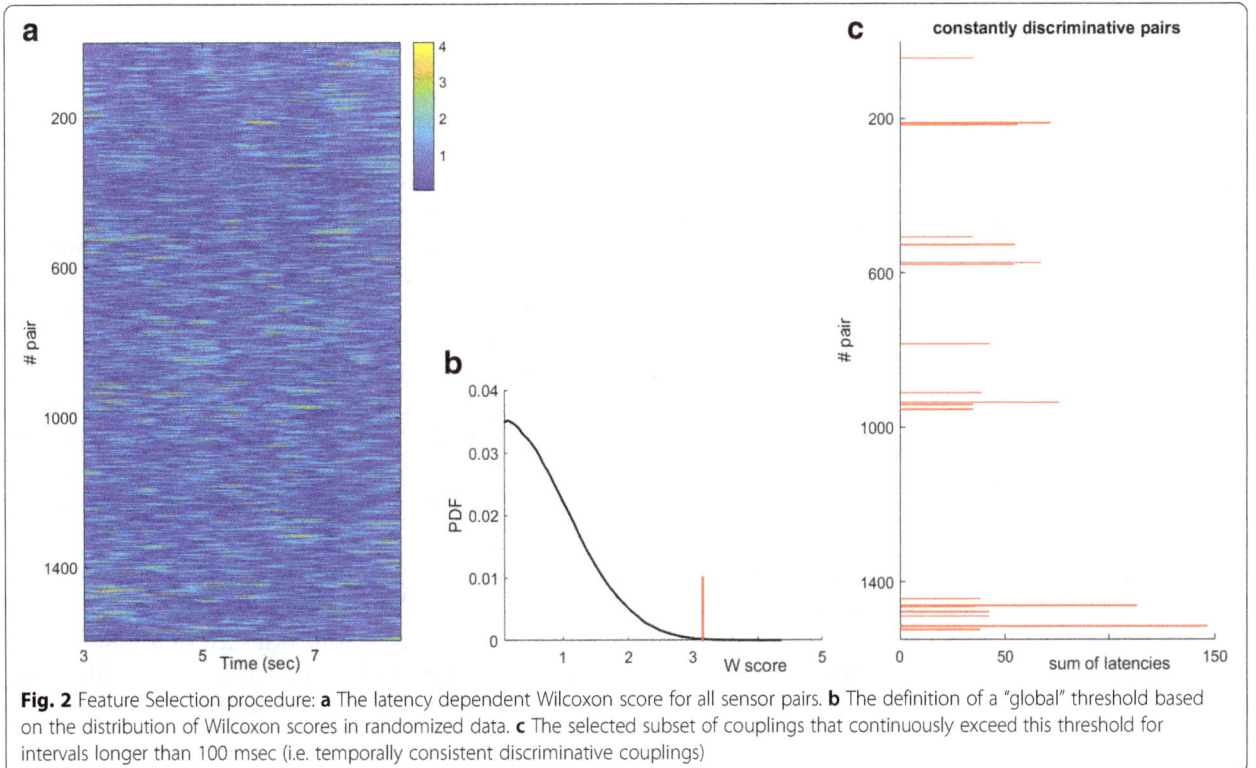

Fig. 2 Feature Selection procedure: **a** The latency dependent Wilcoxon score for all sensor pairs. **b** The definition of a "global" threshold based on the distribution of Wilcoxon scores in randomized data. **c** The selected subset of couplings that continuously exceed this threshold for intervals longer than 100 msec (i.e. temporally consistent discriminative couplings)

reported below, SVM classification had been employed in a "personalized" mode. This trend, that ultimately led to subject-specific brain decoding, was initiated very early during the stage of feature selection. For each trial of an MI movement, the selected discriminative features (depending on subject and brain rhythm) were used to form the input pattern to be used in SVM training and validation.

The performance of the SVM-based binary classification ("left" vs "right") was measured, for each subject independently, under the two different feature-screening procedures, which in turn led to two distinct classification scenarios: one based on static and one based on "instantaneous" connectivity (sub)patterns. Classification performance was expressed in terms of accuracy, and carefully validated using a cross-validation scheme that was dependent on the scenario.

The validation and testing procedure was performed on a single-subject basis. In the reported results (with the exception of the results referred to self-paced MI), a leave-one-out-cross-validation (LOOCV) scheme had been employed to validate the accuracy of the proposed methodology. The use of LOOCV was motivated by the restricted amount of trials available (the sample was not big enough to employ other validation schemes like 70–30% training-test splitting of the dataset). In the LOOCV scheme, $2N_{trial}-1 = 39$ trials were selected as the training-set and the remaining one was used as the unknown sample that the SVM had to associate with a class. The procedure was repeated, cyclically, 40 times and the accuracy was defined based on the 40 predictions obtained from the 40 trials.

We need to clarify here that in the case of static scenario, the feature selection had been embodied in the LOOCV validation scheme (i.e. it was realized 40 times). However, this was not the case for the decoding of time-indexed connectivity patterns (vec($\mathbf{W}[\tau]$)), in which the features should show a consistency across time. In the latter case the feature selection was accomplished outside the LOOCV session of the SVM. Since the number of candidate features (pairwise couplings at multiple instances) was roughly 150 times higher than the available number of trials and therefore the danger of overfitting was even higher than in the case of static connectivity patterns we resorted to bootstrapping [56]. Having in mind to establish a procedure that could also be employed in a potential implementation of a personalized BCI, in which only a small training data-set would be available for crafting the decision function and the overall training should be completed within a reasonable time before the actual use of the BCI system, we proceeded as follows. We repeatedly form (by sampling with replacement) 30 sets of $2N_{trials}$, and the procedure described in eq.(7) was applied to every bootstrap-resample resulting in an ensemble of curves $\{^{boot\_i}Profile(r)\}_{boot\_i = 1:30}$. Feature selection was accomplished, by averaging these profiles and thresholding the obtained average curve.

An SVM-ensemble for self-paced MI decoding

The high performance of the SVM-decoders working with time-resolved connectivity patterns, vec($\mathbf{W}[\tau]$), motivated us to search for a decoding scheme that could operate without the need for an external trigger that would initiate a trial. The original idea was that a "local" SVM tailored to deal with patterns from latency τ_{sel} would show a high confidence level about its prediction only within a time-interval around that latency. Adopting this consideration, connectivity patterns could continuously feed (i.e. as streaming data) to the particular SVM and its decision would be activated only whenever a certain level of confidence was reached. While this idea seemed to work well (after trial-averaging) when applied to the available MI-trials, it had the tendency to produce false-positive detections at the level of single trials (see Fig. 3b). This led us to consider not just one "time-indexed" SVM (the earliest one with the highest performance, that would satisfy the need for a speedy response), but also a sequence of them $\{SVM^i\}$, $i = \tau_{sel\_1}, \tau_{sel\_2}\cdots, \tau_{sel\_M}$ with the scope of making more stringent the decision about detecting an MI event. Assuming a trigger-agnostic scenario, these SVMs will run in parallel resulting in a time-indexed vector $Z(\tau) = [z^1(\tau), z^2(\tau), \ldots, z^M(\tau)]^T$, with entries

$$z^i(\tau) = SVM^i(FeatureExtraction(\text{ vec}(\mathbf{W}[\tau]))),$$
$$i = \tau_{sel_1}, \tau_{sel_2}, \ldots, \tau_{sel_M} \qquad (8)$$

Each entry z^i denotes the confidence of a selected classifier multiplied by the sign of its prediction (+/– is associated with "right"/"left" movement), i.e. a real number within $[-1 \ 1]$. Deviating from the standard approaches for combining classifiers (e.g. voting), in the proposed scheme the classifiers' output are combined based on temporal patterning (that reflects their relative positioning in time, which is associated with the optimal performance in the cued trials). An "instantaneous" classification index is derived by averaging the individual signed confidences after imposing the predefined lags

$$z_{ensemble}(t) = \frac{1}{M} \sum_i^M z^i(t + \tau_{sel_i}) \qquad (9)$$

It is important to note, here, that such an SVM-ensemble formation is feasible and computational tractable, thanks to the prior selection of a unique set of "stable" couplings (via bootstrapping over a small available training set). The suggested SVM-ensemble scheme is supported by two

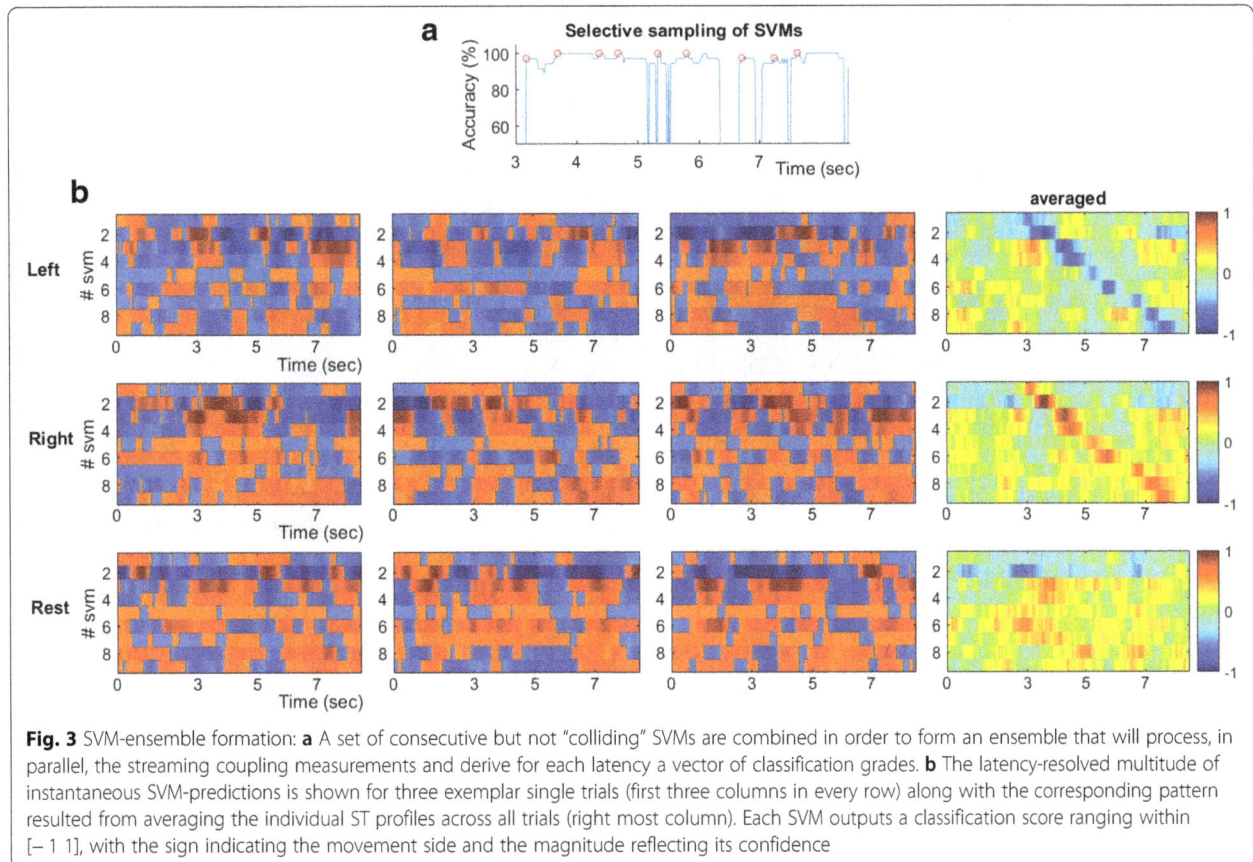

Fig. 3 SVM-ensemble formation: **a** A set of consecutive but not "colliding" SVMs are combined in order to form an ensemble that will process, in parallel, the streaming coupling measurements and derive for each latency a vector of classification grades. **b** The latency-resolved multitude of instantaneous SVM-predictions is shown for three exemplar single trials (first three columns in every row) along with the corresponding pattern resulted from averaging the individual ST profiles across all trials (right most column). Each SVM outputs a classification score ranging within [− 1 1], with the sign indicating the movement side and the magnitude reflecting its confidence

experimental observations. First, the time-indexed accuracy of the locally defined SVMs showed multiple, easy-detectable, peaks (e.g. Figure 3a). This led to an easy automation for selecting the SVMs.[6] Second, there was no pair of SVMs among the selected "local" ones in the ensemble, that showed significant similarity.[7] The latter fact means that all the selected SVMs were defining different separating-hyperplanes in the space of common features.

Results

Group analysis of pairwise couplings

The first part of our analysis was devoted to confirming the hypothesis that there were significant differences between NMD patients and controls regarding the strength of functional couplings. To this end, a single connectivity pattern was first derived (by trial-averaging) for each subject, brain rhythm and recording condition (i.e. "rest", "left", "right"). To facilitate inter-subject comparisons, all the connectivity patterns were confined to the unique set of sensors that were identified as "good" sensors in all subjects. Then, a statistical comparison of the medians (derived at group level) in every pairwise coupling of the connectivity patterns was performed. The Wilcoxon rank sum test was repeatedly applied and the results were corrected for multiple testing, by means of false discovery rate (FDR; $\alpha = 0.05$) [57]. Figure 4,

includes the obtained results for all frequency bands and recording conditions. The statistically significant ($p < 0.05$) pairs stand out as colored entries in the shown matrices. The color in these entries reflect the sign of the observed differences. It was computed based on the medians of the groups $(\text{med}(\{PLV(.)\}^{NMD}) - \text{med}(\{PLV(.)\}^{Control}))$ and clearly indicates (since only red hue is observed) an increased coupling in the patients group compared to the control group, mostly in low and high brain rhythms. It is important to mention here, that increased functional couplings was found in all frequency bands, although not clearly observed when a common color code was used. The topological representation of the statistically significant functional couplings is provided in Additional file 1: Figure S1, with the edge-width reflecting the difference in strength between the group-level medians of each pairwise coupling and the node-size the number of edges that have survived the statistical test ($p < 0.05$) and are incident to the node. It is clear, that the NMD group is characterized by enhanced connectivity even in the resting state. In the two MI-conditions, the majority of nodes being part of the statistical significant couplings follow a distributed pattern, which occasionally includes the primary and supplementary sensory-motor area (for instance, in "left": α_1, β_1 and γ rhythms).

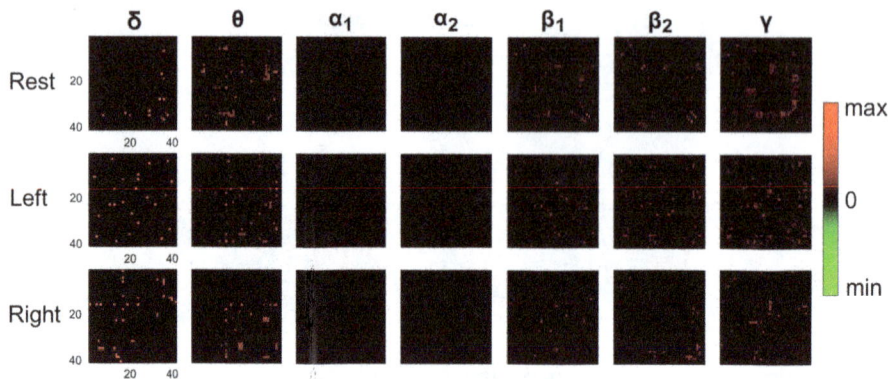

Fig. 4 The results from the statistical comparison (Group-level analysis) of averaged connectivity patterns between patients and controls. Each pairwise coupling was compared independently, for every band and recording condition, by means of Wilcoxon rank sum and the significant ones ($p < 0.05$; corrected for multiple comparisons) are indicated as non-zeroed entries of a "connectivity matrix", with a color code that encapsulates the difference in strength (of the median values in the corresponding groups). Red hue has to be interpreted as higher coupling in patients and green hue as higher coupling in controls, while color intensity reflects the strength of this effect. The absence of green hue in the diagrams clearly indicates the increased coupling in patients group compared to the control group

Group analysis of network metrics

Next, we compared the network organization associated with the functional connectivity patterns as a means to further justify the observed differences between the two groups in terms of pairwise coupling strengths. The three metrics of Strength, GE and LE were first applied at the single-trial level (to "static" **W**s) and then averaged to derive a triad of measurements for each subject, brain rhythm and experimental condition. Figure 5 compares these measurements, after deriving group-medians. The stars in the bars of patients' graphs indicate the statistically significant differences (p-value < 0.01, bonferroni-corrected) in the level of network-metrics, which resulted from the group-analysis of the corresponding measurements (NMD patients vs controls) performed using the Wilcoxon rank sum test. It is easy to observe that despite the lack of statistically significant differences in case of Strength (which practically corresponds to integrating the coupling strength across sensors), the other two metrics regarding the network's efficiency (i.e. GE and LE) depict significant differences for rhythms faster than 8 Hz, where MI spectral activity is expected to be found. The

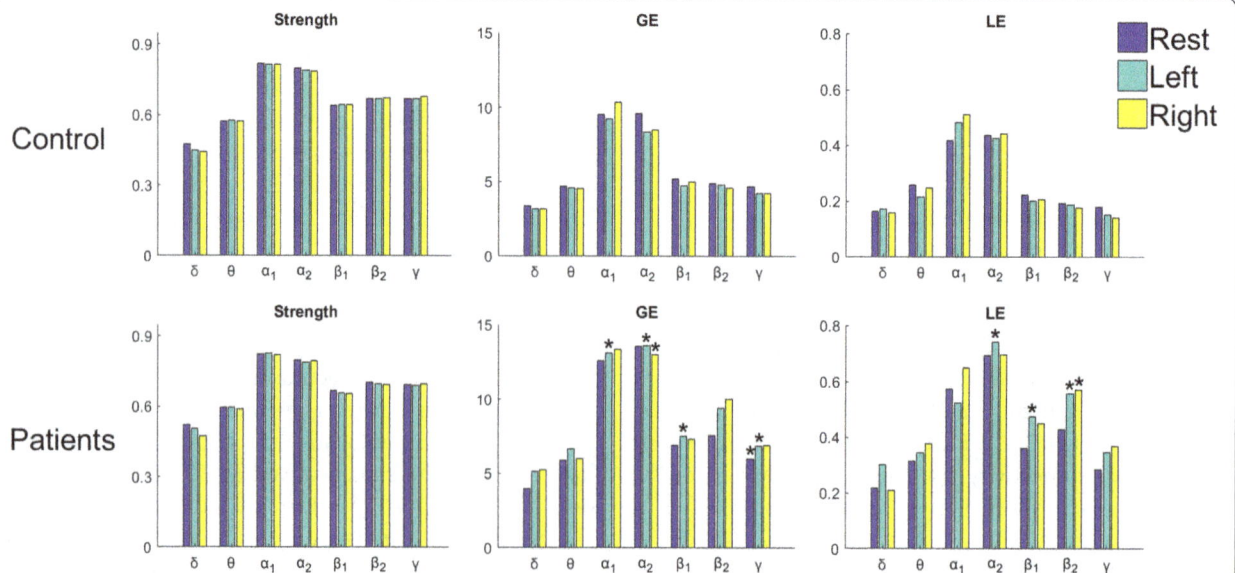

Fig. 5 Contrasting the functional network organization between patients and controls using the standard networks metrics of *strength*, *global-efficiency* (GE) and *local efficiency* (LE). The median values, have been computed across the subjects of each group, and presented for all brain rhythms. Statistically significant differences between the two groups have also been detected (using Wilcoxon rank sum test) and indicated with a star symbol in the corresponding bar of the patients' barplot

observed differences in these two topological metrics (which reflect how efficiently the information flows within the brain network), are related to brain coordination and, hence, can be attributed to the NMD condition itself and the way it affects the patient's brain reorganization during its progression. Interestingly, differences in network organization during MI-tasks were detected in α_2 rhythm, even though the pairwise couplings did not show, individually, any difference between groups based on their PLV-levels (see Fig. 4 and Additional file 1: Figure S1).

Personalized MI decoding – SVM classification based on static patterns

In the third stage of our analysis, we attempted to decode the MI-imagery direction based on the single-trial functional connectivity patterns and compared the performance between the two cohorts. We employed a linear SVM in conjunction with standard, statistical, feature screening. The scope of this screening was to confine the SVM design within the space spanned by the 10 most informative functional couplings. To reduce the possibility of overfitting, this feature selection step had been included in the LOOCV scheme (i.e. it was performed every time an SVM was about to be designed from the set of trials that had been reserved for training). The classification accuracy of the "left vs. right" decoding task for each subject and brain rhythm is shown

in Fig. 6, where it can be justified that working at a personalized level was indeed necessary, since performance (and frequency-band of optimal performance) varied a lot across subjects. It is evident that the accuracy levels for the patients group are significantly higher, with five out of six subjects exceeding 75% accuracy and even the subject with the lowest accuracy (i.e. P3) for this group reaches 65%. It is also interesting to notice that for the NMD group the highest accuracy is associated with $\beta1$ (13–20 Hz) band in four subjects (i.e. P1, P2, P4, P6). On the other hand, half of the control subjects do not surpass the level of 60% accuracy in any of the frequency bands, with subject S5 standing as the best subject for the control group, as it is the only case were 80% of the trials were correctly classified. To confirm rigorously the hypothesis that BCI-naïve patients can perform better than controls in the employed MI tasks, we gathered the highest performance level from each individual in two sets of accuracies, $\{^{NMD}Accuracies\}_{i\,=\,1:6}$ / $\{^{controls}Accuracies\}_{i\,=\,1:6}$, and applied the Wilcoxon rank sum test that revealed a statistical significant difference ($p < 0.05$, one-tailed).

For comparison purposes we have included, as Additional file 1: Figure S2, the results from decoding MI-direction based on power spectral density (PSD) estimates, where the feature screening was applied to the ensemble of PSD measurements (that included the measurements from every sensor and brain rhythm). Overall, the decoding performance stays below 75%

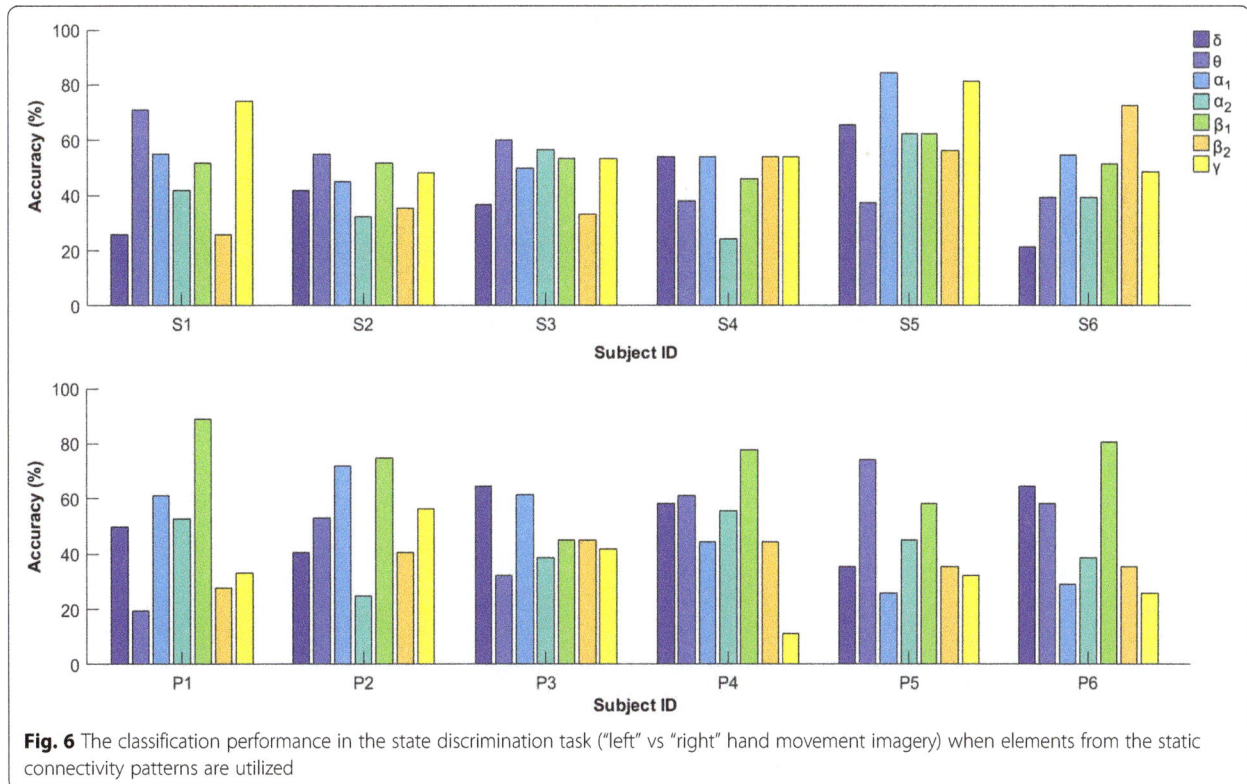

Fig. 6 The classification performance in the state discrimination task ("left" vs "right" hand movement imagery) when elements from the static connectivity patterns are utilized

(except for patient P5), i.e. lower than in the case of PLV measurements. In addition, there is no statistically significant advantage for the NMD group over the controls considering the highest performance level from each individual ($p = 0.43$, one-tailed). Similar trends were obtained from a decoding scheme based on CSPs (see Additional file 1: Figure S3).

Personalized MI decoding – SVM classification based on time-varying patterns

At the expense of increased computations and algorithmic complexity, we then moved to decoding MI-direction from time-varying connectivity patterns for the NMD-patients. Both the beneficial phase-synchrony based representation, for the brain activity in this clinical group, and the fact that MI-BCIs have remained largely unexplored for NMD patients led us to study deeper the relevant dynamic patterns of connectivity. Supporting evidence, regarding the dynamic nature of the underlying phenomena, was offered by the feature screening procedures, since the scores acquired by dynamic patterns were often higher than the ones obtained from static patterns.[8] Working at a personalized level, we first identify the set of functional couplings that showed a stable and highly discriminative behavior (using bootstrapping and eq.(7)). These couplings have been included in Fig. 7. The fixed set of selected entries were extracted, in every single-trial, from the time-indexed connectivity patterns, $\text{vec}(\mathbf{W}[\tau])$, which had been computed with a time-step of 350 ms. The vectors were used to design and evaluate an "instantaneous" SVM (i.e. SVM^τ)

that corresponds to each latency and also follows a LOOCV scheme. The performances of this decoder were estimated by comparing the time-indexed predictions with the class labels of the trials and integrating the results across trials.

Figure 8 shows the corresponding performance curves for the "instantaneous" SVM classification scheme. At every latency the performance was estimated based on the selected couplings (shown in Fig. 7). It is clear, that there is variability among subjects. There are subjects (P1, P3 and P6) reaching the highest accuracy within the first second and maintaining the high performance for the full trial length. On the other hand, subjects P2 and P4 do as well achieve the highest performance levels within the first second but do not maintain it for the trial's full length. Such a trend could be interpreted as declining engagement to the task. Finally, one subject (P5) showed deterioration in performance after the first second. The observed variability can be attributed to the subject's devotion to the task, how he/she performed it, and possibly to the type of NMD. Overall, this classification scheme appears to lead to optimal performance earlier in time.

In quest of self-paced MI decoding

Finally, we explored the possibility of decoding phase-connectivity patterns in a way that could be used in a future implementation of a self-paced MI-BCI, where the user would initiate the MI events at will. Since there were no recordings of self-initiated MI events, we

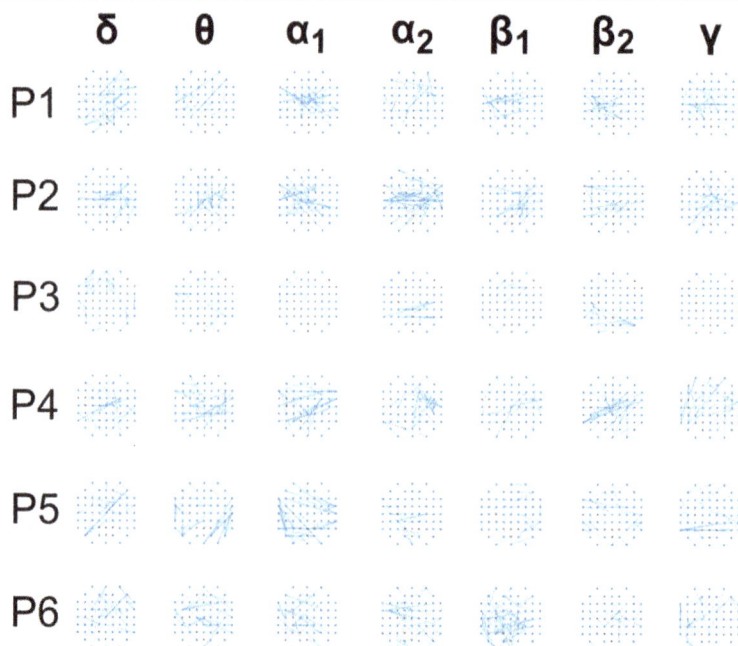

Fig. 7 The statistically significant and temporally consistent couplings as detected by means of a permutation test (random re-labeling of trials), applied for each patient and brain rhythm independently

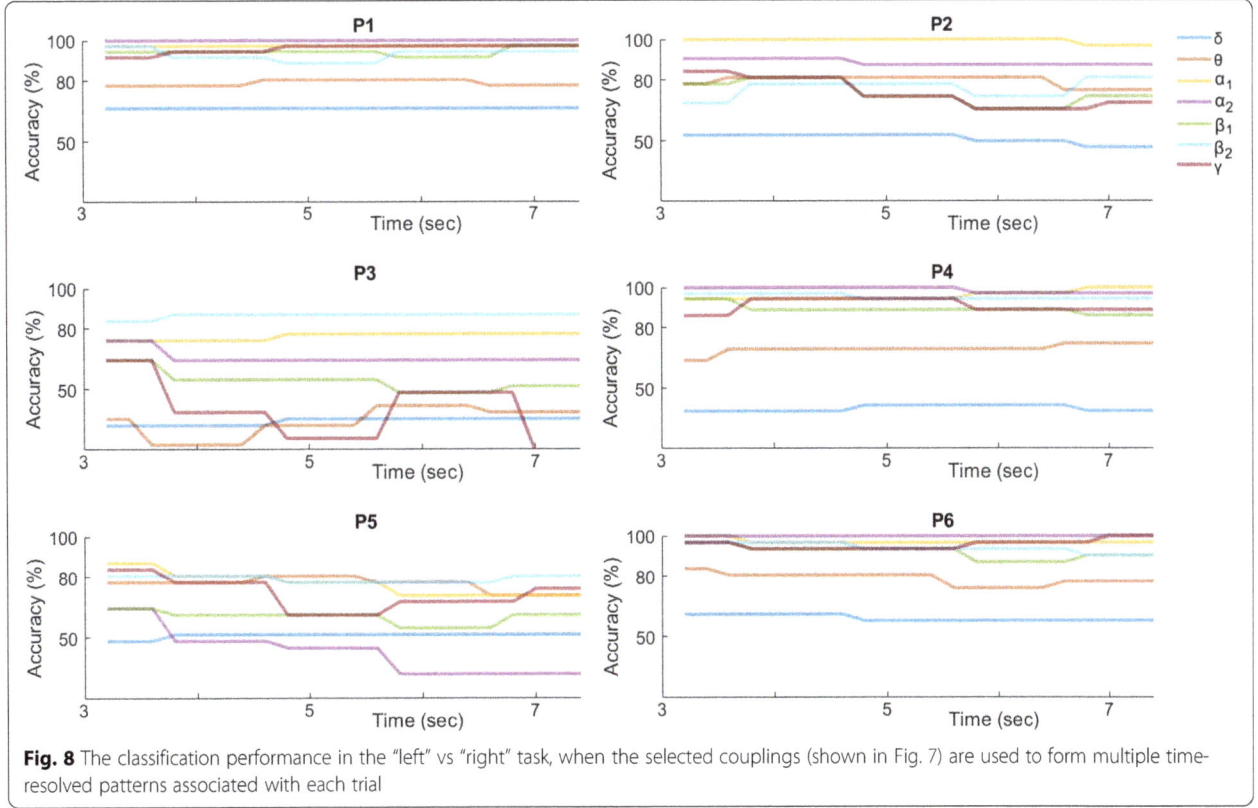

Fig. 8 The classification performance in the "left" vs "right" task, when the selected couplings (shown in Fig. 7) are used to form multiple time-resolved patterns associated with each trial

decided to partially "simulate" the case by exploiting the resting-condition recordings and devising a scheme that would mark a time instance as the beginning of an MI-event ("left" or "right") only when the temporal patterning in the streaming connectivity-data was deviant from the patterning in the baseline (rest) condition. To this end, 20 trials were extracted from each patient's resting-state recording and "baseline" time-resolved connectivity patterns (extending for 8 s) were formed, based on the same signal-analytic pipeline used in the case of MI-trials. Since the purpose of this analysis was the reliable detection of dynamical transitions in brain state (from "idle" to an MI event), the connectivity patterns from resting state and, also, the MI events were derived with high temporal resolution (based on a step of 20 msec), so as to emphasize the temporal aspects of the detection task. To ease the presentation of the results reported in this section, Fig. 9 depicts graphically the employed algorithmic steps.

A training set consisting of 10 trials from each class ("left", "right" and "rest") was formed and utilized in a two-stage data-learning process. During the first-stage, only the MI-related single-trial connectivity patterns ($\{^{left}vec(\mathbf{W}^i[\tau]\}_{i=1:10}$ and $\{^{right}vec(\mathbf{W}^i[\tau]\}_{i=1:10})$ were used for a) the feature-selection, b) the training of all "instantaneous" SVMs, c) the selection among them, of those that populated the ensemble $\{SVM^i\}$. The feature

selection step is exemplified in Fig. 2, for subject P2's connectivity patterns from α_1 rhythm. The selection of SVMs is exemplified in Fig. 3a, while the application of the SVM-ensemble in some trials (from all recording conditions) is demonstrated in Fig. 3b, where the vectors of successive predictions appear as columns in the shown heat-maps. The right-most panels in Fig. 3b includes the corresponding trial-averaged heat-maps, where a "diagonal" pattern is emerging in both cases of "triggered" MI-events but not in the case of resting-state. It was exactly this discrepancy, that the stratified combination of the outputs of the SVMs participating in the ensemble, tried to reveal, in a computationally tractable way, by means of eq.(9).

During the second stage, the temporal traces corresponding to the single-trial "instantaneous" readouts from the SVM-ensemble were derived for the above mentioned MI-related connectivity patterns and, in addition, for the baseline-related ones $\{^{rest}vec(\mathbf{W}^i[\tau]\}_{i=1:10}$. Figure 10 demonstrates the estimated traces of Classification Index, $z_{ensemble}(t)$, in continuation of the example shown previously in Figs. 2 and 3. It is evident that a peak is identifiable, just after the 3rd second (onset), for both the "left" and "right" conditions. On the contrary, the traces derived from the rest condition trials do not illustrate any comparable peak. In an attempt to quantify these observations, and simultaneously complete the design of a totally

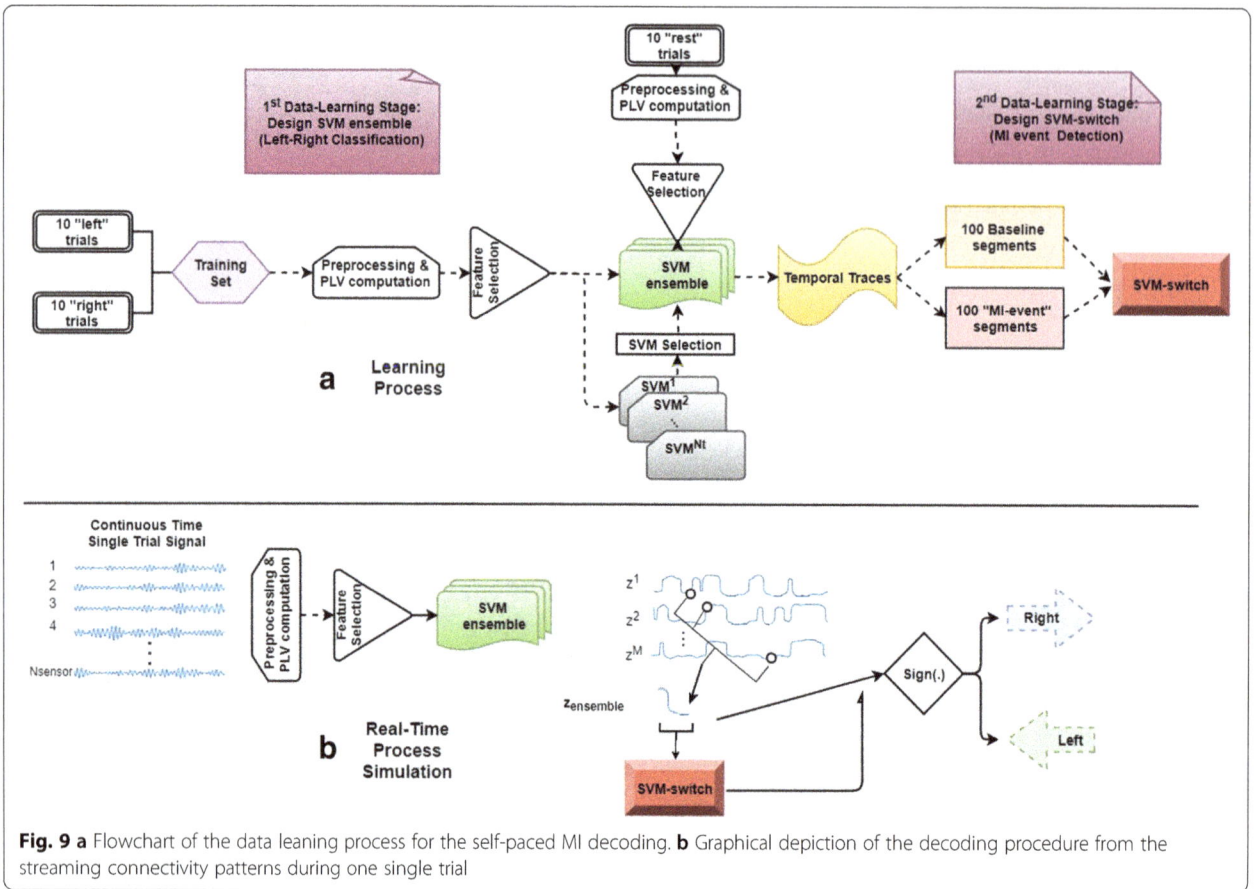

Fig. 9 a Flowchart of the data leaning process for the self-paced MI decoding. **b** Graphical depiction of the decoding procedure from the streaming connectivity patterns during one single trial

self-paced MI-decoding scheme, we used these 30 profiles (as training data) to craft a decision rule, that based on streaming data (a segment of SVM-ensemble readout) would decide if the observed temporal patterning in Classification Index corresponded to baseline condition or to an MI event and, hence, should trigger the command associated with the sign of the trace from the SVM-ensemble. To accomplish the data-learning task, we extracted multiple segments, of 0.5 s width, from the singe-trial traces shown in Fig. 10 and confined within the intervals indicated via vertical dotted lines. These 100 segments were corresponding to the "MI-event" class (regardless direction). An equal number of segments were extracted from the baseline condition, but this time without any restriction about the time interval. These segments constituted the "baseline" class patterns. Both type of segments were used for training a binary-SVM (with a radial basis function kernel) to discriminate an MI event from the baseline state. The trained "SVM-switch", was then fed with the streaming SVM-ensemble readouts,

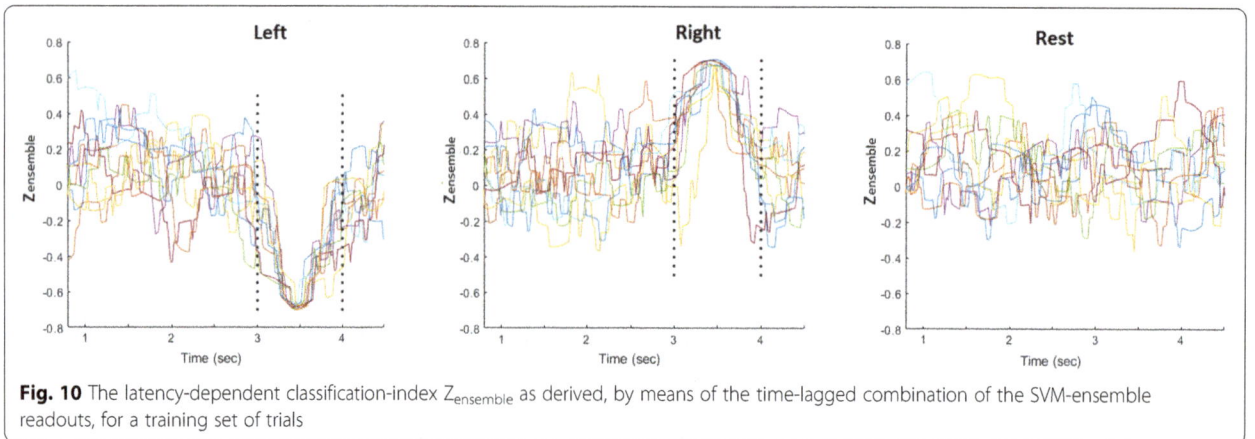

Fig. 10 The latency-dependent classification-index $Z_{ensemble}$ as derived, by means of the time-lagged combination of the SVM-ensemble readouts, for a training set of trials

$z_{ensemble}(t)$, resulted from the underlined testing set of trials. Figure 11, exemplifies this step by first depicting the "instantaneous" single-trial readouts form the SVM-ensemble (formed in Fig. 3a) for the three recording conditions (Fig. 11a) and, then, the corresponding single-trial traces of the instantaneous confidence of the SVM-switch (all the consecutive segments had been fed to this classifier) (Fig. 11b). Using as threshold, the confidence level of 0.5, we obtained only 2 false positive (FP) detections in all three recording conditions (please notice that this would had also been the case if a high confidence level had appeared within the first 3 s interval of a MI trial), and no false negative ones. After referencing these counts to the number of trials, we estimated two probabilistic indices regarding the observed probabilities of FP and FN (here 2/30 and 0/30 respectively).

The overall procedure was repeated after different randomized partitions of the data (i.e. Monte-Carlo cross validation scheme), and the results (after averaging across 100 splits) were tabulated in Table 2. The brain rhythms had been selected according to the performance levels shown in Fig. 8.

The very low probabilities of misdetection and false alarm, in conjunction with the very high performance of the individual MI-decoders participating in the ensemble, make the combined scheme (SVM-ensemble & SVM-switch) potentially suitable for self-paced MI-decoding (see Fig. 9).

Discussion

NMD is a condition that gradually affects the musculature and eventually leads to the loss of any voluntary muscle control. The reflections of NMD on the electroencephalographic brain activity, under the perspective of establishing efficient BCIs, have rarely been studied [42]. It was the scope of this study to examine the differences in the functional brain organization between NMD patients and healthy individuals in a motor-imagery paradigm that, traditionally, is considered fruitful for endogenous BCIs. Rhythm-specific connectivity patterns during motor imagery and resting state were derived and used, first, to contrast the two cohorts in terms of coupling strength and network organization and, then, to explore different possibilities for MI-event decoding and detection schemes, in NMD patients. Special attention was paid to dynamic patterns of functional connectivity in an attempt to identify faster ways to perform MI decoding and relax the dependence of this decoding from external triggering.

Overall, the reported results provide empirical evidence about the hypothesis that NMD patients could perform well in MI tasks, without any training, due to the equivalence, for them, of performing an imagery movement and an actual one; or, equivalently, due to the fact that the disease's progression simulates a long training phase. More specifically, the pairwise phase-coupling was found statistically elevated in NMD patients (Fig. 4 and Additional file 1: Figure S1) and the network organization (associated with faster rhythms) significantly higher (Fig. 5). In addition, MI-decoding, worked out in a personalized manner, was performed more efficiently in patients than in controls (Fig. 6). It is important to notice that Phase-synchrony representation resulted in a more reliable decoding than signal-power representation (compare Fig. 6 with Additional file 1: Figure S2) and CSP approach (Additional file 1: Figure S3).

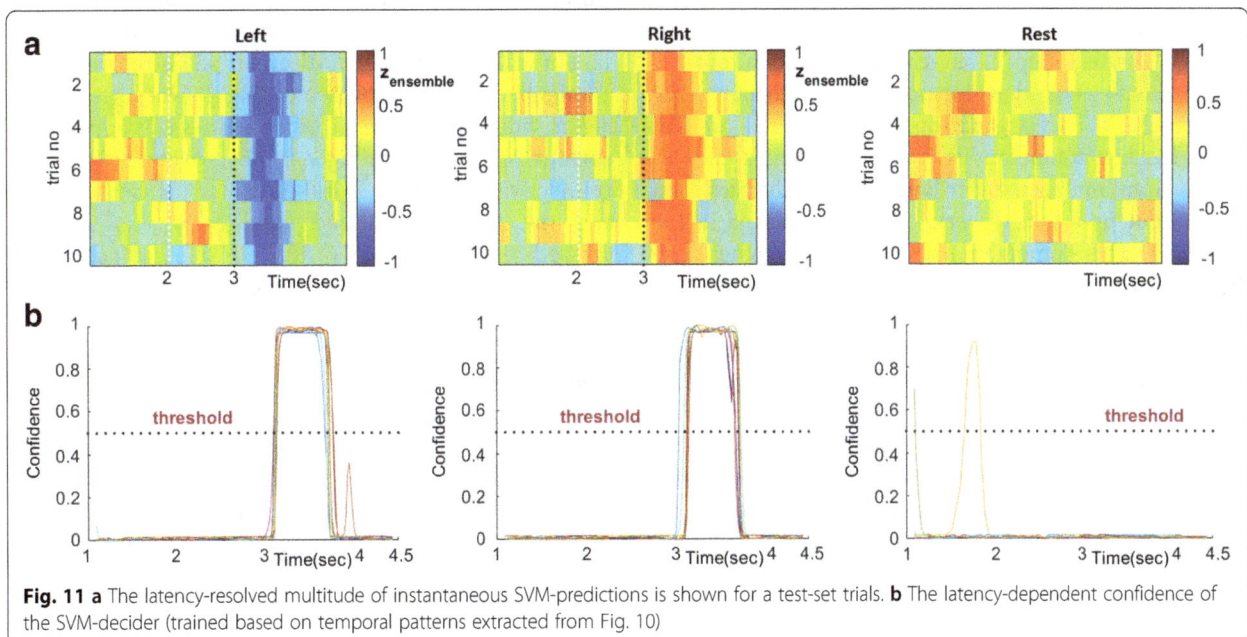

Fig. 11 a The latency-resolved multitude of instantaneous SVM-predictions is shown for a test-set trials. **b** The latency-dependent confidence of the SVM-decider (trained based on temporal patterns extracted from Fig. 10)

Table 2 FP/FN for the SVM-switch

Participant ID	P1	P2	P3	P4	P5	P6
brain rhythm	α_2	α_1	β_2	α_2	α_1	α_2
FP	2.2%	3.5%	7.2%	3.9%	7.2%	2.7%
FN	1.4%	2.0%	5.3%	2.1%	3.3%	1.4%

Moreover, our results also showed that direction decoding can be performed, almost equally well, by training time-indexed SVM-decoders using phase synchrony patterns that are regularly sampled from the post-stimulus time interval (Fig. 8) opening the possibility of reducing the response time in cued MI-based BCIs. This observation led to a lagged combination of distinct SVM-decoders that all operated in the same feature space (Fig. 2) but trained with different time-indexed instantiations of the training set of phase synchrony patterns (Fig. 3a). The introduced combination of SVM-activations acts as an optimal filter that can run in real-time and reliably trigger the recognition of an MI-event (Fig. 11), the direction of which is conveyed by the polarity of the assembled classification-index.

The importance of this work stems from fact that (to the best of our knowledge) there is only one paper that tackles the same problem that is MI-BCI for NMD patients [42]. In line with our work, the authors demonstrate the successful use of BCI. However, MI-decoding is based on time-domain characteristics and requires significant amount of training time (8–12 training sessions).

There are some novelty aspects in this work, that need to be put in the context of contemporary practice in neuroscience research and streaming data analysis. First, we need to underline our choice to work with dynamic phase synchrony patterns, casting new empirical evidence about the benefits of *chronnectomics* ("chronos" = time + "connectomics"), an emerging branch of network neuroscience that focuses on the dynamics of brain-network (self)organization phenomena [58–61]. Phase locking computations can be implemented efficiently from multisite recordings, as already has been pointed out by a recent work [62] and indicated in the Appendix. This computational efficiency, together with the fact that the MI-related network reorganizations are characterized by fast transitions, opens the possibility of prompt MI-detection and decoding in nearly real-time. The second point that deserves further consideration is the SVM-ensemble formation and its use in filtering mode (i.e. its application to streaming connectivity patterns). While such an implementation of SVMs seems rather unusual in EEG-related research, it has already been successfully employed for continuous speech recognition (for instance [63, 64]).

Finally, the main limitations of this study need to be discussed, starting with the restricted number of available trials. Even though precautions were taken (by means of cross-validation) to avoid overfitting, our findings will wait the verification from further studies. Particularly the self-paced MI-decoding scheme was demonstrated and validated using a "crude simulation". This part of our study needs to be treated strictly as a proof-of-concept, since trials from an independent resting state recording were treated as extracts from continuous data interrupted by MI-events. Secondly, although it is common practice in studies with people with disabilities to include a restrained number of participants [35–37, 40], as the recruitment process is not as straightforward as in control population, it would be of great importance to further validate the statistical differences between the groups by encountering higher number of NMD participants in the MI experimental procedure. Thirdly, all the reported results were obtained from off-line analysis, in which "cleaned" data were employed (see Pre-processing section). It remains to show that (whether) the proposed decoding scheme is robust to artifacts like blinks; a possibility that rises since it revolves around phase-descriptor. Alternatively, in a realistic implementation one of the available real-time artifact-removal techniques may be incorporated [65, 66]. Therefore, the evaluation regarding the methodology's performance in terms of challenging, real-time conditions is yet to be explored and is considered to be an intriguing part of any future actions aiming to "build" a self-paced MI BCI. Moreover, a personalized (subject-adaptive) data-learning scheme was pursued for the purpose of MI-decoding. This, inevitably, makes necessary a small training set before a participant can take advantage of the suggested MI-decoding mechanism. While principles of transfer learning maybe useful, we tend to consider as best practice a small training session in which self-initiated MI-events will be embedded in a "relevant" baseline activity recoding (for instance, watching a videoclips sequence and "instruct" skipping the current one by imagining a hand movement). Finally, connectivity patterns were estimated at sensor level and the issue of volume conduction was not addressed since favorable results were obtained readily and the precise modelling was considered beyond the scope of MI-BCIs.

Conclusions

NMD patients appear to possess an inherent advantage, over healthy subjects, in the use of phase-synchrony related MI-BCIs. Patient-specific data-learning procedures have the potential for leading to effective brain decoding schemes from the emerging connectivity patterns, that can be implemented efficiently and, when embedded in patient's daily life, provide a certain level of autonomy.

Endnotes

[1]http://www.who.int/disabilities/world_report/2011/report/en/

[2]http://openvibe.inria.fr/

[3]http://www.ebneuro.biz/en/neurology/ebneuro/galileo-suite/be-plus-ltm

[4]For instance, in the case of δ band ($[f_1, f_2] = [1, 4]$ Hz), and since the sampling frequency was $f_s = 256$ Hz, the size of window was $T_{window} = \frac{CC}{f_1} \times f_s = \frac{3}{1} \times 256 = 768$ *samples*.

[5]https://www.mathworks.com/help/bioinfo/ref/rankfeatures.html

[6]https://www.mathworks.com/help/signal/ref/findpeaks.html

[7]The correlation coefficient $\rho(z^i(t),z^j(t))$, i,j = 1...M, averaged across trials, was lower than 0.2.

[8]i.e. $max_{r,\ \tau}(Score(r, \tau)) > max_r(Score(\tau))$ following the notation of eq.(5) and eq.(6).

Appendix

In the following Matlab-coded implementation of the PLV-computations, the function receives as input the multichannel-signal matrix (row-vectors correspond to sensors) and outputs the square matrix **W** containing all pairwise couplings

function

W=Fast_PLV_for_multichannel_signal(filtered_traces)

% PLV_Matrix = Fast_PLV_for_multichannel_signal(filtered_traces)

% filtered_traces: [N_sensors x N_timepoints] matrix of band-limited signals

% PLV_Matrix: [N_sensors x N_sensors] matrix of pairwise PLVs

[Nsensors,Ntime] = size(filtered_traces);
Phases = angle(hilbert(filtered_signals'))'; Q = (exp(j*Phases));
W = (1/Ntime)*abs(Q * Q')

Additional file

Additional file 1: Figure S1. Topographical representation of the statistically significant functional couplings (shown in Fig. 4). In the emerging graphs, the edge-width reflects the strength of the coupling and the node-size the number of edges incident to that node. The shown results correspond to Group-level analysis and reflect higher connectivity in the NMD patients. **Figure S2.** The classification performance in the state discrimination task ("left" vs "right"), when band-specific power-spectral density estimates are employed. **Figure S3.** The classification performance in the state discrimination task ("left" vs "right"), when the Common Spatial Pattern algorithm is employed in the 8–30 Hz frequency band as described by Fabien Lotte [1]. (ZIP 819 kb)

Abbreviations

ALS: Amyotrophic Lateral Sclerosis; BCI: Brain Computer Interface; CS: Chronic Strokes; CSP: Common Spatial Patterns; EEG: Electroencephalography; ERD/ ERS: Event Related Desynchronization/ Event Related Desynchronization; ERP: Event Related Potentials; FDR: False Discovery Rate; FN: False Negative; FP: False Positive; GE: Global Efficiency; ICA: Independent Component Analysis; LE: Local Efficiency; LOOCV: Leave One Out Cross Validation; MI: Motor Imagery; MS: Multiple Sclerosis; NMD: Neuromuscular Disease; PLV: Phase Locking Value; SCI: Spinal Cord Injury; SMR: Sensorimotor Rhythm; SVM: Support Vector Machines; WHO: World Health Organization

Funding

This work is part of project MAMEM that has received funding from the European Union's Horizon 2020 research and innovation programme under grant agreement No 644780.

Authors' contributions

SN and IK conceived the study; KG collected the physiological data and drafted the paper; KG and NAL performed the data analysis; SN and IK offered critical revisions; all authors reviewed the manuscript. All authors read and approved the final manuscript.

Competing interests

The authors declare that they have no competing interests.

Author details

[1]AIIA lab, Informatics Department, AUTH, Thessaloniki, Greece. [2]Information Technologies Institute (ITI), Centre for Research & Technology Hellas, Thessaloniki-Thermi, Greece. [3]NeuroInformatics.GRoup, AUTH, Thessaloniki, Greece.

References

1. Lebedev MA, Nicolelis MA. Brain-machine interfaces: from basic science to neuroprostheses and neurorehabilitation. Physiol Rev. 2017;97(2):767–837.
2. Nam CS, Nijholt A, Lotte F. Brain–computer interfaces handbook. Technological and Theoretical Advances; 2018. p. 9.
3. Berger H. Über das elektrenkephalogramm des menschen. Archiv für Psychiatrie und Nervenkrankheiten. 1929;87(1):527–70.
4. Liparas D, Dimitriadis SI, Laskaris NA, Tzelepi A, Charalambous K, Angelis L. Exploiting the temporal patterning of transient VEP signals: a statistical single-trial methodology with implications to brain–computer interfaces (BCIs). J Neurosci Methods. 2014;232:189–98.
5. Riechmann H, Finke A, Ritter H. Using a cVEP-based brain-computer Interface to control a virtual agent. IEEE Trans Neural Syst Rehabil Eng. 2016;24(6):692–9.
6. Georgiadis K, Laskaris N, Nikolopoulos S, Kompatsiaris I. Discriminative codewaves: a symbolic dynamics approach to SSVEP recognition for asynchronous BCI. J Neural Eng. 2018;15(2):026008.
7. Xu M, Xiao X, Wang Y, Qi H, Jung TP, Ming D. A brain computer interface based on miniature event-related potentials induced by very small lateral visual stimuli. IEEE Trans Biomed Eng. 2018;65(5):1166–75.
8. Nakayashiki K, Saeki M, Takata Y, Hayashi Y, Kondo T. Modulation of event-related desynchronization during kinematic and kinetic hand movements. J Neuroeng Rehabil. 2014;11(1):90.
9. Andrade J, Cecílio J, Simões M, Sales F, Castelo-Branco M. Separability of motor imagery of the self from interpretation of motor intentions of others at the single trial level: an EEG study. J Neuroeng Rehabil. 2017;14(1):63.
10. Nam CS, Jeon Y, Kim YJ, Lee I, Park K. Movement imagery-related lateralization of event-related (de) synchronization (ERD/ERS): motor-imagery duration effects. Clin Neurophysiol. 2011;122(3):567–77.
11. Solis-Escalante T, Müller-Putz G, Pfurtscheller G. Overt foot movement detection in one single Laplacian EEG derivation. J Neurosci Methods. 2008;175(1):148–53.

12. Ge S, Wang R, Yu D. Classification of four-class motor imagery employing single-channel electroencephalography. PLoS One. 2014;9(6): e98019.

13. Deng S, Srinivasan R, Lappas T, D'Zmura M. EEG classification of imagined syllable rhythm using Hilbert spectrum methods. J Neural Eng. 2010;7(4):046006.

14. Wang L, Zhang X, Zhong X, Zhang Y. Analysis and classification of speech imagery EEG for BCI. Biomed Signal Proc Control. 2013;8(6):901–8.

15. Dimitriadis S, Sun Y, Laskaris N, Thakor N, Bezerianos A. Revealing cross-frequency causal interactions during a mental arithmetic task through symbolic transfer entropy: a novel vector-quantization approach. IEEE Trans Neural Syst Rehabil Eng. 2016;24(10):1017–28.

16. Wang Q, Sourina O. Real-time mental arithmetic task recognition from EEG signals. IEEE Trans Neural Syst Rehabil Eng. 2013;21(2):225–32.

17. Yuan H, He B. Brain–computer interfaces using sensorimotor rhythms: current state and future perspectives. IEEE Trans Biomed Eng. 2014;61(5): 1425–35.

18. Pfurtscheller G, Da Silva FL. Event-related EEG/MEG synchronization and desynchronization: basic principles. Clin Neurophysiol. 1999;110(11):1842–57.

19. Formaggio E, Storti SF, Galazzo IB, Gandolfi M, Geroin C, Smania N, Spezia L, Waldner A, Fiaschi A, Manganotti P. Modulation of event-related desynchronization in robot-assisted hand performance: brain oscillatory changes in active, passive and imagined movements. J Neuroeng Rehabil. 2013;10(1):24.

20. Pfurtscheller G, Brunner C, Schlögl A, Da Silva FL. Mu rhythm (de) synchronization and EEG single-trial classification of different motor imagery tasks. NeuroImage. 2006;31(1):153–9.

21. Ramoser H, Muller-Gerking J, Pfurtscheller G. Optimal spatial filtering of single trial EEG during imagined hand movement. IEEE Trans Rehabil Eng. 2000;8(4):441–6.

22. Ang KK, Chin ZY, Zhang H, Guan C. Filter bank common spatial pattern (FBCSP) in brain-computer interface. InNeural Networks, IJCNN 2008.(IEEE World Congress on Computational Intelligence). IEEE Int Joint Conf. 2008, 2008:2390–7 (pp) IEEE.

23. Robinson N, Guan C, Vinod AP, Ang KK, Tee KP. Multi-class EEG classification of voluntary hand movement directions. J Neural Eng. 2013;10(5):056018.

24. Thomas KP, Guan C, Lau CT, Vinod AP, Ang KK. A new discriminative common spatial pattern method for motor imagery brain–computer interfaces. IEEE Trans Biomed Eng. 2009;56(11):2730–3.

25. Lotte F, Guan C. Regularizing common spatial patterns to improve BCI designs: unified theory and new algorithms. IEEE Trans Biomed Eng. 2011; 58(2):355–62.

26. Brunner C, Scherer R, Graimann B, Supp G, Pfurtscheller G. Online control of a brain-computer interface using phase synchronization. IEEE Trans Biomed Eng. 2006;53(12):2501–6.

27. Caramia N, Lotte F, Ramat S. Optimizing spatial filter pairs for EEG classification based on phase-synchronization. InAcoustics, Speech and Signal Processing (ICASSP), 2014. IEEE Int Conf. 2014:2049–53 IEEE.

28. Stavrinou ML, Moraru L, Cimponeriu L, Della Penna S, Bezerianos A. Evaluation of cortical connectivity during real and imagined rhythmic finger tapping. Brain Topogr. 2007;19(3):137–45.

29. Song L, Gordon E, Gysels E. Phase synchrony rate for the recognition of motor imagery in brain-computer interface. In Advances in Neural Information Processing Systems. 2006:1265–72.

30. Scherer R, Schloegl A, Lee F, Bischof H, Janša J, Pfurtscheller G. The self-paced Graz brain-computer interface: methods and applications. Comput Intell Neurosci. 2007:9.

31. Chae Y, Jeong J, Jo S. Toward brain-actuated humanoid robots: asynchronous direct control using an EEG-based BCI. IEEE Trans Robot. 2012;28(5):1131–44.

32. Leeb R, Friedman D, Müller-Putz GR, Scherer R, Slater M, Pfurtscheller G. Self-paced (asynchronous) BCI control of a wheelchair in virtual environments: a case study with a tetraplegic. Computational intelligence and neuroscience. 2007;1(2007):7.

33. Müller-Putz GR, Kaiser V, Solis-Escalante T, Pfurtscheller G. Fast set-up asynchronous brain-switch based on detection of foot motor imagery in 1-channel EEG. Med Biol Eng comput. 2010;48(3):229–33.

34. Kübler A, Nijboer F, Mellinger J, Vaughan TM, Pawelzik H, Schalk G, McFarland DJ, Birbaumer N, Wolpaw JR. Patients with ALS can use sensorimotor rhythms to operate a brain-computer interface. Neurology. 2005;64(10):1775–7.

35. Bai O, Lin P, Huang D, Fei DY, Floeter MK. Towards a user-friendly brain

36. King CE, Wang PT, Chui LA, Do AH, Nenadic Z. Operation of a brain-computer interface walking simulator for individuals with spinal cord injury. J Neuroeng Rehabil. 2013 Dec;10(1):77.

37. Conradi J, Blankertz B, Tangermann M, Kunzmann V, Curio G. Brain-computer interfacing in tetraplegic patients with high spinal cord injury. Int J Bioelectromagn. 2009;11(2):65–8.

38. Heremans E, Nieuwboer A, Spildooren J, De Bondt S, D'hooge AM, Helsen W, Feys P. Cued motor imagery in patients with multiple sclerosis. Neuroscience. 2012;206:115–21.

39. Allali G, Laidet M, Assal F, Beauchet O, Chofflon M, Armand S, Lalive PH. Adapted timed up and go: a rapid clinical test to assess gait and cognition in multiple sclerosis. Eur Neurol. 2012;67(2):116–20.

40. Leamy DJ, Kocijan J, Domijan K, Duffin J, Roche RA, Commins S, Collins R, Ward TE. An exploration of EEG features during recovery following stroke-implications for BCI-mediated neurorehabilitation therapy. J Neuroeng Rehabil. 2014;11(1):9.

41. Shindo K, Kawashima K, Ushiba J, Ota N, Ito M, Ota T, Kimura A, Liu M. Effects of neurofeedback training with an electroencephalogram-based brain–computer interface for hand paralysis in patients with chronic stroke: a preliminary case series study. J Rehabil Med. 2011;43(10):951–7.

42. Cincotti F, Mattia D, Aloise F, Bufalari S, Schalk G, Oriolo G, Cherubini A, Marciani MG, Babiloni F. Non-invasive brain–computer interface system: towards its application as assistive technology. Brain Res Bull. 2008;75(6):796–803.

43. Nikolopoulos S, Petrantonakis PC, Georgiadis K, Kalaganis F, Liaros G, Lazarou I, Adam K, Papazoglou-Chalikias A, Chatzilari E, Oikonomou VP, Kumar C. A multimodal dataset for authoring and editing multimedia content: the MAMEM project. Data in Brief. 2017;15:1048–56.

44. Delorme A, Sejnowski T, Makeig S. Enhanced detection of artifacts in EEG data using higher-order statistics and independent component analysis. NeuroImage. 2007;34(4):1443–9.

45. Lachaux JP, Rodriguez E, Martinerie J, Varela FJ. Measuring phase synchrony in brain signals. Hum Brain Mapp. 1999;8(4):194–208.

46. Fornito A, Zalesky A, Bullmore E. Fundamentals of brain network analysis. San Diego: Academic Press; 2016.

47. Fallani FD, Richiardi J, Chavez M, Achard S. Graph analysis of functional brain networks: practical issues in translational neuroscience. Phil Trans R Soc B. 2014;369(1653):20130521.

48. Latora V, Marchiori M. Efficient behavior of small-world networks. Phys Rev Lett. 2001;87(19):198701.

49. Dimitriadis SI, Laskaris NA, Tsirka V, Vourkas M, Micheloyannis S, Fotopoulos S. Tracking brain dynamics via time-dependent network analysis. J Neurosci Methods. 2010;193(1):145–55.

50. Dimitriadis SI, Laskaris NA, Tzelepi A. On the quantization of time-varying phase synchrony patterns into distinct functional connectivity microstates (FCμstates) in a multi-trial visual ERP paradigm. Brain Topogr. 2013;26(3): 397–409.

51. Gonuguntla V, Wang Y, Veluvolu KC. Event-related functional network identification: application to EEG classification. IEEE J Selected Topics in Signal Proc. 2016;10(7):1284–94.

52. learning BCMM, recognition p. Information science and statistics. Heidelberg: Springer; 2006.

53. Park C, Looney D, ur Rehman N, Ahrabian A, Mandic DP. Classification of motor imagery BCI using multivariate empirical mode decomposition. IEEE Trans Neural Syst Rehabil Eng. 2013;21(1):10–22.

54. Tam WK, Tong KY, Meng F, Gao S. A minimal set of electrodes for motor imagery BCI to control an assistive device in chronic stroke subjects: a multi-session study. IEEE Trans Neural Sys Rehabil Eng. 2011;19(6):617–27.

55. Platt J. Probabilistic outputs for support vector machines and comparisons to regularized likelihood methods. Advances in Large Margin Classifiers. 1999;10(3):61–74.

56. Efron B, Tibshirani RJ. An introduction to the bootstrap. United States of America: CRC Press; 1994. p. 15.

57. Benjamini Y, Hochberg Y. Controlling the false discovery rate: a practical and powerful approach to multiple testing. J R Stat Soc. 1995;57:289–300.

58. Calhoun VD, Miller R, Pearlson G, Adalı T. The chronnectome: time-varying connectivity networks as the next frontier in fMRI data discovery. Neuron. 2014;84(2):262–74.

59. Liu J, Liao X, Xia M, He Y. Chronnectome fingerprinting: identifying

individuals and predicting higher cognitive functions using dynamic brain connectivity patterns. Hum Brain Mapp. 2018;39(2):902–15.

60. Iakovidou ND, Laskaris NA, Tsichlas C, Manolopoulos Y, Christodoulakis M, Papathanasiou ES, Papacostas SS, Mitsis GD. A symbolic dynamics approach to Epileptic Chronnectomics: Employing strings to predict crisis onset. Theoretical Computer Science. 2018;710:116–25.

61. Mahyari AG, Zoltowski DM, Bernat EM, Aviyente S. A tensor decomposition-based approach for detecting dynamic network states from EEG. IEEE Trans Biomed Eng. 2017;64(1):225–37.

62. Bruña R, Maestú F, Pereda E. Phase Locking Value revisited: teaching new tricks to an old dog. ArXiv preprint arXiv. 2017;1710:08037.

63. Gordan M, Kotropoulos C, Pitas I. A temporal network of support vector machine classifiers for the recognition of visual speech. InHellenic Conference on Artificial Intelligence. Berlin, Heidelberg: Springer; 2002. p. 355–65.

64. Bardideh M, Razzazi F, Ghassemian H. An SVM based confidence measure for continuous speech recognition. InSignal Processing and Communications, 2007. ICSPC 2007. IEEE International Conference 2007 (pp. 1015–1018). IEEE.

65. Hsu SH, Mullen TR, Jung TP, Cauwenberghs G. Real-time adaptive EEG source separation using online recursive independent component analysis. IEEE Trans Neural Syst Rehabil Eng. 2016;24(3):309–19.

66. Yong X, Fatourechi M, Ward RK, Birch GE. Automatic artefact removal in a self-paced hybrid brain-computer interface system. J Neuroeng Rehabil. 2012;9(1):50.

14

Time course of changes in motor-cognitive exergame performances during task-specific training in patients with dementia: identification and predictors of early training response

Christian Werner[1,2]* ⓘ, Rebekka Rosner[3], Stefanie Wiloth[4], Nele Christin Lemke[5], Jürgen M. Bauer[1,2] and Klaus Hauer[1]

Abstract

Background: Some studies have already suggested that exergame interventions can be effective to improve physical, cognitive, motor-cognitive, and psychological outcomes in patients with dementia (PwD). However, little is known about the training volume required to induce such positive effects and the inter-individual differences in training response among PwD. The aim of the study was to analyze the time course of changes in motor-cognitive exergame performances during a task-specific training program and to identify predictors of early training response in PwD.

Methods: Secondary analyses of data from the intervention group (IG) of a randomized, placebo-controlled trial to improve motor-cognitive performances in PwD. Fifty-six geriatric patients with mild-to-moderate dementia randomized to the IG underwent a 10-week, task-specific training program (2×/week) on an exergame-based balance training system (Physiomat®), combining postural control tasks with cognitive tasks of an established neuropsychological test (Trail Making Test). Main outcome was the time required to complete different Physiomat®-Tasks (PTs) assessed at baseline (T1), training session 7 (TS7) and 14 (TS14), and post-intervention after 20 training sessions (T2). Reliable change indices were used to identify early responders from T1 to TS7. A multivariate logistic regression analysis was performed to determine independent predictors of early training response.

Results: Completion time significantly improved already from T1 to TS7 in all PTs ($p \leq .001–.006$), with moderate to very large effect sizes ($r = .38–.52$; Cohen's d = .85–1.45). For most PTs, significant progressive improvements from TS7 to TS14 and TS14 to T2 were not observed. Thirty-one (59.6%) participants were classified as early responders and 21 (40.4%) as non-early responders. Lower baseline exergame performance and lower visuospatial and divided attention abilities were independently associated with early training response.

(Continued on next page)

* Correspondence: christian.werner@bethanien-heidelberg.de
[1]Department of Geriatric Research, Agaplesion Bethanien Hospital Heidelberg, Geriatric Center at the Heidelberg University, Heidelberg, Germany
[2]Center for Geriatric Medicine, Heidelberg University, Heidelberg, Germany
Full list of author information is available at the end of the article

(Continued from previous page)

Conclusions: Substantial task-specific improvements in complex motor-cognitive exergame performances can be obtained within a surprisingly short intervention period in PwD. Our results confirm that not only an excellent training response can be achieved in this patient population, but also that more vulnerable patients with greater deficits in domain-specific cognitive functions associated with fall risk may even reap the most and fastest benefit from motor-cognitive exergame interventions.

Keywords: Dementia, Exergaming, Interactive, Dual-task, Postural control, Balance, Response, Cognition

Background

Attention is the first non-memory cognitive domain to be affected in dementia [1]. Divided attention, which is part of attentional control and the ability that allows individuals to perform two tasks simultaneously (i.e. dual tasks), represents the most affected aspect of attention [2, 3]. Under dual-task conditions, patients with dementia (PwD) or older people with cognitive impairment showed significantly reduced physical functions such as muscle strength [4], gait performance [5], and postural control [6, 7] compared to cognitively healthy older adults. Because everyday life involves many dual-task situations (e.g. walking while talking to someone) and deficits in dual-tasking have been associated with functional decline [8, 9] and falls [10, 11], it has been suggested to incorporate dual-task exercises into preventive or rehabilitative training programs [12–14].

Exergaming

Exergaming represents an emerging and unique form of dual-task training [15, 16], combining physical exercise with cognitively-challenging tasks in an interactive game-based way. In contrast to more traditional motor-cognitive dual-task exercises that combine distinct training tasks (e.g. walking while counting backwards), exergaming typically involves cognitive challenges directly embedded within the physical body movements that need to be performed to complete the game tasks projected onto a display screen [16]. The use of exergames in physical exercise and rehabilitation programs is progressively expanding as their playful character might help to encourage older people to participate in physical activity and to enhance their motivation toward exercise adherence [17, 18].

Potential benefits of exergaming

Recent systematic reviews have shown positive effects of exergaming on physical, cognitive, dual-task and psychosocial outcomes in cognitively healthy older adults [19–26]. Given the growing evidence of its beneficial effects, increasing attention has recently been paid to exergaming also in older people with cognitive impairment and PwD. Some studies have already suggested that exergame interventions can be effective to improve balance and/or gait [27–29], motor-functional status and exercise capacity [30], global cognitive functioning and/or domain-specific cognitive functions (e.g. memory, attention, visuospatial and constructional abilities) [31–33], fear of falling [28, 29], depressive symptoms [31], and exergame performances in these populations [34–36] (for review, see also [37]).

Time course of exergame-induced benefits

General dose-response relationships for traditional physical exercise suggest that untrained individuals may experience significant training benefits from low intensities, frequencies, and/or durations with small increases already during the early training period; however, with increasing performance of individuals, the magnitude of benefit may become less for a similar increase in intensity or amount of activity in the following training period [38, 39]. Although such knowledge is highly relevant for clinicians and practitioners to design time-efficient training protocols, little is yet known about dose-response relationships between exergaming (e.g. total duration of training period, number of training sessions) and its beneficial effects in older people with and without cognitive impairment or PwD [23, 40, 41]. Most frequently, previous studies did not include multiple assessment tests during the intervention period to address this research gap, but tested their participants only before and after the exergame-based training program, with intervention periods ranging widely from 1 to 24 weeks [28–35] (for review, see also [19–26]). Few studies conducted in older patients with Parkinson's disease and healthy elderly [42, 43], older patients with chronic obstructive pulmonary disease [44], older adults with depression [45], or older community-dwelling fallers [46] used mid-term tests (at week 3–6) to assess physical and psychological outcomes after 30% or 50% of the total exergame intervention period (6–12 weeks, 2–5×/week, 30–40 min) [42, 45, 46] or investigated the intersession progression in exergame performances during a 7-week intervention period (2×/week) [43]. Most frequently, these studies observed significant improvements in study outcomes (e.g. balance, depressive symptoms, exergame performance) already after 2 to 4 weeks [42, 43, 46]. To our knowledge, in PwD, a similar study design including not only pre- and post-intervention assessments has been used only in two studies [27, 36].

Padala et al. [27], demonstrated significant balance improvements at post-intervention after 8 weeks but not at the mid-term of their exergame intervention after 4 weeks (5×/week, 30 min); and Fenney and Lee [36], who addressed the intersession changes of exergame performance during a 9-week intervention period (1×/week, 60 min), only described case reports, with heterogeneous results among cases (i.e. both improvements and deteriorations during the early training period), making it difficult to interpret their findings. In all these studies, training-induced changes in outcomes were always evaluated only relative to the pre-intervention assessment. None of them addressed comparisons between mid-term and post-intervention assessments [27, 42, 44–46], nor did they compare other assessment sessions during the intervention period among each other [43], which might have provided an even more detailed insight into the time course of changes in outcomes.

Predictors of exergame training response

In people with cognitive impairment and PwD, effective exergame-based intervention studies have most frequently reported only main effects or mean group differences in changes without addressing inter-individual variability for their outcomes. However, individual differences and the identification of factors associated with training response has high clinical relevance [47]. For example, some persons may respond more favorably to an exergame intervention or the duration of the intervention period necessary to produce significant benefits may differ between persons with specific characteristics. To our knowledge, only Schwenk et al. [28] analyzed predictors of training response to a 4-week exergame-based balance training program in people with cognitive impairment (2×/week, 45 min), suggesting that low baseline performance and a history of falls were associated with greater improvements in balance.

Previous work

We recently evaluated a 10-week, task-specific, motor-cognitive training program with an interactive, exergame-based balance training system (Physiomat®) in PwD. Results of our randomized controlled trial (RCT) demonstrated that, compared to a non-specific, motor placebo activity (unspecific, low-intensity strength and flexibility exercises for the upper body while seated), an exergame intervention significantly improved motor-cognitive performances of PwD in trained and untrained exergame tasks, with partly sustainable effects up to 3 months after training cessation [35]. Training-induced changes during the intervention period and predictors of early training response have not been addressed in this study.

Study aims and hypotheses

The primary aim of these secondary analyses was to provide a more detailed insight into the time course of improvements in motor-cognitive exergame performances during a task-specific training program in patients with mild-to-moderate dementia. A secondary aim was to identify predictive factors associated with early training response. Based on general dose-response relationships for physical exercise [38, 39] and previous findings on predictors of exergame training response in people with cognitive impairment [28], we hypothesized that (1) time course of improvements in exergame performances would also be asymptotic, with the greatest training gains occurring during the early training period and (2) patients with the lowest initial performance would benefit most and the fastest from the exergame intervention.

Methods

Study design

This study presents secondary analyses of a double-blinded, randomized, placebo-controlled intervention trial on the effects of a dementia-specific motor-cognitive training program in patients with mild-to-moderate dementia. Details about the design, intervention, and main analyses of the RCT have been described previously [35, 48, 49]. The secondary analyses involved the motor-cognitive exergame performance of the intervention group (IG) on the Physiomat®, which was assessed at baseline before training (T1), at training session 7 (TS7) and 14 (TS14), and at post-intervention after 20 training sessions (T2) to analyze changes in the Physiomat® performance over the time course of the study period. Baseline patient characteristics were analyzed as potential predictors of early training response from T1 to TS7 for the Physiomat® performance.

Study population

The process of screening, recruitment, enrollment and randomization of participants has been previously described in detail [35]. Inclusion criteria were as follows: ≥ 65 years; Mini-Mental Status Examination (MMSE, [50]) score 17–26; diagnosis of probable dementia based on comprehensive neuropsychological testing (Consortium to Establish a Registry for Alzheimer's Disease [CERAD] test battery, [51]); ability to walk at least 10 m without a walking aid; no severe neurologic, cardiovascular, metabolic, or psychiatric disorders; residence within 15 km of the study center, and written informed consent.

Intervention

Participants took part in an interactive, exergame-based training on the Physiomat® for 10 weeks (2×/week à 10 min; 20 sessions in total) supervised by a qualified trainer experienced in training PwD. The Physiomat®

includes a balance platform moveable in the sagittal, frontal, and transversal plane. By platform-integrated displacement sensors, the three-dimensional movements of the platform are recorded and translated into linear movement of a cursor displayed on a 17-in. computer screen (Fig. 1). To solve a Physiomat® game task shown on the screen, the player must control and move the cursor by bending, tilting, and rotation movements while standing on the platform. A dementia-specific, patient-centered training approach (e.g. verbal instructions and cueing, haptic assistance, verbal praise) [52, 53] was used to train participants in performing a Physiomat®-Follow The Ball Task (FTBT) and more cognitively challenging Physiomat®-Trail Making Tasks (PTMTs) on five different complexity levels as defined by the number of digits to be connected (i.e. 4, 7, 9, 14, or 20 digits). The PTMTs were based on an established neuropsychological test ('Zahlen-Verbindungs-Test' = 'Number-Connection-Test' of the Nuremberg Age Inventory, TMT-NAI, [54], which is a modified version of the Trail Making Test validated for use in PwD.

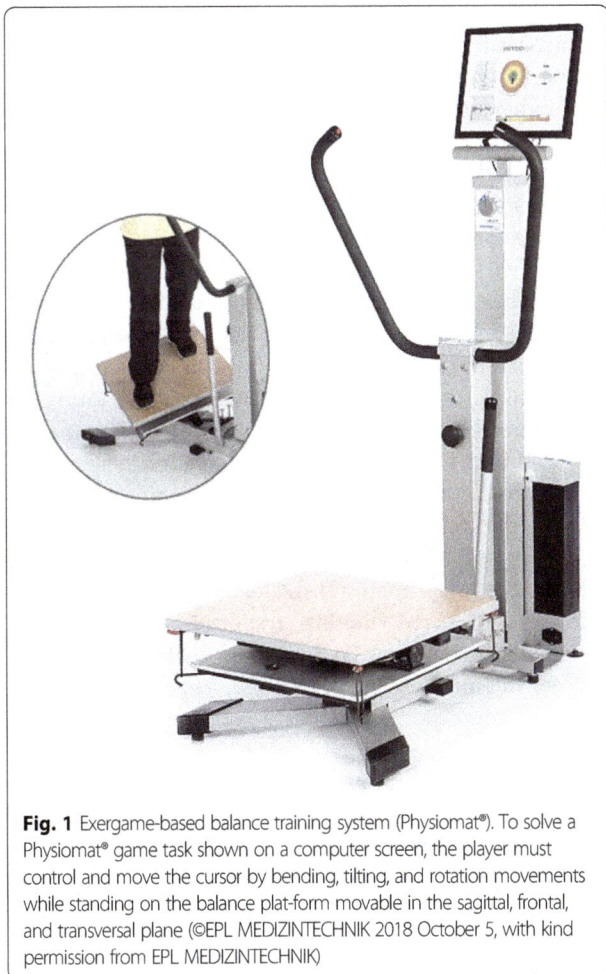

Fig. 1 Exergame-based balance training system (Physiomat®). To solve a Physiomat® game task shown on a computer screen, the player must control and move the cursor by bending, tilting, and rotation movements while standing on the balance plat-form movable in the sagittal, frontal, and transversal plane (©EPL MEDIZINTECHNIK 2018 October 5, with kind permission from EPL MEDIZINTECHNIK)

Participants were instructed to move the cursor on the screen by weight shifting on the platform while holding onto the Physiomat® handles to follow a moving ball on the screen (FTBT) or to connect the digits in ascending order (PTMTs) as fast as possible (for further details on the intervention, see [35]). According to the participants' individual performance level, the complexity of the Physiomat® tasks was successively increased as training progressed. The decision point for increasing the complexity was the ability to complete a Physiomat® task safely without assistance.

Measurements
Outcome variable
The main outcome variable of this study was the Physiomat® performance assessed as the time required to complete the Physiomat® tasks (duration), which was directly derived from the data stream of the Physiomat®-integrated sensors during the gameplay [55]. The tasks included the same FTBT and PTMTs trained during the intervention period, and the same instructions were given as used for the Physiomat® training. No cueing or haptic assistance was provided by test administrator during the assessment. Each test session was started with the FTBT. After successfully completing the FTBT, the PTMT level was successively increased during the assessment until the participant was no longer able to complete a level. Participants performed two trials for each Physiomat® task, where the trial with the shortest duration was used for statistical analysis.

Descriptive and predictor variables
Demographic and clinical characteristics including age, gender, education, comorbidity (number of diagnoses, medications), recent history of falls (previous year), social status (community-dwelling vs. institutionalized), and physiological status for depression (Geriatric Depression Scale, 15-item version [56]) and fear of falling (Falls Efficacy Scale-International, 7-item version [57]) were documented from patient charts or by standardized patient interview.

Motor-functional status was measured by the Performance-Oriented Mobility Assessment (POMA, [58]), the Timed Up and Go [59], and the 5-chair stand test [60].

Cognitive status was screened using the MMSE [50]. Domain-specific cognitive functions were assessed by the CERAD test battery [51], including subtests of verbal fluency, visual naming (Boston Naming Test), verbal episodic memory encoding (word list memory), recall (word list recall) and recognition (word list recognition), visuospatial ability (constructional praxis), non-verbal episodic memory (constructional recall), and phonemic fluency; the modified Trail Making Test (TMT-NAI,

[54]) for speed of information processing; and a Digit-Span Test (DST-NAI, [54]) for working memory. To assess global cognitive functioning, the demographically corrected CERAD total score (CERAD-TS) was calculated [61].

Motor-cognitive dual-task performance (divided attention) was assessed using a simultaneous walking and working memory task. Participants walked along a 5.79 m long GAITRite® instrumented walkway (CIR Systems Inc., Havertown, PA, USA: 4.88 m active area; 120 Hz sampling rate) at a maximum pace while counting backwards as fast as possible in steps of three. Each walk was initiated and terminated 1 m before and after the walkway to account for acceleration and deceleration. To quantify the overall motor-cognitive dual-task performance, the relative dual-task costs (DTC = ([dual task − single task]/single task × 100, [62]) of gait speed ($DTC_{gait\ speed}$) and calculation steps ($DTC_{counting}$) were combined ($DTC_{combined} = (DTC_{gait\ speed} + DTC_{counting})/2$). The dual-task test procedure and data processing as well as the biometrical quality of this dual-task assessment have been previously described in detail [63].

Initial training adherence from T1 to TS7 was documented as the percentage of the first seven training sessions attended relative to the number of the maximum possible training sessions offered in this period in which the participant completed these seven training sessions.

Statistical analysis

Descriptive data were presented as frequencies and percentages for categorical variables, and means, standard deviations (SD) and ranges or medians and ranges for continuous variables as appropriate. To identify significant differences in the Physiomat® performance between the individual test sessions (T1, TS7, TS14, T2), we used one-way repeated-measures analyses of variance (ANOVAs) or Friedman ANOVAs on ranks (for non-normally distributed data) with Bonferroni-adjusted post-hoc paired-samples t-tests and Wilcoxon signed-rank tests, respectively. Effect sizes for post-hoc comparisons were calculated as Cohen's d for paired-samples t-tests ($0.2 \leq d < 0.5$ = small, $0.5 \leq d < 0.8$ = moderate, $0.8 \leq d < 1.3$ = large, $d \geq 1.3$ = very large effect) and as effect size r for the Wilcoxon signed-rank tests ($0.1 \leq r < 0.3$ = small, $0.3 \leq r < 0.5$ = moderate, $0.5 \leq r < 0.7$ = large, $r \geq 0.7$ = very large effect) [64, 65]. Bonferroni-adjusted p-values were reported for the post-hoc multiple comparisons.

Reliable change indices (RCIs [66, 67]) were computed for the duration of each Physiomat® task to identify early responders from T1 to TS7. The RCI can be used to evaluate whether a participant's change in pre- and post-intervention scores is beyond that which might be due to random measurement error, considering the instrument reliability and the sample variability specific for the population of interest. Based on data (i.e.

test-retest reliabilities [r_{tt}]; standard deviations of test [SD_1] and retest [SD_2]) of our previously published study on the biometrical quality of the Physiomat® assessment in PwD [55], the RCI for each Physiomat® task was calculated as follows: (1) standard error of measurement ($SEM_{1/2} = SD_{1/2} \times \sqrt{[1 − r_{tt}]}$); (2) standard error of the difference ($S_{diff} = \sqrt{[SEM_1^2 + SEM_2^2]}$), and (3) reliable change index ($RCI = 1.96 \times S_{diff}$). The calculated RCIs (FTBT: ± 9.5 s; PTMT level 1: ± 5.0 s, level 2: ± 7.5 s, level 3: ± 9.1, level 4: ± 11.0 s, level 5: ± 17.7 s) were used to determine whether a participant's improvement in a specific Physiomat® task was sufficiently large to yield confidence that it was not due to measurement error. Taking into account the participant's individual Physiomat® performance at baseline and the different complex Physiomat® tasks, an early responder (ER) was defined as a participant with an individual decrease in the duration after TS7 that exceeded the RCI either (1) for the most complex Physiomat® task completed at T1 or (2) for at least 50% of the Physiomat® tasks completed at T1. All other participants were defined as "non-early responders" (NER). To identify potential predictive factors associated with early training response, univariate analyses examined differences in participant baseline characteristics between ER and NER using unpaired t-tests, Mann-Whitney U-tests, and χ^2 tests as appropriate. Independent baseline variables included demographic characteristics, comorbidity, psychological and motor-functional status, history of falls, global and domain-specific cognitive functioning, dual-task performance, baseline Physiomat® performances, and initial training adherence (Table 2). For the subsequent analysis, global cognitive functioning was defined by the CERAD-TS, which is regarded as being superior to scores of simplified screening measures such as the MMSE [68], and the baseline Physiomat® performance was defined by the FTBT duration, as the FTBT was the only Physiomat® task with baseline data available for all participants. Variables that showed significant differences in the univariate analyses were entered in a multivariate logistic regression analysis (likelihood ratio-based forward stepwise method) to determine independent predictors of early training response. Results of the regression model were reported as odds ratios (ORs) with 95% confidence intervals (CIs). The goodness-of-fit of the regression model was assessed by the Hosmer-Lemeshow test, and the amount of variance explained by model was expressed as Nagelkerke R^2. Prediction accuracy of the model was defined as the percentage of correctly classified ERs and NERs. A two-sided p-value of ≤ .05 indicated statistical significance. Statistical analyses were performed using IBM SPSS Statistics for Windows, Version 23.0 (IBM Corp., Armonk, NY, USA).

Results

Sample characteristics

The sample for the secondary analyses included the 56 RCT participants allocated to the IG. Participants were multimorbid older patients with mild-to-moderate dementia and impaired motor-functional status (Table 1). Forty-five participants completed all four Physiomat® test sessions (T1, TS7, TS14, T2) over the study period. Four participants dropped out before TS7 due to serious medical events ($n = 2$, 3.6%) or lack of motivation ($n = 2$, 3.6%), and another seven dropped out during the later course of the intervention due to lack of motivation ($n = 4$, 7.1%), injurious falls ($n = 2$, 3.6%), and death ($n = 1$, 1.8%). Participants who dropped out did not differ significantly from those who stayed in the study for any descriptive variable at baseline ($p = .327–.909$) or any parameter for effects of intervention ($p = .235–.933$).

Time course of Physiomat® performance

All 45 participants who stayed in the study successfully completed the rather low cognitively challenging FTBT at all four test sessions; however, the increasing difficulty of the Physiomat® tasks led to gradually decreasing samples sizes for the other, more complex PTMTs (level 1: $n = 43$ to level 5: $n = 13$, Fig. 2) as the participants reached their performance limit at individually different Physiomat® tasks.

Significant differences in the Physiomat® performance between the individual test sessions were found for all Physiomat® tasks ($p < .001$). Post-hoc analyses revealed significant improvements from T1 to TS7 in all Physiomat®

tasks ($p \le .001–.006$), with moderate to very large effect sizes (FTBT, PTMT level 1 & 2: $r = .38–.52$; PTMT level 3–5: $d = .85–1.45$). For 4 out of 6 Physiomat® tasks, the Physiomat® performance did not significantly change between TS7 and TS14 ($p = .359–.999$). During this intermediate phase of the intervention period, significant positive intervention effects were observed only in the PTMT level 2 ($p = .035$) and level 4 ($p = .026$), with moderate effect sizes (level 2: $r = .32$; level 4: $d = .68$). From TS14 to T2, the Physiomat® performance significantly improved only in the PTMT level 1 ($p = .009$) and level 4 ($p = .016$). Effect sizes for these significant improvements were moderate (level 1: $r = .34$; level 4: $d = .74$). For all four other Physiomat® tasks, no significant improvements ($p = .153–.999$) were found during this late phase of the intervention period (TS14 to T2). For each Physiomat® task, the largest effect size between two consecutive test sessions was observed from T1 to TS7 (e.g. PTMT level 3: T1 to TS7: $d = .85$; TS7 to TS14: $d = .34$; TS14 to T2: $d = .22$). Over the last two thirds of the intervention period (TS7 to T2), the Physiomat® performance significantly improved across all Physiomat® tasks ($p \le .001–.036$), with moderate to very large effect sizes (FTBT, PTMT level 1 & 2: $r = .34–.39$; PTMT level 3–5: $d = .53–1.34$) and the largest effect sizes for the most complex Physiomat® tasks (PTMT level 4 & 5: $d = 1.28–1.34$).

Predictors of early training response

Potential predictive factors associated with early training response were analyzed in all the participants who completed the Physiomat® test sessions at T1 and TS7 ($n = 52$). Based on the definition of early training response by the RCIs across the different Physiomat® tasks, 31 (59.6%) participants were classified as ERs and 21 (40.4%) as NERs. The changes of ERs and NERs from T1 to TS7 within the individual Physiomat® tasks were presented in Fig. 3, suggesting that ERs showed lower baseline performance with higher improvements during this early training period up to a performance level at TS7 similar to those of the NERs. At post-intervention (T2), no significant differences in the Physiomat® tasks were found between ERs and NERs ($p = .101–.911$).

Comparisons between the baseline characteristics of two subgroups revealed that ERs initially showed significantly lower Physiomat® performances (FTBT: $p < .001$; PTMT: $p \le .001–.036$) as already indicated in Fig. 3, lower global cognitive functioning (MMSE: $p = .039$; CERAD-TS: $p = .026$), lower visuospatial ability (constructional praxis: $p = .006$), lower speed of information processing (TMT-NAI: $p = .001$), and lower dual-task performance ($DTC_{combined}$: $p = .040$) than NERs (Table 2).

When the variables significantly associated with early training response were entered into the multivariate logistic regression model, baseline Physiomat®

Table 1 Sample characteristics

Variable	Total sample ($n = 56$)
Age, years	82.7 ± 6.2 [65–94]
Females	39 (69.6)
Mini-Mental State Examination, score	22.2 ± 2.8 [17–26]
Education, years	11 [7–20]
Diagnoses	7.7 ± 3.8 [1–18]
Medications	7.6 ± 3.4 [0–14]
Taking cholinesterase inhibitors or memantine	13 (23.2)
Timed Up and Go, s	14.6 [6.5–52.7]
Performance Oriented Mobility Assessment, score	22.4 ± 4.3 [9–28]
5-chair stand test, s	14.8 ± 7.6 [6.8–39.1]
Geriatric Depression Scale, score	2 [0–9]
Falls Efficacy Scale-International, score	8.5 [7–19]
Fall in the previous year	23 (41.1)
Living situation	
Community-dwelling	39 (69.6)
Institutionalized	17 (30.4)

Data are presented as mean ± SD [range], n (%), or median [range]

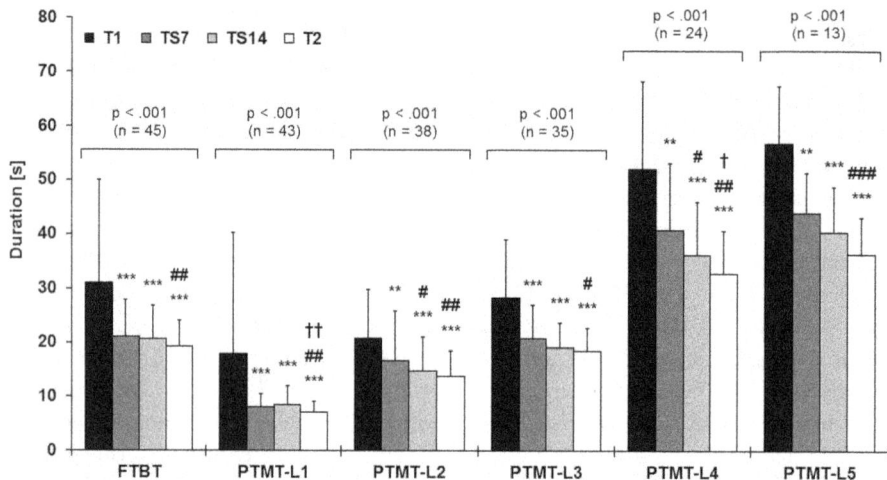

Fig. 2 Performance in the different Physiomat® tasks at baseline (T1, black bars), training session 7 (TS7, dark gray bars) and 14 (TS14, light gray bars), and post- intervention (T2, white bars). Data are given as mean ± SD. FTBT, Physiomat®-Follow The Ball Task; PTMT, Physiomat®-Trail Making Task; L1–5, level 1–5. P-values are given for one-way repeated-measures ANOVAs (PTMT level 3–5) or Friedman ANOVAs on ranks (FTBT, PTMT level 1 & 2). Post-hoc multiple comparisons between the individual test sessions were performed with Bonferroni-adjusted paired t-tests (PTMT level 3–5) or Wilcoxon signed-rank tests (FTBT, PTMT level 1 & 2). Key to statistics: * $p < .05$, ** $p < .01$, *** $p < .001$, in comparison to T1; # $p < .05$, ## $p < .01$, ### $p < .001$, in comparison to TS7; † $p < .05$, †† $p < .01$, in comparison to TS14. Decrease in the duration (in seconds) indicates improvement in the Physiomat® performance

performance (OR = 1.261, $p = .003$), constructional praxis (OR = 0.558, $p = .019$), and dual-task performance (OR = 0.943, $p = .031$), were identified as independent predictors of early training response (Table 3). The regression model was significant ($\chi^2 = 33.96$, df = 3, $p < .001$) and demonstrated goodness-of-fit (Hosmer-Lemeshow-Test: $\chi^2 = 5.45$, df = 8, $p = .709$). It accounted for 64.8% of variance in training response (Nagelkerke $R^2 = .648$) and correctly classified 84.6% participants as ERs or NERs.

Discussion

To the best of our knowledge, the presented study is the first (1) to provide a detailed insight into the time course of changes in motor-cognitive exergame performances during a task-specific training program and (2) to examine potential predictive factors that are associated with early training response in the vulnerable population of multimorbid older patients with mild-to-moderate dementia and impaired motor-functional status.

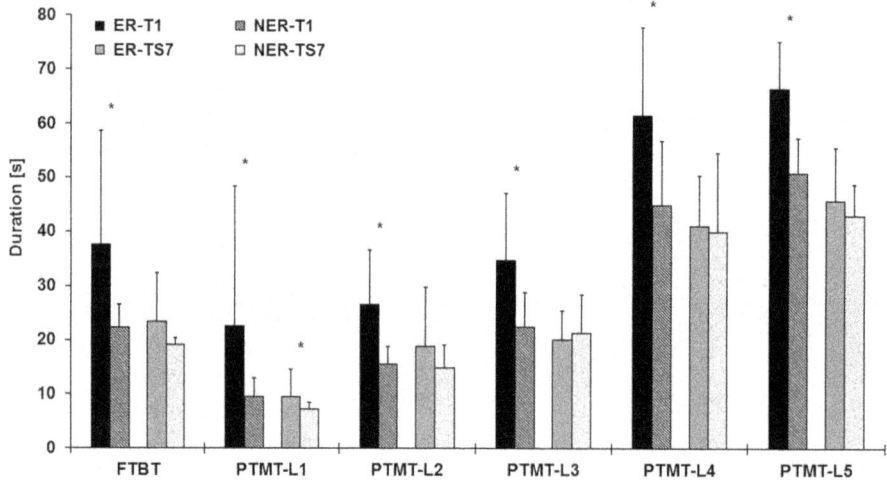

Fig. 3 Performance in the different Physiomat tasks at baseline (T1) and training session 7 (TS7) for early responders (ER) and non-early responders (NER). Data are given as mean ± SD. FTBT, Physiomat®-Follow The Ball Task; PTMT, Physiomat®-Trail Making Task; L1–5, level 1–5. Paired-samples t-tests (PTMT-L3-L5) or Wilcoxon signed-rank tests (FTBT, PTMT-L1/L2) were performed to test differences between ERs and NERs at T1 and TS7, respectively. Key to statistics: * $p < .05$. Decrease in the duration (in seconds) indicates improvement in the Physiomat® performance

Table 2 Baseline comparisons between participant characteristics for early responders and non-early responders

Variable	ERs (n = 31)	NERs (n = 21)	p-value
Age, years[a]	83.5 ± 6.5 [65–93]	82.3 ± 6.0 [70–94]	.514
Females[b]	23 (74.2)	14 (66.7)	.557
Mini-Mental State Examination, score[a]	21.4 ± 2.8 [17–26]	23.0 ± 2.4 [17–26]	.039
Diagnoses[a]	7.5 ± 3.4 [1–17]	7.5 ± 4.1 [1–17]	.994
Medications[a]	7.3 ± 3.3 [0–13]	8.1 ± 3.6 [0–14]	.419
Timed Up and Go, s[c]	14.8 [9.8–52.7]	13.9 [6.5–51.2]	.714
Performance Oriented Mobility Assessment, score[a]	22.2 ± 4.0 [12–28]	23.1 ± 3.9 [15–28]	.405
5-chair stand test, s	14.8 ± 7.6 [6.8–39.1]	13.5 ± 5.1 [7.2–29.4]	.522
Geriatric Depression Scale, score[c]	2 [0–9]	2 [0–8]	.799
Falls Efficacy Scale-International, score[c]	8 [7–13]	8 [7–19]	.826
Fall in the previous year	13 (41.9)	8 (38.1)	.782
CERAD scores[a]			
Total score	70.7 ± 8.7 [54–87]	77.2 ± 12.0 [54–87]	.026
Verbal fluency	9.7 ± 3.7 [3–17]	11.3 ± 3.5 [4–18]	.124
Boston Naming Test	9.9 ± 2.7 [5–15]	11.0 ± 2.4 [5–14]	.150
Word list memory	10.5 ± 3.1 [4–16]	11.2 ± 3.8 [5–16]	.484
Word list recall	2.1 ± 1.8 [0–6]	2.0 ± 1.8 [0–5]	.900
Word list recognition	6.1 ± 2.7 [1–10]	7.1 ± 2.4 [2–10]	.172
Constructional praxis	7.0 ± 2.3 [2–11]	8.7 ± 1.8 [6–11]	.006
Constructional recall	1.7 ± 2.1 [0–7]	2.3 ± 2.2 [0–6]	.337
Phonemic fluency	6.8 ± 3.1 [0–15]	6.7 ± 4.0 [0–16]	.900
TMT-NAI, s[c]	114 [35–300]	57 [32–300]	.001
DST-NAI score[a]	8.6 ± 1.3 [6–11]	9.2 ± 1.0 [7–11]	.098
Dual-task performance (DTC$_{combined}$), %[a]	−36.1 ± 22.3 [− 82.5- -0.4]	−24.0 ± 16.8 [− 54.0- -0.2]	.040
Baseline Physiomat® performance, s			
FTBT[c]	37.6 [18.5–121.1]	21.2 [17.1–31.5]	< .001
PTMT-L1[c,d]	15.6 [5.8–136.1]	8.2 [5.3–19.8]	< .001
PTMT-L2[c,e]	24.7 [10.3–57.3]	15.8 [10.5–21.5]	< .001
PTMT-L3[a,f]	34.7 ± 12.4 [21.6–64.5]	22.4 ± 6.4 [13.2–37.6]	< .001
PTMT-L4[a,g]	61.5 ± 16.2 [37.8–91.4]	44.9 ± 12.0 [31.6–67.5]	.007
PTMT-L5[a,h]	66.4 ± 8.7 [52.6–75.1]	53.7 ± 10.7 [39.1–76.9]	.036
Training adherence at TS7[a]	81.1 ± 20.3 [42.9–100]	76.7 ± 20.9 [33.3–100]	.451

Data are presented as mean ± SD [range], n (%), or median [range]. ERs, early responders; NERs, non-early responders; CERAD, Consortium to Establish a Registry for Alzheimer's Disease, TMT-NAI, Trail Making Test from the Nuremberg Age Inventory; DST-NAI, Digit-Span Test from the Nuremberg Age Inventory; DTC$_{combined}$, combined dual-task costs (i.e. [motor + cognitive dual-tasks costs]/2); FTBT, Physiomat®-Follow The Ball Task; PTMT, Physiomat®-Trail Making Task; L1–5, level 1–5. P-values for [a]t-tests, [b]χ^2 test, and [c]Mann-Whitney U-tests. P-values in bold indicate statistical significance (p ≤ .05). Comparison between [d]n = 30 ERs vs. n = 20 NERs, [e]n = 27 ERs vs. n = 18 NERs, [f]n = 21 ERs vs. n = 18 NERs; [g]n = 12 ERs vs. n = 13 NERs; [h]n = 5 ERs vs. n = 9 NERs

Table 3 Multivariate logistic regression model for predictors of early training response

Variable	β	SEM	OR (95% CI)	P-value
Constructional praxis[a]	−.583	.248	.558 (.344–.907)	.019
Baseline Physiomat® performance[b]	−.232	.079	1.261 (1.081–1.471)	.003
Dual-task performance[c]	−.058	.027	.943 (.895–.995)	.031

Removed from model: TMT-NAI (p = .745), CERAD total score (p = .565). [a]Lower scores indicate lower constructional praxis ability; [b]higher scores indicate lower baseline Physiomat® performance; [c]lower scores indicate lower dual-task performance

Time course of Physiomat® performance

Deficits in motor-cognitive dual-tasking has been repeatedly identified as predictor for functional decline [8, 9] and falls [10, 11], and dual-task abilities have been reported to be reduced in PwD [5–7]. One of the major findings of this study was that in PwD exergame-based dual-task performances can be substantially improved after a surprisingly short period of task-specific interactive motor-cognitive training. We observed significant improvements in all Physiomat® tasks already after 3 weeks.

In older patients with Parkinson's disease and healthy elderly, significant improvements in some but not all Nintendo Wii Fit™ exergames have also been reported after similar durations of task-specific training (2–3 weeks) [43]. In PwD, only a usability study was found, showing that exergame performances can be improved after 4 weeks of task-specific training [34]. However, the frequency and total amount of exercise during the intervention period in this study were substantially higher (4 × 60 min/week = 240 min), and the exergame intervention covered interactive video-sports games with considerably less complex concurrent motor-cognitive tasks (Nintendo Wii Sports™ Bowling and Tennis), compared to our study with a training protocol of two 10 min-exergame sessions per week (3 × 20 min/week = 60 min) on an exergame-based balance platform combining whole-body postural control tasks with complex cognitive tasks of an established neuropsychological test (TMT-NAI, [54]). The prompt training-induced effects on such interactive motor-cognitive dual-task performances have not been previously reported in PwD. These findings suggest that an exergame-based motor-cognitive training program has the potential to represent a time-efficient intervention for improving movement control under cognitive load in PwD, which may contribute to reduced fall risk in this highly vulnerable patient population [14]. Such interactive motor-cognitive training programs might also be associated with more general effects on global cognitive functioning, as previously reported for exergaming [32] or interactive visuomotor game training [69] in cognitively impaired older adults after 10- to 14-week training periods. Based on our findings that improvements in task-specific exergame performances can be made after a much shorter training period, future studies should assess whether potential transfer effects related to exergame interventions can be achieved also after short intervention periods, or even assess the time course of such potential transfer effects.

The time course of improvements in exergame performances seemed to be asymptotic rather than linear, with the greatest part of the total training effects already apparent after the early, 3-week intervention phase (T1 to TS7) across all Physiomat® tasks. After these prompt initial improvements at TS7, the positive effect of the intervention decreased and participants seemed to reach a training plateau during the intermediate intervention phase given the chosen training frequency and intensity. For most of the Physiomat® tasks, the extension of the intervention period by another two training intervals of 3 weeks did not result in significant progressive improvements compared to the corresponding previous test session (TS7 vs. TS14, TS14 vs. T2). However, taking this two training intervals together (TS7 to T2 = 6 weeks), the performance in all Physiomat® tasks significantly improved over the last two thirds of the intervention period. This time course of exergame performances confirmed our hypothesis and is in line with established exercise training principles and general dose-response relationships reported for exercise training [38, 39], suggesting that in training novices and untrained individuals with high potential for improvements, a low training dosage (intensity, frequency, duration) with small increases may already be sufficient to induce significant improvements after a short training period; however, as training duration continues and the performance of individuals increases, the rate of improvements begins to slow down for a similar increase in intensity or amount of activity in the following training period. Thus, a higher rate in the increase of the training parameters (intensity, frequency, and/or duration) is required to provide further effective training stimuli. For each Physiomat® task, we observed significant improvements after the initial intervention phase (T1 to TS7), which in turn may have decreased the participant's potential for improvements within the tasks during the subsequent training period. To achieve further training gains from the increased performance level and this test session on, a training intensification in the following training period seems to have been necessary. The frequency, i.e. the number of training sessions per week, could not be increased in our study due to its design, but we were able to successively further increase the intensity, i.e. the complexity level of the Physiomat® tasks, as participants improved and training progressed. However, for some participants, a higher rate in increase of the intensity was not possible, as the number of available complexity levels of the Physiomat® tasks was limited. For example, the intensity for high-preforming participants that reached the most complex Physiomat® tasks during the early training period could only be further increased by instructions to complete the most complex Physiomat® tasks even more quickly. This rather low rate of further increase in intensity for these participants may have also affected the impact of the intervention during the subsequent training period. Overall, our approach for increasing the intensity might not have been sufficient to induce the same significant improvements observed for the initial 3-week training interval (T1 to TS7) also for the consecutive training intervals of equal length (TS7 to TS14, T14 to T2). Rather, it seemed that the extension of the training duration (TS7 to T2 = 6 weeks) might have played a more important role to further improve participants' performance beyond that reached after the early intervention phase. This finding is also consistent with the idea of the general dose-response principle for exercise training [38], indicating that improvements in some health-related variables may be more related to the volume and amount of exercise than to its intensity.

Over the last two thirds of the intervention period (TS7 to T2) the largest effects were observed for the highest PTMT levels. This might be related to their higher complexity and to the greater sensitivity to detect changes that has been previously reported for these Physiomat® tasks [35]. For the less complex Physiomat® tasks, potential ceiling effects for those participants who completed the higher PTMT levels already at baseline and possibly reached their maximum performance level on the less complex Physiomat® tasks already after the initial training period (T1 to TS7) may have affected the impact of the extended training duration. In the highest PTMT levels, however, there may still have been a higher potential for these high-performing participants to further improve during the subsequent training period, even after initial significant training response, due to the higher complexity of these tasks.

Predictors of early training response

Previous studies in older people with cognitive impairment or PwD identified low baseline performance in primary outcomes (i.e., balance, maximal strength, and/or motor-functional performance) to be independently predictive for positive training response to physical exercise or exergame interventions [28, 52, 70]. Supporting our hypothesis, based on these previous findings, the regression analysis of our study revealed similar results for exergame-based motor-cognitive performances, such that participants with lower initial performance in these outcomes were those who experienced the greatest training gains over the first 3 weeks of the intervention period. The inverse relationship between the magnitude of benefits and the baseline status for an initial training phase was also described in the general dose-response principles for exercise training [38, 39], indicating that those individuals with the lowest performance benefit the most and the fastest from an exercise intervention.

Some studies have found that lower global cognitive functioning negatively influence training response to physical exercise interventions [71–75], whereas other studies have not [28, 52, 70, 76, 77]. Interestingly, and in contrast to all these studies, more severe global cognitive impairment was initially associated with early training

response in the univariate analysis of our study. However, the multivariate analysis suggested that this association might actually be explained by the lower performance in domain-specific cognitive functions, whose effects on trainability have rarely been examined in previous studies [52, 76], rather than by the level of global cognitive functioning, which was not independently associated with early training response in our regression model. In particular, the multivariate analysis revealed that lower visuospatial ability and divided attention were independent predictors of early training response. It is conspicuous that lower performance in these cognitive subdomains was identified to be predictive for early training response as spatial orientation and divided attention were stated to be required and trained on the Physiomat® [35]. Because of their greater deficits in these task-related cognitive functions, ERs may have had more room to improve during the early training period than NERs.

In the univariate analysis, lower performance in speed of information processing as assessed by the TMT-NAI was initially associated with early training response; however, this association was lost in the multivariate analysis, maybe because it was captured by other model covariates, especially by the baseline performance on the Physiomat®, whose game tasks were based also on the TMT-NAI.

Results confirm that not only an excellent training response can be achieved despite cognitive impairment, but also that those participants with greater deficits in training-related, domain-specific cognitive functions of visuospatial ability and divided attention, which both have been associated with fall risk [10, 78], benefit the most and the fastest from the exergame intervention.

Limitations and future research

The present study has some limitations. First, the exergame performance of the control group was only assessed before and at the end of the intervention period. Therefore, the time course of the effects of the exergame intervention in the IG could not be compared to those of the non-specific, motor placebo activity. However, in our previous RCT, we have already demonstrated that improvements in the IG over the entire study period are specifically related to the exergame intervention, with no significant improvements in the control group for exergame-related performances [35]. Second, the increasing difficulty of the Physiomat® tasks during the test sessions led to gradually decreasing sample sizes across the tasks. The statistical analyses of the more complex tasks may therefore be limited by a small sample size. By using increasing difficulty levels for assessment, however, it was ensured that each participant could have been adequately challenged to assess his/her individual maximum performance level ('testing the limits') and to prevent ceiling and floor effects at all test sessions. Third, our results are restricted to patients with mild-to-moderate dementia and so cannot be generalized to those with more severe dementia. Fourth, the small sample size may have affected the results of the regression analysis and limited the precious of our conclusions. Fifth, according to the preplanned study design, potential transfer effects of the exergame intervention (e.g. on balance, cognitive functioning) were not analyzed in this study, representing potential targets for future research.

Conclusions

The present study reveals for the first time that substantial task-specific improvements in complex motor-cognitive performances can be achieved after a surprisingly short exergame-based training program in patients with mild-to-moderate dementia. According to general dose-response relationships for physical exercise, our findings demonstrate that the rate of improvements induced by the exergame intervention decreases as training progresses and that with increasing performance level of individuals a longer training period is required to achieve further improvements. Current findings also highlight the trainability and rehabilitation potential of PwD, especially for more vulnerable patients with low initial performance and more severe impairments in training-related cognitive functions who may even reap the most and fastest benefit from motor-cognitive exergame interventions.

Abbreviations

ANOVA: Analysis of variance; CERAD: Consortium to Establish a Registry for Alzheimer's Disease; CERAD-TS: Total score of the CERAD test battery; CI: Confidence interval; DST-NAI: Digit-Span Test of the Nuremberg Age Inventory; DTC: Dual-task cost; ER: Early responder; FTBT: Physiomat®-Follow The Ball Task; IG: Intervention group; MMSE: Mini-Mental State Examination; NER: Non-early responder; OR: Odds ratio; POMA: Performance Oriented Mobility Assessment; PTMT: Physiomat®-Trail Making Task; PwD: Patients with dementia; RCI: Reliable change index; RCT: Randomized controlled trial; r_{tt}: Test-retest reliability; SD: Standard deviation; SEM: Standard error of measurement; T2: Post-intervention; TMT-NAI: 'Number-Connection-Test' (Trail Making Test) of the Nuremberg Age Inventory; TS14: Training session 14; TS7: Training session 7

Acknowledgements
We thank Michaela Günther-Lange (Agaplesion Bethanien Hospital Heidelberg, Geriatric Center at the Heidelberg University) for her assistance in training and supervision of participants. We also thank the volunteers for their willingness to participate in the study.

Funding
The study was supported by the Dietmar Hopp Foundation, the Robert Bosch Foundation, and the Network of Aging Research (NAR) at the Heidelberg University. The funding sources had no role in the design and conduct of the study; collection, management, analysis, and interpretation of the data; and preparation, review, or approval of the manuscript.

Authors' contributions
CW: Acquisition of participants, study management, statistical analysis and interpretation of data, preparation of manuscript. RR: Analysis and interpretation of data, preparation of manuscript. SW: Acquisition of participants, study management. NCL: Study management, test administration, data collection. JMB: Interpretation of data, preparation of manuscript. KH: Study concept, design and management, supervision of data collection, interpretation of data, and preparation of manuscript. All authors contributed to interpretation of data, drafting the article, and final approval of the manuscript to be published.

Competing interests
The authors declare that they have no competing interests.

Author details
[1]Department of Geriatric Research, Agaplesion Bethanien Hospital Heidelberg, Geriatric Center at the Heidelberg University, Heidelberg, Germany. [2]Center for Geriatric Medicine, Heidelberg University, Heidelberg, Germany. [3]Department of Radiological Diagnostics, Theresien Hospital Mannheim, Mannheim, Germany. [4]Institute of Gerontology, Heidelberg University, Heidelberg, Germany. [5]Network of Aging Research (NAR), Heidelberg University, Heidelberg, Germany.

References
1. Perry RJ, Hodges JR. Attention and executive deficits in Alzheimer's disease. A critical review Brain. 1999;122:383–404.
2. Baddeley AD, Baddeley HA, Bucks RS, Wilcock GK. Attentional control in Alzheimer's disease. Brain. 2001;124:1492–508.
3. Perry RJ, Watson P, Hodges JR. The nature and staging of attention dysfunction in early (minimal and mild) Alzheimer's disease: relationship to episodic and semantic memory impairment. Neuropsychologia. 2000;38(3): 252–71.
4. Hauer K, Marburger C, Oster P. Motor performance deteriorates with simultaneously performed cognitive tasks in geriatric patients. Arch Phys Med Rehabil. 2002;83(2):217–23.
5. Muir SW, Speechley M, Wells J, Borrie M, Gopaul K, Montero-Odasso M. Gait assessment in mild cognitive impairment and Alzheimer's disease: the effect of dual-task challenges across the cognitive spectrum. Gait Posture. 2012; 35(1):96–100.
6. Hauer K, Pfisterer M, Weber C, Wezler N, Kliegel M, Oster P. Cognitive impairment decreases postural control during dual tasks in geriatric patients with a history of severe falls. J Am Geriatr Soc. 2003;51(11):1638–44.
7. Manckoundia P, Pfitzenmeyer P, d'Athis P, Dubost V, Mourey F. Impact of cognitive task on the posture of elderly subjects with Alzheimer's disease compared to healthy elderly subjects. Mov Disord. 2006;21(2):236–41.
8. Lundin-Olsson L, Nyberg L, Gustafson Y. Attention, frailty, and falls: the effect of a manual task on basic mobility. J Am Geriatr Soc. 1998;46(6): 758–61.
9. Faulkner KA, Redfern MS, Rosano C, Landsittel DP, Studenski SA, Cauley JA, et al. Reciprocal influence of concurrent walking and cognitive testing on performance in older adults. Gait Posture. 2006;24(2):182–9.
10. Muir-Hunter SW, Wittwer JE. Dual-task testing to predict falls in community-dwelling older adults: a systematic review. Physiotherapy. 2016;102(1):29–40.
11. Beauchet O, Annweiler C, Dubost V, Allali G, Kressig RW, Bridenbaugh S, et al. Stops walking when talking: a predictor of falls in older adults? Eur J Neurol. 2009;16(7):786–95.
12. Schwenk M, Lauenroth A, Oster P, Hauer K. Effektivität von körperlichem Training zur Verbesserung motorischer Leistungen bei Patienten mit demenzieller Erkrankung. In: Braumann K-M, Stiller N, editors. Bewegungstherapie bei internistischen Erkrankungen. Berlin, Heidelberg: Springer Berlin Heidelberg; 2010. p. 167–84.
13. Ghai S, Ghai I, Effenberg AO. Effects of dual tasks and dual-task training on postural stability: a systematic review and meta-analysis. Clin Interv Aging. 2017;12:557–77.

14. Montero-Odasso M, Speechley M. Falls in cognitively impaired older adults: implications for risk assessment and prevention. J Am Geriatr Soc. 2018; 66(2):367–75.

15. Monteiro-Junior RS, Vaghetti CA, Nascimento OJ, Laks J, Deslandes AC. Exergames: Neuroplastic hypothesis about cognitive improvement and biological effects on physical function of institutionalized older persons. Neural Regen Res. 2016;11(2):201–4.

16. Tait JL, Duckham RL, Milte CM, Main LC, Daly RM. Influence of sequential vs. simultaneous dual-task exercise training on cognitive function in older adults. Front Aging Neurosci. 2017;9:368.

17. van Diest M, Lamoth CJ, Stegenga J, Verkerke GJ, Postema K. Exergaming for balance training of elderly: state of the art and future developments. J Neuroeng Rehabil. 2013;10:101.

18. Molina KI, Ricci NA, de Moraes SA, Perracini MR. Virtual reality using games for improving physical functioning in older adults: a systematic review. J Neuroeng Rehabil. 2014;11:156.

19. Stanmore E, Stubbs B, Vancampfort D, de Bruin ED, Firth J. The effect of active video games on cognitive functioning in clinical and non-clinical populations: a meta-analysis of randomized controlled trials. Neurosci Biobehav Rev. 2017;78:34–43.

20. Schoene D, Valenzuela T, Lord SR, de Bruin ED. The effect of interactive cognitive-motor training in reducing fall risk in older people: a systematic review. BMC Geriatr. 2014;14:107.

21. Skjaeret N, Nawaz A, Morat T, Schoene D, Helbostad JL, Vereijken B. Exercise and rehabilitation delivered through exergames in older adults: an integrative review of technologies, safety and efficacy. Int J Med Inform. 2016;85(1):1–16.

22. Laufer Y, Dar G, Kodesh E. Does a Wii-based exercise program enhance balance control of independently functioning older adults? A systematic review. Clin Interv Aging. 2014;9:1803–13.

23. Chao YY, Scherer YK, Montgomery CA. Effects of using Nintendo Wii exergames in older adults: a review of the literature. J Aging Health. 2015;27(3):379–402.

24. Ogawa EF, You T, Leveille SG. Potential benefits of exergaming for cognition and dual-task function in older adults: a systematic review. J Aging Phys Act. 2016;24(2):332–6.

25. Taylor LM, Kerse N, Frakking T, Maddison R. Active video games for improving physical performance measures in older people: a meta-analysis. J Geriatr Phys Ther. 2018;41(2):108–23.

26. Li J, Theng YL, Foo S. Effect of exergames on depression: a systematic review and meta-analysis. Cyberpsychol Behav Soc Netw. 2016;19(1):34–42.

27. Padala KP, Padala PR, Malloy TR, Geske JA, Dubbert PM, Dennis RA, et al. Wii-fit for improving gait and balance in an assisted living facility: a pilot study. J Aging Res. 2012;2012:597573.

28. Schwenk M, Sabbagh M, Lin I, Morgan P, Grewal GS, Mohler J, et al. Sensor-based balance training with motion feedback in people with mild cognitive impairment. J Rehabil Res Dev. 2016;53(6):945–58.

29. Padala KP, Padala PR, Lensing SY, Dennis RA, Bopp MM, Roberson PK, et al. Home-based exercise program improves balance and fear of falling in community-dwelling older adults with mild Alzheimer's disease: a pilot study. J Alzheimers Dis. 2017;59(2):565–74.

30. Ben-Sadoun G, Sacco G, Manera V, Bourgeois J, Konig A, Foulon P, et al. Physical and cognitive stimulation using an exergame in subjects with normal aging, mild and moderate cognitive impairment. J Alzheimers Dis. 2016;53(4):1299–314.

31. Gonzalez-Palau F, Franco M, Bamidis P, Losada R, Parra E, Papageorgiou SG, et al. The effects of a computer-based cognitive and physical training program in a healthy and mildly cognitive impaired aging sample. Aging Ment Health. 2014;18(7):838–46.

32. Yamaguchi H, Maki Y, Takahashi K. Rehabilitation for dementia using enjoyable video-sports games. Int Psychogeriatr. 2011;23(4):674–6.

33. Weybright E, Dattilo J, Rusch F. Effects of an interactive video game (Nintendo Wii) on older women with mild cognitive impairment. Ther Recreat J. 2010;44(4):271.

34. Legouverneur G, Pino M, Boulay M, Rigaud A-S. Wii sports, a usability study with MCI and Alzheimer's patients. Alzheimers Dement. 2011;7(4):S500–S1.

35. Wiloth S, Werner C, Lemke NC, Bauer J, Hauer K. Motor-cognitive effects of a computerized game-based training method in people with dementia: a randomized controlled trial. Aging Ment Health. 2017:1–12. https://doi.org/10.1080/13607863.2017.1348472.

36. Fenney A, Lee TD. Exploring spared capacity in persons with dementia: what WiiTM can learn. Act Adapt Aging. 2010;34(4):303–13.

37. van Santen J, Droes RM, Holstege M, Henkemans OB, van Rijn A, de Vries R, et al. Effects of exergaming in people with dementia: results of a systematic literature review. J Alzheimers Dis. 2018;63(2):741–60.

38. Haskell WL. J.B. Wolffe Memorial Lecture. Health consequences of physical activity: understanding and challenges regarding dose-response. Med Sci Sports Exerc. 1994;26(6):649–60.

39. Hoffmann J. Physiological aspects of sport training and performance. Champaign, IL: Human Kinetics; 2002.

40. Manera V, Ben-Sadoun G, Aalbers T, Agopyan H, Askenazy F, Benoit M, et al. Recommendations for the use of serious games in neurodegenerative disorders: 2016 Delphi panel. Front Psychol. 2017;8(1243).

41. Manlapaz DG, Sole G, Jayakaran P, Chapple CM. A narrative synthesis of Nintendo Wii fit gaming protocol in addressing balance among healthy older adults: what system works? Games Health J. 2017;6(2):65–74.

42. Esculier JF, Vaudrin J, Beriault P, Gagnon K, Tremblay LE. Home-based balance training programme using Wii fit with balance board for Parkinsons's disease: a pilot study. J Rehabil Med. 2012;44(2):144–50.

43. dos Santos Mendes FA, Pompeu JE, Modenesi Lobo A, Guedes da Silva K, Oliveira Tde P, Peterson Zomignani A, et al. Motor learning, retention and transfer after virtual-reality-based training in Parkinson's disease-effect of motor and cognitive demands of games: a longitudinal, controlled clinical study. Physiotherapy. 2012;98(3):217–23.

44. Albores J, Marolda C, Haggerty M, Gerstenhaber B, Zuwallack R. The use of a home exercise program based on a computer system in patients with chronic obstructive pulmonary disease. J Cardiopulm Rehabil Prev. 2013; 33(1):47–52.

45. Rosenberg D, Depp CA, Vahia IV, Reichstadt J, Palmer BW, Kerr J, et al. Exergames for subsyndromal depression in older adults: a pilot study of a novel intervention. Am J Geriatr Psychiatry. 2010;18(3):221–6.

46. Williams MA, Soiza RL, Jenkinson AM, Stewart A. EXercising with computers in later life (EXCELL) - pilot and feasibility study of the acceptability of the Nintendo® WiiFit in community-dwelling fallers. BMC Res Notes. 2010;3:238.

47. Chmelo EA, Crotts CI, Newman JC, Brinkley TE, Lyles MF, Leng X, et al. Heterogeneity of physical function responses to exercise training in older adults. J Am Geriatr Soc. 2015;63(3):462–9.

48. Werner C, Wiloth S, Lemke NC, Kronbach F, Jansen CP, Oster P, et al. People with dementia can learn compensatory movement maneuvers for the sit-to-stand task: a randomized controlled trial. J Alzheimers Dis. 2017;60(1):107–20.

49. Lemke NC, Werner C, Wiloth S, Oster P, Bauer JM, Hauer K. Transferability and sustainability of motor-cognitive dual-task training in patients with dementia: a randomized controlled trial. Gerontology. 2018:1–16. https://doi.org/10.1159/000490852.

50. Folstein MF, Folstein SE, McHugh PR. "Mini-mental state". A practical method for grading the cognitive state of patients for the clinician. J Psychiatr Res. 1975;12(3):189–98.

51. Morris JC, Mohs RC, Rogers H, Fillenbaum G, Heyman A. Consortium to establish a registry for Alzheimer's disease (CERAD) clinical and neuropsychological assessment of Alzheimer's disease. Psychopharmacol Bull. 1988;24(4):641–52.

52. Hauer K, Schwenk M, Zieschang T, Essig M, Becker C, Oster P. Physical training improves motor performance in people with dementia: a randomized controlled trial. J Am Geriatr Soc. 2012;60(1):8–15.

53. Schwenk M, Oster P, Hauer K. Kraft- und Funktionstraining bei älteren Menschen mit demetieller Erkrankung. Praxis Physiotherapie. 2008;2:59–65.

54. Oswald WD, Fleischmann UM. Das Nürnberger-alters-Inventar (NAI) - Testinventar & NAI-Testmanual und Textband. Göttingen: Hogrefe; 1999.

55. Wiloth S, Lemke N, Werner C, Hauer K. Validation of a computerized, game-based assessment strategy to masure training effects on motor-cognitive functions in people with dementia. JMIR Serious Games. 2016;4(2):e12.

56. Sheikh JI, Yesavage JA. Geriatric depression scale (GDS): recent evidence and development of a shorter version. In: Brink TL, editor. Clinical gerontology: a guide to assessment and intervention. New York, NY: the Haworth press; 1986. p. 165–73.

57. Hauer KA, Kempen GI, Schwenk M, Yardley L, Beyer N, Todd C, et al. Validity and sensitivity to change of the falls efficacy scales international to assess fear of falling in older adults with and without cognitive impairment. Gerontology. 2011;57(5):462–72.

58. Tinetti ME. Performance-oriented assessment of mobility problems in elderly patients. J Am Geriatr Soc. 1986;34(2):119–26.

59. Podsiadlo D, Richardson S. The timed "up & go": a test of basic functional

mobility for frail elderly persons. J Am Geriatr Soc. 1991;39(2):142–8.

60. Guralnik JM, Simonsick EM, Ferrucci L, Glynn RJ, Berkman LF, Blazer DG, et al. A short physical performance battery assessing lower extremity function: association with self-reported disability and prediction of mortality and nursing home admission. J Gerontol. 1994;49(2):M85–94.

61. Chandler MJ, Lacritz LH, Hynan LS, Barnard HD, Allen G, Deschner M, et al. A total score for the CERAD neuropsychological battery. Neurology. 2005; 65(1):102–6.

62. Abernethy B. Dual-task methodology and motor skills research: some applications and methodological constraints. J Hum Mov Stud. 1988;14:101–32.

63. Lemke NC, Wiloth S, Werner C, Hauer K. Validity, test-retest reliability, sensitivity to change and feasibility of motor-cognitive dual task assessments in patients with dementia. Arch Gerontol Geriatr. 2017;70:169–79.

64. Cohen J. Statistical power analysis for the behavioral sciences. New York: Routledge; 1988.

65. Rosenthal JA. Qualitative descriptors of strength of association and effect size. J Soc Serv Res. 1996;21(4):37–59.

66. Jacobson NS, Truax P. Clinical significance: a statistical approach to defining meaningful change in psychotherapy research. J Consult Clin Psychol. 1991; 59(1):12–9.

67. Iverson GL. Interpreting change on the WAIS-III/WMS-III in clinical samples. Arch Clin Neuropsychol. 2001;16(2):183–91.

68. Ehrensperger MM, Berres M, Taylor KI, Monsch AU. Early detection of Alzheimer's disease with a total score of the German CERAD. J Int Neuropsychol Soc. 2010;16(5):910–20.

69. de Boer C, Echlin HV, Rogojin A, Baltaretu BR, Sergio LE. Thinking-while-moving exercises may improve cognition in elderly with mild cognitive deficits: a proof-of-principle study. Dement Geriatr Cogn Dis Extra. 2018:248–58.

70. Schwenk M, Dutzi I, Englert S, Micol W, Najafi B, Mohler J, et al. An intensive exercise program improves motor performances in patients with dementia: translational model of geriatric rehabilitation. J Alzheimers Dis. 2014;39(3):487–98.

71. Uemura K, Shimada H, Makizako H, Doi T, Yoshida D, Tsutsumimoto K, et al. Cognitive function affects trainability for physical performance in exercise intervention among older adults with mild cognitive impairment. Clin Interv Aging. 2013;8:97–102.

72. Ghisla MK, Cossi S, Timpini A, Baroni F, Facchi E, Marengoni A. Predictors of successful rehabilitation in geriatric patients: subgroup analysis of patients with cognitive impairment. Aging Clin Exp Res. 2007;19(5):417–23.

73. Rösler A, Krause T, Niehuus C, von Renteln-Kruse W. Dementia as a cofactor for geriatric rehabilitation-outcome in patients with osteosynthesis of the proximal femur: a retrospective, matched-pair analysis of 250 patients. Arch Gerontol Geriatr. 2009;49(1):e36–9.

74. Morghen S, Gentile S, Ricci E, Guerini F, Bellelli G, Trabucchi M. Rehabilitation of older adults with hip fracture: cognitive function and walking abilities. J Am Geriatr Soc. 2011;59(8):1497–502.

75. Hershkovitz A, Kalandariov Z, Hermush V, Weiss R, Brill S. Factors affecting short-term rehabilitation outcomes of disabled elderly patients with proximal hip fracture. Arch Phys Med Rehabil. 2007;88(7):916–21.

76. Schwenk M, Zieschang T, Englert S, Grewal G, Najafi B, Hauer K. Improvements in gait characteristics after intensive resistance and functional training in people with dementia: a randomised controlled trial. BMC Geriatr. 2014;14:73.

77. Beloosesky Y, Grinblat J, Epelboym B, Weiss A, Grosman B, Hendel D. Functional gain of hip fracture patients in different cognitive and functional groups. Clin Rehabil. 2002;16(3):321–8.

78. Naslund J. Visuospatial ability in relation to fall risk and dementia. Arch Neurol 2010;67(5):643; author reply –4.

15

Vision-based assessment of parkinsonism and levodopa-induced dyskinesia with pose estimation

Michael H. Li[1,2], Tiago A. Mestre[3,4,5,6], Susan H. Fox[3,6] and Babak Taati[1,2,7*]

Abstract

Background: Despite the effectiveness of levodopa for treatment of Parkinson's disease (PD), prolonged usage leads to development of motor complications, most notably levodopa-induced dyskinesia (LID). Persons with PD and their physicians must regularly modify treatment regimens and timing for optimal relief of symptoms. While standardized clinical rating scales exist for assessing the severity of PD symptoms, they must be administered by a trained medical professional and are inherently subjective. Computer vision is an attractive, non-contact, potential solution for automated assessment of PD, made possible by recent advances in computational power and deep learning algorithms. The objective of this paper was to evaluate the feasibility of vision-based assessment of parkinsonism and LID using pose estimation.

Methods: Nine participants with PD and LID completed a levodopa infusion protocol, where symptoms were assessed at regular intervals using the Unified Dyskinesia Rating Scale (UDysRS) and Unified Parkinson's Disease Rating Scale (UPDRS). Movement trajectories of individual joints were extracted from videos of PD assessment using Convolutional Pose Machines, a pose estimation algorithm built with deep learning. Features of the movement trajectories (e.g. kinematic, frequency) were used to train random forests to detect and estimate the severity of parkinsonism and LID. Communication and drinking tasks were used to assess LID, while leg agility and toe tapping tasks were used to assess parkinsonism. Feature sets from tasks were also combined to predict total UDysRS and UPDRS Part III scores.

Results: For LID, the communication task yielded the best results (detection: AUC = 0.930, severity estimation: $r = 0.661$). For parkinsonism, leg agility had better results for severity estimation ($r = 0.618$), while toe tapping was better for detection (AUC = 0.773). UDysRS and UPDRS Part III scores were predicted with $r = 0.741$ and 0.530, respectively.

Conclusion: The proposed system provides insight into the potential of computer vision and deep learning for clinical application in PD and demonstrates promising performance for the future translation of deep learning to PD clinical practices. Convenient and objective assessment of PD symptoms will facilitate more frequent touchpoints between patients and clinicians, leading to better tailoring of treatment and quality of care.

Keywords: Parkinsonism, Levodopa-induced dyskinesia, Computer vision, Deep learning, Pose estimation

* Correspondence: babak.taati@uhn.ca
[1]Toronto Rehabilitation Institute, University Health Network, 550 University Ave, Toronto, ON M5G 2A2, Canada
[2]Institute of Biomaterials and Biomedical Engineering, University of Toronto, 164 College St, Room 407, Toronto, ON M5S 3G9, Canada
Full list of author information is available at the end of the article

Background

Parkinson's disease (PD) is the second most common neurodegenerative disorder after Alzheimer's disease [1], affecting more than 10 million people worldwide [2]. The cardinal features of PD are bradykinesia (slowness of movement), followed by tremor at rest, rigidity, and postural instability [3]. Prevalence of PD increases rapidly over the age of 60 [4], and both global incidence and economic costs associated with PD are expected to rise rapidly in the near future [5, 6]. Since its discovery in the 1960s, levodopa has been the gold standard treatment for PD and is highly effective at improving motor symptoms [7]. However, after prolonged levodopa therapy, 40% of individuals develop levodopa-induced dyskinesia (LID) within 4–6 years [8]. LIDs are involuntary movements characterized by a non-rhythmic motion flowing from one body part to another (chorea) and/or involuntary contractions of opposing muscles causing twisting of the body into abnormal postures (dystonia) [9].

To provide optimal relief of parkinsonism and dyskinesia, treatment regimens must be tailored on an individual basis. While PD patients regularly consult their neurologists to inform treatment adjustments, these consultations occur intermittently and can fail to identify important changes in a patient's condition. Furthermore, the standard clinical rating scales used to record characteristics of PD symptoms require specialized training to perform and are inherently subjective, thus relying on the experience of the rater [10]. Paper diaries have also been used for patient self-reports of symptoms, but patient compliance is low and interpretation of symptoms can differ significantly between patients and physicians [11, 12].

Computerized assessments are an attractive potential solution, allowing automated evaluation of PD signs to be performed more frequently without the assistance of a clinician. The information gathered from these assessments can be relayed to a neurologist to supplement existing clinic visits and inform changes in management. In addition, computerized assessments are expected to provide an objective measurement of signs, and therefore be more consistent than a patient self-report. Computer vision is an appealing modality for assessment of PD and LID: a vision-based system would be completely noncontact and require minimal instrumentation in the form of a camera for data capture and a computer for processing.

To address the inherent subjectivity and inconvenience of current practices in PD assessment, efforts have been made to develop systems capable of objective evaluation of signs. Studies generally involve the recording of motion signals while participants perform tasks from clinical rating scales or execute a predefined protocol of activities of daily living (ADL).

Wearable sensing has thus far been the most popular technology for PD assessment, using accelerometers, gyroscopes, and/or magnetometers to record movements. These sensors are often packaged together as inertial measurement units (IMU). Keijsers et al. continuously monitored participants during a 35 item ADL protocol and predicted dyskinesia severity in one minute time intervals [13]. Focusing on upper limb movements, Salarian et al. attached gyroscopes to the forearms to estimate tremor and bradykinesia severity [14], while Giuffrida et al. used a custom finger mounted sensor to estimate severity of rest, postural, and kinetic tremors [15]. Patel et al. investigated multiple tasks from the Unified Parkinson's Disease Rating Scale (UPDRS) motor assessment to determine the best tasks and movement features for predicting tremor, bradykinesia, and dyskinesia severity [16]. With a single ankle-mounted IMU, Ramsperger et al. were able to identify leg dyskinesias in both lab and home environments [17]. Delrobaei et al. used a motion capture suit comprised of multiple IMUs to track joint angles and generated a dyskinesia severity score that correlated well with clinical scores [18]. Parkinsonian gait has also attracted considerable attention and is the most studied type of gait using wearable sensors [19]. While wearable systems have the potential to be implemented in a discreet and wireless fashion, they still require physical contact with the body. Furthermore, standardization is required regarding the quantity and placement of sensors needed to capture useful movement signals.

In contrast to wearable sensors, vision-based assessment requires only a camera for data capture and computer for processing. These assessments are noncontact, and do not require additional instrumentation to capture more body parts. However, the current state of vision-based assessment for PD and LID is very limited. Multi-colored suits were used for body part segmentation in parkinsonian gait analysis [20, 21], or environments were controlled to simplify extraction of relevant movements [22, 23]. Points on the body were also manually landmarked in video and tracked using image registration to observe global dyskinesia [24]. More complex camera hardware (e.g. Microsoft Kinect) can track motion in 3D with depth sensors and has been used to characterize hand movements [25], as well as analyze parkinsonian gait [26, 27] and assess dyskinesia severity [28] using the Kinect's skeletal tracking capabilities. Multi-camera motion capture systems can capture 3D movements more accurately by tracking the position of reflective markers attached to the points of interest. While they have been explored in the context of PD [29, 30], their prohibitive costs and complicated experimental setup make them impractical outside of research use.

While human pose estimation in video has been actively studied in computer science for several decades, the recent emergence of deep learning has led to substantial improvements in accuracy. Deep learning is a branch of machine learning built on neural networks. These networks, inspired by simplified models of the brain, are composed of layers of neurons that individually perform basic operations, but can be connected and trained to learn complex data representations. One major advantage of deep learning is automatic discovery of useful features, while conventional machine learning approaches use hand engineered features that require domain knowledge to achieve good performance. Convolutional neural networks (CNNs) are a specific deep learning architecture that takes advantage of inherent properties of images to improve efficiency. Toshev and Szegedy were the first to apply deep learning for pose estimation, where they framed joint position prediction as a cascaded regression problem using CNNs as regressors [31]. Chen and Yuille took advantage of the representational power of CNNs to learn the conditional probabilities of the presence of body parts and their spatial relations in a graphical model of pose [32]. Wei et al. iteratively refined joint positions by incorporating long range interactions between body parts over multiple stages of replicated CNNs [33].

The use of deep learning for PD assessment is still in early stages, although a few recent studies have applied deep learning for classification of wearable sensor data [34, 35] as well as extraction of gait parameters [36]. Therefore, an excellent opportunity exists to assess the readiness of deep learning models for vision-based assessment of PD. We have previously shown that features derived from videos of PD assessments using deep learning pose estimation algorithms were correlated to clinical scales of dyskinesia [37]. This paper substantially extends the preliminary results by analyzing additional motor tasks for parkinsonism and by evaluating the predictive power of the chosen feature set.

The key contributions of this paper are as follows:

1. Evaluating the feasibility of extracting useful movement information from 2D videos of Parkinson's assessments using a general purpose deep learning-based pose estimation algorithm
2. Extracting features from movement trajectories and training of a machine learning algorithm for objective, vision-based assessment of motor complications in PD (i.e. parkinsonism and LID)
3. Determining the accuracy of predicting scores of individual tasks in validated, clinical PD assessments using vision-based features as well as predicting total scores of PD assessments using a subset of the full clinical assessment suitable for video analysis

Methods
Dataset
Data was recorded at the Movement Disorders Centre of Toronto Western Hospital with approval from the University Health Network Research Ethics Board and written informed consent from all participants. The primary purpose of the initial study was to determine clinically important changes in parkinsonism and LID rating scales, including the UPDRS and the Unified Dyskinesia Rating Scale (UDysRS). Results of the study and detailed information about the protocol including inclusion/exclusion criteria, demographics, and clinical characteristics of study participants are available in [38]. Participants completed a levodopa infusion protocol that allows a standard assessment of PD and LID severity. Assessments were performed every 15–30 min using tasks from standard clinical rating scales for parkinsonism and LID for a period of 2–4 h. Videos were captured using a consumer grade video camera at 30 frames per second at a resolution of 480×640 or 540×960. The participants were seated and facing the camera in all videos. All videos were rated by two or three neurologists who were blinded to the time elapsed when the video was recorded. The agreement between neurologists was high for the total UPDRS Part III (Krippendorff $\alpha = 0.842$) and the total UDysRS Part III (Krippendorff $\alpha = 0.875$).

Nine participants (5 men, median age 64 years) completed the study. All participants had a diagnosis of idiopathic PD and stable bothersome peak-dose LID for more than 25% of the day, defined as a rating ≥ 2 on UPDRS item 4.1 (Time Spent with Dyskinesias) and a rating ≥ 1 on the Lang-Fahn Activities of Daily Living Dyskinesia Scale. The UDysRS Part III was used to rate the severity of dyskinesia and the UPDRS Part III was used to rate the severity of parkinsonism. Participants had a median score of 28.5 (IQR 24.2–34.8) on the UPDRS Part III in off state and a median score of 14 (IQR 11–16) on the UDysRS Patient Dyskinesia Questionnaire (Part 1b) [38]. A subset of tasks was selected for automated assessment based on perceived feasibility of vision-based analysis and on correlation to the total validated assessment score. The tasks selected were:

- Communication (UDysRS Part III) – the participant describes an image, engages in discussion with the examiner, mental math or recall
- Drinking from a cup (UDysRS Part III)
- Leg agility (UPDRS Part 3.8) – stomping of the leg vertically with as much speed and amplitude as possible
- Toe tapping (UPDRS Part 3.7)

The tasks of interest were manually segmented from the complete assessment videos. While the camera was positioned on a tripod, occasional adjustments were made by the experimenter, thus introducing camera motion. Videos containing severe occlusions or camera motion were removed. Video information can be found in Table 1. The UDysRS Part III contains seven scores for each task for different parts of the body from 0 (no dyskinesia) to 4 (incapacitating dyskinesia). The seven parts of the body rated are the face, neck, left and right arm/shoulder, left and right leg/hip, and trunk. The total validated score is the sum of the seven highest scores for each body part across all tasks. The UPDRS Part III also uses a five-point scale for severity in each task, and body parts may be rated separately depending on the task. For leg agility and toe tapping, there are ratings for the left and right sides of the body, and these tasks are designed to capture lower body parkinsonism. The total validated score for the UPDRS Part III is the sum of 28 available item scores. Due to practical reasons, it was not possible to perform certain items in the assessments and thus, they are not part of the total score calculation. The dressing task was omitted from the UDysRS and the rigidity assessment was omitted from the UPDRS.

Trajectory extraction

Pose estimation was conducted using Convolutional Pose Machines (CPM) [33]. The CPM library can be found at https://github.com/shihenw/convolutional-pose-machines-release. CPM is a state-of-the-art deep learning-based pose estimation algorithm that iteratively refines heatmaps of joint predictions using long range dependencies between joints. CPM was pre-trained on the MPII Human Pose Dataset, which contained 25,000 images with annotated body joints and covered over 400 human activities [39]. To assist pose estimation, a bounding box was annotated around the participant in the first frame of each video. Video frames were resized and padded to 368×368 before being input to CPM. The output of CPM was a 14-point skeleton with annotation of the head, neck, shoulders, elbows, wrists, hips, knees, and ankles. Joint trajectories were extracted independently for each frame. Sample detections are shown in Fig. 1. As tasks captured different facets of PD and LID, preprocessing strategies were tailored for each task. Preprocessing, feature extraction, and evaluation were performed using Python 2.7 with OpenCV 2.4.9 and scikit-learn 0.17.0.

Communication and drinking

Both communication and drinking tasks were rated using the UDysRS Part III, which contains seven subscores for dyskinesia of the face, neck, arms, trunk, and legs. The face dyskinesia subscore was not considered as it requires more complex modelling than available through pose estimation.

a. *Camera shake removal* – Camera motion was isolated by tracking the movement of stationary points in the scene. This was done by detecting and tracking points outside the bounding box where the person was identified using the Kanade-Lucas-Tomasi (KLT) tracker [40]. A maximum of 500 points were tracked, and the median of the frame-to-frame motions was taken as the camera trajectory. Joint trajectories were stabilized by subtracting the camera trajectory.

b. *Discontinuity removal* – Due to the frame-by-frame nature of the pose estimation approach, temporarily poor estimation can introduce large discontinuities in the joint trajectories. To identify discontinuities, a threshold was placed on the 2D frame-to-frame motion of the joint trajectories. The threshold was half of the head length, so that the threshold would be invariant to the distance of the participant from the camera. Joint trajectories were split when the threshold was exceeded, creating multiple temporal segments. The goal of grouping temporal segments is to identify segments that were similarly located spatially and to reject outliers. Grouping of segments proceeded as a forward temporal pass of the entire trajectory. For the current segment, the separation distance between the start of the segment and the end of the existing segment groups was computed. The current segment was added to the group with the minimum separation distance provided the distance was less than the threshold. If this constraint could not be satisfied, the segment became a new group. The confidence of pose estimations from CPM was used to determine which group of segments was most likely to reflect the actual movement. The confidence was the height of the maximum on the heatmap produced by CPM indicating the joint location. The group of segments with the highest median confidence was selected, and

Table 1 Video durations for each task

Task	# of videos	Total duration (h:mm:ss)	Average duration (s)
Communication	134	1:13:26	32.9
Drinking	124	15:20	7.4
Leg agility	134	24:05	10.8
Toe tapping	134	21:17	9.5

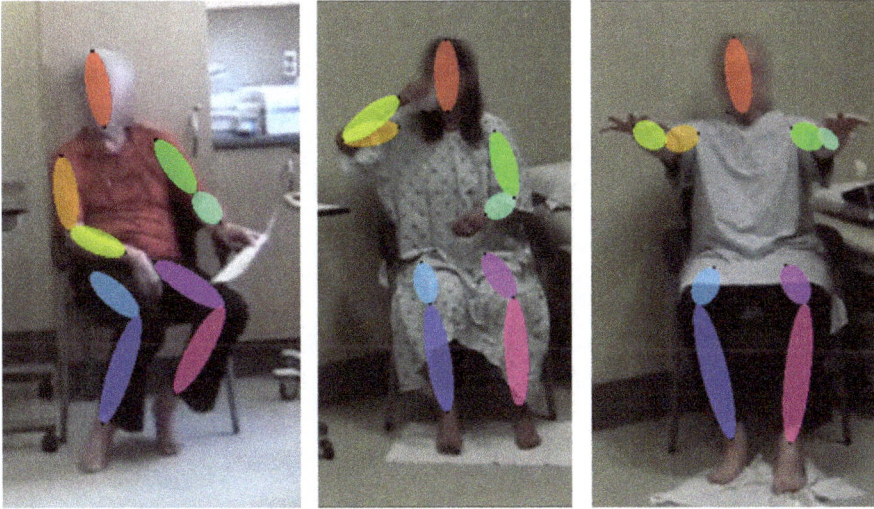

Fig. 1 Examples of poses from the dataset estimated using Convolutional Pose Machines

gaps between segments were filled using linear interpolation. Segments that did not span the entire signal were truncated at the segment end points.

c. *Face tracking* - Although the skeleton from CPM contains a head annotation, it is located on the top of the head and was therefore unsuitable for tracking head turning. To resolve this, a bounding box was placed on the face, which was tracked using the MEEM object tracker [41]. The bounding box was initialized as a square centered at the midpoint between the head and neck annotations, where the side length was the vertical distance between the head and neck. The bottom two thirds and middle 50% horizontally of the square are used as the final bounding box. The bounding box was tracked over time using MEEM and the motion of the center of the bounding box was taken as the face trajectory. By tracking salient facial features such as the eyes, nose, and mouth, the object tracker was able to track head turning as the bounding box stayed centered on the nose. The face trajectory replaced the head and neck trajectories from CPM.

Leg agility

Leg agility parkinsonism was assessed using the UPDRS Part 3.8, containing two item scores for the left and right side. Camera shake removal was the same as for the communication and drinking tasks. Due to the wide range in leg movement amplitudes for varying levels of parkinsonism, it was not possible to define a threshold suitable for all leg agility videos. Therefore, in lieu of discontinuity removal, a low pass filter was used for smoothing. The filter was a 5th order Butterworth filter with a cut-off frequency of 5 Hz, selected to preserve leg movements while removing high frequency jitter caused by frame-to-frame detection noise.

Toe tapping

Toe tapping parkinsonism was assessed using the UPDRS Part 3.7, which contains two item scores for the left and right feet. As the skeleton from CPM included ankle locations and not the feet, dense optical flow was used to capture the toe tapping movements [42]. It was assumed that the participant was sitting upright with their feet flat on the floor, such that there was no significant ankle motion and the foot was located directly below the ankle. Therefore, the median ankle position in the video was used to infer the area of the foot. A square bounding box was positioned below the ankle, such that the ankle was at the center of the top edge. As the head length provided an approximation of the scale of the person in the image, it was used as the side length of the bounding box. The bounding box was truncated if it extended beyond the video frame.

Given a set of frame-to-frame optical flows, the aggregate toe tapping velocity was computed as the median of non-zero optical flows. Flow velocities greater than 5.0×10^{-4} pixels/frame were considered non-zero. Discontinuity removal was not required as optical flow uses adjacent frames to infer motion. As a result, the aggregate velocity signal does not have the discontinuities present in frame-by-frame pose estimation. A schematic of the process for extracting the velocities from toe tapping is shown in Fig. 2.

Feature extraction

A total of 13 joint trajectories exist after CPM and preprocessing. These trajectories are the left and right shoulders, elbows, wrists, hips, knees, ankles from the

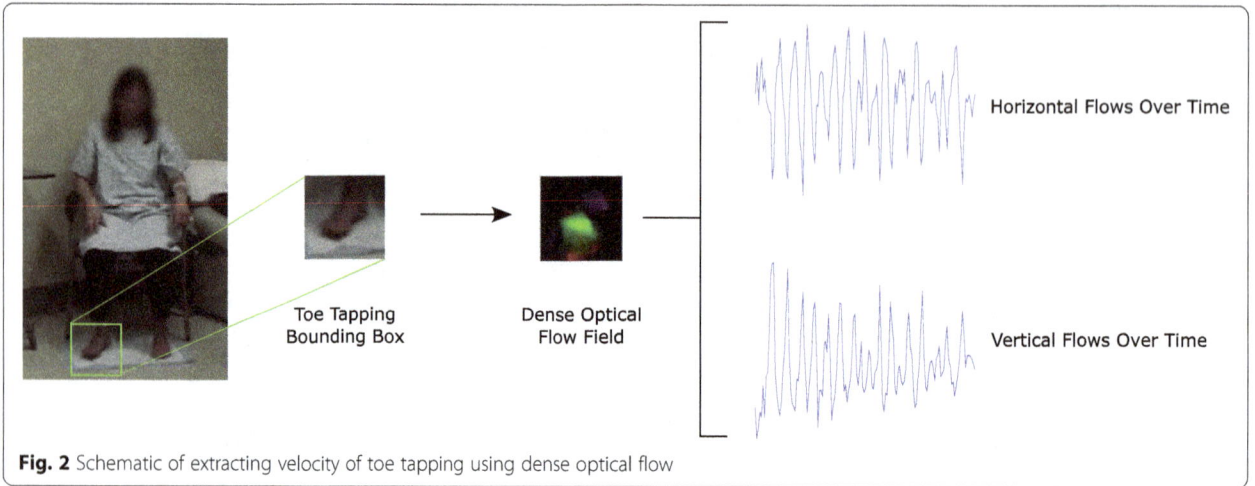

Fig. 2 Schematic of extracting velocity of toe tapping using dense optical flow

CPM skeleton and the face trajectory from MEEM. Trajectories were normalized by head length to ensure features were comparable across videos. A Savitzky-Golay filter (polynomial order = 3, window length = 11 samples) was used for smoothing and for computing signal derivatives. As each task rating contains subscores that are focused on different anatomical regions, only relevant joint trajectories were used for each subscore. Table 2 provides a legend of the abbreviations used to refer to each joint, while the joints used for each task are shown in Table 3.

For all tasks besides toe tapping, 32 features were extracted per joint trajectory. There were 15 kinematic features: the maximum, median, mean, standard deviation, and interquartile range of the speed, magnitude of acceleration, and magnitude of jerk. Scalar kinematic features were used as the magnitude of movement was more important than the direction. The inclusion of higher order

kinematics was inspired by measures of movement smoothness in stroke recovery [43]. Spectral features were computed from the Welch power spectral density (PSD) of the displacement and velocity signals. The horizontal and vertical components of the movement signal were combined as a complex signal before spectral estimation to produce an asymmetric spectrum. Afterwards, the positive and negative halves of the full spectrum were summed. There was a total of 16 spectral features: the peak magnitude, entropy, total power, half point (i.e. frequency that divides spectral power into equal halves), and power bands 0.5–1 Hz, > 2 Hz, > 4 Hz, > 6 Hz for both the displacement and velocity PSDs. The PSDs were normalized before computing power bands such that they were relative to the total power. The final feature was the convex hull, which quantifies the area that a joint moved within.

Since the signal for the toe tapping task was an aggregate velocity, the feature extraction approach was modified. Kinematic features were computed separately for

Table 2 Abbreviations for annotated joints

Joint	Abbreviation
Face	Face
Left shoulder	Lsho
Left elbow	Lelb
Left wrist	Lwri
Left hip	Lhip
Left knee	Lkne
Left ankle	Lank
Right shoulder	Rsho
Right elbow	Relb
Right wrist	Rwri
Right hip	Rhip
Right knee	Rkne
Right ankle	Rank

Table 3 Joint trajectories for each task

Task	Subscore	Joints used
Communication/Drinking (UDysRS)	Neck	Face
	Rarm	Rsho, Relb, Rwri
	Larm	Lsho, Lelb, Lwri
	Trunk	Rsho, Lsho
	Rleg	Rhip, Rkne, Rank
	Lleg	Lhip, Lkne, Lank
Leg agility (UPDRS)	Right	Rhip, Rkne, Rank
	Left	Lhip, Lkne, Lank
Toe tapping (UPDRS)	Right	Rank[a]
	Left	Lank[a]

[a]For the toe tapping task, ankle locations were used to create a bounding box for motion extraction

the total speed and for the horizontal and vertical velocities. In addition to the 15 features used for the other tasks, measures of distribution shape (skew and kurtosis) were also computed for velocity, acceleration, and jerk, yielding 21 features per signal for a total of 63 kinematic features. As there was no displacement signal, spectral features were only extracted from the velocity signal. The horizontal and vertical components of the aggregate velocity were used to compute four velocity PSDs: combined horizontal and vertical as a complex signal, horizontal only, vertical only, and magnitude of velocity. Each PSD had eight features, for a total of 32 spectral features. Convex hull could not be computed without a displacement signal. Overall, there were 95 features per joint for the toe tapping task.

As the communication task involved multiple subtasks, transitions between subtasks often contained voluntary movements or the video was cut by the examiner. Therefore, the communication task was divided into subtasks, features were computed for each subtask and then averaged to get the overall communication task features.

Evaluation

All experiments (i.e. binary classification, regression, and multiclass classification) were performed using leave-one-subject-out cross-validation and random forest. Specific implementation details and metrics are described in the following sections. Random forest hyperparameters were selected using 200 iterations of randomized search. Possible values for hyperparameters are given in Table 4 (m = number of features).

Binary classification

Binary classification can be framed as the detection of pathological motion, whether PD or LID. For each subscore of the UDysRS and UPDRS, ratings were on a scale of 0–4, where 0 indicated normal motion and 4 indicated severe impairment. The rating for each task was the average of multiple ratings from neurologists who scored the same video. Score thresholds for binarization were selected to balance classes. For the communication and drinking tasks, a threshold of 0.5 was used for binarizing scores, where average scores equal to or less than

0.5 were considered normal motion. For the leg agility and toe tapping tasks, there were fewer low ratings so thresholds of 1 and less than 2 (not inclusive) were selected, respectively, for binarization of scores. Metrics used were the F1-score and area under the curve (AUC).

Regression

The goal of regression is prediction of the clinical rating of PD or LID severity based on movement features. While these rating scales have been validated based on clinimetric properties, the single items that comprise the scales have not been validated as standalone measures. Therefore, in addition to predicting scores on single items, performance is also evaluated for prediction of total scores using pooled features from the relevant rating scales. The communication and drinking tasks were used to predict their respective UDysRS Part III item scores, while the leg agility and toe tapping tasks were used to predict their UPDRS Part III item scores. The total validated score for the UDysRS Part III contains the highest subscores for each body part across all tasks (0–4) and the sum of subscores (0–28), while the total validated score for the UPDRS Part III was the sum of all task scores (0–112). For the UDysRS Part III, features were combined from the communication and drinking tasks. For the UPDRS Part III, features were combined from the communication, leg agility, and toe tapping tasks. While the communication task is not an item in the UPDRS Part III, the involuntary movements could be a useful proxy of other items, such as 3.14 - global spontaneity of movement. Since the UPDRS Part III also describes upper body movements, all recorded joints from the leg agility task were included, not only those in Table 3. Metrics used were the RMS error and Pearson correlation between predictions and clinician ratings. Mean correlations were computed using Fisher z-transformation [44].

Multiclass classification

There are three possible classifications of motions – PD, PD with LID, or normal. For tasks to be suitable, they require ratings for both PD and LID. Although the communication task does not explicitly have a rating for PD,

Table 4 Possible hyperparameter choices for random forest. Ranges are integer intervals

Hyperparameter	Possible values	
	Classification (Binary/Multiclass)	Regression
Max features to try	$[1, ..., \lfloor\sqrt{m}\rfloor]$	$[1, ..., \lfloor m/3 \rfloor]$
Min samples to split node	$[1, ..., 11]$	
Min samples to be leaf node	$[1, ..., 11]$	
Number of trees	$[25, ..., 50]^a$	
Impurity criterion	Gini index/Entropy	N/A

[a]except UPDRS Part III total score, $[64, ..., 128]$

the UPDRS Part 3.14 (global spontaneity of movement) is used as a replacement as it is a global rating of PD. Ratings were averaged across all applicable body part subscores to generate a single severity score. Given ratings of both PD and LID, if neither score was greater than 1, the motion was considered normal. Otherwise, the motion was assigned the label corresponding to the higher score. If ratings were equal and greater than 1, the motion was omitted as it could not be definitively considered PD or LID. The metric used to assess performance was accuracy.

Results

Binary classification and regression results for communication and drinking tasks are shown in Table 5, while results for the leg agility and toe tapping tasks are given in Table 6. Errors provided are the standard deviation of results when cross-validation was run multiple times. For binary classification, the number of ratings binarized to the negative class (i.e. "no dyskinesia" or "no parkinsonism") is denoted by n_0 and informs if the classification task was well balanced. There are some disparities between the number of videos (Table 1) and the number of samples shown in Tables 5 and 6, as some videos did not have all possible ratings available.

Binary classification of communication task features achieved a mean AUC of 0.930, while drinking task performance had a mean AUC of 0.634. For the leg agility task, the mean AUC was 0.770, while the AUC for the toe tapping task was 0.773. The mean correlation between LID severity predictions and ground truth ratings for the communication task was 0.661, compared to

0.043 for the drinking task. For PD severity predictions, the mean correlations were 0.618 and 0.372 for the leg agility and toe tapping tasks, respectively.

For multiclass classification, the overall accuracy on the communication task was 71.4%. Sensitivity and specificity for each class are provided in Table 7. For predicting the total validated scores on the UDysRS Part III and UPDRS Part III, the results are given in Table 8. The correlation between predicted and ground truth ratings was 0.741 and 0.530 for the UDysRS and UPDRS, respectively.

Discussion

The purpose of this study was to determine if features derived from PD assessment videos using pose estimation could be used for detection and severity estimation of parkinsonism and dyskinesia. Random forest classifiers and regressors were trained for the communication, drinking, leg agility, and toe tapping tasks. The task with the best performance was the communication task. This was not surprising, as it is well-known clinically that the communication task elicits involuntary movements [45]. Despite the RMS error appearing similar for the drinking task, the correlation of 0.043 shows performance was poor in comparison to the communication task. This was because most ratings for the drinking task were between 0 and 2, thus emphasizing that both RMS and correlation are necessary to accurately portray performance. However, the mean AUC greater than 0.5 indicates that features from the drinking task still had slight discriminative power for detecting dyskinesia, even though they were inconsistent for measuring the severity of dyskinesia. Drinking task arm subscore performance

Table 5 Results for communication and drinking tasks (UDysRS)

Communication ($n = 128$)							
Binary Classification	Neck $n_0 = 48$	Rarm $n_0 = 60$	Larm $n_0 = 54$	Trunk $n_0 = 60$	Rleg $n_0 = 57$	Lleg $n_0 = 59$	Mean
F1	0.941 ± 0.003	0.920 ± 0.004	0.929 ± 0.014	0.960 ± 0.009	0.819 ± 0.007	0.865 ± 0.007	0.906 ± 0.002
AUC	0.935 ± 0.006	0.957 ± 0.004	0.946 ± 0.005	0.983 ± 0.002	0.852 ± 0.007	0.907 ± 0.005	0.930 ± 0.001
Regression	Neck	Rarm	Larm	Trunk	Rleg	Lleg	Mean
RMS	0.559 ± 0.008	0.399 ± 0.008	0.465 ± 0.011	0.513 ± 0.011	0.579 ± 0.009	0.590 ± 0.011	0.518 ± 0.005
r	0.712 ± 0.017	0.760 ± 0.022	0.645 ± 0.029	0.760 ± 0.024	0.522 ± 0.021	0.490 ± 0.024	0.661 ± 0.011
Drinking ($n = 118$)							
Binary Classification	Neck $n_0 = 61$	Rarm $n_0 = 79$	Larm $n_0 = 81$	Trunk $n_0 = 60$	Rleg $n_0 = 70$	Lleg $n_0 = 66$	Mean
F1	0.711 ± 0.026	0.148 ± 0.054	0.289 ± 0.068	0.643 ± 0.013	0.594 ± 0.046	0.617 ± 0.020	0.500 ± 0.015
AUC	0.774 ± 0.007	0.418 ± 0.033	0.557 ± 0.015	0.687 ± 0.014	0.673 ± 0.027	0.696 ± 0.012	0.634 ± 0.005
Regression	Neck	Rarm	Larm	Trunk	Rleg	Lleg	Mean
RMS	0.724 ± 0.003	0.737 ± 0.005	0.575 ± 0.005	0.701 ± 0.008	0.586 ± 0.008	0.622 ± 0.009	0.657 ± 0.003
r	0.075 ± 0.008	−0.150 ± 0.015	−0.003 ± 0.018	0.099 ± 0.020	0.087 ± 0.026	0.147 ± 0.025	0.043 ± 0.008

Table 6 Results for leg agility and toe tapping tasks (UPDRS)

	Leg agility (n = 75)			Toe tapping (n = 76)		
Binary Classification	Right $n_0 = 43$	Left $n_0 = 36$	Mean	Right $n_0 = 39$	Left $n_0 = 36$	Mean
F1	0.538 ± 0.012	0.725 ± 0.036	0.631 ± 0.022	0.755 ± 0.018	0.694 ± 0.027	0.725 ± 0.019
AUC	0.699 ± 0.017	0.842 ± 0.028	0.770 ± 0.007	0.842 ± 0.006	0.704 ± 0.015	0.773 ± 0.010
Regression	Right	Left	Mean	Right	Left	Mean
RMS	0.648 ± 0.024	0.462 ± 0.023	0.555 ± 0.013	0.614 ± 0.014	0.615 ± 0.014	0.614 ± 0.009
r	0.504 ± 0.049	0.710 ± 0.058	0.618 ± 0.029	0.383 ± 0.034	0.360 ± 0.032	0.372 ± 0.022

was noticeably worse than for other subscores, which was likely due to inability to discern voluntary from involuntary movements, as well as increased occlusion of upper limbs during movement. Multiclass classification of the communication task had poor sensitivity (< 10%) in detecting normal movements. The class that was best discriminated was LID. Intuitively, the communication task does not prompt participants to move voluntarily, therefore the slowness or absence of movement in PD and the lack of voluntary movement in the normal class can be confused with each other. This contrasts with the larger involuntary movements present in LID, which are easily identifiable.

Although only features from a subset of the full assessments were used to predict the total UPDRS Part III and UDysRS Part III scores, predictions had moderate to good correlation with total scores. This implies that this technology could use an abbreviated version of these clinical scales, although further analyses with a larger population would be required for validation. Previous studies have used measures derived from simple tasks such as the timed up and go [46] and a touchscreen finger tapping and spiral drawing test [47] to achieve moderate to good correlation with the total UPDRS Part III score. While the RMS error for the total UPDRS Part III appears much larger than the RMS error for the UDysRS Part III, this is consistent with the range of possible values for each scale. The UPDRS Part III had a range of 0–112 compared to the UDysRS Part III's range of 0–28. It may be possible to improve performance on task subscores by using joints from the entire body. It is likely that motor complications in one part of the body will be correlated to motor complications elsewhere. However, these correlations would be unlikely to generalize across a population, as each person's PD will manifest

differently. Likewise, only features extracted from a specific task were used for predicting the task's rating despite possible performance boost from using additional task features. Each task was included in their respective rating scales to capture different facets of motor complications, and the correlations between these tasks would be unique to each individual.

No explicit feature selection was performed despite having many features compared to samples. Although the random forest algorithm is generally resistant to overfitting, feature selection can often still reduce features that are not useful. However, after evaluating several feature selection methods, no performance boost was observed compared to applying random forest with all features. Dimensionality reduction methods were not tested as feature transformation would reduce interpretability, thus making further analysis more difficult. Likewise, more complex algorithms that learn feature representations were not considered as discovered features may not have been clinically useful. While the emphasis of this analysis was on model accuracy, the parity of performance even after feature selection indicates that future models could be built with comparable performance and a smaller set of features. Identification of features that consistently perform well or poorly is the next step towards deployment of more lightweight models.

The use of 2D pose estimation was motivated by visual inspection of motor complications during Parkinson's assessments and observation of gross movements. It was hypothesized that 2D pose estimation would be successful at extracting movement information accurate enough to infer the severity of motor complications. While the results indicate that features derived from CPM pose estimation could capture clinically relevant information

Table 7 Multiclass classification results for communication task

	n	Sensitivity	Specificity
LID	26	96.2% ± 3.8%	95.7% ± 0.9%
Normal	17	9.4% ± 3.2%	89.7% ± 3.0%
PD	34	83.5% ± 4.5%	68.4% ± 1.3%
Overall Accuracy	77	71.4% ± 2.8%	

Table 8 Results for prediction of validated scores. UDysRS Part III is predicted using features from the communication and drinking tasks, while UPDRS Part III is predicted using features from the communication, leg agility (all joints) and toe tapping tasks

Regression	UDysRS Part III (n = 118)	UPDRS Part III (n = 74)
RMS	2.906 ± 0.084	7.765 ± 0.154
r	0.741 ± 0.033	0.530 ± 0.026

from videos, this serves as an indirect measure of the accuracy of pose estimation. In preliminary testing, a benchmark made of frames of video from the dataset was used to assess CPM. All body parts were well-detected except for the knees. Knee detection was complicated due to the hospital gowns worn by participants, which resulted in insufficient texture to discern knee location. This means that the involuntary opening and closing motions of the knees were poorly tracked, which may explain why leg subscore predictions were the worst in the communication task. However, ankles were well-tracked so this is not expected to have significantly affected performance on the leg agility task.

As the MPII dataset that CPM was trained with contained images of individuals sitting, the model could generalize to the PD assessment videos. A further evaluation by Trumble et al. supports the accuracy of CPM, as a CPM-based 3D pose estimation with multiple views performed well in comparison to other vision-based and wearable algorithms when validated against motion capture data [48]. The quality of trajectories generated using CPM and derived features should generalize well to other studies of PD assessments, as the video recording quality is consistent with recommended recording protocols and videos used for initial validation of the UDysRS [49, 50]. However, the CPM model pre-trained on MPII is limited by inability to track head turning and does not detect feet and hands. In the future, an improved model could be trained specifically with images more representative of clinical or home environments, as well as augmented datasets that include head orientation, foot, and hand positions. Models that impose biomechanical restrictions on joint positioning [51] or integrate video information for 3D pose estimation [52] could also improve performance.

The optical flow-based method for extracting motion from toe tapping took advantage of the foot being anchored by the heel. The algorithm may not be transferrable to other applications as it relied on assumptions of foot location with respect to the ankle. For example, upper body measures of parkinsonism such as hand open/close and pronation/supination often involved significant arm motion and video motion blur, which would not be feasible to track accurately using the optical flow-based method without a more complicated approach. Furthermore, generalizability to other toe tapping applications could be limited by differences in recording conditions. While this toe tapping algorithm cannot be directly evaluated by its accuracy at tracking foot motion, it is possible to compare its relative performance against other studies that have assessed toe tapping. Heldman et al. used an accelerometer heel-clip mounted to the person's shoe while Kim et al. used a gyrosensor mounted on the top of the foot

[53, 54]. Heldman et al. achieved $r = 0.86$ and RMS of 0.44 and Kim et al. achieved $r = 0.72–0.81$ for different features when compared against the UPDRS toe tapping score. There is a gap in performance as the vision-based method presented is less accurate at tracking the motion. However, the tradeoff is convenience for accuracy, as vision-based is still easier to use than wearables due to lack of special hardware requirements and attachment of sensors.

Due to differing experimental conditions and rating scales used in past studies, it is difficult to perform a direct comparison in terms of system performance. The closest study in terms of experimental protocol was Rao et al., who analyzed videos of the communication task and tracked manually landmarked joint locations to develop a dyskinesia severity score [24]. They report good correlation between their score and the UDysRS Part IV (single rating of disability) score (Kendall tau-b correlation 0.68–0.85 for different neurologists). Their study used non-rigid image registration for tracking, which was not able to infer joint positions if occluded and could not recover if the joint position was lost. In contrast, deep learning-based pose estimation learns the structure of the human body after seeing training data and can often make accurate predictions of joint locations even when the joints are not visible. Dyshel et al. leveraged the Kinect's skeletal tracking to extract movement parameters from tasks from the UPDRS and Abnormal Involuntary Movement Scale (AIMS) [28]. They trained a classifier to detect dyskinesia with an AUC of 0.906 and quantified the dyskinesia severity based on the percent of a movement classified as dyskinetic. This quantitative measure had good correlation with AIMS scores (general correlation coefficient 0.805). In wearable sensing, Patel et al. reported classification errors of 1.7% and 1.2% for parkinsonism and dyskinesia, respectively, using tasks from the UPDRS [16]. Tsipouras et al. detected dyskinesia with 92.51% accuracy in a continuous recording of multiple ADLs [55]. Eskofier et al. used CNNs on accelerometer recordings of the pronation/supination and hand movements tasks and achieved parkinsonism classification accuracy of 90.9% [34]. In our work, the best performance for binary classification of dyskinesia was in the communication task, with an AUC of 0.930. This is comparable with other studies, including those using wearables, although the difficulty of classification is highly dependent on the length of the motion segments to be classified and the type of motion performed. For parkinsonism, the best binary classification performance was for the toe tapping task, with an AUC of 0.773. This is not as high as dyskinesia classification performance and can likely be attributed to the distribution of ratings. In the communication task, 30–40% of ratings for subscores were at the lower limit of the scale (i.e. 0), whereas for the leg agility and toe tapping tasks, this percentage was much smaller (less than 3%). Threshold selection for binarizing scores was based on balancing classes, and therefore may not have been optimal with respect to clinical definitions. Ideally, the solution would be to gather sufficient data to represent all ratings and to select thresholds either based on clinical supervision or by discovery of an optimal separation between groups.

Limitations

As the videos from this dataset were not captured for subsequent computer vision analysis, there were recording issues that introduced noise, including different camera angles and zoom. Despite these concerns, the videos are representative of the quality of videos used by clinicians for PD assessment, and the availability of the data outweighed the unnecessary burden on participants required to perform a new experiment. However, manual intervention was required for task segmentation and person localization. For this feasibility study, the videos were of sufficient quality; however, standardization of recording protocols to eliminate camera shake should improve algorithm performance and consistency. Future studies could use deep learning algorithms that take advantage of temporal information in videos for more accurate pose estimation [52]. In addition, CPM's accuracy for pose estimation was limited by the resolution of the input video (368×368). Performance could be improved with algorithms accepting a higher resolution video or by applying refinements for subpixel accuracy. Calibrating cameras to a known distance in advance would enable movement amplitudes to be measured in a unit of length comparable to other studies (e.g. metres). Although single-camera systems offer the possibility of convenient, non-contact measurement of PD motor complications, occlusions and the fixed nature of cameras can limit use cases, especially in outdoor environments. Resolving human pose in 3D is also significantly more difficult and inaccurate without using multiple cameras. The optical flow-based method used for toe tapping has not been validated in the context of foot motion estimation. It will be important to define the scope of applications to mitigate these limitations.

The recruitment criteria selected individuals with moderate levels of dyskinesia. Therefore, the study population reflects only a segment of the patient population. The small sample size should also be increased in follow-up studies to ensure generalizability of results. In addition, a small number of tasks from the UPDRS and UDysRS were not assessed for practical reasons. While adjustments of rating scales are common practice, studies have shown that the UPDRS and UDysRS retain validity despite multiple missing items [56, 57]. Future studies should also include healthy participants as controls.

Regression performance is reported using correlation; however, it is unclear what would be a clinically useful level of agreement. Furthermore, while a high correlation may indicate that a method is able to mimic clinicians, validation based on agreement with clinical ratings does not provide insight into whether such technologies can achieve better sensitivity to clinically important changes than subjective rating scales. Additional investigation is required to compare the sensitivity of the proposed system to validated clinical measures.

Conclusion

This paper presents the first application of deep learning for vision-based assessment of parkinsonism and LID. The results demonstrate that state-of-the-art pose estimation algorithms can extract meaningful information about PD motor signs from videos of Parkinson's assessments and provide a performance baseline for future studies of PD with deep learning. The long-term goal for this system is deployment in a mobile or tablet application. For home usage, the application could be used by patients to perform regular self-assessments and relay the information to their doctor to provide objective supplemental information for their next clinic visit. An automated system capable of detecting changes in symptom severity could also have major impact in accelerating clinical trials for new therapies.

Acknowledgements
The authors greatly appreciate the support of Drs. Isabelle Beaulieu-Boire, Camila C. Aquino, and Nicolas Phielipp for providing clinical ratings of patients in this study.

Funding
Research was supported by the Natural Sciences and Engineering Research Council of Canada (NSERC), the Toronto Rehabilitation Institute–University Health Network, and the Toronto Western Hospital Foundation.

Authors' contributions
MHL analyzed the data and drafted the manuscript. TAM and SHF conceived the initial project, collected the dataset, and revised the manuscript. BT conceived the study and revised the manuscript.

Competing interests

In the preceding 12 months, SH Fox has received:

Consultancies	Avanir, Biotie, Britannia, C2N, Cynapsus, Kyowa, Orion, Sunovion, Zambon
Honoraria	International Parkinson and Movement Disorder Society, CHDI, American Academy of Neurology
Research funding	Michael J. Fox Foundation for Parkinson's Disease Research, NIH, Parkinson Canada, Toronto Western Hospital Foundation
Salary	UHN Department of Medicine Practice Plan

TA Mestre has received:

Consultancies	Abbvie, CHDI Foundation/Management
Honoraria	Abbvie, International Parkinson and Movement Disorder Society, American Academy of Neurology, University of Ottawa
Research funding	Parkinson Canada, Parkinson Research Consortium, Parkinson's Disease Foundation, Parkinson's Study Group
Salary	University of Ottawa Medical Associates

MH Li and B Taati have no competing interests to disclose.

Author details

[1]Toronto Rehabilitation Institute, University Health Network, 550 University Ave, Toronto, ON M5G 2A2, Canada. [2]Institute of Biomaterials and Biomedical Engineering, University of Toronto, 164 College St, Room 407, Toronto, ON M5S 3G9, Canada. [3]Edmond J. Safra Program in Parkinson's Disease, Toronto Western Hospital, University Health Network, 399 Bathurst St, Toronto, ON M5T 2S8, Canada. [4]The Ottawa Hospital Research Institute, 1053 Carling Ave, Ottawa, ON K1Y 4E9, Canada. [5]Division of Neurology, Department of Medicine, 1053 Carling Ave, Ottawa, ON K1Y 4E9, Canada. [6]Division of Neurology, University of Toronto, Suite RFE 3-805, 200 Elizabeth St, Toronto, ON M5G 2C4, Canada. [7]Department of Computer Science, University of Toronto, 10 King's College Road, Room 3302, Toronto, ON M5S 3G4, Canada.

References

1. Nussbaum RL, Ellis CE. Alzheimer's disease and Parkinson's disease. N Engl J Med. 2003;348:1356–64.
2. Statistics on Parkinson's - Parkinson's Disease Foundation (PDF). [cited 2017 Mar 28]. Available from: http://parkinson.org/Understanding-Parkinsons/Causes-and-Statistics/Statistics.
3. Jankovic J. Parkinson's disease: clinical features and diagnosis. J Neurol Neurosurg Psychiatry. 2008;79:368–76.
4. Van Den Eeden SK, Tanner CM, Bernstein AL, Fross RD, Leimpeter A, Bloch DA, et al. Incidence of Parkinson's disease: variation by age, gender, and race/ethnicity. Am J Epidemiol. 2003;157:1015–22.
5. Dorsey ER, Constantinescu R, Thompson JP, Biglan KM, Holloway RG, Kieburtz K, et al. Projected number of people with Parkinson disease in the most populous nations, 2005 through 2030. Neurology. 2007;68:384–6.
6. Findley LJ. The economic impact of Parkinson's disease. Parkinsonism Relat Disord. 2007;13(Supplement):S8–12.
7. National Collaborating Centre for Chronic Conditions (UK). Parkinson's Disease: National Clinical Guideline for Diagnosis and Management in Primary and Secondary Care. London: Royal College of Physicians (UK); 2006 [cited 2015 Nov 28]. Available from: http://www.ncbi.nlm.nih.gov/books/NBK48513/
8. Ahlskog JE, Muenter MD. Frequency of levodopa-related dyskinesias and motor fluctuations as estimated from the cumulative literature. Mov Disord. 2001;16:448–58.
9. Zis P, Chaudhuri KR, Samuel M. Phenomenology of Levodopa-Induced Dyskinesia. In: Fox SH, Brotchie JM, editors. Levodopa-Induc Dyskinesia Park Dis. London: Springer; 2014. p. 1–16.
10. Post B, Merkus MP, de Bie RMA, de Haan RJ, Speelman JD. Unified Parkinson's disease rating scale motor examination: are ratings of nurses, residents in neurology, and movement disorders specialists interchangeable? Mov Disord. 2005;20:1577–84.
11. Stone AA, Shiffman S, Schwartz JE, Broderick JE, Hufford MR. Patient compliance with paper and electronic diaries. Control Clin Trials. 2003;24:182–99.
12. Goetz CG, Leurgans S, Hinson VK, Blasucci LM, Zimmerman J, Fan W, et al. Evaluating Parkinson's disease patients at home: utility of self-videotaping for objective motor, dyskinesia, and ON–OFF assessments. Mov Disord. 2008;23:1479–82.
13. Keijsers NLW, Horstink MWIM, Gielen SCAM. Automatic assessment of levodopa-induced dyskinesias in daily life by neural networks. Mov Disord. 2003;18:70–80.
14. Salarian A, Russmann H, Wider C, Burkhard PR, Vingerhoets FJG, Aminian K. Quantification of tremor and bradykinesia in Parkinson's disease using a novel ambulatory monitoring system. IEEE Trans Biomed Eng. 2007;54:313–22.
15. Giuffrida JP, Riley DE, Maddux BN, Heldman DA. Clinically deployable Kinesia™ technology for automated tremor assessment. Mov Disord. 2009;24:723–30.
16. Patel S, Lorincz K, Hughes R, Huggins N, Growdon J, Standaert D, et al. Monitoring motor fluctuations in patients with Parkinson's disease using wearable sensors. IEEE Trans Inf Technol Biomed. 2009;13:864–73.
17. Ramsperger R, Meckler S, Heger T, van Uem J, Hucker S, Braatz U, et al. Continuous leg dyskinesia assessment in Parkinson's disease –clinical validity and ecological effect. Parkinsonism Relat Disord. 2016;26:41–6.
18. Delrobaei M, Baktash N, Gilmore G, McIsaac K, Jog M. Using Wearable Technology to Generate Objective Parkinson's Disease Dyskinesia Severity Score: Possibilities for Home Monitoring. IEEE Trans Neural Syst Rehabil Eng. 2017;PP:1.
19. Chen S, Lach J, Lo B, Yang G. Toward pervasive gait analysis with wearable sensors: a systematic review. IEEE J Biomed Health Inform. 2016;20:1521–37.
20. Green RD, Guan L, Burne JA. Video analysis of gait for diagnosing movement disorders. J Electron Imaging. 2000;9:16–21.
21. Lee H, Guan L, Lee I. Video analysis of human gait and posture to determine neurological disorders. EURASIP J Image Video Process. 2008;2008:380867.
22. Cho C-W, Chao W-H, Lin S-H, Chen Y-Y. A vision-based analysis system for gait recognition in patients with Parkinson's disease. Expert Syst Appl. 2009;36:7033–9.
23. Khan T, Nyholm D, Westin J, Dougherty M. A computer vision framework for finger-tapping evaluation in Parkinson's disease. Artif Intell Med. 2014;60:27–40.
24. Rao AS, Dawant BM, Bodenheimer RE, Li R, Fang J, Phibbs F, et al. Validating an objective video-based dyskinesia severity score in Parkinson's disease patients. Parkinsonism Relat Disord. 2013;19:232–7.
25. Dror B, Yanai E, Frid A, Peleg N, Goldenthal N, Schlesinger I, et al. Automatic assessment of Parkinson's Disease from natural hands movements using 3D depth sensor. 2014 IEEE 28th Conv Electr Electron Eng Isr IEEEI. 2014:1–5.
26. Procházka A, Vyšata O, Vališ M, Ťupa O, Schätz M, Mařík V. Use of the image and depth sensors of the Microsoft Kinect for the detection of gait disorders. Neural Comput Appl. 2015;26:1621–9.
27. Rocha AP, Choupina H, Fernandes JM, Rosas MJ, Vaz R, Cunha JPS. Kinect v2 Based System for Parkinson's Disease Assessment. 2015 37th Annu Int Conf IEEE Eng Med Biol Soc EMBC. 2015;2015:1279–82.
28. Dyshel M, Arkadir D, Bergman H, Weinshall D. Quantifying Levodopa-Induced Dyskinesia Using Depth Camera. Proc IEEE Int Conf Comput Vis Workshop. 2015:119–26.
29. Roiz Rde M, EWA C, Pazinatto MM, Reis JG, Cliquet A Jr. Barasnevicius-Quagliato EMA Gait analysis comparing Parkinson's disease with healthy elderly subjects. Arq Neuropsiquiatr. 2010;68:81–6.
30. Das S, Trutoiu L, Murai A, Alcindor D, Oh M, De la Torre F, et al. Quantitative measurement of motor symptoms in Parkinson's disease: A study with full-body motion capture data. 2011 Annu Int Conf IEEE Eng Med Biol Soc EMBC. 2011:6789–92.

31. Toshev A, Szegedy C. DeepPose: human pose estimation via deep neural networks. IEEE Conf Comput Vis Pattern Recognit. 2014;2014.

32. Chen X, Yuille A. Articulated Pose Estimation by a Graphical Model with Image Dependent Pairwise Relations. Adv Neural Inf Process Syst NIPS 2014. 2014;1:1736–44.

33. Wei SE, Ramakrishna V, Kanade T, Sheikh Y. Convolutional Pose Machines. 2016 IEEE Conf Comput Vis Pattern Recognit CVPR. 2016. p. 4724–4732.

34. Eskofier BM, Lee SI, Daneault JF, Golabchi FN, Ferreira-Carvalho G, Vergara-Diaz G, et al. Recent machine learning advancements in sensor-based mobility analysis: Deep learning for Parkinson's disease assessment. 2016 38th Annu Int Conf IEEE Eng Med Biol Soc EMBC. 2016:655–8.

35. Hammerla NY, Fisher J, Andras P, Rochester L, Walker R, Ploetz T. PD Disease State Assessment in Naturalistic Environments Using Deep Learning. Twenty-Ninth AAAI Conf Artif Intell. 2015.

36. Hannink J, Kautz T, Pasluosta CF, Gaßmann K, Klucken J, Eskofier BM. Sensor-based gait parameter extraction with deep convolutional neural networks. IEEE J Biomed Health Inform. 2017;21(1):85–93.

37. Li MH, Mestre TA, Fox SH, Taati B. Automated Vision-Based Analysis of Levodopa-Induced Dyskinesia with Deep Learning. 2017 39th Annu Int Conf IEEE Eng Med Biol Soc EMBC. 2017;2017:3377–80.

38. Mestre TA, Beaulieu-Boire I, Aquino CC, Phielipp N, Poon YY, Lui JP, et al. What is a clinically important change in the unified dyskinesia rating scale in Parkinson's disease? Parkinsonism Relat Disord. 2015;21:1349–54.

39. Andriluka M, Pishchulin L, Gehler P, Schiele B. 2D Human Pose Estimation: New Benchmark and State of the Art Analysis. 2014 IEEE Conf Comput Vis Pattern Recognit. 2014:3686–93.

40. Tomasi C, Kanade T. Detection and tracking of point features. Pittsburgh: School of Computer Science, Carnegie Mellon UnivPittsburgh; 1991.

41. Zhang J, Ma S, Sclaroff S. MEEM: Robust Tracking via Multiple Experts Using Entropy Minimization. In: Fleet D, Pajdla T, Schiele B, Tuytelaars T, editors. Comput Vis–ECCV 2014. Springer International Publishing; 2014. p. 188–203.

42. Farnebäck G. Two-frame motion estimation based on polynomial expansion. In: Bigun J, Gustavsson T, editors. Image Anal. Berlin Heidelberg: Springer; 2003. p. 363–70.

43. Balasubramanian S, Melendez-Calderon A, Roby-Brami A, Burdet E. On the analysis of movement smoothness. J NeuroEngineering Rehabil. 2015;12:112.

44. Silver NC, Dunlap WP. Averaging correlation coefficients: should Fisher's z transformation be used? J Appl Psychol. 1987;72:146–8.

45. Hoff JI, van Hilten BJ, Roos RA. A review of the assessment of dyskinesias. Mov Disord Off J Mov Disord Soc. 1999;14:737–43.

46. Zampieri C, Salarian A, Carlson-Kuhta P, Aminian K, Nutt JG, Horak FB. The instrumented timed up and go test: potential outcome measure for disease modifying therapies in Parkinson's disease. J Neurol Neurosurg Psychiatry. 2010;81:171–6.

47. Memedi M, Nyholm D, Johansson A, Palhagen S, Willows T, Widner H, et al. Validity and responsiveness of at-home touch-screen assessments in advanced Parkinson's disease. IEEE J Biomed Health Inform. 2015;PP:1.

48. Trumble M, Gilbert A, Malleson C, Hilton A, Collomosse J. Total Capture: 3D Human Pose Estimation Fusing Video and Inertial Sensors. Proc 28th Br Mach Vis Conf. London, UK; 2017 [cited 2018 Sep 7]. p. 1–13. Available from: https://bmvc2017.london/proceedings/

49. Barton B, Cubo E. In: Falup-Pecurariu C, Ferreira J, Martinez-Martin P, Chaudhuri KR, editors. How to record a video of a movement disorder patient. Vienna: Springer Vienna; 2017. p. 59–63. Available from: https://doi.org/10.1007/978-3-7091-1628-9_7.

50. Goetz CG, Nutt JG, Stebbins GT. The unified dyskinesia rating scale: presentation and clinimetric profile. Mov Disord. 2008;23:2398–403.

51. Akhter I, Black MJ. Pose-Conditioned Joint Angle Limits for 3D Human Pose Reconstruction. Boston: MA; 2015. p. 1446–55.

52. Zhou X, Zhu M, Leonardos S, Derpanis KG, Daniilidis K. Sparseness Meets Deepness: 3D Human Pose Estimation From Monocular Video. Proc IEEE Conf Comput Vis Pattern Recognit. 2016:4966–75.

53. Heldman DA, Filipkowski DE, Riley DE, Whitney CM, Walter BL, Gunzler SA, et al. Automated motion sensor quantification of gait and lower extremity bradykinesia. Conf Proc Annu Int Conf IEEE Eng Med Biol Soc IEEE Eng Med Biol Soc Annu Conf. 2012;2012:1956–9.

54. Kim J-W, Kwon Y, Kim Y-M, Chung H-Y, Eom G-M, Jun J-H, et al. Analysis of lower limb bradykinesia in Parkinson's disease patients. Geriatr Gerontol Int. 2012;12:257–64.

55. Tsipouras MG, Tzallas AT, Rigas G, Tsouli S, Fotiadis DI, Konitsiotis S. An automated methodology for levodopa-induced dyskinesia: assessment based on gyroscope and accelerometer signals. Artif Intell Med. 2012; 55:127–35.

56. Goetz CG, Luo S, Wang L, Tilley BC, LaPelle NR, Stebbins GT. Handling missing values in the MDS-UPDRS. Mov Disord Off J Mov Disord Soc. 2015; 30:1632–8.

57. Luo S, Ren X, Han W, Goetz CG, Stebbins GT. Missing Data in the Unified Dyskinesia Rating Scale (UDysRS). Mov Disord Clin Pract. 2018 [cited 2018 Sep 9]; Available from: https://onlinelibrary.wiley.com/doi/abs/10.1002/mdc3.12642

16

Regenerative peripheral nerve interfaces for real-time, proportional control of a Neuroprosthetic hand

Christopher M. Frost[1†], Daniel C. Ursu[1,2*†] ⓘ, Shane M. Flattery[3], Andrej Nedic[1], Cheryl A. Hassett[1], Jana D. Moon[1], Patrick J. Buchanan[1], R. Brent Gillespie[2], Theodore A. Kung[1], Stephen W. P. Kemp[1,4], Paul S. Cederna[1,4] and Melanie G. Urbanchek[1]

Abstract

Introduction: Regenerative peripheral nerve interfaces (RPNIs) are biological constructs which amplify neural signals and have shown long-term stability in rat models. Real-time control of a neuroprosthesis in rat models has not yet been demonstrated. The purpose of this study was to: a) design and validate a system for translating electromyography (EMG) signals from an RPNI in a rat model into real-time control of a neuroprosthetic hand, and; b) use the system to demonstrate RPNI proportional neuroprosthesis control.

Methods: Animals were randomly assigned to three experimental groups: (1) Control; (2) Denervated, and; (3) RPNI. In the RPNI group, the extensor digitorum longus (EDL) muscle was dissected free, denervated, transferred to the lateral thigh and neurotized with the residual end of the transected common peroneal nerve. Rats received tactile stimuli to the hind-limb via monofilaments, and electrodes were used to record EMG. Signals were filtered, rectified and integrated using a moving sample window. Processed EMG signals (iEMG) from RPNIs were validated against Control and Denervated group outputs.

Results: Voluntary reflexive rat movements produced signaling that activated the prosthesis in both the Control and RPNI groups, but produced no activation in the Denervated group. Signal-to-Noise ratio between hind-limb movement and resting iEMG was 3.55 for Controls and 3.81 for RPNIs. Both Control and RPNI groups exhibited a logarithmic iEMG increase with increased monofilament pressure, allowing graded prosthetic hand speed control ($R^2 = 0.758$ and $R^2 = 0.802$, respectively).

Conclusion: EMG signals were successfully acquired from RPNIs and translated into real-time neuroprosthetic control. Signal contamination from muscles adjacent to the RPNI was minimal. RPNI constructs provided reliable proportional prosthetic hand control.

Keywords: Peripheral nerve Interface, Prosthetics, Regenerative medicine, Amputees

* Correspondence: danursu@umich.edu
†Christopher M. Frost and Daniel C. Ursu contributed equally to this work.
[1]University of Michigan Department of Surgery, Section of Plastic Surgery, 570 MSRB II Level A, 1150 W. Medical Center Drive, Ann Arbor, MI 48109-5456, USA
[2]University of Michigan Department of Mechanical Engineering, Ann Arbor, MI, USA
Full list of author information is available at the end of the article

Introduction

Approximately 185,000 individuals suffer limb loss annually in the United States [1]. The growing rate of amputees and technological advancements have greatly improved human-neuroprosthetic interfacing [2]. A comprehensive literature review on the needs and priorities of prostheses users performed by Cordella et al. in 2016 revealed that an estimated 75% of upper prosthetic users wore functional prostheses for at least 8 h per day, compared with only 45% of cosmetic prosthesis owners [3]. A functional prosthesis was more likely to be worn the higher the level of amputation, and especially during dynamic activities of daily living, such as work, driving and sports [3]. Importantly, upper arm amputees who tested both conventional (body powered or myoelectric arms) and the DEKA Gen 3 advanced myoelectric prosthesis found conventional prostheses performed faster, and with smoother motions and less movement deviation than the advanced DEKA prosthetic device [4]. This finding is largely attributed to a lack of an intuitive, functional neural interface that can provide high fidelity control signals to actualize the functionality of advanced neuroprosthetic devices.

Advanced anthropomorphic modular prosthetic arm systems have only become commercially available in the last 5 years, in large part due to technology developed with DARPA's funding of the Revolutionizing Prosthetics Program in 2006 [5]. Currently, multi-electrode-based prosthetic devices, such as the DEKA arm (DEKA, Manchester, NH), i-Limb (TouchBionics, Touch Bionics, Mansfield, MA), the Johns Hopkins Modular Prosthetic Limb (MPL, Johns Hopkins University Applied Physics Lab, Baltimore, MD), and Ottobock (Otto Bock HealthCare, Duderstadt, Germany), provide increased ranges of motion, dexterity and control options, and are capable of up to five-finger movements and 20 degrees of freedom [6, 7]. However, a limitation in controlling these advanced robotic prostheses is the need for an appropriate neural interface that can extract clear multifunctional signal information at a speed that matches naturalistic human motion [8, 9].

Neural interfaces, i.e. the use of electrodes to record physiological signals for voluntary prosthetic control, come in different forms and all have unique advantages and challenges. All prostheses require either nerve or muscle electrodes as part of the neural interface [6], and consequently, interfacing electrodes vary in size (standard pad to microelectrodes), shape (multipolar cuff, fine wire, sieve), number of electrode sites (bipolar or multi-array), and location (transverse intrafascicular multichannel nerve, longitudinal intrafascicular nerve, epimysial, intramysial and intracortical microelectrode arrays placed in the cortex) [9–12]. Cuff electrodes circumferentially envelope peripheral nerves and nerve fascicles, and have shown promising results in signal transduction; however, long term signal fidelity may be compromised due to epineurial inflammation and scarring [13–15]. Both intrafascicular electrodes and sieve electrodes allow for nerve and signal specificity, but are hampered by long-term signal loss due to biofouling [16–18]. Epimysial and intramysial electrodes can be larger in size, are physically more robust, are less compromised by fibrosis, and transduce myoelectric signals with less impedance [19].

The most successful form of neural interfacing to date is Targeted Muscle Reinnervation (TMR) [20]. TMR is an FDA-approved procedure to surgically construct additional EMG control sites using residual nerves [21]. Remaining nerves from the amputated limb are transferred to expendable regions of residual muscle in or near the residual limb; commonly, the ipsilateral pectoral muscle is denervated and used for this purpose. The nerves reinnervate the "target" and produce additional EMG signal sites for prosthetic control. Ideally, TMR is performed during the initial amputation procedure, which has been proven to reduce neuroma formation [22–24]. TMR uses external skin surface electrodes to transduce EMG signals, thus avoiding the build-up of connective tissue on electrodes due to a foreign body reaction. Yet a disadvantage of surface EMG electrode systems is their lack of robustness to variance caused by donning, fatigue, perspiration, and other conditions that cause positional and physiological changes in the electrical characteristics of the signal sites [21]. Moreover, the reinnervation of the whole pectoral muscle with up to three nerves, each of which is responsible for specific and distinct functions in the arm, requires the implementation of complex pattern classification and feature extraction algorithms, such that the overlapping neural signals acquired from the EMG electrode array can be decoded and assigned to their intended control targets [25].

Despite the advancements that have benefitted human-prosthetic interfacing, a need remains for a neural interface that can provide real-time, long-term, contamination free, signal fidelity for optimal prosthetic activation and control. In this study, we use the Regenerative Peripheral Nerve Interface (RPNI) as a strategy for neural interfacing. RPNIs are neuromuscular biological interfaces surgically constructed from free muscle grafts (3 × 1 cm.) obtained from expendable skeletal muscle in the residual limb or from a distant site. The residual peripheral nerves are dissected into single nerve fascicles, or groups of fascicles, to create functional units. The muscle grafts are then neurotized by the terminal branches of the residual nerves. Revascularization, regeneration, and eventually reinnervation allows the RPNI to mature in 3 to 4 months [26, 27]. This technique reduces the amount of neural manipulation and risk of iatrogenic nerve damage. Previous studies in our laboratory have shown that RPNIs transduce evoked muscle potentials for up to 18 months, prevent neuroma formation, and amplify motor nerve signaling [28, 29]. Thus, RPNI technology takes advantage of the signal from individual muscles that can be recorded via intramuscular EMG signals generated from the RPNI, obviating the need for signal decoding of multi-nerve motor features via classification algorithms [21].

There have been few investigations into the fine motor control of neuroprosthetic devices using the RPNI technique. As such, the purposes of this study were to: a) build and validate an algorithm for translating EMG signals from RPNIs for real-time control of a myoelectrically actuated neuroprosthetic hand; and b) use this algorithm to demonstrate the ability of RPNIs to provide proportional neuroprosthesis control. It was hypothesized that both Control and RPNI groups would demonstrate reliable and proportional control of the myoelectric hand, while the Denervated group would not activate the neuroprosthesis.

Methods
Animal model
All procedures were approved by the University of Michigan, Institutional Animal Care and Use Committee, and were in strict accordance with the National Research Council's *Guide for the Care and Use of Laboratory Animals* (1996) [30]. Retired F344 male breeder rats (Charles River, Wilmington, MA) weighing 300 to 420 g were anesthetized with weight-based Pentobarbital and administered Buprenorphine-HCl as analgesia.

Regenerative peripheral nerve Interface surgery
The study design consisted of three separate groups, Control ($n = 2$), Denervated ($n = 1$), and RPNI ($n = 3$). In each group, all rats underwent a proximal and distal tenotomy of the extensor digitorum longus (EDL) muscle. In the Control group, no additional interventions were performed. In the Denervated and RPNI groups, the common peroneal nerve was divided and the free EDL muscle graft was transferred to the lateral thigh. In the RPNI group, the proximal end of the divided peroneal nerve was implanted into the EDL skeletal muscle graft to create an RPNI. In the Denervated group, the proximal end of the peroneal nerve was reflected proximally to prevent EDL skeletal muscle graft reinnervation (Fig. 1).

Two stainless steel electrodes made of Cooner wire (Cooner Wire Co., Chatsworth, CA) were sutured onto the EDL epimysium, with electrodes separated longitudinally by 1.5 cm. The EDL muscle was then covered by a single-layer of acellular porcine intestinal submucosa scaffold (SIS) (Surgisis, Cook Biotech, West Lafayette, IN). The leading ends and connecting cables of the electrodes were tunneled, coiled, and buried subcutaneously within the dorsum of each rat between the scapulae.

Testing protocol
Five months following implantation, the free ends of the implanted electrode cables were exposed through a dorsal incision. EMG signals were then recorded, amplified to 1000x and band-pass filtered (1–500 Hz) on a custom-built analog bipolar instrumentation amplifier. Signal amplitudes were calibrated using a function generator (B&K Precision, Model 4075, B&K Precision Corporation, Yorba Linda, CA) and oscilloscope

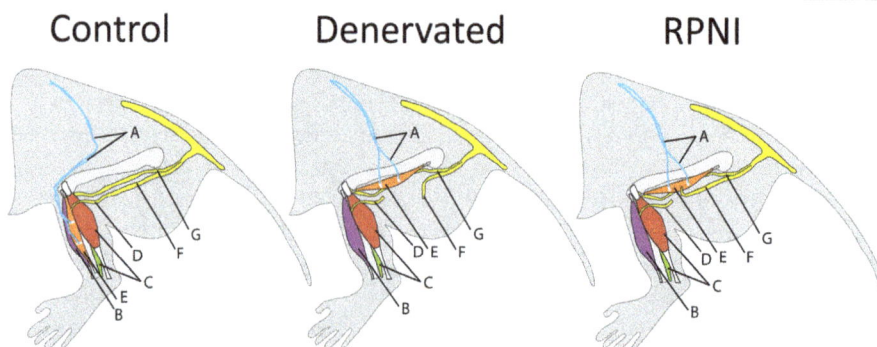

Fig. 1 Left: Control group with primary repair of the extensor digitorum longus muscle (EDL) tenotomies without denervation of the muscle. Center: Denervated group with free EDL muscle graft performed to the lateral thigh. Neurotization and reinnervation was not performed, leaving the EDL muscle graft without innervation. Electrode placement was identical to the Control group. Right: Regenerative Peripheral Nerve Interface (RPNI) group with free EDL muscle graft performed to the lateral thigh. Neurotization and reinnervation were implemented using the peroneal nerve. Each rat received bipolar epimysial electrodes (white), whose wires (blue) were tunneled subcutaneously to the upper dorsum. **a.** bipolar electrode cables. **b.** *tibialis* anterior muscle; **c.** soleus and gastrocnemius muscles; **d.** distal end of common peroneal nerve; **e.** EDL muscle; **f.** proximal common peroneal nerve; **g.** tibial nerve

(Agilent InfiniiVision Model MSO-X 2012-A, Agilent Technologies, Santa Clara, CA). The amplified and filtered signals were acquired at a 3 kHz sampling rate using a data acquisition card (NI BNC 2120, National Instruments, Austin, TX) using LabVIEW software (National Instruments, Austin, TX). During post processing, the signals were digitally rectified and zero-phase low-pass filtered to 50 Hz.

A von Frey monofilament testing protocol was initiated to evoke reflex anterior compartment dorsiflexion of the hind paw, and activation of the EDL or RPNI muscle [31]. During testing, each rat was placed in a $4 \times 5 \times 8$ in.^{3} Plexiglas® box with a wire mesh bottom. Monofilament fibers were applied to the left experimental ankle to induce a voluntary muscle reflex leg movement. Monofilament pressure was initiated at 4 g of force, and monofilament fibers of up to 100 g were randomly administered to the ankle. Four cycles lasting five minutes were performed at each monofilament force level. All rats were free to ambulate while connected to the myoelectric prosthesis to correct for

the possibility of EMG signaling from other muscles. To avoid habituation, 1–2 min of rest was allowed between each testing cycle. Rats in each group were evaluated for 3 days with 2 days of rest between each evaluation period. The monofilament testing lasted no longer than 2 h per day. Post-evaluation, all rats were sacrificed and their hind limb dissected in order to assess the amount of scar tissue and vascularity in the repaired EDL (Control group) and free grafted muscles in the lateral thigh (RPNI and Denervated groups). Prosthetic activation and hind limb movement were video recorded at 120 frames per second using a high-speed, high-definition camera (GoPro Hero2, San Mateo, CA). Rectified EMG and prosthetic activation were synchronized and recorded using the LabVIEW software (Fig. 2).

Algorithm design

A computer algorithm was written using LabVIEW to allow interpretation of the EMG activity and prosthetic control. The rectified and filtered EMG signals were divided into 300 millisecond intervals. Each 300 millisecond interval was then integrated with respect to time and a mean value iEMG was calculated in units of mV × sec. A running threshold was calculated by averaging all previous intervals, giving 50% weight to the immediately prior interval. Activation of the prosthesis occurred when the real-time iEMG was greater than the running threshold by at least one standard deviation (Fig. 3).

Graded control of the prosthesis was achieved by modulation of the output voltage to the "DMC + Hand" (Otto Bock Healthcare, Vienna, Austria) using an Arduino Uno R3 prototyping board (Arduino LLC. Cambridge, MA) equipped with a motor-driving amplifier (SparkFun Electronics, Niwot, CO). Output voltage to the hand was increased with larger iEMG values by calculating the number of standard deviations above the running threshold for each iEMG interval (Eq. 1).

$$V_{Output} = V_{Max} - \frac{V_{Max}}{1 + (SD_{Above\ Threshold})} \qquad (1)$$

Data analysis

Video recordings of each testing period were analyzed to determine interface performance. Sensitivity and specificity were each calculated based on appropriate activation of the prosthesis during hind limb movement and non-activation during periods of rest, respectively. The number of recorded prosthetic movements during each 4-min testing period was compared to the total number of observed leg movements to determine sensitivity (Eq. 2). The number of errant

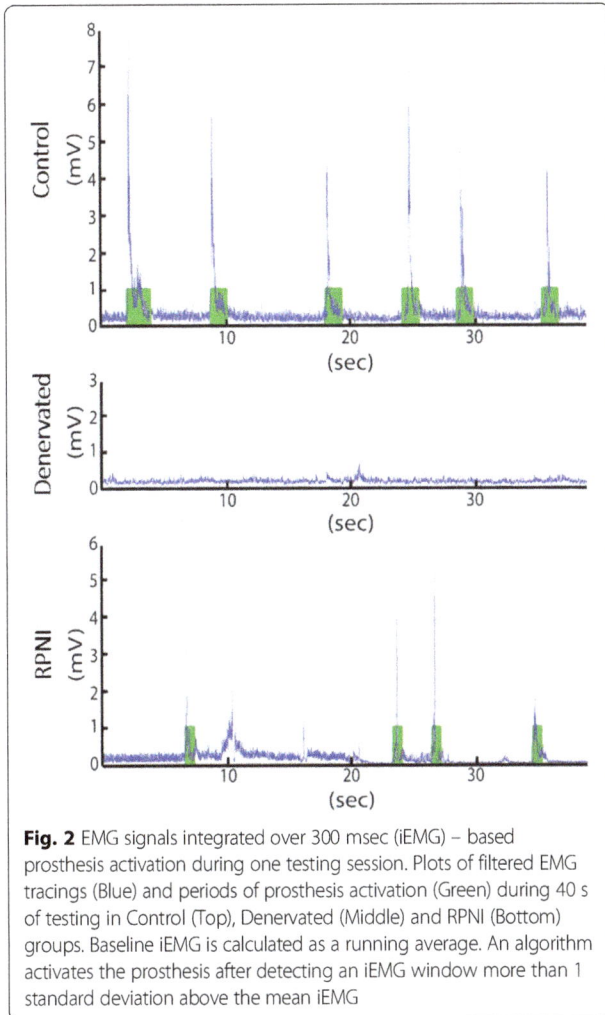

Fig. 2 EMG signals integrated over 300 msec (iEMG) – based prosthesis activation during one testing session. Plots of filtered EMG tracings (Blue) and periods of prosthesis activation (Green) during 40 s of testing in Control (Top), Denervated (Middle) and RPNI (Bottom) groups. Baseline iEMG is calculated as a running average. An algorithm activates the prosthesis after detecting an iEMG window more than 1 standard deviation above the mean iEMG

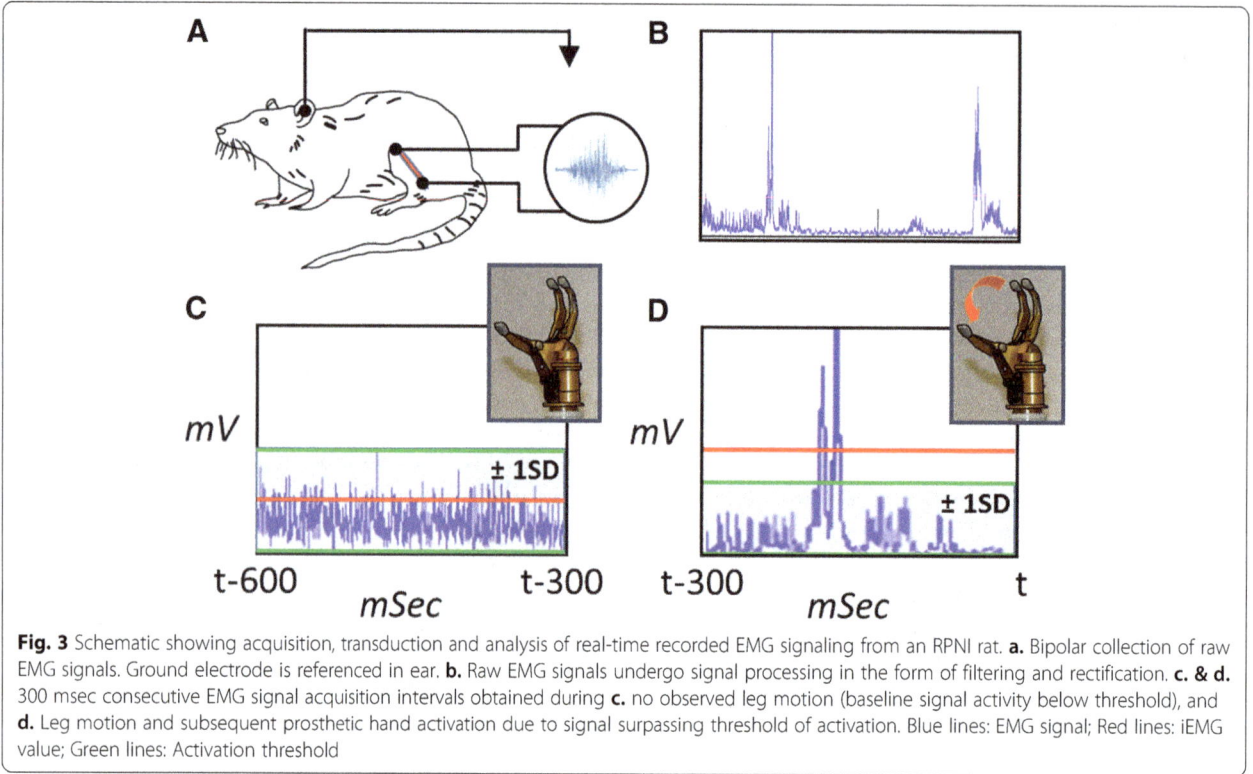

Fig. 3 Schematic showing acquisition, transduction and analysis of real-time recorded EMG signaling from an RPNI rat. **a.** Bipolar collection of raw EMG signals. Ground electrode is referenced in ear. **b.** Raw EMG signals undergo signal processing in the form of filtering and rectification. **c. & d.** 300 msec consecutive EMG signal acquisition intervals obtained during **c.** no observed leg motion (baseline signal activity below threshold), and **d.** Leg motion and subsequent prosthetic hand activation due to signal surpassing threshold of activation. Blue lines: EMG signal; Red lines: iEMG value; Green lines: Activation threshold

activations of the prosthesis during rest intervals with no hind limb movement was calculated to determine specificity (Eq. 3). Within group Student's T-Test statistical computations were performed using SPSS Statistics 22, (SPSS, IBM Inc., 2013, Armonk, NY). Significance levels were set to $\alpha = 0.05$.

$$Sensitivity = \frac{Prosthetic\ activations\ after\ hindlimb\ movement}{Total\ number\ of\ hindlimb\ movements} \tag{2}$$

$$Specifity = \frac{Total\ rest\ intervals - prosthetic\ activations\ during\ rest\ intervals}{Total\ rest\ intervals} \tag{3}$$

Results

Accuracy of Neuroprosthesis activation

In total, 1040 Control group hind limb movements in 208 min and 876 RPNI group hind limb movements in 172 min were captured. (see Video, Additional file 1: Video S1, which demonstrates prosthesis activation in response to monofilament stimulation on the volar side of the hind paw) Significantly reduced hind paw movements were recorded during 51 min within the Denervated group, likely resulting from the lack of peroneal nerve innervation to the lateral compartment musculature of the lower hind limb (see Video, Additional file 2: Video S2, which demonstrates no prosthesis

activation in response to monofilament stimulation on the volar side of the hind paw in a Denervated rat).

The iEMG activation signals were significantly higher in both the Control and RPNI groups when compared to the baseline signals obtained during the between-trial resting periods, indicating that the calculated threshold denoting prosthesis activation (Eq. 1) was successfully defined. The calculated sensitivity (ability to detect prosthetic activation after stimulation) and specificity (ability to prevent unwanted activation during rest) values for prosthesis activation are reported in Table 1. Signal to noise ratio means and standard deviations between iEMG resulting in initial hind limb movement, (i.e. iEMG acquired during the lowest monofilament stimulus resulting in paw retraction, and therefore prosthesis activation) and resting iEMG was 3.55 ± 0.38 and 3.81 ± 0.52 for the Control and RPNI groups, respectively.

Table 1 Summary Data of EMG Translation System

Dependent variables	SURGICAL GROUPS		
	Control (n = 2 rats)	Denervated (n = 1 rat)	RPNI (n = 3 rats)
Mass (g) on test day	420	397	302
Sensitivity	0.902 (0.06)	[a]	0.879 (0.08)
Specificity	0.998 (0.004)	1.0 (0.0)	0.988 (0.02)

Values are means (± 1 SD). Sensitivity and specificity were excellent across all three groups. [a] Denervated group as expected did not show activity during rat movement; therefore no sensitivity was calculated

Proportional control of the Neuroprosthesis

Proportional control of a neuroprosthesis requires the ability to distinguish variations in EMG peak recordings from volitional behavior. Using this tenet, EMG amplitude was mapped 1:1 to the speed of prosthetic hand movement [32]. Increasing von Frey monofilament pressure led to an observable increase in rat hind limb movement intensity. Rats in the Control and RPNI groups had a positive logarithmic correlation between von Frey filament forces (intensity of stimulus), EMG amplitude, and therefore the instantaneous voltage used to actuate the prosthetic hand. This positive correlation enabled a pre-programmed, graded control of the prosthetic hand speed ($R^2 = 0.802$, $p < 0.05$ and $R^2 = 0.758$, p < 0.05, respectively) (Fig. 4).

As expected, no significant correlations were found between resting "baseline" iEMG activity and the monofilament pressure subsequently used for either the Control or RPNI groups ($R^2 = 0.12$ and $R^2 = 0.19$, respectively). This is expected, as changes in "baseline" iEMG activity results from biologic and electronic variation, whereas increased iEMG activity during activation is due to increased muscle activation, contraction, and movement, not random variation (Fig. 5).

Discussion

Regenerative peripheral nerve interfaces (RPNI) provide a biologic connection to peripheral nerves to amplify efferent motor action potentials producing high-fidelity motor control signals and favorable signal to noise ratios. In this study, we have demonstrated reliable RPNI signal transduction in real-time EMG signals obtained during voluntary muscle activation. To date, this is the first study to demonstrate both real time and proportional control of a myoelectric prosthesis using an RPNI.

The amplitude based direct control algorithm strategy determined for this study was modelled using simple linear regression. While there are many means of quantifying muscle activity using myoelectric signals [33], integrated EMG was chosen as the proportional input to the controller, as it has been shown to be a reliable quantifier of muscle force [34]. In order to reset the integration to zero, a 300 millisecond acquisition window was employed; the window timespan was chosen to ensure that at maximum opening velocity (300 mm/s), the prosthetic hand does not exceed its opening width (100 mm) [35]. To ensure that the prosthetic gripper's activation does not occur as a result of background noise or previous myoelectric activity, a running threshold was computed using a weighted average of the myoelectric signals recorded during previous acquisition windows. Consequently, the prosthetic hand was actuated only if the integrated EMG signal obtained during the current sampling window was one standard deviation above threshold [25];

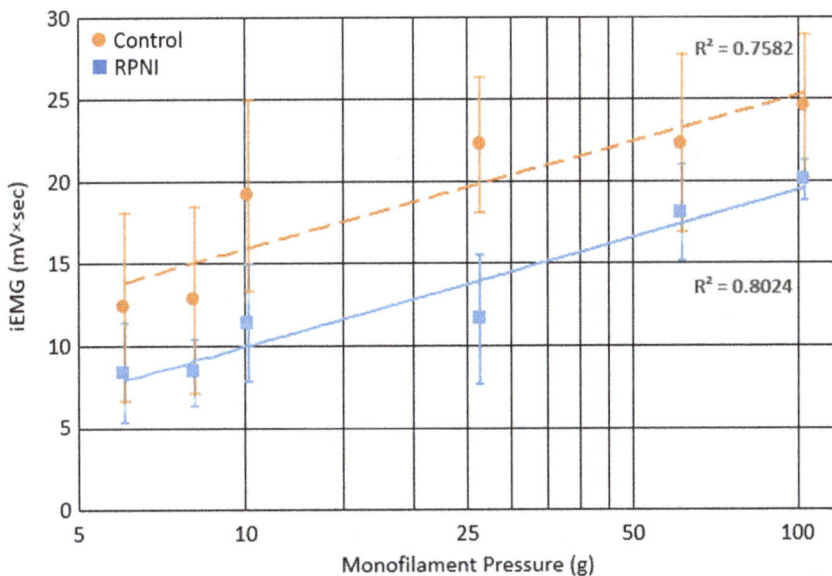

Fig. 4 A semi-logarithmic relationship between monofilament pressure applied and iEMG recorded during four testing blocks. Each block lasted 5 min for each increment of pressure increase in RPNI and Control groups (blue and orange, respectively). Monofilament pressure is graphed logarithmically to linearize each graph. Each represents the mean ± 1 SD for the average of 54 leg movements for control and 51 leg movements for RPNI per increment of pressure. Positive trends in both RPNI and Control groups imply RPNI transduced EMG signals of proportional intensity similar to that of an in situ Control

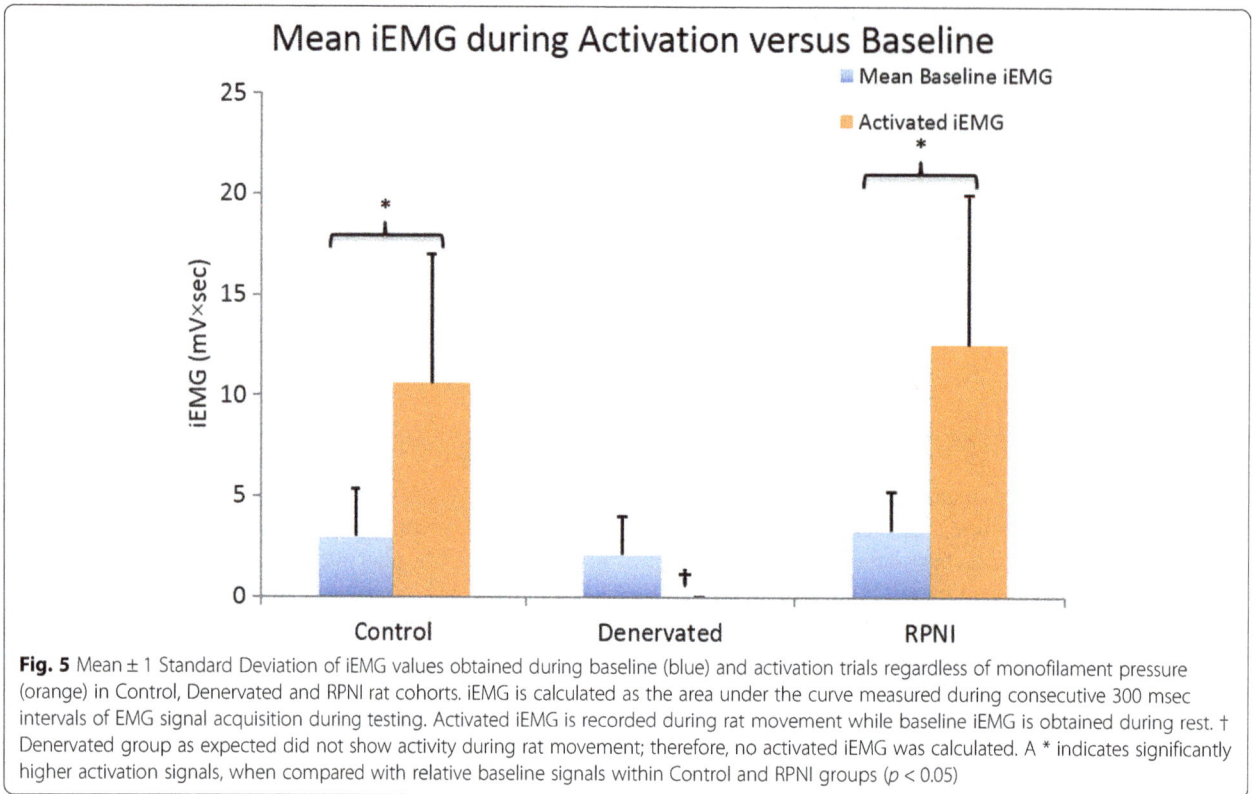

Fig. 5 Mean ± 1 Standard Deviation of iEMG values obtained during baseline (blue) and activation trials regardless of monofilament pressure (orange) in Control, Denervated and RPNI rat cohorts. iEMG is calculated as the area under the curve measured during consecutive 300 msec intervals of EMG signal acquisition during testing. Activated iEMG is recorded during rat movement while baseline iEMG is obtained during rest. † Denervated group as expected did not show activity during rat movement; therefore, no activated iEMG was calculated. A * indicates significantly higher activation signals, when compared with relative baseline signals within Control and RPNI groups ($p < 0.05$)

during actuation, the gripper's velocity was proportional to the amount of discrete standard deviations that iEMG lay above threshold.

An important criterion in patient satisfaction resides in the reaction time of the prosthetic device [24, 36–38]. The algorithm in this study integrated EMG signals over 300 millisecond intervals, building an acceptable 300 millisecond delay into the prosthesis activation time. Integrating EMG signals over this period reduced errant prosthetic activation due to random variation in baseline EMG. Future studies utilizing RPNI interfaces with alternative methods for prosthesis activation can reduce this built-in delay. In the present study, prosthetic hand speed was increased with increasing amplitude of iEMG signals. A strong, positive correlation existed between iEMG signal amplitude and the monofilament force applied to the rat's limb (i.e. the experimental stimulus). This is pivotal, as adjusting both speed and directional movement of a prosthetic device restores greater functionality to the amputee.

One of the primary challenges in neural interfaces is long-term durability in performance. The current study shows that RPNIs were safe and effective in the rat hind limb. As expected, post-experimental gross evaluation of the lateral thigh compartment revealed that the free muscle grafts were healthy in RPNI group rats, but were severely atrophic in the Denervated group. Furthermore, the consistently low EMG signals

derived from the Denervated group signify that RPNI EMG activity is not affected by motion artifact or crosstalk from neighboring muscles.

The implantation procedures were well tolerated, consistent with previous RPNI implantation surgeries [27–29, 39]. Within the lifespan of the rat, we have observed minimal to no signal degradation over at least 7 months post implantation [29]. The electrodes implanted in the RPNI in this study were stainless steel, and interfaced directly with transferred skeletal muscle, thereby avoiding direct contact with the peripheral nerve and corresponding biofouling of the electrode, possible neural inflammation and injury. While muscle tissue tolerates the presence of epi- or intra-muscular electrodes fairly well, electrode materials and designs are currently being investigated to continue to minimize the inflammatory response. [40, 41]

The study's purposes included proof that signals transduced from only one RPNI are suitable to control a one degree of freedom (DOF) myoelectric hand. RPNI technology with multiple implanted RPNIs would also be applicable for prostheses capable of many DOFs. As devised, each RPNI is anatomically "hard-wired" from select motor control areas of the brain through peripheral nerves to individual RPNIs. Consequently, multiple RPNI EMG signals, or co-activation, could be decoded using linear regression control or parallel multi-site control as accomplished with signals available in TMR [42]. Control strategies such as amplitude based direct control, as well as sequential and simultaneous pattern recognition have been studied with able bodied and TMR patients [32]. Those who study efficient control may find that providing several strategies may allow a neuroprosthesis user to achieve fine actuation with direct control, and larger movements with simultaneous control [42].

There are inherent limitations to demonstrating the feasibility of myoelectric prosthesis control using a rat model. Limiting RPNI implantation to one RPNI per one rat hind limb allows for only a simple model which limits prosthetic functionality to single axis actuation. RPNIs are currently being implanted in humans, on multiple individual nerve branches, to provide numerous independent DOF. In this manner, each RPNI will contribute to several movements of a prosthesis when the transduced EMG signals are processed using pattern recognition.

Finally, in this study, we valuated outcomes 135 days after RPNI surgery with electrode implantation. This time-point was selected based on previous studies showing RPNI revascularization, muscle fiber regeneration, and reinnervation occurring at 120 days [29]. Future longitudinal studies of RPNI control of a neuroprosthetic device are currently assessing the lifetime efficacy of RPNI signal transduction.

Conclusion
This study validated an algorithm for translating EMG signals from RPNIs for real-time control of a neuroprosthetic hand. Signal contamination from muscles adjacent to the RPNI was minimal. The EMG signals were successfully acquired from RPNIs and translated into real-time neuroprosthetic control via an algorithm that allowed for concrete demonstration that RPNIs provide reliable proportional control of the neuroprosthesis. RPNI myoelectric hand control was both sensitive and specific.

Acknowledgements
We thank Nicholas B. Langhals, PhD for technical assistance.

Funding
This work was sponsored by the Defense Advanced Research Projects Agency (DARPA) MTO through the Space and Naval Warfare Systems Center, Pacific Grant/Contract No. N66001-11-C-4190 and National Institutes of Health, National Institute of General Medical Sciences, T32 GM008616.

Authors' contributions
CF and DU oversaw and ran the animal experiments, programmed the data acquisition software and analyzed the data. In addition, DU constructed the electrical apparatus used to control the movement of the prosthetic hand along with the control algorithm. SF and AN assisted in running the animal experiments and categorizing the data for analysis. CH, JM, and PB performed the animal surgeries. RBG, TK, and SK along with PC and MU provided valuable mentorship and extensive help with preparing and revising the manuscript. All authors contributed to the manuscript's preparation and revision. All authors read and approved the final manuscript.

Competing interests
The authors declare that they have no competing interests.

Author details
[1]University of Michigan Department of Surgery, Section of Plastic Surgery, 570 MSRB II Level A, 1150 W. Medical Center Drive, Ann Arbor, MI 48109-5456, USA. [2]University of Michigan Department of Mechanical Engineering, Ann Arbor, MI, USA. [3]Vassar College, Poughkeepsie, NY, USA. [4]Department of Biomedical Engineering, University of Michigan, Ann Arbor, MI, USA.

References
1. Ziegler-Graham K, et al. Estimating the prevalence of limb loss in the United States: 2005 to 2050. Arch Phys Med Rehabil. 2008;89(3):422–9.
2. Cloutier A, Yang J. Design, control, and sensory feedback of externally powered hand prostheses: a literature review. Crit Rev Biomed Eng. 2013;41(2):161–81.
3. Cordella F, et al. Literature review on needs of upper limb prosthesis users. Front Neurosci. 2016;10:209.
4. Cowley J, Resnik L, Wilken J, Smurr Walters L, Gates D. Movement quality of conventional prostheses and the DEKA Arm during everyday tasks. Prosthet Orthot Int. 2017;41:33–40.
5. Miranda RA, et al. DARPA-funded efforts in the development of novel brain-computer interface technologies. J Neurosci Methods. 2015;244:52–67.
6. Biddiss EA, Chau TT. Upper limb prosthesis use and abandonment: a survey of the last 25 years. Prosthetics Orthot Int. 2007;31(3):236–57.
7. Ryait HS, Arora AS, Agarwal R. Study of issues in the development of surface EMG controlled human hand. J Mater Sci Mater Med. 2009; 20(Suppl 1):S107–14.
8. Engdahl SM, et al. Surveying the interest of individuals with upper limb loss in novel prosthetic control techniques. J NeuroEng Rehabil. 2015;12:53.
9. Navarro X, et al. A critical review of interfaces with the peripheral nervous system for the control of neuroprostheses and hybrid bionic systems. J Peripher Nerv Syst. 2005;10(3):229–58.
10. Gilja V, et al. Clinical translation of a high-performance neural prosthesis. Nat Med. 2015;21(10):1142–5.
11. Badia J, et al. Spatial and functional selectivity of peripheral nerve signal recording with the transversal Intrafascicular multichannel electrode (TIME). IEEE Trans Neural Syst Rehabil Eng. 2016;24(1):20–7.
12. Castro F, Negredo P, Avendano C. Fiber composition of the rat sciatic nerve and its modification during regeneration through a sieve electrode. Brain Res. 2008;1190:65–77.
13. Larsen JO, et al. Degeneration and regeneration in rabbit peripheral nerve with long-term nerve cuff electrode implant: a stereological study of myelinated and unmyelinated axons. Acta Neuropathol. 1998;96(4):365–78.
14. Thil MA, et al. Time course of tissue remodelling and electrophysiology in the rat sciatic nerve after spiral cuff electrode implantation. J Neuroimmunol. 2007;185(1–2):103–14.
15. Tan DW, et al. A neural interface provides long-term stable natural touch perception. Sci Transl Med. 2014;6(257):257ra138.

16. Yoshida K, Stieglitz T, Shaoyu Q. Bioelectric interfaces for the peripheral nervous system. In: Engineering in Medicine and Biology Society (EMBC), 2014 36th Annual International Conference of the IEEE; 2014.

17. Thota AK, et al. A system and method to interface with multiple groups of axons in several fascicles of peripheral nerves. J Neurosci Methods. 2015; 244:78–84.

18. Jia X, et al. Residual motor signal in long-term human severed peripheral nerves and feasibility of neural signal-controlled artificial limb. J Hand Surg. 2007;32(5):657–66.

19. Hargrove L, et al. The effect of ECG interference on pattern-recognition-based myoelectric control for targeted muscle reinnervated patients. IEEE Trans Biomed Eng. 2009;56(9):2197–201.

20. Kuiken TA, et al. Targeted muscle reinnervation for real-time myoelectric control of multifunction artificial arms. JAMA. 2009;301(6):619–28.

21. Ohnishi K, Weir RF, Kuiken TA. Neural machine interfaces for controlling multifunctional powered upper-limb prostheses. Expert Rev Med Devices. 2007;4(1):43–53.

22. Zhou P, et al. Decoding a New Neural–Machine Interface for Control of Artificial Limbs. J Neurophysiol. 2007;98:2974–82.

23. Cheesborough JE, et al. Targeted muscle reinnervation in the initial management of traumatic upper extremity amputation injury. Hand (New York). 2014;9(2):253–7.

24. Resnik L, Klinger SL, Etter K. The DEKA arm: its features, functionality, and evolution during the veterans affairs study to optimize the DEKA arm. Prosthetics Orthot Int. 2014;38(6):492–504.

25. Jiang N, Englehart KB, Parker PA. Extracting simultaneous and proportional neural control information for multiple-DOF prostheses from the surface electromyographic signal. IEEE Trans Biomed Eng. 2009;56(4):1070–80.

26. Kubiak CA, Kemp SWP, Cederna PS. The regenerative peripheral nerve interface for neuroma management. JAMA Surg. 2018;153(7):681–2.

27. Baldwin J, et al. Abstract 99: Early Muscle Revascularization and Regeneration at the Regenerative Peripheral Nerve Interface. Plast Reconstr Surg. 2012;130(1S):73.

28. Urbanchek MG, et al. Long-Term Stability of Regenerative Peripheral Nerve Interfaces (RPNI). Plast Reconstr Surg. 2011;128(4S):88–9.

29. Kung TA, et al. Regenerative peripheral nerve interface viability and signal transduction with an implanted electrode. Plast Reconstr Surg. 2014;133(6):1380–94.

30. Guide for the Care and Use of Laboratory Animals. Nat'l Research Council (US) Committee for the Update of the Guide for the Care and Use of Laboratory Animals. 8th ed. Washington (DC): Guide for the Care and Use of Laboratory Animals; 2011.

31. Nedic A, Moon JD, Kung TA, et al. Von Frey monofilament testing successfully discriminates between sensory function of mixed nerve and sensory nerve regenerative peripheral nerve interfaces. 6th International IEEE/EMBS Conference on Neural Engineering (NER); 2013. p. 255–8.

32. Wurth SM, Hargrove LJ. A real-time comparison between direct control, sequential pattern recognition control and simultaneous pattern recognition control using a Fitts' law style assessment procedure. J NeuroEng Rehabil. 2014;11(1):1–13.

33. Geethanjali P. Myoelectric control of prosthetic hands: state-of-the-art review. Med Devices (Auckl). 2016;9:247–55.

34. Metral S, Cassar G. Relationship between force and integrated EMG activity during voluntary isometric anisotonic contraction. Eur J Appl Physiol Occup Physiol. 1981;46(2):185–98.

35. Ottobock USA, SensorHand Speed Myoelectric Prosthesis Technical Data. Pamphlet. 2018. https://www.ottobockus.com/prosthetics/upper-limb-prosthetics/solution-overview/myoelectric-devices-speedhands/.

36. Belter JT, et al. Mechanical design and performance specifications of anthropomorphic prosthetic hands: a review. J Rehabil Res Dev. 2013; 50(5):599–618.

37. Yao J, et al. Sensory cortical re-mapping following upper-limb amputation and subsequent targeted reinnervation: a case report. Neuroimage Clin. 2015;8:329–36.

38. Alshammary NA, Dalley SA, Goldfarb M. Assessment of a multigrasp myoelectric control approach for use by transhumeral amputees. Conf Proc IEEE Eng Med Biol Soc. 2012;2012:968–71.

39. Hu Y, et al. Muscle graft volume for regenerative peripheral nerve interfaces as optimized by electrical signal capacity for Neuroprosthetic control. Plast Reconstr Surg. 2015;136(2):443.

40. Micera S, Navarro X. Bidirectional interfaces with the peripheral nervous system. Int Rev Neurobiol. 2009;86:23–38.

41. Vasudevan S, Patel K, Welle C. Rodent model for assessing the long term safety and performance of peripheral nerve recording electrodes. J Neural Eng. 2017;14(1):016008.

42. Smith LH, Kuiken TA, Hargrove LJ. Evaluation of Linear Regression Simultaneous Myoelectric Control Using Intramuscular EMG. IEEE Trans Biomed Eng. 2016;63:737–46.

17

Reliability, validity, and clinical feasibility of a rapid and objective assessment of post-stroke deficits in hand proprioception

Mike D. Rinderknecht[1]* (iD), Olivier Lambercy[1] (iD), Vanessa Raible[2], Imke Büsching[2,3], Aida Sehle[2,3], Joachim Liepert[2,3] and Roger Gassert[1] (iD)

Abstract

Background: Proprioceptive function can be affected after neurological injuries such as stroke. Severe and persistent proprioceptive impairments may be associated with a poor functional recovery after stroke. To better understand their role in the recovery process, and to improve diagnostics, prognostics, and the design of therapeutic interventions, it is essential to quantify proprioceptive deficits accurately and sensitively. However, current clinical assessments lack sensitivity due to ordinal scales and suffer from poor reliability and ceiling effects. Robotic technology offers new possibilities to address some of these limitations. Nevertheless, it is important to investigate the psychometric and clinimetric properties of technology-assisted assessments.

Methods: We present an automated robot-assisted assessment of proprioception at the level of the metacarpophalangeal joint, and evaluate its reliability, validity, and clinical feasibility in a study with 23 participants with stroke and an age-matched group of 29 neurologically intact controls. The assessment uses a two-alternative forced choice paradigm and an adaptive sampling procedure to identify objectively the difference threshold of angular joint position.

Results: Results revealed a good reliability ($ICC(2,1) = 0.73$) for assessing proprioception of the impaired hand of participants with stroke. Assessments showed similar task execution characteristics (e.g., number of trials and duration per trial) between participants with stroke and controls and a short administration time of approximately 12 min. A difference in proprioceptive function could be found between participants with a right hemisphere stroke and control subjects ($p < 0.001$). Furthermore, we observed larger proprioceptive deficits in participants with a right hemisphere stroke compared to a left hemisphere stroke ($p = 0.028$), despite the exclusion of participants with neglect. No meaningful correlation could be established with clinical scales for different modalities of somatosensation. We hypothesize that this is due to their low resolution and ceiling effects.

Conclusions: This study has demonstrated the assessment's applicability in the impaired population and promising integration into clinical routine. In conclusion, the proposed assessment has the potential to become a powerful tool to investigate proprioceptive deficits in longitudinal studies as well as to inform and adjust sensorimotor rehabilitation to the patient's deficits.

Keywords: Difference threshold, MCP, Metacarpophalangeal joint, Parameter Estimation by Sequential Testing, Psychophysics, Quantitative measurements, Robot-assisted assessment, Somatosensory function

*Correspondence: mike.rinderknecht@hest.ethz.ch
[1] Rehabilitation Engineering Laboratory, Department of Health Sciences and Technology, ETH Zurich, Zurich, Switzerland
Full list of author information is available at the end of the article

Background

Proprioception is of great importance for the control of fine and coordinated movements of the upper limb [1–4], and thus for activities of daily living [5–9]. Neurological injuries can affect proprioceptive function, and despite highly variable prevalence reported in the literature, it is estimated that about half of stroke patients suffer from impaired proprioception [10–15]. As there is growing evidence that somatosensory impairment leads to a poor prognosis for post-stroke functional recovery in patients with severe and persistent somatosensory dysfunction [16–19], proprioception in stroke patients has been receiving increased attention. Furthermore, proprioception has been shown to be a relevant predictor for the level of independence patients achieve at discharge [20, 21].

In order to investigate and better understand the role of proprioception in the recovery of neurological patients, for diagnosis as well as the design of therapeutic approaches, accurate and sensitive assessments are essential. Only very few assessments for proprioception are clinically used (e.g., up-down test [22, 23], dual joint position test [24], positional mimicry and finger finding [22, 25]), as, in contrast to other approaches, they are quick and easy to administer in a clinical setting. Unfortunately, these assessments are known to be highly subjective, use dichotomous or ordinal scales, and suffer from large variability due to the lack of standardized protocols and manual administration. This results in low inter-rater reliability, as well as ceiling effects [22, 26, 27]. Thus, they may be suitable for screening patients but not for assessing functional improvements [28]. According to the results of a cross-sectional survey, more than 50% of a sample of 172 occupational and physiotherapists agreed that current methods to assess somatosensory deficits should be improved [29], and assessments with finer degrees of movement (i.e., better controlled movements and finer grading) are required [30].

More quantitative approaches have been proposed, for example using simple apparatuses still requiring manual intervention of the examiner (e.g., using protractor scales [31–34] or objects to discriminate by grasping [35]). Furthermore, a large number of robotic approaches taking advantage of today's actuation, control and sensing technology for better stimulus control [36] and using different assessment paradigms have been developed (e.g., matching and movement reproduction methods [14, 37–50], detection of passive motion [51–53] or perturbations [54–56], as well as difference threshold assessments [57–59]). An essential step when developing a new assessment is the evaluation of its psychometric and clinimetric properties (e.g., reliability, validity, sensitivity, feasibility, and clinical utility) and its potential confounds. To increase clinical acceptance, set-up and testing time, as well as the complexity and cost of the robotic devices should be reduced as much as possible. While some of these properties have been evaluated for matching and perturbation assessments, mostly targeting proximal joints such as shoulder and elbow (e.g., [38, 54, 60]), assessments estimating proprioceptive difference thresholds at finger joints have not been sufficiently optimized and evaluated so far.

The aim of our work is to investigate the reliability, feasibility, and validity of an existing robot-assisted assessment providing a quantitative outcome measure of the metacarpophalangeal (MCP) joint proprioception on a ratio scale [58] in participants with stroke and in an age-matched group of neurologically intact controls (NIC). The assessment is based on an objective two-interval two-alternative forced choice (2AFC) paradigm [61] and Parameter Estimation by Sequential Testing (PEST) [62], an adaptive sampling procedure used to determine perception thresholds. We examine the test-retest reliability for the impaired and unimpaired hands in participants with stroke, and evaluate the clinical feasibility and usability by investigating different task execution properties, such as duration, number of trials by comparing participants with stroke to NIC subjects, and confounds such as memory and inattention. We acknowledge that the terms inattention and neglect are often used interchangeably in the clinical realm. In the present manuscript we defer to how the term "inattention" is used in psychophysical testing and where it represents a time period of distraction from the task. Further, we use the term neglect to represent the common condition that occurs post-stroke and is characterized by a reduced sensory awareness of the side of the body and environment contralateral to the lesion. As a subanalysis, the differences between perception thresholds of participants with left hemisphere stroke (LHS), participants with right hemisphere stroke (RHS), and NIC subjects, and between both hands within participants with stroke (ipsilesional versus contralesional) and NIC subjects (dominant versus non-dominant) are compared (construct validity). Based on findings from other studies [14, 47, 63], we hypothesize that participants with stroke will have decreased proprioceptive performance compared to NIC subjects, and that the proportion of more severely affected participants with stroke may be larger in the RHS group than in the LHS group. Such findings could be related to existing evidence for a non-preferred arm advantage for proprioceptive feedback processing in neurologically intact subjects [40, 42, 64–67]. Furthermore, the robotic outcome measure is correlated to different clinical scales for somatosensation (concurrent validity). This study further discusses the potential of this assessment of proprioceptive deficits in participants with stroke for successful integration and use in a clinical setting.

Methods

Subjects

Twenty-three participants with stroke were recruited and enrolled in this study. They had to be > 2 weeks after their first clinical stroke (without an upper limit on post-stroke weeks). Participants with stroke were recruited on a patient-by-patient basis among the patients receiving an inpatient neurological rehabilitation at the Kliniken Schmieder Allensbach, Germany. Exclusion criteria for the participants with stroke were inability to detect any manually applied large passive finger movements. Other exclusion criteria regarding somatosensory deficits were not defined in this exploratory study to have a heterogeneous sample population with potentially a wide range of levels of proprioceptive deficits. Additional exclusion criteria were severe hand edema, high muscle tone—particularly in the flexor digitorum superficialis muscle and the flexor digitorum profundus muscle—evaluated with the Modified Ashworth Scale [68], or pain preventing the use of the robotic assessment tool, severe cognitive impairment, aphasia, and neglect. If participants with stroke had difficulties with understanding the goal of the study and the instructions, the Montreal Cognitive Assessment (MoCA) [69] was performed as a screening cognitive exam. In case of a value below 26 points on the MoCA scale, the participant was excluded. The presence of neglect symptoms was assessed by clinical observation. In case neglect was suspected, the Bells Test [70] was performed. Twenty-nine neurologically intact control (NIC) subjects within the same age range served as a control group. Only self-reported right handed subjects were included to avoid a handedness confound when comparing proprioceptive performance between the dominant and non-dominant hands in participants with LHS and RHS. Handedness was assessed with the Edinburgh Handedness Inventory (left handed: score < -40, right handed: score > 40, ambidextrous otherwise) [71]. Participants with stroke were asked to evaluate their post-stroke handedness retrospectively. The study was approved by the institutional ethics committee of the University of Konstanz. All subjects gave signed, written informed consent in accordance with the Declaration of Helsinki before participating in the experiment.

Robotic assessment of proprioception

Apparatus

The improved version of the Robotic Sensory Trainer was used in this study [58] (Fig. 1) to assess the proprioceptive difference threshold or limen (DL) in joint angle position of the MCP joint of the index finger. This robotic tool can provide well-controlled, passive MCP joint angle displacements in flexion and extension (Fig. 1a and b). The finger is inserted and attached to a sliding finger carriage mounted on a remote-center-of-motion mechanism allowing for a biomechanically correct movement around the MCP joint when the joint location is aligned with the prolongation of the black arrow on the device (Fig. 1a). The hand and forearm of the subject can be strapped to an adjustable support structure using Velcro® bands, in an attempt to maximize comfort in any pathological hand and arm posture required by the tested subject. The flexion and extension displacements are controlled by software (LabVIEW, National Instruments, Austin, TX, USA) running on an all-in-one touchscreen computer covering the tested hand (Fig. 1c). The program not only runs the psychophysical protocol but also provides a subject interface on which the feedback (i.e., subject's responses after each trial) can be provided.

Adaptive psychophysical procedure

A two-interval, 2AFC paradigm [61] in combination with the logarithmic version of the adaptive stimulus placement method PEST [62] were used as proposed and previously tested in a pilot study [58]. 2AFC should lead to more objective, sensitive and almost bias-free threshold estimates [61, 72]. PEST was selected among different stimulus placement methods due to its fast adaptation over a wide range of stimuli values resulting in an efficient assessment, which converges rapidly towards the desired threshold [58].

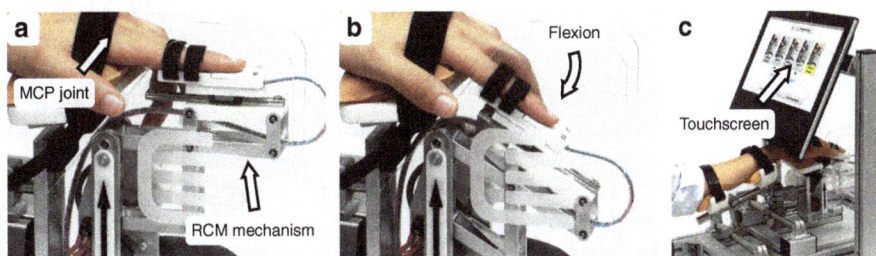

Fig. 1 Robotic Sensory Trainer. **a** Rest position of the index finger. Side view on the remote-center-of-motion (RCM) mechanism of the apparatus used to apply passive movements around the metacarpophalangeal (MCP) joint. **b** Flexed position of the index finger. **c** Experimental setup with a touchscreen, covering the tested hand, for instructions and post-trial subject feedback on perceived stimuli

Each trial consisted of two consecutive passive index finger movements to different MCP joint flexion angles applied by the robotic apparatus. Each movement sequence (i.e., interval) started at a horizontal finger position (referred to as rest position) as depicted in Fig. 1a. Each flexion movement lasted 1 s and the finger was kept at the MCP flexion angle for 1.5 s before moving back to resting position. Each movement followed a natural minimum jerk trajectory [73]. After the two intervals, the subject was asked to indicate on the touchscreen (Fig. 1c) which of the two angular movements was perceived as larger (2AFC paradigm).

The angular difference (referred to as stimulus level x) between the two presented angles of one trial was always defined as positive and determined by the PEST algorithm [62] taking past responses into account. The two angles were symmetrically arranged around a reference angle of 20° MCP flexion and presented in randomized order. The range of x was limited to flexion movements and, by the mechanical constraints of the device, to [0°, 40°]. As starting parameters of the PEST algorithm, a start level x_0 and a start step of 5.5° and 2°, respectively, were chosen. The other PEST parameters $W = 1$ and $P_t = 0.75$ were chosen for the Wald sequential likelihood-ratio test [74] leading to a convergence towards 75% correct responses. This set of parameters was successfully tested in a previous pilot study with young NIC subjects [58]. The robotic assessment was terminated as soon as one of the three termination conditions were fulfilled: (i) minimum step of ±0.1°, (ii) 20 consecutive trials at same level, or (iii) a maximum number of trials defined in the experimental protocol reached.

Primary outcome measure: difference limen estimation

In theory, PEST should directly provide the difference limen (DL, in the literature sometimes also referred to as difference threshold or just-noticeable difference) by convergence. According to the original concept, the level (at which no trials are actually run) called for by the last small step can be used as the threshold estimate [62]. However, depending on the choice of termination criteria and parameters, it can occur that PEST does not converge within the given number of maximum trials. Furthermore, it is possible that periods of lack of attention towards the end of the assessment may lead to partial divergence from the threshold, resulting in poorer estimates. These issues can be partly addressed by using hybrid procedures: determining the test levels with the PEST algorithm and estimating the final threshold estimate from a parametrized psychometric function fitted on the data of the entire PEST sequence [75]. It could be shown in our previous work that the DL at the MCP joint estimated by this fitting method strongly correlated with the converged values provided by PEST [58] with

the advantage of being more robust and providing also reasonable estimates in the above mentioned cases.

Loss of attention during psychophysical assessments, in particular in those using two-interval 2AFC, can be a confound leading to considerable bias, due to altered perception, especially as attention deficits are likely to be present in the stroke population [76, 77]. To address this issue, a method was developed allowing to identify the onset and end of sustained inattention periods in PEST sequences, to exclude this interval of biased data before fitting the psychometric function and calculating the outcome measure [78]. This method can significantly reduce estimation errors by up to around 75%, even in sequences of less than 100 trials, as demonstrated in computer simulations and tested on behavioral data [78]. Thus, before estimating the DL in the present study, this method was applied *post-hoc* to each recorded PEST sequence.

In the present work, the following sigmoidal psychometric function $\psi(x)$ was fitted to the proportion of correct responses at stimulus levels x using a Maximum Likelihood criterion [79]:

$$\psi(x; \alpha, \beta, \gamma, \lambda) = \gamma + (1 - \gamma - \lambda) F(x; \alpha, \beta) . \quad (1)$$

In this work, the generic sigmoid function $F(x; \alpha, \beta)$ of the equation above corresponded to a cumulative Gaussian function $F_{Gauss}(x; \mu, \sigma)$. The parameter μ corresponds to the inflection point of $\psi(x)$ and σ is inversely proportional to the slope at the inflection point. According to the 2AFC paradigm, the guessing rate γ was set to 0.5. The lapse rate λ (taking into account stimulus-independent errors also referred to as lapses) was allowed to vary within $[0, 0.1]$, in order to reduce estimation bias [80]. Since the inflection point μ depends on the lapse rate λ, the DL was defined as outcome measure at $x_T = \psi^{-1}(0.75)$.

Clinical assessments

Proprioceptive function was assessed based on the up-down test described by [22]. The distal phalanx of the index finger was moved up or down, 5 times each, in random order. Participants with stroke reported the direction of the movement verbally in absence of vision of the tested finger. The final score (0–10) consisted of the number or correctly identified movement directions.

In addition, other somatosensory modalities were tested. Topesthesia (localization of touch) was tested by manually stroking the dorsal side of the fingers (2x per finger, random order). The outcome measure was the number of correctly identified fingers (0–10). Von Frey hairs (OptiHair$_2$, MARSTOCKnervtest, Schriesheim, Germany) were used to assess the absolute tactile perception threshold on the fingertip of the index finger. The score was computed by taking the geometric mean of the reverse values (5 suprathreshold and 5 subthreshold) of the descending staircase according to [81], on a scale from 1 (0.25 mN) to 12 (512 mN). Pallesthesia (sensation of mechanical vibration) was assessed using a 64 Hz, graduated Rydel-Seiffer tuning fork (Martin, Tuttlingen, Germany) [82] on the MCP joint of the index finger. The sensibility was scored from 0–8 in steps of one with 0 corresponding to no sensation at all. Stereognosis (ability to recognize objects by using only tactile information) was assessed with the subscale of the Nottingham Sensory Assessment [22]. The outcome was the number of correctly identified objects (0–10).

Attention and working memory were assessed using the backward recitation condition of the Digit Span subtest of the Wechsler Adult Intelligence Scale® - Third Edition (WAIS®-III) [83], where participants with stroke were asked to recite an auditorily presented series of digits backwards. Two trials with random numbers were consecutively performed for each digit span (2–6 numbers, in increasing order). The total score consisted of the total number of correctly recited digit spans ranging from 0–12.

Experimental protocol

Both, participants with stroke and NIC subjects performed the robotic proprioception assessment of both hands (randomized order) in one session. For the participants with stroke, the maximum number of trials for the PEST algorithm was set to 60 trials, which should correspond to an assessment duration of around 15 min according to a pilot study in young NIC subjects [58]. This number of trials was selected to allow a future integration of the assessment into clinical routine, and because longer assessments could be too strenuous for participants with stroke due to the cognitive demand (e.g. attention to the task). As these points were less critical for NIC subjects, the maximum number of PEST trials was set to 120 trials. This allowed evaluating the appropriateness of the chosen parameters of the PEST procedure. To investigate test-retest reliability, the robotic test was conducted in participants with stroke in a second session not more than 4 days after the first session. For a subset of 10 of the 23 recruited participants with stroke, clinical assessments (of both hands where applicable) were performed in a separate session by a different therapist. The therapists were blinded to the outcomes of the other assessments. No clinical assessments were conducted in NIC subjects due to ceiling effects. All assessments took place at the Kliniken Schmieder Allensbach, Germany.

Data analysis

To evaluate the test-retest reliability (in participants with stroke), the intraclass correlation coefficient $ICC(2, 1)$ (two-way layout with random effects for absolute agreement) [84], as well as its 95% confidence interval

(CI), standard error of measurement SEM, and smallest real difference SRD (sometimes referred to as minimal detectable change MDC) were computed according to [85] and [86]. Systematic bias was analyzed by calculating the mean difference $\bar{d}$ between the two test occasions and its 95% CI, and by visualization in a Bland-Altman plot [85]. The reliability analysis was performed separately for the impaired and unimpaired hand.

To compare the outcome measures of NIC subjects to participants with stroke and to create models of neurologically intact performance, the PEST sequences of the NIC subjects were truncated to 60 trials to be of same length as for the participants with stroke. Furthermore, outliers in the NIC group were identified according to Tukey's rule and excluded from all statistical analysis.

Outcome measures from the robotic assessment were compared between the left and right hand of NIC subjects (paired test), between the impaired hand of the participants with stroke and the corresponding hand in NIC subjects (two unpaired tests for LHS and RHS), and between the unimpaired hand of the participants with stroke and the corresponding hand in NIC subjects (two unpaired tests for LHS and RHS). For participants with stroke, the average of both test and retest outcomes was used. Two-sample t-tests or Wilcoxon rank sum tests, respectively paired-sample t-tests or paired Wilcoxon signed rank tests, were conducted depending on whether data (or their differences for paired testing) were normally distributed or not. Normality was tested with the Shapiro–Wilk or the Shapiro–Francia test, depending on the kurtosis. To correct for multiple comparisons, a Šidák-correction was used. To compare the effect of a LHS versus a RHS on proprioceptive function of the impaired hand (as well as unimpaired hand), their differences to NIC baseline of the corresponding hand were compared in an unpaired test. As NIC baseline the median was used, as the distributions of the left and right DL in NIC subjects were not both normally distributed. Again, the test-retest average was used for the participants with stroke.

Subjects in this study were not age-matched on an individual basis but on a group level by including subjects within the same age range. In return, the sample size of NIC subjects was chosen to be larger, which should improve the estimated distribution of DLs for the same age range. To model neurologically intact performance in elderly, log–normal (semi-infinite positive support) probability density functions were fitted on the DL data of NIC subjects for the right (dominant) and left (non-dominant) hand separately. The 95th percentile was used to characterize impairment in participants with stroke. The CI for the 95th percentile cutoff were calculated by bootstrapping.

The trial duration of the robotic assessment was compared between impaired and unimpaired hands of participants with stroke (averaged test-retest, paired-sample *t*-test or paired Wilcoxon signed rank test, depending on normality of the paired differences), and between NIC subjects (mean of both hands for each subject) and the impaired, respectively unimpaired hand of participants with stroke (averaged test-retest, two-sample *t*-test or Wilcoxon rank sum test, depending on normality of the two distributions). The Šidák-correction method was used to correct for multiple comparisons.

Spearman's rank-order correlations were calculated for the impaired hand between the DL (test-retest average) and the outcome measures of the clinical scales (i.e., up-down, localization, Von Frey hair, vibration, stereognosis, working memory). As the up-down test also measures proprioception, the correlation with the robotic assessment could be regarded as a test for concurrent validity. The clinical scores for the impaired hand and the working memory test were also compared between the participants with RHS and LHS with two-sample *t*-tests and Wilcoxon rank sum tests, respectively.

The influence of sex on the proprioceptive outcome measures was tested by separately comparing the robotic outcome measures for the dominant as well as the non-dominant hand in male versus female NIC subjects, and for the impaired as well as the unimpaired hand in participants with stroke (two-sample *t*-test or Wilcoxon rank sum test, depending on normality of the distributions).

Significance levels were set to $\alpha = 0.05$. Probability values $p < 0.05$ and $p < 0.01$ are marked as * and **. Descriptive statistics are reported as mean $\pm$ SD, unless otherwise stated. For non-parametric statistics the median and interquartile range (IQR) was reported. All statistical analyses were performed in MATLAB R2014a (MathWorks, Natick, MA, USA).

Results

Twenty-one participants with stroke completed the two sessions of robotic assessments, and two participants with stroke dropped out of the study (P1 was not able to perceive any movements applied by the robotic device, and P6 prematurely quit the study). As reported by the therapist conducting the robotic assessments, one of the 21 participants with stroke (P13) was not able to correctly follow the task instructions and showed severe concentration problems. Therefore, this participant was excluded from all statistical analyses. Of the 20 participants with stroke (65.9 $\pm$ 8.3 years, range: [55, 79] years, 12 male, 8 female, pre-stroke handedness: 18 right handed, 2 ambidextrous), 10 suffered from a LHS and 10 from a RHS. Participants with stroke were 43.7 $\pm$ 118.8 weeks post lesion (range: [4, 517] weeks). For one chronic participant with stroke (P17) only the year but not the exact lesion date

was known. Average number of days between the test and retest of the robotic assessment in participants with stroke was 2 $\pm$ 1 days (range: [1, 4] days), and between the clinical assessment and the first robotic assessment was 4 $\pm$ 4 days (range: [0, 13] days). The demographics of all the 23 recruited participants with stroke can be found in Table 1. One of the 29 NIC subjects was excluded according to Tukey's rule. The average age of the remaining 28 NIC subjects (13 male, 15 female, all right handed) was 63.2 $\pm$ 6.6 years (range: [55, 80] years).

The outcomes of the robotic assessment for all groups (NIC, LHS, and RHS) are illustrated for both hands in Fig. 2. Performance of NIC subjects in the robotic proprioception assessment averaged at 1.82° $\pm$ 0.77° (median: 1.70°, IQR: [1.31°, 2.40°]) for the right (dominant) hand, and 1.62°$\pm$ 0.78° (median: 1.39°, IQR: [0.98°, 2.08°]) for the left (non-dominant) hand. There was no statistically significant difference between the two hands ($t(27) = 1.046, p = 0.838$). No significant effect of sex on the DL was found in NIC subjects (all *p*-values > 0.4). Participants with LHS averaged at 2.35°$\pm$ 0.94° (median: 2.31°, IQR: [2.12°, 2.65°]) for the impaired (right) hand, and 2.43°$\pm$ 0.80° (median: 2.27°, IQR: [1.87°, 2.84°]) for the unimpaired (left) hand. Participants with RHS averaged at 3.95°$\pm$ 2.36° (median: 3.21°, IQR: [2.17°, 5.10°]) for the impaired (left) hand, and 3.31°$\pm$ 2.66° (median: 2.19°, IQR: [1.79°, 4.81°]) for the unimpaired (right) hand. No significant effect of sex on the DL was found in participants with stroke (all *p*-values > 0.2). For participants with LHS, there was no significant difference between their impaired (right) hand and the right hand of NIC subjects ($t(36) = 1.747, p = 0.373$). However, there was a significant difference between their unimpaired (left) hand and the left hand of NIC subjects ($Z = 2.7, p = 0.038$). For participants with RHS, proprioception of the impaired (left) hand was significantly worse than the left hand of NIC subjects ($t(36) = 4.656, p < 0.001$), whereas the unimpaired (right) hand was not significantly different ($Z = 1.8, p = 0.307$). The difference from baseline for the impaired hand in participants with RHS was significantly larger compared to participants with LHS ($t(18) = -2.384, p = 0.028$). There was no significant difference between the unimpaired hand in participants with RHS compared to participants with LHS ($Z = -0.9, p = 0.385$). The two log–normal models for neurologically intact proprioception were DL $\sim$ Lognormal(μ, σ^2) with $\mu = 0.493$ and $\sigma = 0.508$ for the right, dominant hand and $\mu = 0.381$ and $\sigma = 0.455$ for the left, non-dominant hand. The 95th percentile of NIC subjects was 3.78° (CI: [3.03°, 5.32°]) for the right and 3.10° (CI: [2.47°, 4.01°]) for the left hand. The DL of the left hand was higher than the 95th percentile for 2 NIC subjects. The test-retest average outcome value of the unimpaired (left) hand of participants with LHS was above the impairment

Table 1 Demographics of the participants with stroke

Participant with stroke	Age [years]	Gender	Handedness (pre-stroke)	Lesion side	Post lesion [weeks]	Stroke type and location
P1 (D)	74	M	R	LHS	11	Infarction of the left MCA
P2	56	M	R	RHS	6	ICH in the right frontotemporal region
P3	68	M	R	LHS	5	Hemorrhage in the left basal ganglia
P4	60	F	A	RHS	14	Partial infarction of the right MCA
P5	79	M	R	LHS	4	Hemorrhage in the left basal ganglia with intraventricular extension
P6 (D)	67	M	R	RHS	12	Infarction of the right MCA, with emphasis on the dorsal and cranial aspects and involvement of the basal ganglia
P7	57	F	A	LHS	20	Left ACA SAH and cerebral vasospasms with partial infarction in the left MCA- and ACA-territory
P8	67	M	R	RHS	6	Infarction of the right MCA
P9	55	M	R	LHS	8	Hemorrhage in left basal ganglia
P10	57	F	R	LHS	14	Left pontine infarction
P11	70	F	R	RHS	6	Right cerebellar infarction
P12	79	M	R	RHS	7	Infarction of the right MCA
P13 (E)	55	M	R	RHS	14	Partial infarction of the right MCA
P14	79	F	R	RHS	517	Hemorrhage in the right basal ganglia
P15	75	F	R	LHS	144	Infarction of the left MCA
P16	62	M	R	RHS	7	Infarction in the right medulla oblongata
P17	72	M	R	LHS	197–249	Left ICH
P18	67	M	R	LHS	6	Hemorrhage in the left basal ganglia
P19	57	F	R	RHS	10	Mixed SAH and ICH of the right ACA
P20	73	M	R	RHS	15	Multiple ischemia in the right MCA-territory
P21	58	F	R	LHS	5	Multiple ischemia in the left MCA- and PCA-territory
P22	67	M	R	LHS	14	Cerebellar (both sides) and left pontine nucleus infarctions
P23	60	M	R	RHS	23	Ischemic infarction in the right vertebrobasilar territory

One participant with stroke (P13) was excluded due to inability to concentrate and follow the task instructions correctly. For participant P17 only the lesion year was known.
Abbreviations: *D* dropout, *E* excluded, *M* male, *F* female, *R* right handed, *A* ambidextrous, *RHS* right hemisphere stroke, *LHS* left hemisphere stroke, *ACA* anterior cerebral artery, *ICH* intracerebral hemorrhage, *MCA* middle cerebral artery, *PCA* posterior cerebral artery, *SAH* subarachnoid hemorrhage

cutoff value for 1 participant. Based on a single assessment, 2 (test), respectively 1 (retest), additional participants with stroke would have been considered as impaired. In 5 participants with RHS both test and retest assessments of the impaired (left) hand were above the cutoff value. For the DL of the right hand, this was the case for 1 participant with LHS (impaired hand). The average DLs of the unimpaired (right) hand were above the cutoff in 3 participants with RHS. In one of these participants only the result of one assessment (test) would be considered as impaired. Based on a single assessment, 1 (retest) additional participant with stroke would have been considered as impaired. In 2 participants with RHS both impaired and unimpaired hands were above the 95th percentile.

The values of test-retest reliability for the impaired and unimpaired hand were 0.73 and 0.16, respectively. The detailed descriptive statistics for the DL of the test and

retest, reliability, *SEM* characterizing the measurement variability, and *SRD* for evaluating changes are summarized in Table 2.

There were no systematic biases between test and retest, as can be seen by $\bar{d}$ and its 95% CI in the Bland-Altman plot (Fig. 3).

The average number of trials, convergence rate of the PEST algorithm, duration of the assessment, and duration per trial are reported in Table 3. There was no statistically significant difference for the duration per trial between assessments of the impaired and unimpaired hand in participants with stroke ($Z = 1.6, p = 0.272$), nor between assessments in NIC subjects and the impaired ($Z = 0.4, p = 0.963$) or unimpaired ($Z = 1.4, p = 0.416$) hand of participants with stroke, respectively. The inattention detection rate (percentage of cases) based on the psychophysical data and resulting number of excluded trials (around one third of the trials in participants with

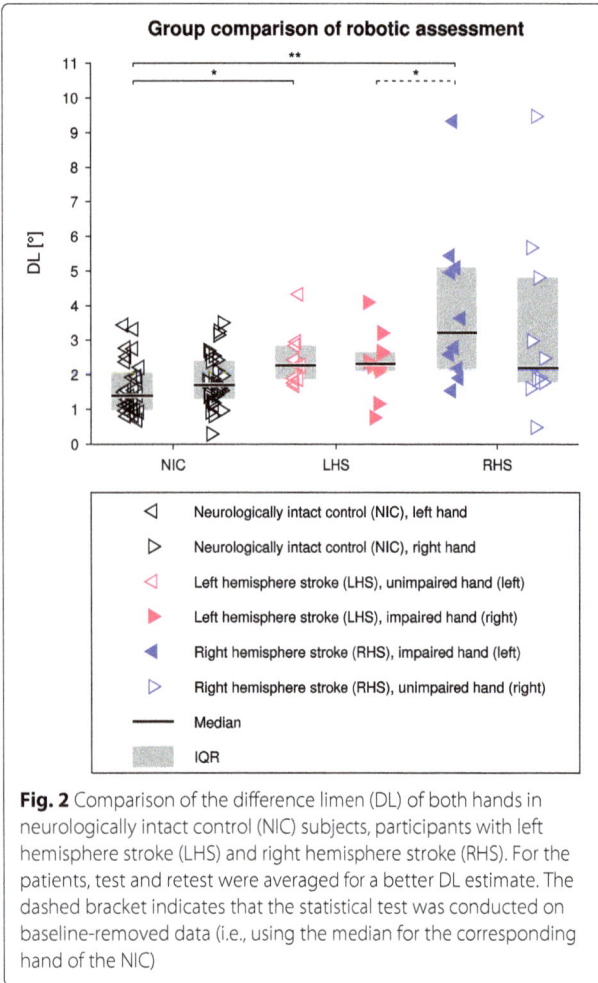

Fig. 2 Comparison of the difference limen (DL) of both hands in neurologically intact control (NIC) subjects, participants with left hemisphere stroke (LHS) and right hemisphere stroke (RHS). For the patients, test and retest were averaged for a better DL estimate. The dashed bracket indicates that the statistical test was conducted on baseline-removed data (i.e., using the median for the corresponding hand of the NIC)

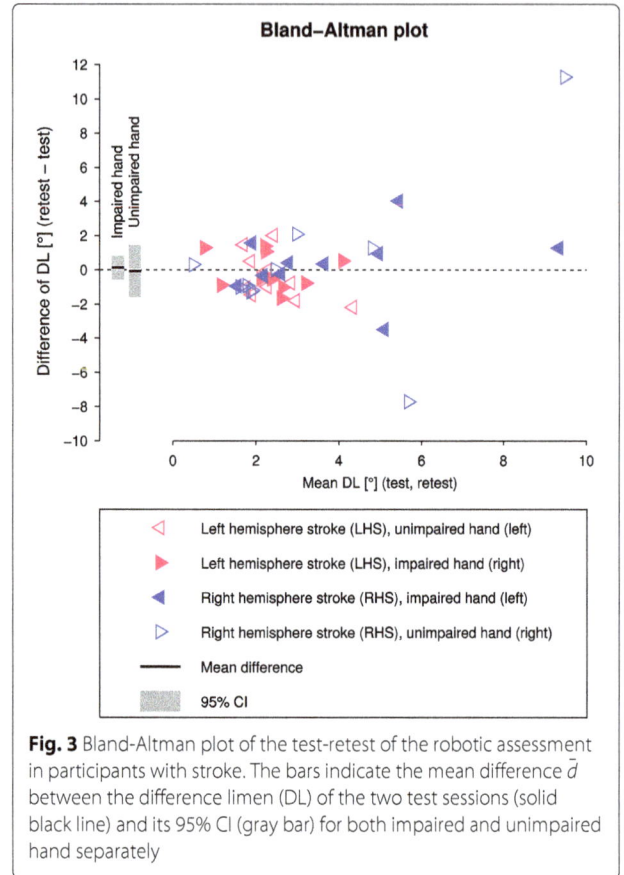

Fig. 3 Bland-Altman plot of the test-retest of the robotic assessment in participants with stroke. The bars indicate the mean difference $\bar{d}$ between the difference limen (DL) of the two test sessions (solid black line) and its 95% CI (gray bar) for both impaired and unimpaired hand separately

stroke and one sixth in NIC subjects) are also summarized in Table 3.

All Spearman's rank-order correlations between the robotic outcome measure and the clinical scales were weak to fair and not statistically significant (see Table 4). Many clinical assessments showed either floor or ceiling effects, with up to 90% of the data. In particular, in the up-down test, which is the most relevant of the clinical scales as it measures proprioception, all except one participant with stroke reached the highest possible score showing no proprioceptive deficits. Statistical tests did not show any

significant differences between participants with RHS and LHS for the clinical assessments (neither for tests assessing the impaired hand ($p > 0.325$) nor for the working memory test ($p = 0.121$)).

Discussion

The aim of this study was to evaluate the psychometric and clinimetric properties (reliability, validity, and clinical feasibility and usability) of a robot-assisted assessment of MCP proprioception, using a 2AFC approach and the adaptive sampling procedure PEST providing the angular joint position DL, in a stroke population. The study demonstrated a good reliability for the contralesional hand in participants with stroke, a difference in proprioceptive function between participants with stroke

Table 2 Reliability analysis

	DL Test		DL Retest				
	Mean ± SD	Range	Mean ± SD	Range	ICC(2, 1) [CI]	SEM	SRD
Impaired	3.08° ± 1.93°	[0.12°, 8.70°]	3.21° ± 2.22°	[0.73°, 9.97°]	0.73 [0.44, 0.89]	1.07°	2.95°
Unimpaired	2.90° ± 1.94°	[0.33°, 9.53°]	2.84° ± 3.11°	[0.65°, 15.11°]	0.16 [0.00, 0.56]	2.33°	6.45°

Summary of the reliability analysis for the outcome measure of the robotic assessment (i.e., difference limen (DL)) of the impaired and unimpaired hand, respectively. Reported are descriptive statistics for the DL for both test and retest, reliability (ICC(2, 1) and its 95% CI), standard error of measurement (SEM), and smallest real difference (SRD)

Table 3 Task execution characteristics and inattention

	Max trials	Trials	Converged	Duration	Duration/trial	Inattention	Trials excluded
Impaired	60	55 ± 5	35%	12.3 ± 1.7 min	13.4 ± 1.6 s	10%	20 ± 8
Unimpaired	60	53 ± 7	45%	11.3 ± 1.8 min	12.8 ± 0.8 s	18%	16 ± 9
NIC, both hands	120	65 ± 18	91%	14.1 ± 3.8 min	13.1 ± 0.7 s	13% (7%)	14 ± 9 (8 ± 2)

Summary of the properties of the PEST sequences, as well as percentage of cases where sustained inattention (distraction from the task) was detected (according to [78]) and resulting number of excluded trials, for participants with stroke (impaired and unimpaired hand) and neurologically intact controls (NIC). For trial- and duration-related results, test and retest were averaged for each participant with stroke, whereas in the case of NIC subjects their left and right hand were averaged. For the results regarding inattention, test and retest were pooled for the participants with stroke, and left and right hand were pooled for the NIC subjects. The values in parentheses correspond to the percentage of cases where sustained inattention was detected and resulting number of excluded trials after truncating the sequences to a maximum of 60 trials

and NIC subjects, and that participants with RHS may be more affected compared to participants with LHS. Only weak correlations between the robotic outcome measure and clinical scales were obtained, among others due to ceiling effects of the latter. The assessment duration of around 12 min, demonstrated high feasibility of the assessment in an impaired population.

Test-retest reliability

According to general reliability recommendations (excellent: > 0.75, fair to good: $0.4–0.75$, poor: < 0.4) [87], the intraclass correlation analysis revealed a good reliability for the impaired hand in participants with stroke and a poor reliability for the unimpaired hand. The poor reliability for the unimpaired limb may result from the distribution of data, with LHS and RHS having more similar means and LHS and RHS combined having a smaller IQR compared to the impaired side, as inter-subject variability has an influence on reliability [88]. Therefore, we can recommend to use the proposed assessment as a reliable tool for the impaired, contralesional hand of stroke patients.

Studies evaluating other assessment approaches using various matching paradigms for different upper limb joints [14, 31, 32, 34, 35, 38, 41, 50, 54, 56, 60] or similar joint position DL estimation methods [34, 59] reported coefficients of reliability ranging from fair to excellent for most outcome measures. However, it is difficult to compare results, as other approaches may measure different aspects of proprioception, or because some studies investigated the reliability in NIC subjects instead of in the target population, which may

lead to non-representative results, due to different inter- and intra-subject variabilities [88]. Several studies also used inappropriate time intervals between the test and retest (e.g., right after each other without a time interval long enough to prevent recall bias) or suboptimal methods for calculating reliability. In comparison to robotic approaches, the kinaesthetic subscales of the Nottingham Sensory Assessment (finger finding, positional mimicry, and up-down test) have a poor inter-rater agreement (Cohen's κ from 0.26 to 0.39) for the hand [22, 26]. This may originate among others from the nature of the manually applied stimuli which are not well-controlled (e.g., amplitude of movement) and thus may vary across raters.

The Bland-Altman plot showed that there was no systematic bias from test to retest. However, it revealed two outlier data points for the unimpaired hand according Tukey's outlier test (difference of test-retest $> 4.08°$ or $< -4.41°$). Visual inspection of the PEST sequences showed that for both outliers in one of their two test-retest sequences there was a period of divergence from the threshold, possibly due to inattention (i.e., distraction from the task), which failed to be detected by the inattention detection algorithm [78]. Removing these two outliers from the reliability analysis improved the reliability for the assessment of the unimpaired hand and resulted in a fair reliability ($ICC(2, 1)$ [CI]: $r = 0.41$ [0.00, 0.73]).

It should be noted that the $ICC(2, 1)$ is very sensitive and directly depends on the intra- and inter-subject variability. As a matter of fact, removing participants with stroke P8 with an average DL of 9.33° (test: 8.70°, retest: 9.97°) for

Table 4 Clinical assessments and correlations

	Up-down	Localization	Von Frey hair	Vibration	Stereognosis	Working memory
Mean $\pm$ SD	9.80 ± 0.63	9.30 ± 1.89	3.72 ± 1.79	7.00 ± 0.94	8.60 ± 0.97	5.15 ± 1.92
Range	[8.00, 10.00]	[4.00, 10.00]	[1.41, 8.27]	[5.00, 8.00]	[8.00, 10.00]	[3.00, 8.00]
Floor/ceiling	0%/90%	0%/80%	0%/0%	0%/30%	0%/30%	0%/0%
Spearman $r_s(8)$	-0.41	0.34	0.16	-0.09	0.34	-0.09
Spearman p	0.24	0.34	0.65	0.81	0.33	0.81

Descriptive statistics of the clinical assessments and Spearman's rank-order correlation (r_s, $n = 10$) with the average of the difference limen (DL) of test and retest provided by the robotic assessment. Reported correlations are for the impaired (contralesional) side

the impaired hand, would reduce the test-retest reliability $(ICC(2,1)$ [CI]: $r = 0.49$ [$0.04, 0.77$]). This shows that reporting the CI for the reliability is also important. Indeed, the reliability without P8 still remains within the CI reported in Table 2. By including also sub-acute participants with stroke in a future cross-sectional study with a larger sample size, we would expect more participants with stroke with high DLs, confirming a good test-retest reliability.

Construct validity and proprioceptive consequences of stroke

Hypothesis-based comparisons between NIC subjects and participants with stroke, as well as between participants with RHS and LHS could give some indication of validity of the assessment (i.e., construct validity). As a matter of fact, the robotic assessments of proprioception of the present study revealed worse proprioception (around 2.3 times larger DL) in the impaired (left) hand of the RHS group compared to NIC subjects. This is comparable to the results showing a fingertip position DL (flexion–extension) three times larger in participants with stroke compared to the control group when using a Same-Different paradigm [89]. The existence of post-stroke proprioceptive deficits could also be established with various matching studies [14, 31, 47, 90] and studies using other types of proprioceptive measures [54]. While one would also expect the impaired (right) hand of participants with LHS to have a significantly larger DL, this was not the case in our study. When modeling NIC performance, half of the 10 participants with RHS were above the 95th percentile of NIC performance, compared to one out of 10 participants with LHS. This can be due to various reasons. Since this was an exploratory study including participants with stroke suffering from different levels of impairment, some of the included participants with stroke may not have presented important proprioceptive deficits, resulting in a reduced difference between the NIC and stroke groups. The high rate of ceiling effects in the clinical scales (e.g., in the up-down test) would support this hypothesis. Other reasons could be the inclusion of participants with stoke within a broad range of time after stroke, as proprioceptive impairments after stroke can reduce with time [91], lack of sub-acute participants with stroke, and the exclusion of participants with stroke who were not able to detect any manually applied large passive finger movements, which reduces the reported prevalence of proprioceptive deficits. Another hypothesis for this RHS/LHS difference could be that in the right handed participants with RHS, the non-dominant (left) hand is impaired which could potentially suffer more from non-use, compared to the dominant (right) hand which is affected in right handed participants with LHS.

Another reason for more severe proprioceptive deficits in participants with RHS could be the higher ratio of participants with RHS with a cortical stroke when compared to participants with LHS. This could potentially explain a minor neglect or somatosensory deficit in participants with RHS. It is possible that with the screening procedure for neglect some participants with stroke with minor or declining neglect might have also been included in the study. Furthermore, cortical LHS may lead more often to aphasia [92], which could also explain the smaller ratio of participants with LHS with a cortical stroke, as aphasia is an exclusion criterion. When inspecting the stroke type and location, it can be noticed that participants who suffered from ischemia or infarction of the MCA (middle cerebral artery) or in the MCA-territory tend to have among the highest DLs for the impaired hand. All participants with RHS among these fall beyond the 95th percentile of healthy performance. This could be explained by the fact that the majority of the somatosensory cortex is supplied by the MCA [93]. Participants with only partial infarctions of the MCA or in the MCA-territory did not present such high DLs.

While there are several studies with NIC subjects [43, 48, 64, 66, 67] suggesting a left arm/right hemisphere advantage for the processing of proprioceptive inputs in right handed subjects and vice versa for left handed subjects [48, 67], no statistical significant dominance in proprioceptive performance could be shown for the non-dominant hand in NIC subjects of the present study. However, as the values for the mean as well as the median DL were lower for the non-dominant limb, the results tend to support this evidence. This proprioceptive dominance of the non-dominant limb may be attributed to an imbalance of body side representations in the different hemispheres, which, in case of a stroke, could lead to an asymmetric incidence of proprioceptive deficits [94] and more severe proprioceptive deficits when the non-dominant limb is affected. For this reason, when comparing between the performance of the impaired limbs of participants with LHS and RHS in this study, the trend for better proprioception of the non-dominant limb was accounted for by removing the baseline (i.e., the median for the corresponding hand of the NIC). Indeed, our study revealed a significant difference between the impaired limbs of participants with LHS and RHS (all right handed with two exceptions being ambidextrous), the latter showing more severe proprioceptive deficits in accordance to our hypothesis. These findings are in line with other studies showing similar tendencies in different proprioceptive outcome measures in stroke patients [14, 47, 63], and thus may endorse the validity of this assessment.

Our study also showed that the unimpaired hand can be affected after stroke: The group analysis revealed a significant difference for the unimpaired (left) hand of participants with LHS, and three of the participants with RHS had DLs larger than the 95th percentiles of the corresponding hand in NIC subjects. The first could be explained by the fact that LHS subjects had similar medians for both hands, but the NIC subjects showed a trend towards better proprioception in the left hand. In contrast to the impaired hand, no significant difference was found between participants with LHS and RHS for the unimpaired hand. However, there were more participants with RHS with DLs above the 95th percentile compared to participants with LHS. This is in line with the aforementioned hemispheric dominance for proprioception and with existing evidence revealing deficits in the "unimpaired" ipsilesional limb after unilateral cortical lesions [95–97]. Thus, it would be more correct to refer to this limb as "less affected" instead of "unimpaired". As a consequence, proprioceptive performance of the impaired hand and its recovery progress throughout therapy should be compared to the NIC population instead of to the ipsilesional limb of the participant with stroke.

Concurrent validity

From all correlations with clinical scales, the best correlation was found between the proprioceptive DL provided by the robotic assessment and the clinical outcome measure of the proprioceptive up-down test. However, since a ceiling effect occurred on the up-down test for all but one participants with stroke (9/10 participants with stroke scored the maximum points), the correlation for this clinical scale should not be over-interpreted. Correlations with all other clinical assessments (not directly targeting proprioception) were also weak to fair. Thus, no concurrent validity could be established by correlating the robotic outcome measure with the clinical scales. This clearly demonstrates the limitations of clinical assessments, unable to sensitively quantify and differentiate proprioceptive deficits, and points out the need for finer-graded proprioceptive assessments as gold standards [30]—a need also identified by therapists [29]. As a consequence of these results, it is not surprising that when comparing the clinical scores between participants with RHS and LHS, no statistically significant differences could be found.

Similar as for the construct validity, the concurrent validity analysis would benefit from the inclusion of sub-acute participants with stroke with more severe proprioceptive deficits. In a future study, different sensitive outcome measures of robotic proprioception assessments using different paradigms but assessing the same proprioceptive aspects could be correlated to circumvent the common problem of coarse clinical scales and further investigate concurrent validity.

Clinical feasibility and confounds: duration, number of trials, inattention, and memory

The similarity of unconstrained trial duration (i.e., without time limit) between participants with stroke and NIC subjects proves the feasibility of the assessment concept and response interface in participants with stroke (independently of whether the contralesional or ipsilesional hand was tested). The convergence of PEST (around trial 65 in NIC subjects) shows that a maximum number of 60 trials and other termination criteria for PEST are adequately chosen for a clinical application in patients. Since the DL estimate is based on the fit of the psychometric function using data from the full sequence, it is not imperative to obtain convergence of the PEST algorithm to compute the outcome measure. Around 60 PEST trials requiring in total less than 15 min is a good compromise between precision and accuracy of the outcome measures and clinical feasibility, as assessments should be quick to administer [29, 98].

While there exist some position matching assessments which are reported to be more rapid (e.g., [14, 50]), the duration of the assessment should be put into relation with the information content of the outcome measures and the reliability of the assessment. Nevertheless, the present assessment is relatively quick to administer, comparable to recently developed perturbation detection assessments taking 10–15 min [55, 56] and much faster than other assessments using a 2AFC paradigm requiring around 45 min [59].

The results with NIC subjects in Table 3 show that periods of inattention to the task are more frequent in a longer assessment, resulting in the potential collection of biased data and unreliable estimates of proprioception. However, despite the reduction of the assessment time, NIC subjects and participants with stroke still showed periods of inattention. Moreover, the prevalence of inattention was higher in participants with stroke, which is in line with the literature [76, 77]. The inattention confound could be addressed successfully by using the inattention detection algorithm [78]. This is also reflected in the reliability: When not using the algorithm to reduce the introduced bias from inattention to the task, the reliability decreases ($ICC(2,1)$ [CI]: $r = 0.63$ [0.28, 0.84], for the impaired hand). Furthermore, differences between NIC subjects and participants with stroke (partially due to the inattention confound) would increase and could lead to misleading interpretation. Thus, the results presented here (i.e., when using the inattention detection algorithm) are more conservative and should more accurately represent differences in proprioception.

The lack of correlation between the robotic outcome measures and the working memory test, as well as the Bland-Altman analysis and a previously conducted mixed-effects-model on 30 elderly NIC subjects [99] demonstrate the robustness of the assessment against memory, learning, and fatigue confounds, as there were no systematic biases originating from multiple measurements, number of trials, or order of hands assessed.

Robot-assisted assessment paradigm

Using the 2AFC paradigm with passively presented proprioceptive stimuli makes the proposed method a purely proprioceptive assessment independent of motor function, in contrast to most ipsi- or contralateral matching assessments. Furthermore, it relies neither on interhemispheric transfer for the comparison of stimuli nor on the sensorimotor function of the ipsilesional "unimpaired" limb, which is an advantage, as the central integration of proprioceptive information across the limbs and the ipsilesional limb may also be affected by a cerebral lesion [96, 100], as also found in the present study. This paradigm for the assessment of single-joint proprioception also allows the use of more cost-effective and simpler robotic devices with only one actuated degree-of-freedom, in contrast to sophisticated robotic multi-limb devices or actuated planar end-effector platforms (e.g., [101, 102]) used for other types of proprioceptive assessments [14, 54]. Furthermore, there exists some evidence that after stroke there is a high agreement of somatosensory deficits in neighboring body parts [103], which could render the assessment of multiple joints redundant in many cases.

Compared to other psychophysical paradigms (e.g., Yes-No or Same-Different), 2AFC is more robust against decision criteria (i.e., response bias) [61, 72], is suggested to help directing the subject's attention to the task [95], and allows measurements of sensitivity to smaller thresholds [61]. In addition, PEST can adapt and converge over a wide range of angle differences without prior knowledge about the subject's DL, while converging rapidly towards the DL. This leads to shorter assessments with data points covering the regions of interest of the psychometric function.

Presenting passive movements with different amplitudes but same trajectory duration leads to varying peak velocity. Therefore, the subject may partly not only rely on the perception of angular joint position but also movement velocity. This is preferable to a time confound, as primary endings of muscle spindles respond both to the length change and rate of length change of the muscle [104]. As a consequence, the proposed robotic assessment remains a purely proprioceptive test and assesses both subparts of proprioception: limb position sense (sense of stationary position) and kinaesthesia (sense of limb movement) [23]. Other solutions such as using movement velocities below detection threshold [37] would not be feasible in

a clinical setting as they would result in an increased assessment duration.

Limitations of the study

One limitation of the present study is the lack of a sensitive clinical scale as a reference for proprioceptive function. Therefore, some participants with stroke did not present detectable proprioceptive deficits according to the up-down test (as suggested by the high ceiling rate). On the other hand, participants with stroke with the inability to detect any large passive movement were excluded, as they would not be able to perform the robotic assessment. Both of these factors limit the severity range of deficits. As a consequence, the stroke group was more similar to the control group. These points negatively affected the concurrent validity analysis and hypothesis testing (e.g., when comparing participants with stroke to NIC subjects).

Age-matching is important, as proprioception declines with age [33, 35, 37, 40, 42, 48, 52, 53, 99, 105, 106]. By individually age-matching subjects instead of age-matching on a group level, the statistical power could be increased by using paired tests comparing participants with stroke and NIC subjects. On the other hand, age-matching on a group level allows increasing the sample size of the NIC group when creating normative models. The width of the CIs of the 95th percentiles of healthy performance show, however, that a future study would benefit from a larger sample size for better estimates of cutoff values. Thus, the number of participants with stroke suffering from deficits based on the present cutoff value are only indicative and should be interpreted with care.

The reliability analysis would also benefit from a larger sample size [107]. Nevertheless, this exploratory study already demonstrated good reliability when testing the impaired (contralesional) hand of participants with stroke. Based on this promising finding, a new cross-sectional study with a larger sample size can be conducted, including also left handed subjects.

Conclusion

The evaluation of psychometric and clinimetric properties in this exploratory study including participants with stroke and a group of neurologically intact subjects demonstrated good reliability, validity, and high feasibility of the proposed robot-assisted adaptive assessment of finger proprioception. While existing clinical scales that do not require any tools may be appropriate for some fast preliminary screening of neurological patients, this robotic assessment has the potential to sensitively and accurately quantify proprioceptive deficits. Together with its good usability and short administration time, which facilitate its integration into clinical routine, it becomes a powerful tool for more standardized assessments, for understanding the role of proprioceptive deficits in the functional recovery process, as well as for improving diagnostics, prognostics, monitoring, and planning of sensorimotor rehabilitation programs in patients after neurological injuries.

Abbreviations
2AFC: Two-alternative forced choice; A: Ambidextrous; ACA: Anterior cerebral artery; CI: Confidence interval; D: Dropout; DL: Difference limen; E: Excluded; F: Female; ICC: Intraclass correlation coefficient; ICH: Intracerebral hemorrhage; IQR: Interquartile range; LHS: Left hemisphere stroke; M: Male; MCA: Middle cerebral artery; MCP: Metacarpophalangeal; NIC: Neurologically intact controls; PCA: Posterior cerebral artery; PEST: Parameter Estimation by Sequential Testing; R: Right handed; RHS: Right hemisphere stroke; SAH: Subarachnoid hemorrhage

Acknowledgements
The authors would like to thank J.-C. Metzger, W. L. Popp, and K. Leuenberger for inspiring and profitable discussions.

Funding
This research was supported by the ETH Zurich Foundation in collaboration with Hocoma AG, the Janggen–Pöhn Foundation, the Schmieder Foundation for Science and Research, and the Swiss National Science Foundation through project 320030L_170163.

Authors' contributions
MR, OL, JL, and RG designed the study, VR, IB and AS participated in subject recruitment and data collection, MR performed the analysis, interpreted the results, and drafted the manuscript. All authors revised the manuscript and approved the final version.

Competing interests
The authors declare that they have no competing interests.

Author details
[1]Rehabilitation Engineering Laboratory, Department of Health Sciences and Technology, ETH Zurich, Zurich, Switzerland . [2]Department of Neurorehabilitation, Kliniken Schmieder, Allensbach, Germany . [3]Lurija Institut, Konstanz, Germany .

References
1. Hasan Z. Role of proprioceptors in neural control. Curr Opin Neurobiol. 1992;2(6):824–9.
2. Sober SJ, Sabes PN. Multisensory integration during motor planning. J Neurosci. 2003;23(18):6982–92.
3. Butler AJ, Fink GR, Dohle C, Wunderlich G, Tellmann L, Seitz RJ, Zilles K, Freund H-J. Neural mechanisms underlying reaching for remembered targets cued kinesthetically or visually in left or right hemispace. Hum Brain Mapp. 2004;21(3):165–77. https://doi.org/10.1002/hbm.20001.
4. Konczak J, Corcos DM, Horak F, Poizner H, Shapiro M, Tuite P, Volkmann J, Maschke M. Proprioception and motor control in Parkinson's disease. J Mot Behav. 2009;41(6):543–52. https://doi.org/10.3200/35-09-002.
5. Jeannerod M, Michel F, Prablanc C. The control of hand movements in a case of hemianaesthesia following a parietal lesion. Brain. 1984;107 (Pt 3):899–920.
6. Ghez C, Gordon J, Ghilardi MF, Christakos CN, Cooper SE. Roles of proprioceptive input in the programming of arm trajectories. Cold Spring Harb Symp Quant Biol. 1990;55:837–47.
7. Gentilucci M, Toni I, Chieffi S, Pavesi G. The role of proprioception in the control of prehension movements: a kinematic study in a peripherally deafferented patient and in normal subjects. Exp Brain Res. 1994;99(3):483–500.
8. Carey LM. Somatosensory Loss after Stroke. Critical Reviews™ in Physical and Rehabilitation Medicine. 1995;7(1):51–91.
9. Sarlegna FR, Sainburg RL. The roles of vision and proprioception in the planning of reaching movements. Adv Exp Med Biol. 2009;629:317–35.
10. Reding MJ, Potes E. Rehabilitation outcome following initial unilateral hemispheric stroke. Life table analysis approach. Stroke. 1988;19:1354–8.
11. Shah SK. Deficits affecting the function of the paralysed arm following hemiplegia. Aust Occup Ther J. 1978;25(2):12–19. https://doi.org/10.1111/j.1440-1630.1978.tb00656.x.
12. Sullivan JE, Hedman LD. Sensory dysfunction following stroke: Incidence, significance, examination, and intervention. Top Stroke Rehabil. 2008;15(3):200–17.
13. Schabrun SM, Hillier S. Evidence for the retraining of sensation after stroke: a systematic review. Clin Rehabil. 2009;23(1):27–39. https://doi.org/10.1177/0269215508098897.
14. Dukelow SP, Herter TM, Moore KD, Demers MJ, Glasgow JI, Bagg SD, Norman KE, Scott SH. Quantitative assessment of limb position sense following stroke. Neurorehabil Neural Repair. 2010;24(2):178–87. https://doi.org/10.1177/1545968309345267.
15. Kessner SS, Bingel U, Thomalla G. Somatosensory deficits after stroke: a scoping review. Top Stroke Rehabil. 2016;23(2):136–146. https://doi.org/10.1080/10749357.2015.1116822.
16. Kusoffsky A, Wadell I, Nilsson BY. The relationship between sensory impairment and motor recovery in patients with hemiplegia. Scand J Rehab Med. 1982;14:27–32.
17. Feys H, De Weerdt W, Nuyens G, van de Winckel A, Selz B, Kiekens C. Predicting motor recovery of the upper limb after stroke rehabilitation: value of a clinical examination. Physiother Res Int. 2000;5(1):1–18.
18. Han L, Law-Gibson D, Reding M. Key neurological impairments influence function-related group outcomes after stroke. Stroke. 2002;33(7):1920–4.
19. Abela E, Missimer J, Wiest R, Federspiel A, Hess C, Sturzenegger M, Weder B. Lesions to primary sensory and posterior parietal cortices impair recovery from hand paresis after stroke. PloS ONE. 2012;7(2):31275.
20. Smith DL, Akhtar AJ, Garraway WM. Proprioception and spatial neglect after stroke. Age Ageing. 1983;12(1):63–69.
21. Prescott RJ, Garraway WM, Akhtar AJ. Predicting functional outcome following acute stroke using a standard clinical examination. Stroke. 1982;13(5):641–7.
22. Lincoln NB, Crow JL, Jackson JM, Waters GR, Adams SA, Hodgson P. The unreliability of sensory assessments. Clin Rehabil. 1991;5(4):273–82. https://doi.org/10.1177/026921559100500403.
23. Gilman S. Joint position sense and vibration sense: anatomical organisation and assessment. J Neurol Neurosurg Psychiatry. 2002;73(5):473–7.
24. Beckmann YY, Çiftçi Y, Ertekin C. The detection of sensitivity of proprioception by a new clinical test: the dual joint position test. Clin Neurol Neurosurg. 2013;115(7):1023–7. https://doi.org/10.1016/j.clineuro.2012.10.017.
25. Hirayama K, Fukutake T, Kawamura M. 'Thumb localizing test' for detecting a lesion in the posterior column-medial lemniscal system. J Neurol Sci. 1999;167(1):45–49.
26. Lincoln N, Jackson J, Adams S. Reliability and revision of the Nottingham Sensory Assessment for stroke patients. Physiotherapy. 1998;84(8):358–65.
27. Winward CE, Halligan PW, Wade DT. Current practice and clinical relevance of somatosensory assessment after stroke. Clin Rehabil. 1999;13(1):48–55.
28. Hillier S, Immink M, Thewlis D. Assessing Proprioception: A Systematic Review of Possibilities. Neurorehabil Neural Repair. 2015;29(10):933–49. https://doi.org/10.1177/1545968315573055.

29. Pumpa LU, Cahill LS, Carey LM. Somatosensory assessment and treatment after stroke: An evidence-practice gap. Aust Occup Ther J. 2015;62(2):93–104. https://doi.org/10.1111/1440-1630.12170.

30. Suetterlin KJ, Sayer AA. Proprioception: where are we now? A commentary on clinical assessment, changes across the life course, functional implications and future interventions. Age Ageing. 2014;43(3): 313–8. http://doi.org/10.1093/ageing/aft174.

31. Carey LM, Oke LE, Matyas TA. Impaired limb position sense after stroke: a quantitative test for clinical use. Arch Phys Med Rehabil. 1996;77(12): 1271–8.

32. Wycherley AS, Helliwell PS, Bird HA. A novel device for the measurement of proprioception in the hand. Rheumatol (Oxford). 2005;44(5):638–41. http://doi.org/10.1093/rheumatology/keh568.

33. Schmidt L, Depper L, Kerkhoff G. Effects of age, sex and arm on the precision of arm position sense—left-arm superiority in healthy right-handers. Front Hum Neurosci. 2013;7:915. https://doi.org/10.3389/fnhum.2013.00915.

34. Hoseini N, Sexton BM, Kurtz K, Liu Y, Block HJ. Adaptive Staircase Measurement of Hand Proprioception. PLoS ONE. 2015;10(8):0135757. https://doi.org/10.1371/journal.pone.0135757.

35. Kalisch T, Kattenstroth J-C, Kowalewski R, Tegenthoff M, Dinse HR. Age-related changes in the joint position sense of the human hand. Clin Interv Aging. 2012;7:499–507. https://doi.org/10.2147/CIA.S37573.

36. Scott SH, Dukelow SP. Potential of robots as next-generation technology for clinical assessment of neurological disorders and upper-limb therapy. J Rehabil Res Dev. 2011;48(4):335–53.

37. Ferrell WR, Crighton A, Sturrock R. D. Age-dependent changes in position sense in human proximal interphalangeal joints. Neuroreport. 1992;3(3):259–61.

38. Lönn J, Crenshaw AG, Djupsjöbacka M, Johansson H. Reliability of position sense testing assessed with a fully automated system. Clin Physiol. 2000;20(1):30–37.

39. Lönn J, Crenshaw AG, Djupsjöbacka M, Pedersen J, Johansson H. Position sense testing: influence of starting position and type of displacement. Arch Phys Med Rehabil. 2000;81(5):592–7.

40. Adamo DE, Martin BJ, Brown SH. Age-related differences in upper limb proprioceptive acuity. Percept Mot Skills. 2007;104(3 Pt 2):1297–309. https://doi.org/10.2466/pms.104.4.1297-1309.

41. Juul-Kristensen B, Lund H, Hansen K, Christensen H, Danneskiold-Samsøe B, Bliddal H. Test-retest reliability of joint position and kinesthetic sense in the elbow of healthy subjects. Physiother Theory Pract. 2008;24(1):65–72. https://doi.org/10.1080/09593980701378173.

42. Adamo DE, Alexander NB, Brown SH. The influence of age and physical activity on upper limb proprioceptive ability. J Aging Phys Act. 2009;17(3):272–93.

43. Adamo DE, Martin BJ. Position sense asymmetry. Exp Brain Res. 2009;192(1):87–95. https://doi.org/10.1007/s00221-008-1560-0.

44. Dukelow SP, Herter TM, Bagg SD, Scott SH. The independence of deficits in position sense and visually guided reaching following stroke. J Neuroeng Rehabil. 2012;9:72. https://doi.org/10.1186/1743-0003-9-72.

45. Gay A, Harbst K, Kaufman KR, Hansen DK, Laskowski ER, Berger RA. New method of measuring wrist joint position sense avoiding cutaneous and visual inputs. J Neuroeng Rehabil. 2010;7:5. https://doi.org/10.1186/1743-0003-7-5.

46. Squeri V, Zenzeri J, Morasso P, Basteris A. Integrating proprioceptive assessment with proprioceptive training of stroke patients. In: Rehabilitation Robotics (ICORR), 2011 IEEE International Conference On. Zurich; 2011. p. 1–6. https://doi.org/10.1109/ICORR.2011.5975500.

47. Semrau JA, Herter TM, Scott SH, Dukelow SP. Robotic identification of kinesthetic deficits after stroke. Stroke. 2013;44(12):3414–21. https://doi.org/10.1161/STROKEAHA.113.002058.

48. Herter TM, Scott SH, Dukelow SP. Systematic changes in position sense accompany normal aging across adulthood. J Neuroeng Rehabil. 2014;11(1):43. https://doi.org/10.1186/1743-0003-11-43.

49. Nomura Y, Ito T. Posture-Angle Perception and Reproduction Characteristics with Wrist Flexion/Extension Motions. In: International Conference on Advances in Computer-Human Interactions (ACHI), 2014. Barcelona, Spain; 2014. p. 154–159.

50. Rinderknecht MD, Popp WL, Lambercy O, Gassert R. Reliable and Rapid Robotic Assessment of Wrist Proprioception Using a Gauge Position Matching Paradigm. Front Hum Neurosci. 2016;10(316):. https://doi.org/10.3389/fnhum.2016.00316.

51. Kokmen E, Bossemeyer Jr R, Williams WJ. Quantitative evaluation of joint motion sensation in an aging population. J Gerontol. 1978;33(1):62–67.

52. Wright ML, Adamo DE, Brown SH. Age-related declines in the detection of passive wrist movement. Neurosci Lett. 2011;500(2):108–12. https://doi.org/10.1016/j.neulet.2011.06.015.

53. Ingemanson ML, Rowe JB, Chan V, Wolbrecht ET, Cramer SC, Reinkensmeyer DJ. Use of a robotic device to measure age-related decline in finger proprioception. Exp Brain Res. 2015;234(1):83–93. https://doi.org/10.1007/s00221-015-4440-4.

54. Simo L, Botzer L, Ghez C, Scheidt RA. A robotic test of proprioception within the hemiparetic arm post-stroke. J Neuroeng Rehabil. 2014;11:77. https://doi.org/10.1186/1743-0003-11-77.

55. Bourke TC, Coderre AM, Bagg SD, Dukelow SP, Norman KE, Scott SH. Impaired corrective responses to postural perturbations of the arm in Individuals with subacute stroke. J Neuroeng Rehabil. 2015;12:7. https://doi.org/10.1186/1743-0003-12-7.

56. Mrotek LA, Bengtson M, Stoeckmann T, Botzer L, Ghez CP, McGuire J, Scheidt RA. The Arm Movement Detection (AMD) test: a fast robotic test of proprioceptive acuity in the arm. J NeuroEngineering Rehabil. 2017;14(1):64. https://doi.org/10.1186/s12984-017-0269-3.

57. Lambercy O, Juárez Robles A, Kim Y, Gassert R. Design of a robotic device for assessment and rehabilitation of hand sensory function. In: Rehabilitation Robotics (ICORR), 2011 IEEE International Conference on. Zurich; 2011. p. 1–6. https://doi.org/10.1109/ICORR.2011.5975436. http://dx.doi.org/10.1109/ICORR.2011.5975436.

58. Rinderknecht MD, Popp WL, Lambercy O, Gassert R. Experimental Validation of a Rapid, Adaptive Robotic Assessment of the MCP Joint Angle Difference Threshold. In: Auvray M, Duriez C, editors. Haptics: Neuroscience, Devices, Modeling, and Applications. Lecture Notes in Computer Science. Berlin: Springer; 2014. p. 3–10.

59. Cappello L, Elangovan N, Contu S, Khosravani S, Konczak J, Masia L. Robot-aided assessment of wrist proprioception. Front Hum Neurosci. 2015;9:198. https://doi.org/10.3389/fnhum.2015.00198.

60. Semrau JA, Herter TM, Scott SH, Dukelow SP. Inter-rater reliability of kinesthetic measurements with the KINARM robotic exoskeleton. J NeuroEngineering Rehabil. 2017;14(1):42. https://doi.org/10.1186/s12984-017-0260-z.

61. Macmillan NA, Douglas Creelman C. Detection Theory: A User's Guide. New Jersey: Lawrence Erlbaum Associates; 2005.

62. Taylor MM, Douglas Creelman C. PEST: Efficient estimates on probability functions. The Journal of the Acoustical Society of America. 1967;41:782.

63. Sterzi R, Bottini G, Celani MG, Righetti E, Lamassa M, Ricci S, Vallar G. Hemianopia, hemianaesthesia, and hemiplegia after right and left hemisphere damage. A hemispheric difference. J Neurol, Neurosurg Psychiatry. 1993;56(3):308–10. https://doi.org/10.1136/jnnp.56.3.308. http://jnnp.bmj.com/content/56/3/308.full.pdf.

64. Goble DJ, Lewis CA, Brown SH. Upper limb asymmetries in the utilization of proprioceptive feedback. Exp Brain Res. 2006;168(1-2): 307–11. https://doi.org/10.1007/s00221-005-0280-y.

65. Goble DJ, Brown SH. The biological and behavioral basis of upper limb asymmetries in sensorimotor performance. Neurosci Biobehav Rev. 2008;32(3):598–610. https://doi.org/10.1016/j.neubiorev.2007.10.006.

66. Goble DJ, Brown SH. Upper limb asymmetries in the matching of proprioceptive versus visual targets. J Neurophysiol. 2008;99(6):3063–74. https://doi.org/10.1152/jn.90259.2008.

67. Goble DJ, Noble BC, Brown SH. Proprioceptive target matching asymmetries in left-handed individuals. Exp Brain Res. 2009;197(4): 403–8. https://doi.org/10.1007/s00221-009-1922-2.

68. Bohannon RW, Smith MB. Interrater reliability of a modified Ashworth scale of muscle spasticity. Phys Ther. 1987;67(2):206–7.

69. Nasreddine ZS, Phillips NA, Bédirian V, Charbonneau S, Whitehead V, Collin I, Cummings JL, Chertkow H. The Montreal Cognitive Assessment, MoCA: A Brief Screening Tool For Mild Cognitive Impairment. J Am Geriatr Soc. 2005;53(4):695–9. https://doi.org/10.1111/j.1532-5415.2005.53221.x.

70. Gauthier L, Dehaut F, Joanette Y. The Bells Test: A quantitative and qualitative test for visual neglect. International Journal of Clinical Neuropsychology. 1989;11(2):49–54.

71. Oldfield RC. The assessment and analysis of handedness: the Edinburgh inventory. Neuropsychologia. 1971;9(1):97–113.

72. Gescheider G. Psychophysics: method, theory, and applications. New Jersey: Lawrence Erlbaum Associates; 1985.

73. Hogan N. Adaptive control of mechanical impedance by coactivation of antagonist muscles. Autom Control, IEEE Trans. 1984;29(8):681–90. https://doi.org/10.1109/TAC.1984.1103644.

74. Wald A. Sequential Analysis. New York: Wiley; 1947, pp. 88–105196199.

75. Hall JL. Hybrid adaptive procedure for estimation of psychometric functions. J Acoust Soc Am. 1981;69:1763.

76. Tuhrim S. Medical therapy of ischemic stroke. In: Gordon WA, editor. Advances in Stroke Rehabilitation. London: Andover Medical Publishers; 1993. p. 3–15. Chap. Medical therapy of ischemic stroke.

77. Rinne P, Hassan M, Goniotakis D, Chohan K, Sharma P, Langdon D, Soto D, Bentley P. Triple dissociation of attention networks in stroke according to lesion location. Neurology. 2013;81(9):812–20. https://doi.org/10.1212/WNL.0b013e3182a2ca34.

78. Rinderknecht MD, Ranzani R, Popp WL, Lambercy O, Gassert R. Algorithm for improving psychophysical threshold estimates by detecting sustained inattention in experiments using PEST. Attention Perception Psychophysics. 2018;1943-393X:1–17. https://doi.org/10.3758/s13414-018-1521-z.

79. Prins N, Kingdom FAA. Palamedes: Matlab routines for analyzing psychophysical data. 2009. http://www.palamedestoolbox.org. Accessed 7 Jan 2013.

80. Wichmann FA, Hill NJ. The psychometric function: I, Fitting, sampling, and goodness of fit. Percept Psychophys. 2001;63(8):1293–313.

81. Rolke R, Magerl W, Campbell KA, Schalber C, Caspari S, Birklein F, Treede R-D. Quantitative sensory testing: a comprehensive protocol for clinical trials. Eur J Pain. 2006;10(1):77–77. https://doi.org/10.1016/j.ejpain.2005.02.003.

82. Rydel A, Seiffer W. Untersuchungen über das Vibrationsgefühl oder die sog. "Knochensensibilität" (Pallästhesie). Eur Arch Psychiatry Clin Neurosci. 1903;37(2):488–536.

83. Wechsler D. WAIS-III: Administration and Scoring Manual: Wechsler Adult Intelligence scale. San Antonio: Psychological Corporation; 1997.

84. Shrout PE, Fleiss JL. Intraclass correlations: uses in assessing rater reliability. Psychol Bull. 1979;86(2):420–8.

85. Lexell JE, Downham DY. How to assess the reliability of measurements in rehabilitation. Am J Phys Med Rehabil. 2005;84(9):719–23.

86. de Vet HCW, Terwee CB, Knol DL, Bouter LM. When to use agreement versus reliability measures. J Clin Epidemiol. 2006;59(10):1033–9. https://doi.org/10.1016/j.jclinepi.2005.10.015.

87. Fleiss JL. Reliability of Measurement. The Design and Analysis of Clinical Experiments. Hoboken: Wiley; 1999, pp. 1–32. https://doi.org/10.1002/9781118032923.ch1. http://dx.doi.org/10.1002/9781118032923.ch1.

88. Streiner DL, Norman GR. Health Measurement Scales: a Practical Guide to Their Development and Use. USA: Oxford university press; 2008.

89. Brewer BR, Klatzky R, Matsuoka Y. Visual feedback distortion in a robotic environment for hand rehabilitation. Brain Res Bull. 2008;75(6):804–13.

90. Kattenstroth J-C, Kalisch T, Kowalewski R, Tegenthoff M, Dinse HR. Quantitative assessment of joint position sense recovery in subacute stroke patients: a pilot study. J Rehabil Med. 2013;45(10):1004–9. https://doi.org/10.2340/16501977-1225.

91. Semrau JA, Herter TM, Scott SH, Dukelow SP. Examining Differences in Patterns of Sensory and Motor Recovery After Stroke With Robotics. Stroke. 2015;46(12):3459–69. https://doi.org/10.1161/STROKEAHA.115.010750.

92. Pedersen PM, Stig Jørgensen H, Nakayama H, Raaschou HO, Olsen TS. Aphasia in acute stroke: incidence, determinants, and recovery. Ann Neurol. 1995;38(4):659–66.

93. Gray H, Standring S, Anand N, Birch R, Collins P, Crossman A, Gleeson M, Jawaheer G, Smith AL, Spratt JD, et al. Gray's Anatomy: the Anatomical Basis of Clinical Practice. Amsterdam: Elsevier; 2016.

94. Vallar G, Antonucci G, Guariglia C, Pizzamiglio L. Deficits of position sense, unilateral neglect and optokinetic stimulation. Neuropsychologia. 1993;31(11):1191–200.

95. Dannenbaum RM, Jones LA. The assessment and treatment of patients who have sensory loss following cortical lesions. J Hand Ther. 1993;6(2):130–8.

96. Carey LM, Matyas TA. Frequency of discriminative sensory loss in the hand after stroke in a rehabilitation setting. J Rehabil Med. 2011;43(3):257–63. https://doi.org/10.2340/16501977-0662.

97. Jones RD, Donaldson IM, Parkin PJ. Impairment and recovery of ipsilateral sensory-motor function following unilateral cerebral infarction. Brain. 1989;112(1):113–32.

98. Gresham G, Duncan P, Stason W, Adams H, Adelman A, Alexander D, Bishop D, Diller L, Donaldson N, Granger C, Holland A, Kelly-Hayes M, McDowell F, Myers L, Phipps M, Roth E, Siebens H, Tarvin G, Trombly C. Post-stroke rehabilitation: Assessment, referral, and patient management. Quick Reference Guide for Clinicians, Number 16. J Pharmacoepidemiol. 1996;5(2):35–63.

99. Rinderknecht MD, Lambercy O, Raible V, Liepert J, Gassert R. Age-based model for metacarpophalangeal joint proprioception in elderly. Clin Interv Aging. 2017;12:635–43. https://doi.org/10.2147/CIA.S129601.

100. Schaefer SY, Haaland KY, Sainburg RL. Ipsilesional motor deficits following stroke reflect hemispheric specializations for movement control. Brain. 2007;130(Pt 8):2146–58. http://doi.org/10.1093/brain/awm145.

101. Scott SH. Apparatus for measuring and perturbing shoulder and elbow joint positions and torques during reaching. Journal of Neuroscience Methods. 1999;89(2):119–27. http://doi.org/10.1016/s0165-0270(99)00053-9.

102. Scheidt RA, Lillis KP, Emerson SJ. Visual, motor and attentional influences on proprioceptive contributions to perception of hand path rectilinearity during reaching. Exp Brain Res. 2010;204(2):239–54. https://doi.org/10.1007/s00221-010-2308-1.

103. Connell LA, Lincoln NB, Radford KA. Somatosensory impairment after stroke: frequency of different deficits and their recovery. Clin Rehabil. 2008;22(8):758–67. https://doi.org/10.1177/0269215508090674.

104. Proske U, Gandevia SC. The proprioceptive senses: their roles in signaling body shape, body position and movement, and muscle force. Physiol Rev. 2012;92(4):1651–97. https://doi.org/10.1152/physrev.00048.2011.

105. Stelmach G, Sirica A. Aging and proprioception. AGE. 1986;9(4):99–103. https://doi.org/10.1007/BF02432281.

106. Fry-Welch D, Campbell J, Foltz B, Macek R. Age-Related Changes in Upper Extremity Kinesthesis. Physical & Occupational Therapy in Geriatrics. 2003;20(3-4):137–54.

107. Hopkins WG. Measures of reliability in sports medicine and science. Sports Med. 2000;30(1):1–15.

18

Reliability, validity and discriminant ability of the instrumental indices provided by a novel planar robotic device for upper limb rehabilitation

Marco Germanotta[1]*[iD], Arianna Cruciani[1], Cristiano Pecchioli[1], Simona Loreti[1,2], Albino Spedicato[1], Matteo Meotti[1], Rita Mosca[1], Gabriele Speranza[1], Francesca Cecchi[3], Giorgia Giannarelli[1], Luca Padua[1,4] and Irene Aprile[1]

Abstract

Background: In the last few years, there has been an increasing interest in the use of robotic devices to objectively quantify motor performance of patients after brain damage. Although these robot-derived measures can potentially add meaningful information about the patient's dexterity, as well as be used as outcome measurements after the rehabilitation treatment, they need to be validated before being used in clinical practice. The present work aims to evaluate the reliability, the validity and the discriminant ability of the metrics provided by a novel robotic device for upper limb rehabilitation.

Methods: Forty-eight patients with sub-acute stroke and 40 age-matched healthy subjects were involved in this study. Clinical evaluation included: Fugl-Meyer Assessment for the upper limb, Action Research Arm Test, and Barthel Index. Robotic evaluation of the upper limb performance consisted of 14 measures of motor ability quantifying the dexterity in performing planar reaching movements. Patients were evaluated twice, one day apart, to assess the reliability of the robotic metrics, using the Intraclass Correlation Coefficient. Validity was assessed by analyzing the correlation of the robotic metrics with the clinical scales, by means of the Spearman's Correlation Coefficient. Finally, the ability of the robotic metrics to distinguish between patients with stroke and healthy subjects was investigated with t-tests and the Effect Size.

Results: Reliability was found to be excellent for 12 measures and from moderate to good for the remaining 2. Most of the robotic indices were strongly correlated with the clinical scales, while a few showed a moderate correlation and only one was not correlated with the Barthel Index and weakly correlated with the remain two. Finally, all but one the provided metrics were able to discriminate between the two groups, with large effect sizes for most of them.

Conclusion: We found that all the robotic indices except one provided by a novel robotic device for upper limb rehabilitation are reliable, sensitive and strongly correlated both with motor and disability clinical scales. Therefore, this device is suitable as evaluation tool for the upper limb motor performance of patients with sub-acute stroke in clinical practice.

Keywords: Stroke, Upper limb, Robot-mediated evaluation, Reliability, Validity, Discriminant ability

* Correspondence: mgermanotta@dongnocchi.it
[1]IRCCS Fondazione Don Carlo Gnocchi, Piazzale Morandi 6, 20121 Milan, Italy
Full list of author information is available at the end of the article

Background

In the last years, Robot – Mediated Therapy has represented one of the most promising approach to restore motor function of upper limb after brain damage [1] mainly because it enables, in comparison with conventional treatment approaches, highly intensive trainings in specifically designed tasks, for extended periods of time [2]. Along with their use as rehabilitation tools, the robotic devices can also act as evaluation tools in order to objectively quantify motor performance of patients after brain damage. In fact, because of their built-in technology in terms of sensors and actuators, the robotic devices are able to acquire data about kinematics and kinetics of patients' upper limb which are processed to obtain quantitative indices related to the upper-extremity movement quality. According to Sivan et al. [3], these robotic indices are appropriate as a tool to describe bodily functions on all phases of stroke recovery and, therefore, can be effectively used to assess both the level of impairment as well as the improvement after therapy. Robotic indices are therefore increasingly used to assess patients' dexterity (where loss of dexterity refers to an inability to coordinate muscle activity in the performance of a motor task [4]) with the aim of overcoming, at least partially, the intrinsic limitations of the clinical scale, such as a low rate of reproducibility, low resolution, lack of sensitivity, as well as floor and ceiling effects [5].

Even though most of the studies involve patients with stroke [6–14], robotic evaluations are also used in neurological diseases as Multiple Sclerosis [15], Cerebral Palsy [16, 17], or Ataxia [18].

On their review, Nordin et al. [19] identified more than fifty different kinematic metrics currently used in robot-assisted rehabilitation researches. Usually, the evaluated movement is a reaching task, and more specifically center-out point-to-point movement, since it is important to perform in many activities of daily life. Less often, different tasks, such as shape drawing/tracing tasks, are also analyzed.

Although these new robot-derived measures can potentially add meaningful information about the patient's performance, their properties in terms of reliability, validity and responsiveness should be assessed, before their use in clinical practice. In fact, in order to be brought into the clinical field, they have to be stable, sensitive and clinically meaningful measures. The review of Maciejasz et al. [20] identified more than 120 robotic devices for upper limb rehabilitation and most of them allow measuring kinematic and/or kinetic parameters which describe the motor ability of patients. If one considers the amount of robots for the upper limb that are currently available, few studies have investigated the psychometric properties of the robotic indices [7, 18, 21]

and, except for a few cases, a complete analysis of their metric characteristics and concurrent validity with clinical scales is missing [19]. In addition, it is mandatory to validate the metrics provided by the specific device of interest. In fact, the robotic structure and the provided support can be different among devices, affecting the validity and sensitivity of the results [7]. As suggested by Nordin et al. [19], the mechanical structure of the robot, as well as its control scheme, play an important role in providing assessment data. As an example, data obtained from end-effector robots cannot be directly compared with those provided by exoskeletons, since the degree of interaction between patients and robot is different in terms of support and mechanical interface and this could affect the patient's performance. The results obtained with a specific device cannot be arbitrarily extended to a different one, since they likely have a different conception. Therefore, for each device it is necessary to verify the validity and sensitivity of the instrumental outcome measures.

Recently, a novel type of haptic interface was proposed, which is fully portable and employs onboard sensors and electronics to solve accurate localization and also uses motors for force feedback generation [22]. This end-effector device has been designed for application in neuro-rehabilitation protocols and it adopts specific mechanical, electrical and control solutions in order to cope with patient requirements. Along with several therapeutic scenarios, it also qualifies as an evaluation tool providing some indices about the patients' sensor-motor skills, similar to those already described in literature.

To the best of our knowledge, however, the quantitative indices provided by this device have not yet been validated in terms of their psychometric properties. Therefore, the goal of the present work is to evaluate, within a multicenter study aimed to compare a traditional and a robotic rehabilitation approach, the reliability, the concurrent validity and the discriminant ability of the indices provided by a novel rehabilitation device during an unassisted reaching task.

Methods
Participants

Forty-eight consecutive patients with subacute stroke (both inpatient and outpatients) were enrolled in 4 different rehabilitation centers of the Fondazione Don Carlo Gnocchi for this study. Inclusion criteria were: (1) first-ever stroke (cerebral infarction or hemorrhage), confirmed by either brain CT or MRI findings (2) age between 40 and 85 years; (3) time latency since stroke ranging from 2 weeks to 6 months; (4) cognitive and language abilities sufficient to understand the experiments and follow instructions. Exclusion criteria were:

(1) upper extremity Fugl-Meyer score > 58; (2) behavioral and cognitive disorders and/or reduced compliance that would interfere with active therapy; (3) fixed contraction deformity in the affected limb that would interfere with active therapy (ankylosis, Modified Ashworth Scale = 4); (4) inability to discriminate distinctly the images showed on a 22″ monitor placed at the eye level of each subject at a distance of about 50 cm, even with corrective glasses. Forty age-matched subjects without neurological or other relevant medical conditions served as a reference population. Demographic and characteristics of the participants are shown in Table 1.

This study is a cross-sectional objective analysis of baseline data collected as part of a larger clinical trial, approved by the institutional ethics committee (FDG_6.4. 2016) and registered at clinicaltrials.gov with identifier number (NCT02879279). All participants gave informed consent according to the Declaration of Helsinki.

Clinical assessment

Patients were clinically evaluated using the upper limb part Fugl-Meyer Assessment of Motor Recovery after Stroke (FMA), the Action Research Arm test (ARAT) and the Barthel Index (BI).

The FMA evaluates recovery in post-stroke hemiplegic patients and it is one of the most widely used quantitative measures of motor impairment [23]. It is characterized by a high inter-rater reliability [24, 25] and validity [26]. This measure includes five domains (motor function, sensory function, balance, joint range of motion, joint pain) to assess synergistic and voluntary movement after stroke. A three-point ordinary scale is used to assess movement (0 = unable; 1 = partial; 2 = performs fully) in each item. In this research we used the upper limb section in the motor function domain (FMA-UL).

The score ranges from 0 (most severe impairment) to 66 (no impairment).

The ARAT [27] assesses upper limb function using observational methods and consists of 19 items organized in 4 sections: Grasp, Grip, Pinch and Gross movements. The performance of each task is scored on a 4-point ordinal scale (0 = unable to complete any part of the task, 1 = the task is only partially completed, 2 = the task is completed but with great difficulty and/or in an abnormally long time, and 3 = the movement is performed normally). The maximum ARAT score is 57 points, which means normal upper limb function.

The BI [28] assesses the ability of an individual with a neuromuscular or musculoskeletal disorder to take care of him/herself, and consists of 10 items, evaluating both personal care (feeding, dressing, hygiene) and mobility activities (transferring, walking/wheeling). Possible values range from 0 to 100, with lower scores representing greater dependency.

Equipment and robotic assessment

The robotic assessment of upper limb motor performance was conducted by means of MOTORE (MObile roboT for upper limb neurOrtho Rehabilitation, Humanware, Italy), see Fig. 1. This is a planar end-effector device designed for application in neuro-rehabilitation protocols and it adopts specific mechanical, electrical and control solutions in order to meet the requirements of neuro-rehabilitation. MOTORE is equipped with an onboard computing unit, an odometry system (based on encoders) and a specifically designed global localization system (which recognizes patterns on the working surface). In fact, the device moves by means of transwheels on the planar working surface and it uses a 2DOF load cell in the handle to measure the interaction force with the patient. The device has 3 DC motors so that it can (a) help the patient when he/she is not able to

Table 1 Demographic and clinical characteristics of the sample

	Patients with stroke ($n = 48$)	Healthy subjects ($n = 40$)
Sex M/F	33/15	26/14
Age, mean ± SD (years)	64 ± 11	65 ± 13
Classification		
Cerebral ischemia (N)	28	–
Cerebral hemorrhage (N)	20	–
Time from lesion, mean ± SD (days)	88 ± 42	–
FMA-UL, mean ± SD	29 ± 18	–
ARAT, mean ± SD	15 ± 18	–
BI, mean ± SD	40 ± 24	–

SD Standard Deviation, *FMA-UL* Fugl-Meyer Assessment for the Upper Limb, *ARAT* Action Research Arm Test, *BI* Barthel Index

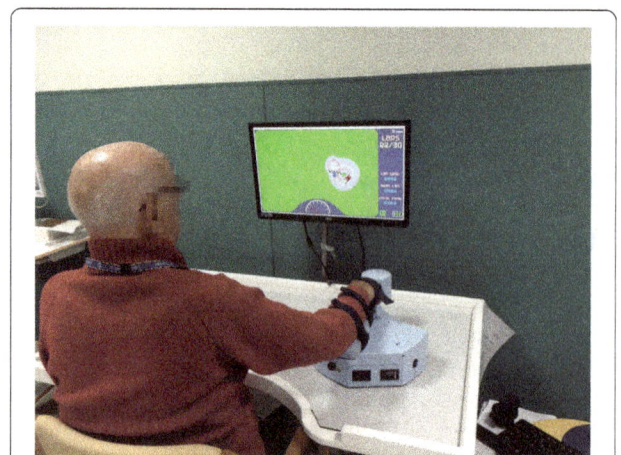

Fig. 1 Patient engaged in a rehabilitation session with MOTORE

accomplish the task, (b) prevent movements different from the ideal trajectories, (c) provide different weight and viscosity behaviors, (d) maintain a proper orientation on the plane. The device generates force feedback without any intermediate link to the ground or frame, thanks to the motion of the wheels and using the information obtained from the load cell. A Bluetooth connection links the device to a PC unit, where a software shows targets to be reached and trajectories to be followed as well as a user/therapist interface for the selection of the exercise parameters. The robot is controlled in admittance mode: forces measured by the load cell are used to determine the linear velocity of the device, on the basis of two parameters (M, that is the apparent mass of the device, and b, that is the nominal viscosity) that can be modified to change the robot behavior [29]. Compared with other similar robotic systems, it is characterized by its portability, being specifically conceived for teleoperation applications. During the rehabilitation session, ambulatory subjects are comfortably seated on a chair, while non-ambulatory patients are seated on their wheelchair, in front of a height-adjustable table. The center of the workspace is located in front of the subject at the midline of the body. Subject's forearm is supported by the device, with his/her hand grasping the handle of the robot.

Similar to other devices, together with several rehabilitation exercises (based both on tracking or occupational-like exercises) it provides an Evaluation Task, based on a center-out point-to-point reaching activity: following a visual feedback, subjects are asked to move the device from the center to a peripheral target and come back to the center, starting at the "East" position and proceeding clockwise, making a total of 16 reaching movements. During the Evaluation Task, both the position of the robot (a white ball) and of the target to be reached (a yellow circle) are shown on the screen. The provided visual feedback, the target location and the movement sequence are shown in Fig. 2. Once the test is completed, several indices are computed by the device and displayed to give a feedback to the patient about her/his performance. These indices are summarized in Table 2. During the Evaluation Task, the apparent mass M and nominal viscosity b are set to the minimum, to minimizing the inertia of the device and, therefore, to allow the patient to move it with the least possible effort.

Experimental protocol

In our study, each participant was asked to perform the Evaluation Task provided by the device three times, making a total of 48 reaching movements (i.e., three nonconsecutive reaching movements for each direction). The participants were not asked to perform the task with a specific time constraint and, then, the movement

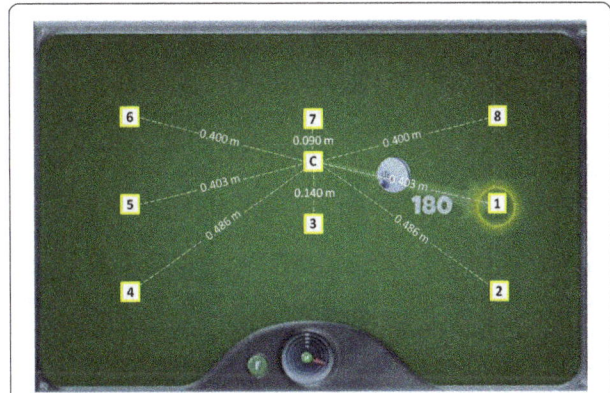

Fig. 2 The evaluation task of MOTORE. In figure is showed the visual feedback showed to the patients on the screen, together with the position of each target. The white ball indicates the position of the end-effector; the yellow circle indicates the target to be reached. The yellow squares, not showed to the patient during the task, indicate the position of the targets: C is the central target, while the numbers from 1 to 8 indicate the external targets with the sequence of the center-out movements. In addition, the distance of each target from the center is reported

accuracy was implicitly a task requisite [18, 30]. When a patient or a healthy subject was unable to reach a target (due to the upper limb impairment, or to the wide investigated workspace), he/she was asked to move the robot as far as possible toward the target. For each subject, a session (three repetitions of the Evaluation Task) lasted between 5 and 10 min, depending on the patient's impairment.

All the patients and a subgroup of healthy subjects were tested twice, 1 day apart, to assess the test-retest reliability of the provided outcome measures. For both test sessions, the value of each metric obtained in the three repetition was recorded and their mean value was computed and used for the statistical analysis.

Table 2 Outcome measures provided by MOTORE

Index	Description
Duration	Time required to complete the task
Velocity$_{mean}$	Average velocity of the device during the test
Length$_{tot}$	Global length of the path travelled by the subject during center-out movements; it ranges from 0 (no movement) to 2.808 m (patient can fully perform the entire task)
Length$_i$	Length of the path travelled by the subject toward the i-th target ($i = 1:8$)
Score	Mean of the ratios between the actual distance covered by the patients and the required distance to be travelled, computed for each required movement. It ranges from 0 (no movement) to 10 (the patient can fully perform the required task)
Work$_{tot}$	Line integral of the force along the path described by the patient
Work$_{tan}$	The amount of total work directed towards the target

Statistical analysis

All statistical analyses were performed using MedCalc (version 17, MedCalc Software, Ostend, Belgium) and SPSS (version 20, SPSS Inc., Chicago IL, USA).

Test-retest reliability

Relative test-retest reliability was assessed based on data obtained from patients at the two test sessions by using the Intraclass Correlation Coefficient (ICC), using a two-way random effect, absolute agreement, multiple measurements model. Reliability was classified as excellent (ICC > 0.90), good (0.75 < ICC ≤ 0.90), moderate (0.5 < ICC ≤ 0.75) or poor otherwise [31]. Absolute test-retest reliability was analyzed comparing for each index data obtained during the two test sessions by mean of paired t-tests and Bland-Altman plots.

Intra-session reliability was investigated in stroke patients comparing the data obtained in the three repetitions, for each session separately, by using a repeated measure ANOVA test. For each index, if the test was significant, a post-hoc analysis with Bonferroni correction was carried out.

Concurrent validity

To assess the concurrent validity of the robotic indices, the correlations between the robotic parameters and the clinical scales (FMA-UL and ARAT) were investigated using the Spearman's rank correlation coefficients. The same analysis was used to investigate the relationships between robotic indices and impairment in the activities of daily living, as measured by the BI. The coefficient values were interpreted as follows [32]: 0.0–0.2 little if any; 0.2–0.4 weak; 0.4–0.7 moderate; 0.7–1.0 strong.

Discriminant ability

The ability of the robotic indices to discriminate stroke patients from healthy subjects was evaluated by means of unpaired t tests; for each index, the effect size was also evaluated through the Cohen's d coefficient (small ≥0.20, medium ≥0.50, large ≥0.80 [33]).

For all the statistical analysis, a p value less than 0.05 was deemed significant.

Results

Test-retest reliability

ICCs and 95% confidence intervals, as well as the results of the statistical analysis of the comparison of the two assessments, are shown in Table 3.

Referring to the relative test-retest reliability, Duration, Velocity$_{mean}$, Length$_{tot}$, Length$_1$, Length$_4$, Length$_5$, Length$_6$, Length$_7$, Length$_8$, Score, Work$_{tot}$ and Work$_{tan}$ displayed an excellent reliability (ICC > 0.9), while a good (ICC ≥ 0.75) and a moderate (ICC ≥ 0.5) reliability was shown by Length$_2$ and Length$_3$ respectively. With

respect to the absolute reliability, we found a statistically significant reduction of Duration ($p = 0.004$) and a statistically significant increase of Velocity$_{mean}$ ($p < 0.001$), when data obtained at the first test session were compared with those obtained 1 day after (see Figs. 3 and 4 for Bland-Altman analysis).

Finally, the intra-session reliability showed, during the test, a significant decrease of the Duration ($p = 0.05$), and a significant increase of the Velocity$_{mean}$ ($p < 0.001$) and the Score ($p = 0.045$), while, during the retest, only a significant increase of the Velocity$_{mean}$ was found ($p = 0.001$). With respect all the remaining indices, no differences between repetitions were found (see Figs. 5 and 6).

With respect to the healthy subjects, we found that the relative test-retest reliability was excellent for the Duration, good for the Velocity$_{mean}$ and the Work$_{tan}$, and moderate to poor for all the remaining indices (Table 4). The absolute reliability showed that a significant decrease of the Duration (p < 0.001) and a significant increase of the Velocity$_{mean}$ ($p = 0.014$) and the Work$_{tan}$ ($p = 0.04$).

Concurrent validity

The results of the correlation analysis between the robotic indices and the clinical scale are shown in Table 5. Most of the robotic indices showed a strong correlation with the FM, with Length$_2$ e Length$_3$ being moderately correlated and Work$_{tot}$ weakly correlated with the FM. When examining correlations between robotic indices and the ARAT, we observed similar results to those obtained with the FM, with slightly lower correlation coefficients overall. Finally, all the provided indices but the Work$_{tot}$ were moderately correlated (11 indices) to strongly correlated (2 indices, namely Length$_{tot}$ and Score) with the BI. It is worthy to note that almost all the correlations are significant wit a p level lower than 0.001 and, therefore, they remain significant even after a Bonferroni correction (i.e., with an alpha set to 0.05/42 = 0.0012, where 42 is the number of analyzed correlations). The results of the correlation analysis between the robotic indices are provided as Additional file 1: Table S1.

Discriminant ability

The expected ability of the robotic indices to distinguish between patients with subacute stroke and age-matched healthy subjects was confirmed by the results of the statistical analysis. In fact, all the robotic indices but the Work$_{tot}$ obtained from patients with sub-acute stroke were statistically different from those of controls (see Table 6). The analysis of the effect size showed that the discriminant ability was medium for the Work$_{tan}$ and large for all the remaining indices, being ES higher than 1 for 8 of them.

Table 3 Test-retest reliability in stroke patients ($n = 48$)

	Test mean (SD)	Retest mean (SD)	ICC	95% CI		Paired t test (P)
				Lower bound	Upper bound	
Duration (s)	193.7 (107.30)	176.8 (111.90)	0.962	0.922	0.980	**0.004**
Velocity$_{mean}$ (m/s)	0.05 (0.04)	0.07 (0.04)	0.914	0.756	0.962	**< 0.001**
Length$_{tot}$ (m)	1.80 (0.92)	1.84 (1.01)	0.951	0.912	0.972	0.495
Lenght$_1$ (m)	0.25 (0.16)	0.25 (0.18)	0.930	0.876	0.960	0.784
Lenght$_2$ (m)	0.38 (0.14)	0.35 (0.17)	0.804	0.652	0.890	0.149
Lenght$_3$ (m)	0.13 (0.03)	0.13 (0.02)	0.693	0.456	0.828	0.542
Lenght$_4$ (m)	0.34 (0.18)	0.36 (0.17)	0.917	0.851	0.953	0.113
Lenght$_5$ (m)	0.24 (0.17)	0.25 (0.18)	0.907	0.834	0.948	0.551
Lenght$_6$ (m)	0.20 (0.17)	0.22 (0.18)	0.917	0.852	0.953	0.13
Lenght$_7$ (m)	0.05 (0.04)	0.06 (0.04)	0.957	0.924	0.976	0.188
Lenght$_8$ (m)	0.21 (0.17)	0.22 (0.18)	0.934	0.883	0.963	0.467
Score	7.91 (2.20)	7.99 (2.45)	0.972	0.949	0.984	0.477
Work$_{tot}$ (J)	19.88 (12.75)	20.79 (15.45)	0.908	0.837	0.949	0.446
Work$_{tan}$ (J)	10.22 (8.65)	11.26 (0.18)	0.957	0.922	0.976	0.061

Intraclass Correlation Coefficient (ICC) with 95% Confidence Interval (CI), and result of the t tests. Bold values indicated statistical significance, with p value less than 0.05

Discussion

In this study we assessed for the first time the intra-session and the between-day test-retest reliability, and the validity of the outcome measures provided by a novel planar robot for upper limb rehabilitation, in a sample of patients with sub-acute stroke, and their ability to differentiate patients from a group of age-matched healthy subjects. The abovementioned outcome measures assess the ability of patients in performing a planar reaching task. Similar protocols are provided by several robotic devices and extensively used to assess the residual motor ability of the upper limb in patients with stroke [6–14], or other neurological diseases [15, 16, 34]. However, the specific mechanical, electrical and control solutions adopted in the device requires a validation of the provided measures, since the results obtained from different devices cannot be simply extended [7]. In fact, because each robot differ from the others in terms of

Table 4 Test-retest reliability in healthy subjects ($n = 19$)

	Test mean (SD)	Retest mean (SD)	ICC	95% CI		Paired t test (P)
				Lower bound	Upper bound	
Duration (s)	107.3 (56.30)	83.96 (50.02)	0.914	0.336	0.977	**0.000**
Velocity$_{mean}$ (m/s)	0.08 (0.04)	0.10 (0.06)	0.81	0.437	0.931	**0.014**
Length$_{tot}$ (m)	2.64 (0.29)	2.68 (0.21)	0.593	−0.064	0.844	0.484
Lenght$_1$ (m)	0.39 (0.03)	0.39 (0.03)	0.627	−0.002	0.858	0.966
Lenght$_2$ (m)	0.46 (0.08)	0.47 (0.09)	0.93	0.822	0.973	0.309
Lenght$_3$ (m)	0.14 (0.01)	0.14 (0.00)	§	§	§	0.331
Lenght$_4$ (m)	0.46 (0.10)	0.48 (0.01)	0.01	−1.511	0.615	0.273
Lenght$_5$ (m)	0.38 (0.06)	0.39 (0.03)	0.087	−1.446	0.652	0.458
Lenght$_6$ (m)	0.35 (0.07)	0.35 (0.09)	0.722	0.260	0.894	0.870
Lenght$_7$ (m)	0.09 (0.01)	0.09 (0.00)	§	§	§	0.358
Lenght$_8$ (m)	0.38 (0.04)	0.38 (0.06)	0.814	0.512	0.929	0.729
Score	9.68 (0.58)	9.78 (0.37)	0.522	−0.249	0.816	0.453
Work$_{tot}$ (J)	17.62 (10.29)	19.84 (8.21)	0.695	0.227	0.882	0.296
Work$_{tan}$ (J)	13.17 (7.38)	15.42 (6.61)	0.868	0.632	0.950	**0.040**

Intraclass Correlation Coefficient (ICC) with 95% Confidence Interval (CI), and result of the t tests. Bold values indicated statistical significance, with p value less than 0.05. The symbol § indicate null variance in the data

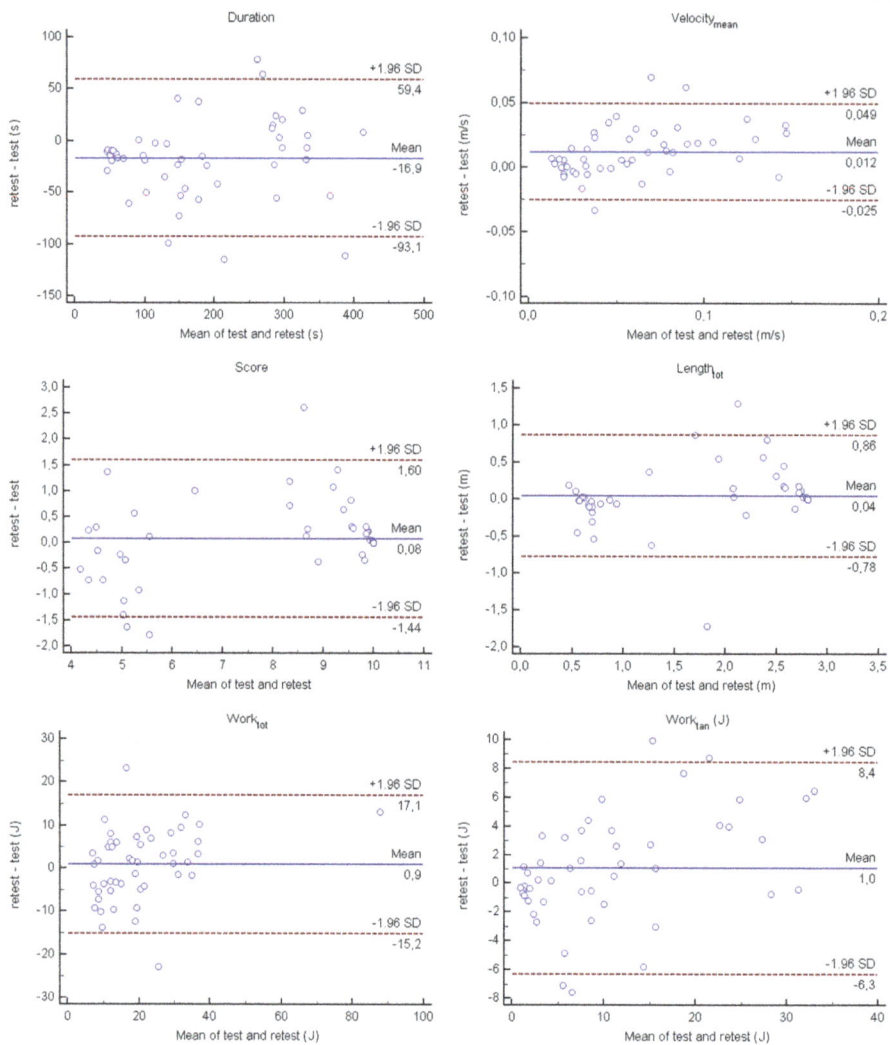

Fig. 3 Bland-Altman plots of the robotic indices assessing the whole task

provided support, mechanical structure and control algorithm, the validity and the sensitivity of similar metrics could be different among different devices [7].

Differently from clinical scales, that are worldwide recognized and easy to administered in any rehabilitation center, robotic outcome measures can be used only in center equipped with similar devices, and the obtained results are hard to share among centers. However, the metrological characteristic of these measures are often superior to those of clinical scales and, therefore, they can be a very powerful tool to monitor the improvement of the patients, at least in centers where similar devices are installed. Moreover, the increasing data sharing capacity, as well as the spread of these devices, may improve in the future diffusion and use of these data among centers.

With respect to the relative reliability, as assessed by the ICCs, we found that almost all the provided indices

exhibited good to excellent reliability across the two separate testing days, in patients with sub-acute stroke. These results are in accordance with previous works, where a high reliability was shown by similar indices provided by other upper limb robotic devices [8, 13, 35] in stroke patients. It is worth noting that several indices showed an ICC value higher than 0.9, meaning that they could be used for intra-individual comparisons (i.e. for individual decision-making) and not just for group-level comparisons (i.e. for the evaluation of a whole large group of patients), where an ICC value of 0.7 level is acceptable.

With respect to the absolute reliability, an unexpected result was the significant decrease of the duration and the significant increase of the $Velocity_{mean}$ in the second evaluation (retest), when compared with the first (test). It is likely that in the first test session patients were more cautious in performing the required task, moving

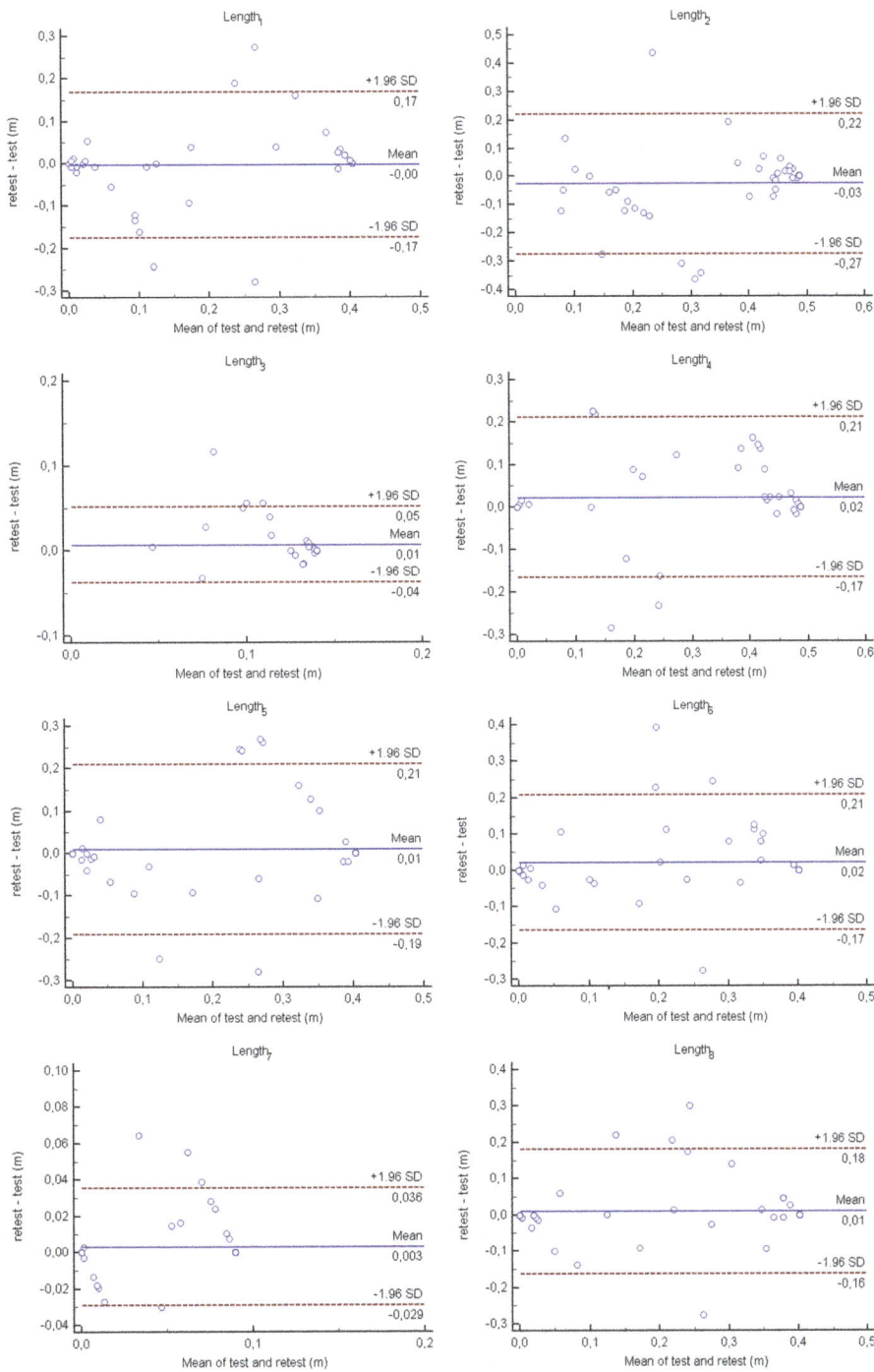

Fig. 4 Bland-Altman plots of the robotic indices assessing the path length travelled by stroke patients towards each target

the robot in a slower way, if compared to the second test session. These results would have probably been different if patients had performed a practice test before the first evaluation, in order to familiarize with the device. In fact, it must be highlighted that we have deliberately chosen not to perform a practice test before the first evaluation. Analyzing the data coming from each repetition in the first day of evaluation, we found a significant trend in both indices that, in the second day was absent for the Duration and less evident for the Velocity$_{mean}$. Therefore, our results support the hypothesis that, at least with respect to these two indices (Duration and Velocity$_{mean}$), in clinical practice as well as in research study, some familiarization trials, before the actual

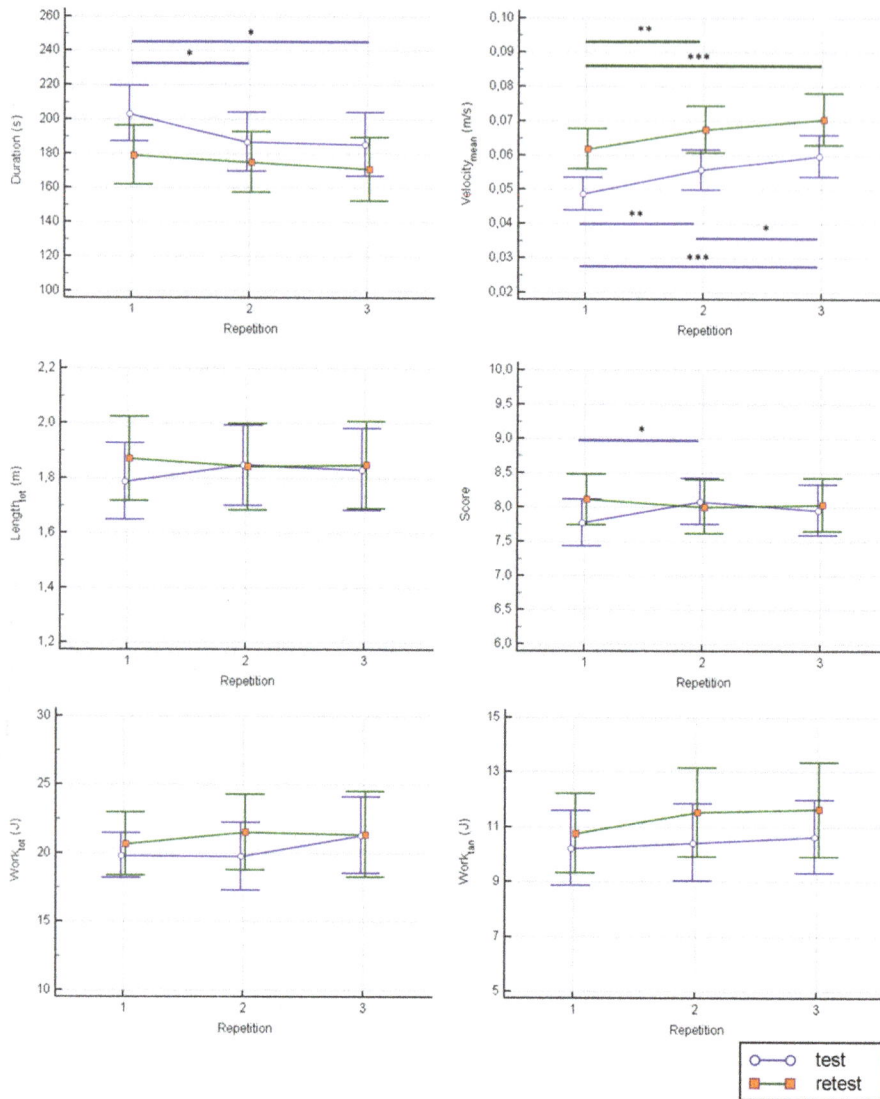

Fig. 5 Intra-session reliability analysis in stroke patients: robotic indices assessing the whole task. Blue lines represent the statistical analysis of the first session (test), while green lines represent the statistical analysis of the second session (retest). The symbols *, ** and *** represent a statistically significant difference between repetitions, with a p value less than 0.05, 0.01 and 0.001, respectively

evaluation, should be performed. This is particularly true because both Duration and Velocity$_{mean}$ are hallmarks of the upper limb impairment following a stroke [36] and they have to be evaluated in a robotic assessment.

On the contrary, no other indices showed significant differences in the two evaluations confirming their absolute reliability, meaning that patients did not change the travelled path or the mechanical work produced to move the hand/robot.

With respect to the healthy subjects, similar or slightly lower ICC values were found for the indices independent from the travelled distance (i.e., the Duration, the Velocity$_{mean}$ and the Work$_{tan}$), while we obtained very low ICC values for almost all the metrics related to the travelled distance. This can be easily explained with the very low

to null between-subject variance in the data. Similar to the stroke patients, a learning effect was detected, as showed by the statistical significant differences in Duration, Velocity$_{mean}$ and Work$_{tan}$ between the two evaluations.

The validity study showed that all investigated indices were significantly correlated with the Fugl-Meyer assessment and the Action Research Arm Test. This led us to confirm the concurrent validity of the robotic indices against common clinical scale of upper limb impairment, implying that they provide meaningful information from a clinical point of view. Compared to the clinical scales, the robotic assessment can be obtained quickly and recorded at several time-points during the rehabilitation path. The relation between the FM and the robotic

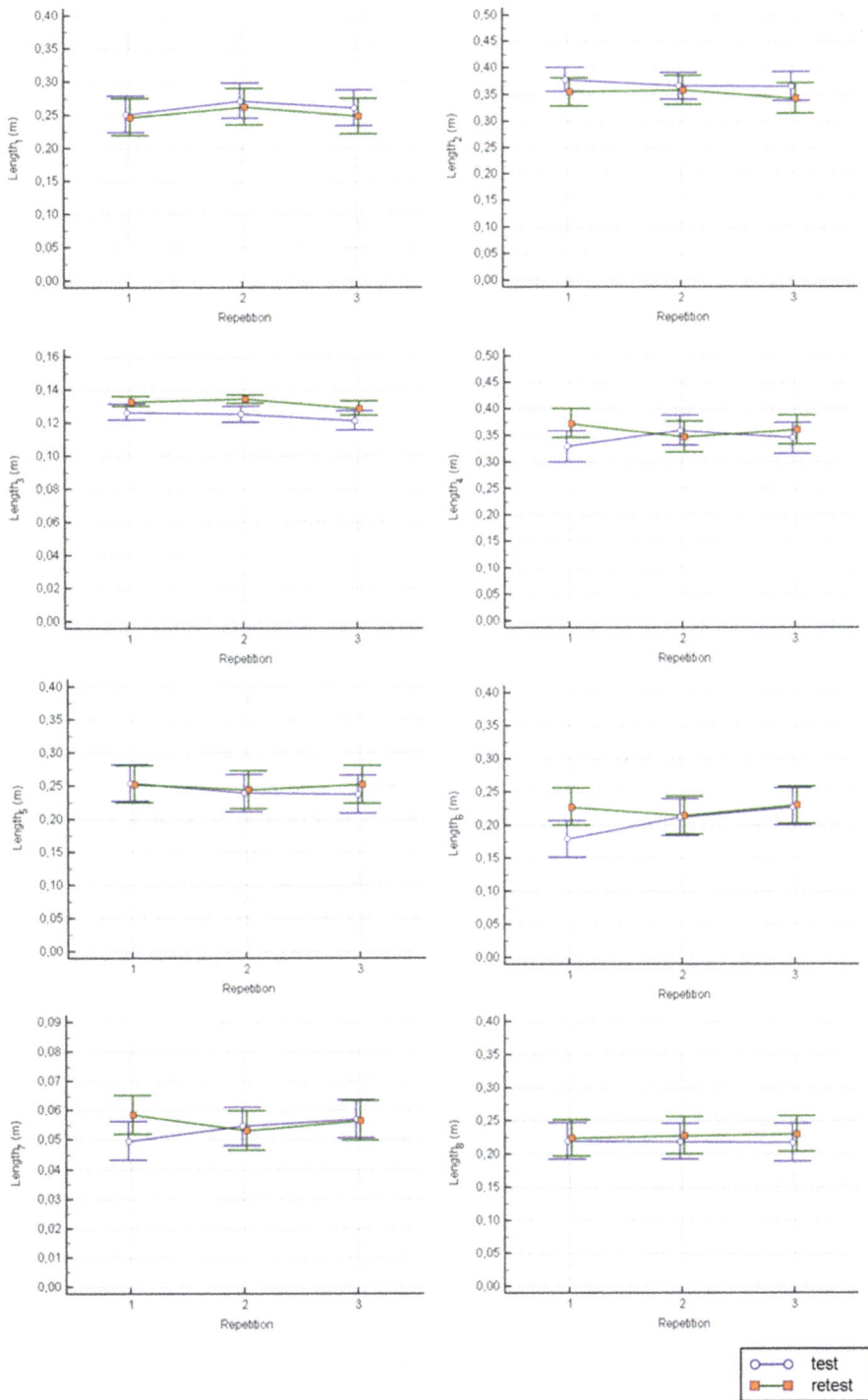

Fig. 6 Intra-session reliability analysis in stroke patients: robotic indices assessing the path length travelled towards each target. Blue lines represent the statistical analysis of the first session (test), while green lines represent the statistical analysis of the second session (retest)

assessment has been largely studied, being the FM the most commonly used clinical scale used in trial involving robotic devices [3]. Generally, the robotic indices were found to be correlated with the FM with similar or lower correlation coefficient [5, 7, 10, 11, 21, 37–39], when compared with those obtained with MOTORE. Similar results were found in the correlation with the ARAT. This result is not surprising, since the FM and the ARAT were found to be highly correlated to each other [40, 41]. The correlation coefficients we found were

Table 5 Validity

	FMA-UL	ARAT	BI
Duration	-0.8507^{***}	-0.7716^{***}	-0.6738^{***}
$Velocity_{mean}$	0.8227^{***}	0.7587^{***}	0.6340^{***}
$Length_{tot}$	0.8551^{***}	0.7268^{***}	0.7139^{***}
$Lenght_1$	0.7700^{***}	0.6273^{***}	0.6423^{***}
$Lenght_2$	0.6259^{***}	0.5904^{***}	0.4419^{**}
$Lenght_3$	0.5093^{***}	0.4613^{***}	0.4195^{**}
$Lenght_4$	0.7172^{***}	0.5689^{***}	0.6021^{***}
$Lenght_5$	0.8047^{***}	0.6666^{***}	0.6638^{***}
$Lenght_6$	0.8026^{***}	0.7075^{***}	0.6914^{***}
$Lenght_7$	0.8267^{***}	0.6979^{***}	0.6404^{***}
$Lenght_8$	0.8584^{***}	0.7196^{***}	0.6241^{***}
Score	0.8443^{***}	0.7384^{***}	0.7417^{***}
$Work_{tot}$	0.3472^{**}	0.3672^{**}	0.1700
$Work_{tan}$	0.8188^{***}	0.6942^{***}	0.6564^{***}

Spearman's correlation coefficient between the robotic indices and the following clinical scale: Upper limb subscale of the Fugl-Meyer Assessment (FMA-UL), Action Research Arm Test (ARAT), and Barthel Index (BI). The symbols **, and *** indicate a p value less than 0.01 and 0.001 respectively

generally higher, when compared to other studies [42]. A possible explanation could be the greater variability in patient's disability in our study, when compared to that of other studies (see, for example, [7, 12, 37]). In fact, it is known that the value of the correlation coefficient is greater if there is more variability among the observations [43]. Of particular interest is the result about the correlation between the robotic measures and the BI, being the BI a global measure of disability rather than a motor assessment scale. This means that the upper limb

motor performance, even if measured in a simple planar reaching task but in instrumental way, could, at least partially, reflect the ability in the activities of daily living.

The differences we have found between the different directions in terms of validity can be related to the different level of difficulty of the required movement. In fact, higher correlation coefficients were found for the movements towards the targets farther from the subject's body (i.e., 6, 7 and 8), while lower coefficients were found for the movements towards the targets nearer the subject's body (i.e., 2, 3 and 4). These differences can be explained by considering some clinical aspects about the upper limb motor recovery in patients with stroke. In most cases, stroke patients are facilitated to perform flexion elbow movements and, therefore, to lead their arm toward the body. In other words, harder movements can better differentiate the level of impairment of patient and, therefore, can show higher correlations with the clinical scales. With respect to the ICC analysis, the lower value we found for the $Length_3$ can be mainly related to the lower variance between patients. Referring to the discriminant ability, it should be underlined that all the robotic indices but the $Work_{tot}$ were significantly different between patients with sub-acute stroke and healthy subjects, with a strong effect size (a moderate effect size was observed only for $Work_{tan}$). With respect to the Duration, our results are in accordance to those obtained, for example, by Otaka et al. [7], or Coderre et al. [13], where higher time necessary to complete planar task were detected in patients with stroke, when compared to healthy subjects. Similarly, with respect to the $Velocity_{mean}$, a reduction of speed in patients with stroke was detected in several studies [6, 12].

Table 6 Discriminant ability

Robotic indices	Patients with stroke (N = 48) Mean (SD)	Healthy subjects (N = 40) Mean (SD)	Unpaired t test (P)	Effect Size
Duration (s)	193.7 (107.30)	93.30 (53.50)	< 0.001	1.18
$Velocity_{mean}$ (m/s)	0.05 (0.04)	0.09 (0.05)	< 0.001	0.86
$Length_{tot}$ (m)	1.80 (0.92)	2.67 (0.24)	< 0.001	1.30
$Lenght_1$ (m)	0.25 (0.16)	0.39 (0.03)	< 0.001	1.17
$Lenght_2$ (m)	0.38 (0.14)	0.46 (0.08)	0.001	0.75
$Lenght_3$ (m)	0.13 (0.03)	0.14 (0.01)	0.004	0.62
$Lenght_4$ (m)	0.34 (0.18)	0.47 (0.07)	< 0.001	0.98
$Lenght_5$ (m)	0.24 (0.17)	0.39 (0.04)	< 0.001	1.20
$Lenght_6$ (m)	0.20 (0.17)	0.35 (0.08)	< 0.001	1.17
$Lenght_7$ (m)	0.05 (0.04)	0.09 (0.00)	< 0.001	1.31
$Lenght_8$ (m)	0.21 (0.17)	0.38 (0.05)	< 0.001	1.33
Score	7.91 (2.20)	9.74 (0.47)	< 0.001	1.16
$Work_{tot}$ (J)	19.88 (12.75)	19.03 (9.11)	0.717	–
$Work_{tan}$ (J)	10.22 (8.65)	14.62 (6.98)	0.010	0.56

Descriptive statistics for the robotic indices in patients with stroke (N = 48) and healthy subjects (N = 40). Comparison is assessed by means of t tests. For significant differences, the Effect Size is also reported

A statistically significant difference between the two groups was also found for all the Length and Score parameters, that are related to the ability of the patients to travel the distance toward the target with the impaired arm. Usually these parameters are not assessed in point-to-point reaching tasks performed in a transversal plan, since the patient's ability to reach the target is a mandatory requirement to be included in the evaluation (see, for example, Otaka et al. [7]). However, a decreased movement distance in reaching task is evident in patients with stroke [44] and, therefore, in our opinion, an evaluation of this aspect could add meaningful information about the patient's dexterity and the course of the therapy.

Finally, referring to the work-related parameters, to the best of our knowledge, ours is the first study that evaluates the differences between patients with stroke and healthy subject with similar metrics. We found that $Work_{tan}$ was significantly different between the two groups, while the $Work_{tot}$ was not. Zollo et al. [12] employed both total and useful work (similar to the $Work_{tan}$), to assess the effect of the rehabilitation intervention, rather than the motor skills of patients with stroke. Interestingly, Zollo et al. found that the total work did not change after therapy while the useful work increased after the robotic treatment. Their results, along with us, suggest to employ only the useful work, i. e. the work spent to move towards the target, rather than the total work, as a work-related measure of motor impairment in patients with stroke. In our opinion, the $Work_{tot}$ did not differ between stroke patients and healthy individuals because it counts the entire work performed by the subject; with respect to the patients it takes into account the work done to move the robot in a curved path, considering both the "physiological part of the movement" (toward the target) and the "pathological part of the movement" (perpendicular to the correct direction). Therefore, it is combined by two factors, one reducing because of the impairment, and one increasing because of the impairment. This could also affect the correlations with the clinical scales.

A limitation of this study is the absence of robotic measurement assessing movement smoothness. In fact, movement smoothness, quantified by means of several parameters based on velocity or more commonly jerk, was found to be an hallmark of severity in patients with stroke [37]. It is worth noting that, almost the totality of the studies obtained these parameters after a data reduction, starting from the raw data provided by the robot. MOTORE, as well as providing the investigated parameters, allow the access to raw data, and, therefore, allow to compute smoothness parameter. Obviously, this is more time-consuming, and likely, more suitable for use in research rather than in clinical practice. Since this study is especially designed to assess the properties of the provided robotic indices for a routine clinical use, we decided not to consider indices computed from raw data. In fact, the goal of this study is to use these measures to obtain a frequent evaluation during the treatment, with the aim of calibrating the treatment on patient's needs, ability, and motor changes, in order to design patient-tailored rehabilitation programs. Future work should be addressed to analyze the properties of the measure of smoothness, obtained from raw data.

Finally, the design of this study is cross-sectional. A longitudinal design is needed to measure responsiveness of the robotic parameters after rehabilitation.

Conclusion

We found that all the robotic indices but the $Work_{tot}$ provided by a novel robotic device for the upper limb rehabilitation, are reliable, sensitive and strongly correlated both with motor and disability clinical scales. Therefore, they are suitable as an evaluation tool for the upper limb motor performance of patients with sub-acute stroke in clinical practice. The instrumental outcome measures are very important to have an objective but also easy evaluation, as well as to define the best treatment for the patient. In fact, the recovery of the upper limb can vary greatly from patient to patient and in this perspective, instrumental and objective data could be a guide to address the treatment path.

Acknowledgements
The Authors wish to thank Eugenio Ialungo, Caterina Felici, Gaetanina Competiello and Antonietta Chiusano for their help in data acquisition; Manuele Barilli and Lucia Avila for their help in patients' recruitment; and Valerio Gower and Marta Beorchia for their technical support.

Authors' contributions
MG: Concept and design, acquisition of data, analysis and interpretation of data, preparation of manuscript; AC, CP, SL, AS, MM, RM and GG: acquisition of data, analysis and interpretation of data; GS and FC: analysis and interpretation of data; LP: Concept and design, analysis and interpretation of data; IA: Concept and design, analysis and interpretation of data, preparation of manuscript. All authors read and approved the final manuscript.

Competing interests
The authors declare that they have no competing interests.

Author details
[1]IRCCS Fondazione Don Carlo Gnocchi, Piazzale Morandi 6, 20121 Milan, Italy. [2]Physical Medicine and Rehabilitation Unit, Sant'Andrea Hospital, "Sapienza"

University of Rome, Via di Grottarossa, 1035, 00189 Rome, Italy. [3]IRCCS Fondazione Don Carlo Gnocchi, Via di Scandicci, 269, 50143 Florence, Italy. [4]Department of Geriatrics, Neurosciences and Orthopaedics, Università Cattolica del Sacro Cuore, Largo Francesco Vito 1, 00168 Rome, Italy.

References

1.   Loureiro RCV, Harwin WS, Nagai K, Johnson M. Advances in upper limb stroke rehabilitation: a technology push. Med Biol Eng Comput. 2011;49:1103–18.

2.   Volpe BT, Krebs HI, Hogan N. Is robot-aided sensorimotor training in stroke rehabilitation a realistic option? Curr Opin Neurol. 2001;14:745–52.

3.   Sivan M, O'Connor RJ, Makower S, Levesley M, Bhakta B. Systematic review of outcome measures used in the evaluation of robot-assisted upper limb exercise in stroke. J Rehabil Med. 2011;43:181–9.

4.   Canning CG, Ada L, O'Dwyer NJ. Abnormal muscle activation characteristics associated with loss of dexterity after stroke. J Neurol Sci. 2000;176:45–56.

5.   Krabben T, Molier BI, Houwink A, Rietman JS, Buurke JH, Prange GB. Circle drawing as evaluative movement task in stroke rehabilitation: an explorative study. J Neuroeng Rehabil. 2011;8:15.

6.   Longhi M, Merlo A, Prati P, Giacobbi M, Mazzoli D. Instrumental indices for upper limb function assessment in stroke patients: a validation study. J Neuroeng Rehabil. 2016;13:52.

7.   Otaka E, Otaka Y, Kasuga S, Nishimoto A, Yamazaki K, Kawakami M, Ushiba J, Liu M. Clinical usefulness and validity of robotic measures of reaching movement in hemiparetic stroke patients. J Neuroeng Rehabil. 2015;12:66.

8.   Gilliaux M, Lejeune T, Detrembleur C, Sapin J, Dehez B, Selves C, Stoquart G. Using the robotic device REAplan as a valid, reliable, and sensitive tool to quantify upper limb impairments in stroke patients. J Rehabil Med. 2014;46:117–25.

9.   Debert CT, Herter TM, Scott SH, Dukelow S. Robotic assessment of sensorimotor deficits after traumatic brain injury. J Neurol Phys Ther. 2012;36:58–67.

10. Celik O, O'Malley MK, Boake C, Levin HS, Yozbatiran N, Reistetter TA. Normalized movement quality measures for therapeutic robots strongly correlate with clinical motor impairment measures. IEEE Trans Neural Syst Rehabil Eng. 2010;18:433–44.

11. Zollo L, Rossini L, Bravi M, Magrone G, Sterzi S, Guglielmelli E. Quantitative evaluation of upper-limb motor control in robot-aided rehabilitation. Med Biol Eng Comput. 2011;49:1131–44.

12. Zollo L, Gallotta E, Guglielmelli E, Sterzi S. Robotic technologies and rehabilitation: new tools for upper-limb therapy and assessment in chronic stroke. Eur J Phys Rehabil Med. 2011;47:223–36.

13. Coderre AM, Amr Abou Zeid AA, Dukelow SP, Demmer MJ, Moore KD, Demers MJ, Bretzke H, Herter TM, Glasgow JI, Norman KE, Bagg SD, Scott SH. Assessment of upper-limb sensorimotor function of subacute stroke patients using visually guided reaching. Neurorehabil Neural Repair. 2010;24:528–41.

14. Bosecker C, Dipietro L, Volpe B, Igo Krebs H. Kinematic robot-based evaluation scales and clinical counterparts to measure upper limb motor performance in patients with chronic stroke. Neurorehabil Neural Repair. 2010;24:62–9.

15. Casadio M, Sanguineti V, Morasso P, Solaro C. Abnormal sensorimotor control, but intact force field adaptation, in multiple sclerosis subjects with no clinical disability. Mult Scler. 2008;14:330–42.

16. Frascarelli F, Masia L, Di Rosa G, Petrarca M, Cappa P, Castelli E. Robot-mediated and clinical scales evaluation after upper limb botulinum toxin type a injection in children with hemiplegia. J Rehabil Med. 2009;41:988–94.

17. Masia L, Frascarelli F, Morasso P, Di Rosa G, Petrarca M, Castelli E, Cappa P. Reduced short term adaptation to robot generated dynamic environment in children affected by cerebral palsy. J Neuroeng Rehabil. 2011;8:28.

18. Germanotta M, Vasco G, Petrarca M, Rossi S, Carniel S, Bertini E, Cappa P, Castelli E. Robotic and clinical evaluation of upper limb motor performance in patients with Friedreich's Ataxia: an observational study. J Neuroeng Rehabil. 2015;12:41.

19. Nordin N, Xie SQ, Wünsche B. Assessment of movement quality in robot-assisted upper limb rehabilitation after stroke: a review. J Neuroeng Rehabil. 2014;11:137.

20. Maciejasz P, Eschweiler J, Gerlach-Hahn K, Jansen-Troy A, Leonhardt S. A survey on robotic devices for upper limb rehabilitation. J Neuroeng Rehabil. 2014;11:3.

21. McKenzie A, Dodakian L, See J, Le V, Quinlan EB, Bridgford C, Head D, Han

VL, Cramer SC. Validity of robot-based assessments of upper extremity function. Arch Phys Med Rehabil. 2017;98(10):1969–76.

22. Avizzano CA, Satler M, Cappiello G, Scoglio A, Ruffaldi E, Bergamasco M. MOTORE: a mobile haptic interface for neuro-rehabilitation. In 2011 RO-MAN. IEEE; 2011:383–88. https://doi.org/10.1109/ROMAN.2011.6005238.

23. Gladstone DJ, Danells CJ, Black SE. The fugl-meyer assessment of motor recovery after stroke: a critical review of its measurement properties. Neurorehabil Neural Repair. 2002;16:232–40.

24. Duncan PW, Propst M, Nelson SG. Reliability of the Fugl-Meyer assessment of sensorimotor recovery following cerebrovascular accident. Phys Ther. 1983;63(10):1606.

25. Sanford J, Moreland J, Swanson LR, Stratford PW, Gowland C. Reliability of the Fugl-Meyer assessment for testing motor performance in patients following stroke. Phys Ther. 1993;73:447–54.

26. De Weerdt WJG, Harrison MA. Measuring recovery of arm-hand function in stroke patients: a comparison of the Brunnstrom-Fugl-Meyer test and the action research arm test. Physiother Canada. 1985;37:65–70.

27. Lyle RC. A performance test for assessment of upper limb function in physical rehabilitation treatment and research. Int J Rehabil Res. 1981;4:483–92.

28. Collin C, Wade DT, Davies S, Horne V. The Barthel ADL index: a reliability study. Int Disabil Stud. 1988;10:61–3.

29. Ruffaldi E, Satler M, Papini GPR, Avizzano CA: A flexible framework for mobile based haptic rendering. In 2013 IEEE RO-MAN IEEE; 2013:732–37. https://doi.org/10.1109/ROMAN.2013.6628400.

30. Pellegrino L, Coscia M, Muller M, Solaro C, Casadio M. Evaluating upper limb impairments in multiple sclerosis by exposure to different mechanical environments. Sci Rep. 2018;8:2110.

31. Koo TK, Li MY. A guideline of selecting and reporting Intraclass correlation coefficients for reliability research. J Chiropr Med. 2016;15:155–63.

32. Guilford JP. Fundamental Statistics in Psychology and Education. New York (330 West 42nd Street): McGraw-Hill Book Company; 1956. p. 565. P. $6.25. Sci Educ 1957, 41:244–244

33. Cohen J. Statistical power analysis for the behavioral sciences (revised ed.). Hillsdale: Lawrence Erlbaum Associates, Inc; 1977.

34. Germanotta M, Vasco G, Petrarca M, Rossi S, Carniel S, Bertini E, Cappa P, Castelli E. Robotic and clinical evaluation of upper limb motor performance in patients with Friedreich's Ataxia: an observational study. J Neuroeng Rehabil. 2015;12(1):41.

35. Colombo R, Cusmano I, Sterpi I, Mazzone A, Delconte C, Pisano F. Test-retest reliability of robotic assessment measures for the evaluation of upper limb recovery. IEEE Trans Neural Syst Rehabil Eng. 2014;22:1020–9.

36. Aprile I, Rabuffetti M, Padua L, Di Sipio E, Simbolotti C, Ferrarin M. Kinematic analysis of the upper limb motor strategies in stroke patients as a tool towards advanced neurorehabilitation strategies: a preliminary study. Biomed Res Int. 2014;2014:636123.

37. Rohrer B, Fasoli S, Krebs HI, Hughes R, Volpe B, Frontera WR, Stein J, Hogan N. Movement smoothness changes during stroke recovery. J Neurosci. 2002; 22:8297–304.

38. Colombo R, Pisano F, Micera S, Mazzone A, Delconte C, Carrozza MC, Dario P, Minuco G. Robotic techniques for upper limb evaluation and rehabilitation of stroke patients. IEEE Trans Neural Syst Rehabil Eng. 2005;13:311–24.

39. Dipietro L, Krebs HI, Fasoli SE, Volpe BT, Stein J, Bever C, Hogan N. Changing motor synergies in chronic stroke. J Neurophysiol. 2007;98:757–68.

40. Rabadi MH, Rabadi FM. Comparison of the action research arm test and the Fugl-Meyer assessment as measures of upper-extremity motor weakness after stroke. Arch Phys Med Rehabil. 2006;87:962–6.

41. Hsieh YW, Wu CY, Lin KC, Chang YF, Chen CL, Liu JS. Responsiveness and validity of three outcome measures of motor function after stroke rehabilitation. Stroke. 2009;40:1386–91.

42. Do Tran V, Dario P, Mazzoleni S. Kinematic measures for upper limb robot-assisted therapy following stroke and correlations with clinical outcome measures: a review. Med Eng Phys. 2018;53:13–31.

43. Goodwin LD, Leech NL. Understanding correlation: factors that affect the size of r. J Exp Educ. 2006;74:249–66.

44. Kamper DG, McKenna-Cole AN, Kahn LE, Reinkensmeyer DJ. Alterations in reaching after stroke and their relation to movement direction and impairment severity. Arch Phys Med Rehabil. 2002;83:702–7.

19

Reference values for gait temporal and loading symmetry of lower-limb amputees can help in refocusing rehabilitation targets

Andrea Giovanni Cutti[*], Gennaro Verni, Gian Luca Migliore, Amedeo Amoresano and Michele Raggi

From Second World Congress hosted by the American Orthotic & Prosthetic Association (AOPA)
Las Vegas, NV, USA. 06-09 September 2017

Abstract

Background: The literature suggests that optimal levels of gait symmetry might exist for lower-limb amputees. Not only these optimal values are unknown, but we also don't know typical symmetry ratios or which measures of symmetry are essential. Focusing on the symmetries of stance, step, first peak and impulse of the ground reaction force, the aim of this work was to answer to three methodological and three clinical questions. The methodological questions wanted to establish a minimum set of symmetry indexes to study and if there are limitations in their calculations. The clinical questions wanted to establish if typical levels of temporal and loading symmetry exist, and change with the level of amputation and prosthetic components.

Methods: Sixty traumatic, K3-K4 amputees were involved in the study: 12 transfemoral mechanical knee users (TFM), 25 C-leg knee users (TFC), and 23 transtibial amputees (TT). Ninety-two percent used the Ossur Variflex foot. Ten healthy subjects were also included. Ground reaction force from both feet were collected with the Novel Pedar-X. Symmetry indexes were calculated and statistically compared with regression analyses and non-parametric analysis of variance among subjects.

Results: Stance symmetry can be reported instead of step, but it cannot substitute impulse and first peak symmetry. The first peak cannot always be detected on all amputees. Statistically significant differences exist for stance symmetry among all groups, for impulse symmetry between TFM and TFC/TT, for first peak symmetry between transfemoral amputees altogether and TT. Regarding impulse symmetry, 25% of TFC and 43% of TT had a higher impulse on the prosthetic side. Regarding first peak symmetry, 59% of TF and 30% of TT loaded more the prosthetic side.

Conclusions: Typical levels of symmetry for stance, impulse and first peak change with the level of amputation and componentry. Indications exist that C-leg and energy-storage-and-return feet can improve symmetry. Results are suggestive of two mechanisms related to sound side knee osteoarthritis: increased impulse for TF and increased first peak for TT. These results can be useful in clinics to set rehabilitation targets, understand the advancements of a patient during gait retraining, compare and chose components and possibly rehabilitation programs.

Keywords: Gait, Ground reaction force, Symmetry, Rehabilitation, Amputees, Prosthesis, Osteoarthritis, C-leg, Microprocessor controlled knees, Energy storage and return feet

* Correspondence: ag.cutti@inail.it
INAIL Prosthetic Center, Via Rabuina 14, 40054 Vigorso di Budrio, BO, Italy

Background

Lower-limb amputees tend to walk asymmetrically when looking at gait temporal and loading parameters, with more time spent and load exerted on the intact limb [1–9]. Temporal asymmetry is typically measured based on step or stance duration; loading asymmetry based the magnitude of the first peak of the vertical ground reaction force (GRF), and the impulse of GRF [2, 3, 6, 10].

Temporal and loading asymmetries were associated to several comorbidities [5]: increased falls [11], osteoarthritis of the sound limb [10, 12–15], osteoporosis of the contralateral limb [15, 16], back pain [17–20]. In addition, walking in public with noticeable asymmetries attracts the general attention [21], which can be very uncomfortable for some prosthesis users. With this background, it is not surprising that a common, almost unquestioned [22], goal for rehabilitation is to regain a symmetric walking [9, 23].

However, the literature does not clearly indicate that striving for perfect symmetry is really and always the best option. Already in 1998, Winter & Sienko [1] stated that "human system with major structural asymmetries in the neuromuscular skeletal system cannot be optimal when gait is symmetrical. Rather, a new non-symmetrical optimal is probably being sought by the amputee within the constraints of his residual system and the mechanics of his prosthesis". Later in 2005, Schmid and co-workers [3] compared the center of pressure trajectories under the sound and prosthetic foot of transfemoral amputees and concluded that the longer stance on the sound side can be ascribed to the greater ability of the sound leg to advance the step and maintain balance until the prosthetic limb can sustain the body weight. Hof et al. [4] corroborated this explanation in the theoretical framework of the "extrapolated center of mass" [24], concluding that stance time asymmetry is a "sensible adaptation" of experienced transfemoral amputees to improve stability during walking, to overcome the missing lateral ankle strategy of prosthetic feet. More recently, Adamczyk & Kuo [8], with a theoretical and experimental approach involving transtibial amputees, concluded that "some asymmetry may be unavoidable in cases of unilateral limb loss" due to the reduced ankle plantar flexion of the ankle, with direct consequences on stance duration, greater collision work at the sound side, greater work overall, and increased peak force at loading response [25–27]. Imposing symmetry can actually be detrimental, as also observed by [27, 28].

The evidences from the literature, therefore, indicate that optimal symmetry ratios might exist, to obtain a compromise among stability, forward progression, preservation of body structures and perception of a "normal and symmetric biped locomotion" [21]. Unfortunately, at present not only optimal symmetry ratios are unknown, but we also don't know typical symmetry ratios or which measures of symmetry are essential and which are redundant.

In our opinion, 3 methodological and 3 clinical questions should be answered to clarify these open issues. The *methodological* questions are:

- Q1: do all amputees show the typical M-shaped pattern of the GRF [29], with presence and appropriate timing of its two peaks? In case of a negative answer, the measure of loading symmetry based on the first peak of GRF will be restrict to patients presenting the M-shaped pattern;
- Q2: can we limit the study of temporal symmetry to stance, leaving out step symmetry? We will give a positive answer if stance and step symmetries are very strongly correlated for all amputees, with a coefficient of determination $R^2 > 0.64$ [30];
- Q3: can we further limit the study of gait symmetry to just stance symmetry, leaving out loading symmetry, whose measure requires more cumbersome and expensive equipment? We will give a positive answer if stance symmetry is very strongly correlated ($R^2 > 0.64$) with the symmetry of the first peak and impulse of GRF.

The *clinical* questions are:

- Q4: does gait symmetry depend on the level of amputation? In case of a positive answer, typical ranges of symmetry should be established, which can be used to understand how far a new patient is from well adapted prosthesis users in terms of percentiles;
- Q5: do advanced prosthetic components improve temporal and loading symmetry? In particular, do C-leg users have better results than mechanical knee users of the same mobility level?
- Q6: is it always true that amputees overload the sound side both in terms of first peak and impulse of GRF, thus contributing to the development of osteoarthritis?

Unfortunately, at present it is difficult to answer to these questions based on the available literature, because there are no studies that considered, *at the same time* 1) both temporal and loading asymmetries, 2) both transfemoral and transtibial amputees treated at the *same* prosthetic & rehabilitation center, 3) mechanical and electronic knees, 4) energy-storage-and-return feet instead of the SACH (Solid-Ankle Cushion-Heel) foot. Moreover, the number of patients included is typically limited to 8, both for studies on transtibial and transfemoral amputees. Finally, no studies addressed the correlation between temporal and loading parameters.

The aim of this study was to overcome these limitations and answer to questions Q1-Q6 on three groups of well-adapted, traumatic, K3-K4 amputees: transfemoral amputees using a restricted set of mechanical knees (TFM), transfemoral amputees using the C-leg (TFC), transtibial amputees using energy-storage-and-return feet (TT). A additional group of healthy control subjects ("Controls" in short), was also included to highlight general trends.

Methods
Subjects
Sixty K3-K4 lower-limb amputees participated in the study after signing an informed consent: 12 mechanical knee users (TFM, 46 ± 10 y.o.), 25 C-leg users (TFC, 48 ± 13 y.o), 23 transtibial amputees (TT, 44 ± 14 y.o.), with no statistically significant differences in term of age (ANOVA, $p > 0.62$). Ten controls were also included (28 ± 2 y.o.). All amputees had completed a 3-week, intense gait training program at the same specialized prosthetic & rehabilitation center, with the support of the same rehabilitation team. The clinical center has ISO 9001 treatment pathways for amputees and provides over 800 transfemoral and 1200 transtibial prostheses every year. Following training, all patients had been successfully using their prostheses for at least 1 month at the time of testing.

The components provided to patients are summarized in Table 1. Almost 92% of patients used either the Variflex or Variflex LP foot. Mechanical knees were selected to match the activity level of the C-leg, and are consistent with knees selected for comparison with the C-leg in previous studies [31, 32].

Measurements
After standing still for 10 s, subjects walked along a long indoor hall at self-selected speed, that was noted. During this trial, the GRF was measured on each side through instrumented insoles (Pedar-X, Novel, D), sampling at 100 Hz [33, 34].

Data processing
For each subject, GRF data were export to MATLAB. Based on the 10 s' orthostatic posture, body weight was calculated. Assuming a foot-floor contact threshold at 10% body weight, we detected heel-strike and toe-off

events for the two sides. We isolated the steady state condition by considering the central 10 strides.

Calculation of temporal symmetry
For each stride, we calculated the step and stance duration. Then, for each couple of consecutive sound-affected gait cycles, we calculated the following indexes of symmetry:

- Step Symmetry (SPS): Step Duration $_{SOUND}$ / Step Duration $_{AFFECTED}$
- Stance Symmetry (SNS): Stance Duration $_{SOUND}$ / Stance Duration $_{AFFECTED}$

For Controls, ratios were right over left side. A value of 1 represents perfect symmetry. For each index of symmetry, we calculated the subject's median value over the trial. Finally, we obtained the distribution of the median values for the two indexes over TFM, TFC, TT and Controls.

Calculation of loading symmetry
For each gait cycle, the integral over the stance period of GRF was calculated, i.e. the *impulse of GRF*, as previously reported by [2]. Then, for each couple of consecutive sound-affected gait cycles, we calculated the index of symmetry:

- Impulse Symmetry (IMS): Impulse $_{SOUND}$ / Impulse $_{AFFECTED}$

A value of 1 represents perfect symmetry. Right over left side was used for Controls.

Afterward, the GRF profile of each gait cycle was checked to verify the presence of the first peak within the 0–40% of the gait cycle, and of a second peak within the 60–100%. Subjects reporting both peaks in more than half of the trials formed the "*Two-Peaks*" subgroup.

For the subjects in *Two-Peaks* we operated as follows. For each couple of consecutive sound-affected gait cycles, we calculated the following index:

- First Peak Symmetry (P1S): First peak $_{SOUND}$ / First peak $_{AFFECTED}$

P1S provides a measure of peak force asymmetry at loading response, while IMS provides a measure of the asymmetry in cyclic loading. These are two different mechanism of osteoarthritis development [10, 35–37].

For each index of symmetry, we calculated the subject's median value over the trial. Finally, we obtained the distribution of the median values for the two indexes over TFM, TFC, TT and Controls.

Table 1 Prosthetic components used and associated quantities

	TFM	TFC	TT
Foot	Variflex LP: 10 1C40: 2	Variflex LP: 25	Variflex: 18 Variflex LP: 2 Truestep: 1 Esprit: 1 1C40: 1
Knee	TotalKnee 2100: 5 3R60: 2 Mauch: 2	C-leg: 25	

Statistical analysis

The distribution of the four indexes of symmetry (SPS, SNS, IMS and P1S) was checked for normality within each group (TFM, TFC, TT and Controls) and over all subjects, both visually with the Normal Probability Plot and with the Lilliefors test. This last failed for SPS_{TFM} and $P1S_{TT}$ and there were doubts about IMS in general.

The relationship between SNS and the three indexes SPS, IMS and P1S was evaluated with regression methods with the MATLAB Curve Fitting Toolbox. The strength of the relationship was primarily evaluated in terms of R^2. This statistical parameter, multiplied by 100, is usually interpreted as the variance of "y" accounted for by "x", where in this case "y" is SPS or IMS or P1S, and "x" is SNS. In addition, the root-mean-square error (RMSE) of the residuals was also reported.

Distributions were reported in terms of median and interquartile range [3], with box plots. For each symmetry index, the Kruskal-Wallis test ($\alpha = 0.05$) was adopted to check for overall statistically significant differences among TFM, TFC, TT and Controls. In identifying pairwise differences, the Tukey-Kramer "HSD" correction was applied within the MATLAB "multcompare" function.

Results

Gait speed was compared among TFM (1.12 ± 0.13 m/s), TFC (1.17 ± 0.12 m/s), TT (1.23 ± 0.19 m/s) and Controls (1.41 ± 0.21 m/s). ANOVA did not show statistically significant differences among amputees ($p = 0.14$), but only between Controls and amputees ($p = 0.0005$).

Further results are reported hereinafter based on their relevance for questions Q1-Q6.

Question Q1

Figure 1 reports the number of subjects in subgroups *Two-Peaks*, which decreases from TT (20/23), to TFM (7/12) to TFC (10/25). The number of TFC with non-standard GRF is remarkably high (60%); these patients report a consistent "alternative" pattern (example provided in Fig. 1b). Based on these results, the answer to Q1 was negative and the calculation of the symmetry index P1S was restricted to the subjects in *Two-Peaks*.

Question Q2

Figure 2 reports the regression analysis for SPS vs SNS considering the whole set of patients and Controls ("ALL" in brief). R^2 and RMSE values for each group

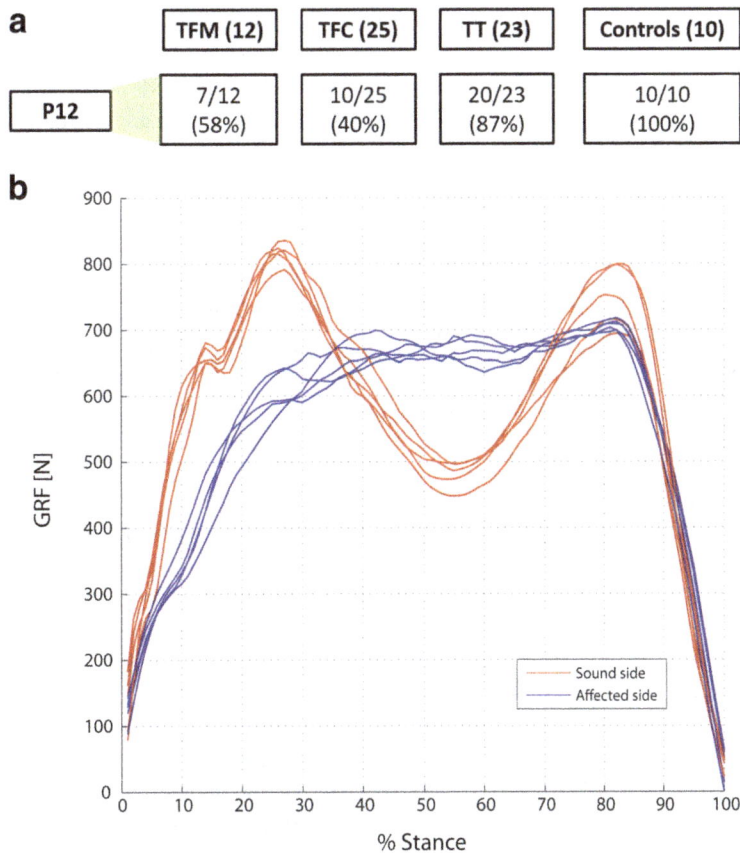

Fig. 1 a Number of subjects in subgroup *Two-Peaks* for TFM (transfemoral mechanical knee users), TFC (transfemoral C-leg users), TT (transtibial amputees), and Controls: b typical alternative vertical ground reaction force pattern shown by TFC patients not included in *Two-Peaks*

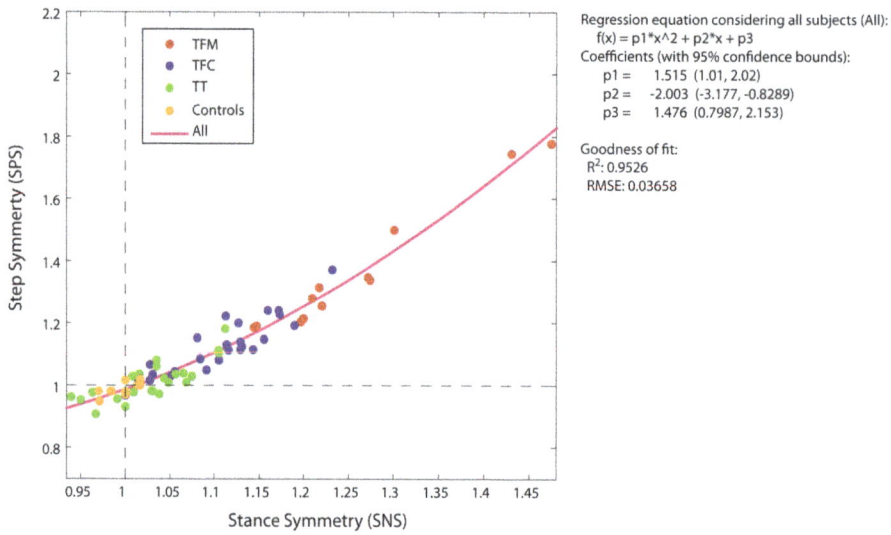

Fig. 2 Step symmetry index (SPS) vs Stance symmetry index (SNS). Each dot represents one subject. Subjects of the same group feature the same color (see legend in the plot). The purple parabolic line is the regression line for ALL subjects together. The equation of the fitting is reported on the right, with the fitting quality parameters R^2 (coefficient of determination) and RMSE (Root Mean Squared Error)

(TFM, TFC, TT, Controls) and ALL are reported in Table 2. R^2 was at least 0.70 for all amputees, with RMSE < 0.042. Therefore, the answer to Q2 was positive and only SPS was further considered.

Question Q3

Figure 3a and b report the regression analysis for IMS vs SNS and P1S vs SNS, respectively, for ALL. R^2 and RMSE values for each group (TFM, TFC, TT, Controls) and ALL are reported in Table 2. For IMS vs SNS, R^2 was lower than 0.64 for TT, with RMSE > 0.128. For P1S vs SNS, R^2 was lower than 0.2 for all amputees. Therefore, the answer to Q3 was negative and IMS, P1S and SPS were separately considered in all subsequent analyses.

Table 2 Quality of fit of the regressions for step (SPS), impulse (IMS) and first peak symmetry (P1S) indexes vs stance symmetry index (SNS)

	SPS vs SNS		IMS vs SNS		P1S vs SNS	
	R^2	RMSE	R^2	RMSE	R^2	RMSE
TFM	**0,97**	**0,042**	**0,81**	**0,137**	*0,06*	*0,154*
TFC	**0,81**	**0,042**	**0,69**	**0,090**	*0,04*	*0,177*
TT	**0,70**	**0,036**	0,37	0,128	*0,20*	*0,289*
CONTROLS	0,51	0,017	0,47	0,040	*0,05*	*0,038*
ALL	**0,95**	**0,037**	**0,79**	**0,103**	*0,00*	*0,247*

The coefficient of determination (R^2), and the Root Mean Squared Error (RMSE) are reported for every group (*TFM* transfemoral mechanical knee users, *TFC* transfemoral C-leg users, *TT* transtibial amputees, Controls), and for all subjects altogether (ALL). Bold: $R^2 > 0.64$, Regular: $0.36 < R^2 < 0.64$, Italic: $R^2 < 0.36$ [30]

Questions Q4-Q6

Figures 4a, 5a and 6a report the distribution of SNS, IMS and P1S for TFC, TFC, TT and Controls. Numerical values are reported in Table 3.

For SNS and IMS, the Kruskal-Wallis test showed statistically significant differences among the medians of the groups ($p < 0.0001$) (Figs. 4b and 5b). The pairwise analyses for:

- SNS (Fig. 4c) showed that all amputee groups are different among each other, supporting a positive answer for *Q4 and Q5*;
- IMS (Fig. 5c) showed a statistically significant difference between TFM and all other groups, with all TFM values > 1 as opposed to TFC and TT. This supports a partially positive answer to *Q4*, a positive answer to *Q5* and a negative answer to *Q6*.

For P1S, the Kruskal-Wallis test reported a statistically significant difference in the medians among groups ($p = 0.0443$) (Fig. 6b). The pairwise comparison did not show differences (Fig. 6c). This is a very possible situation for three reasons:

- the Kruskal-Wallis and pairwise comparisons try to negate different hypotheses;
- we applied a quite conservative multiple comparison strategy (HSD);
- the statistical power is reduced by the decreased number of transfemoral amputees (TF) within *Two-Peaks*.

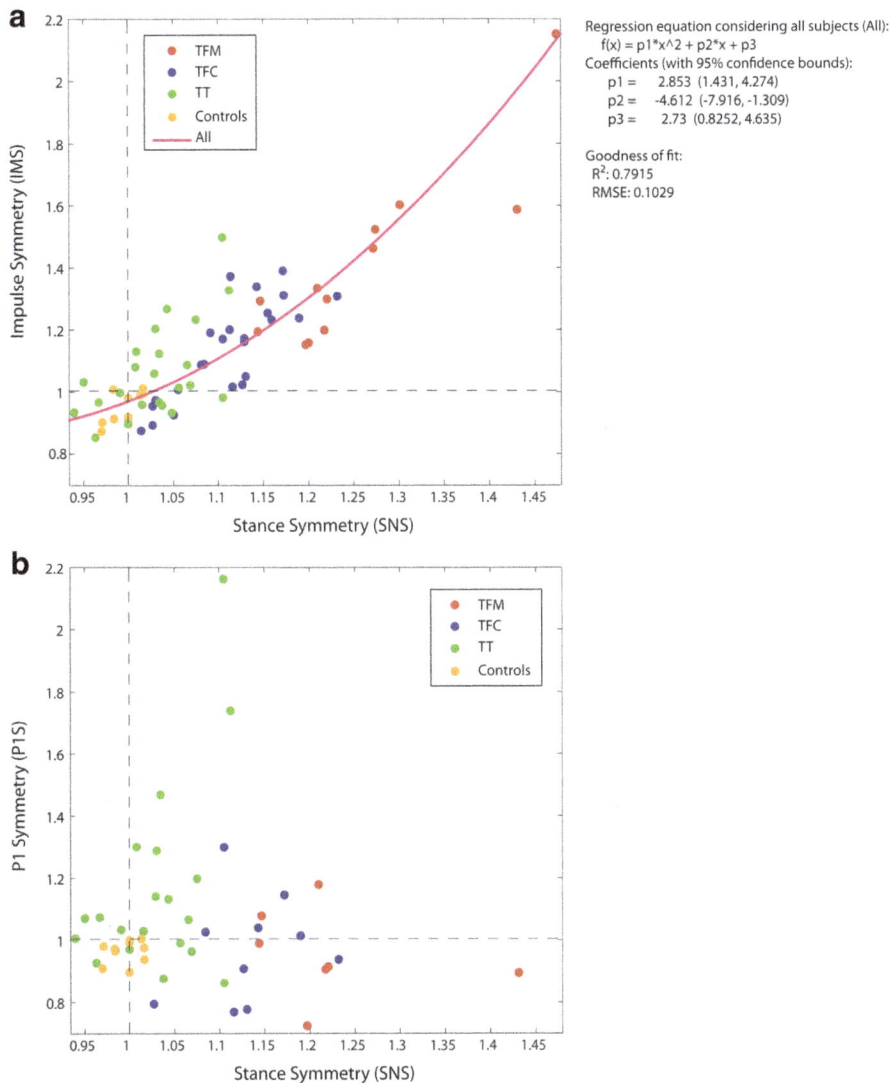

Fig. 3 a Impulse symmetry index (IMS) vs Stance symmetry index (SNS) and **b** First peak symmetry index (P1S) vs SNS. Each dot represents a subject. Subjects of the same group feature the same color (see legend in the plot). In (**a**), the purple parabolic line is the regression line for ALL subjects together. The equation of the fitting is reported on the right, with the fitting quality parameters R^2 (coefficient of determination) and RMSE (Root Mean Squared Error). No valid regression was found for P1S vs SNS. TFM: transfemoral mechanical knee users, TFC: transfemoral C-leg users, TT: transtibial amputees

For this reason, we grouped subjects per level of amputation (TFM and TFC together), and results are reported in Fig. 7a. The Kruskal-Wallis test now shows a stronger significance among groups ($p = 0.0186$) and the pairwise analysis shows a statistically significant difference between TF and TT. The variability in P1S is much higher in amputees than in Controls (Bartlett's test for equal variances, $p = 0.001$). These results support a negative answer to Q6.

Discussion

In this study, we addressed three methodological and three clinical questions regarding the temporal and loading symmetry of transfemoral amputees (both mechanical and C-leg users) and transtibial amputees, to support in the

development of more targeted rehabilitation goals, that are particularly needed [9, 38].

As a general consideration, the self-selected walking speed was not statistically different among amputees, despite a slight increase in the median from TFM, to TFC, to TT toward Controls. Absolute values compare well with previously reported data [2, 7, 39].

For the sake of clarity, results are discussed below for each question, in comparison with the available literature whenever possible.

Question Q1

Question Q1 asked if all amputees show the typical M-shaped pattern of the GRF, with presence and

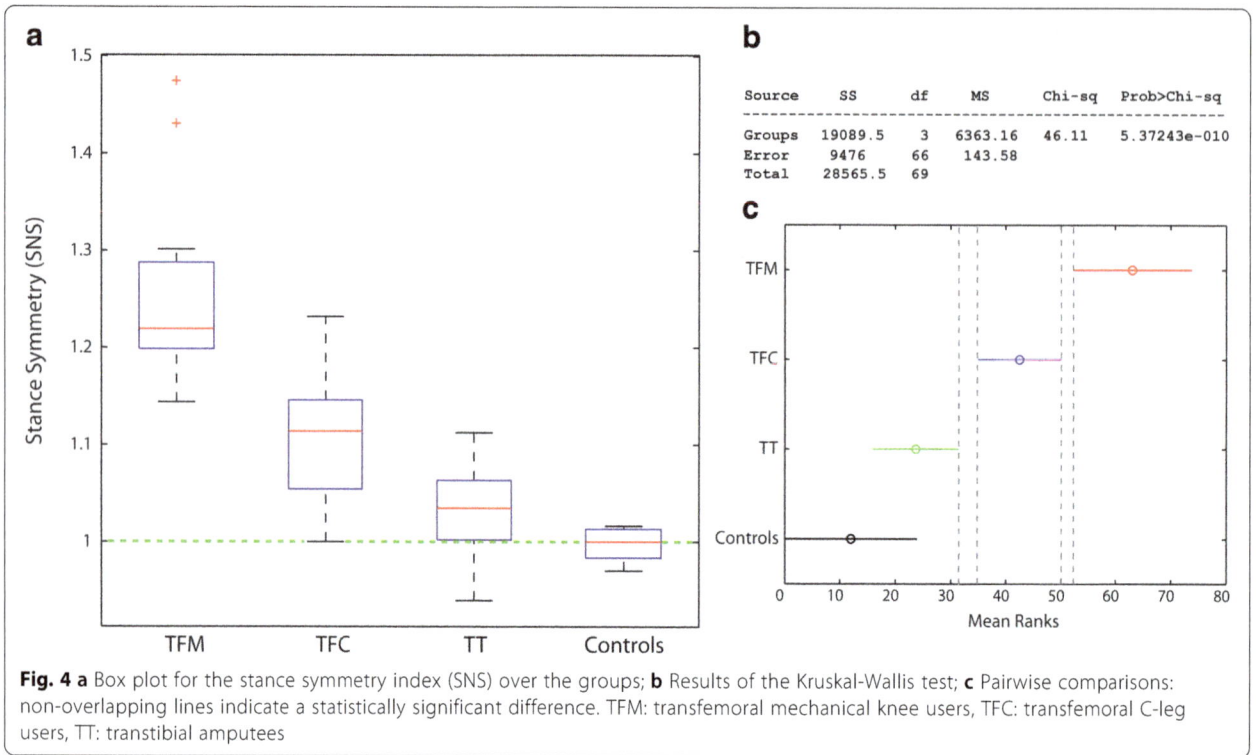

Fig. 4 a Box plot for the stance symmetry index (SNS) over the groups; **b** Results of the Kruskal-Wallis test; **c** Pairwise comparisons: non-overlapping lines indicate a statistically significant difference. TFM: transfemoral mechanical knee users, TFC: transfemoral C-leg users, TT: transtibial amputees

appropriate timing of its two peaks. Results support a negative answer.

As previously noted, this is particularly evident for TFC, who presented a consistent "alternative" pattern: after a steep rise (initial contact/loading response), GRF shows a

further (almost) monotonical increase (midstance), after which it drops (terminal stance/pre-swing). TFM falling out of *Two-Peaks* did not present this pattern, and were typically not included in *Two-Peaks* due to a delayed P1 after 40% of the stance phase. Since no kinematic and

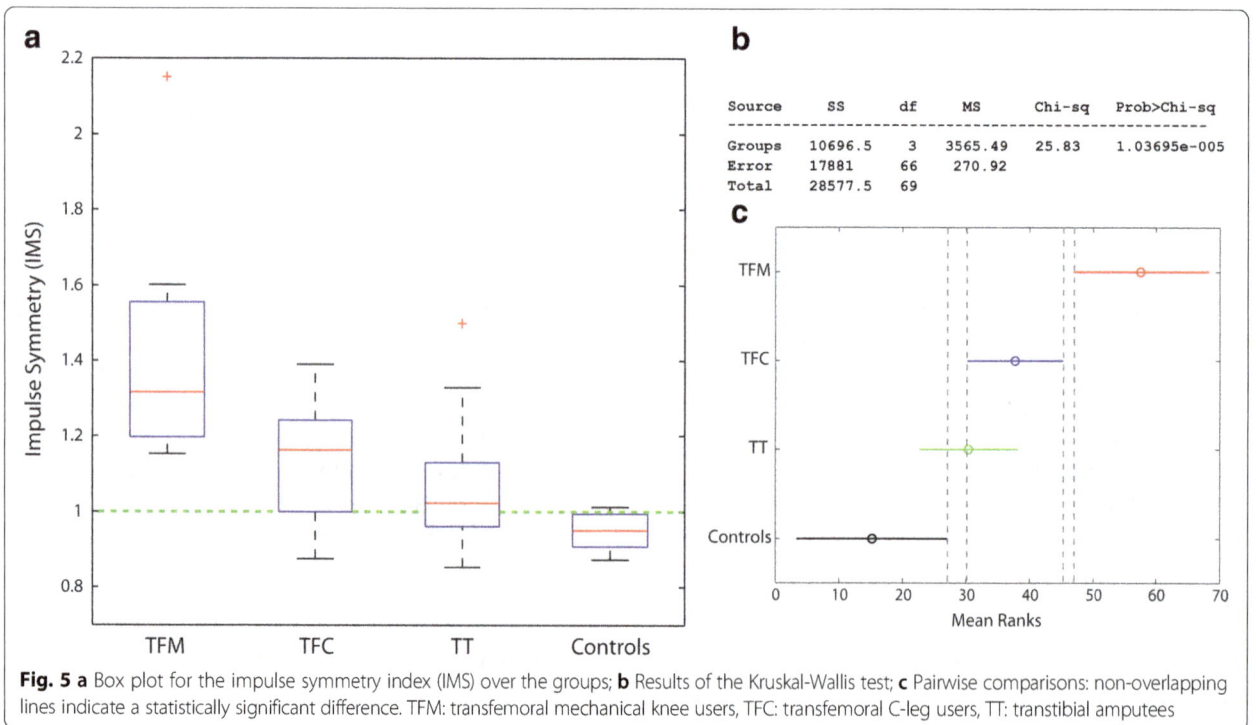

Fig. 5 a Box plot for the impulse symmetry index (IMS) over the groups; **b** Results of the Kruskal-Wallis test; **c** Pairwise comparisons: non-overlapping lines indicate a statistically significant difference. TFM: transfemoral mechanical knee users, TFC: transfemoral C-leg users, TT: transtibial amputees

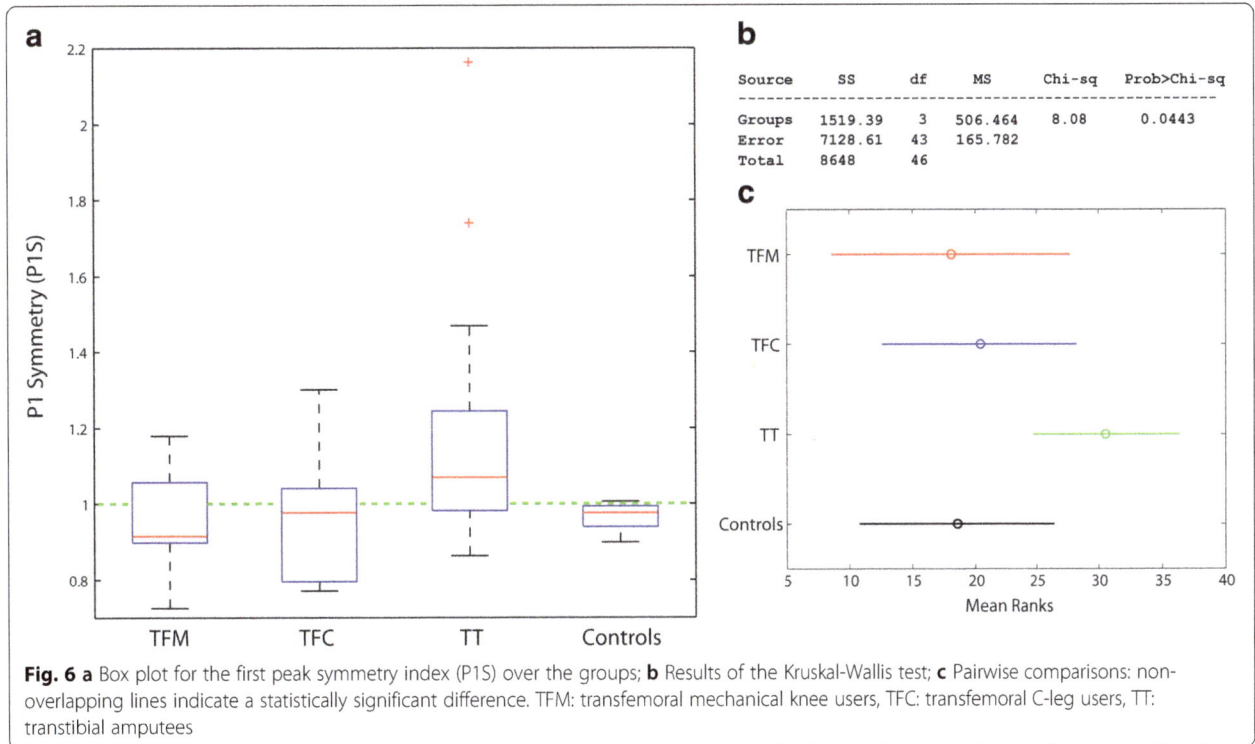

Fig. 6 a Box plot for the first peak symmetry index (P1S) over the groups; **b** Results of the Kruskal-Wallis test; **c** Pairwise comparisons: non-overlapping lines indicate a statistically significant difference. TFM: transfemoral mechanical knee users, TFC: transfemoral C-leg users, TT: transtibial amputees

kinetic data were collected, we can just speculate that this TFC pattern is the combined effect of:

- the Variflex behavior, with strong energy storage in loading response [25, 26];
- C-leg knee flexion in loading response [40];
- the confidence gained by this group of amputees on the capacity of the C-leg to sustain them at heel-strike and loading response, with no need to force extension.

The ultimate effect for this pattern is a "soft landing" on the prosthetic side, which might increase comfort [32]. These speculations require future experimental confirmations, but match well with previous evidences that only a fraction of transfemoral amputees can fully

rely on C-leg stability despite knee flexion during early stance [32, 40]. This might be the effect of a specialized rehabilitation.

Question Q2

Question Q2 asked if we can limit the study of temporal symmetry to stance leaving out step symmetry. Results support a positive answer.

The regression of SPS vs SNS for each group and for ALL was quadratic, with excellent fits.

SNS explained from 70 to 97% of the variance in SPS data in amputees (R^2, as reported in Table 2). Even for Controls, who feature a very small peak-to-peak SNS (.97 to 1.01), the explained SPS variance is 50% with a RMSE as small as 0.017.

Table 3 Numerical values for the indexes of symmetry SNS (stance), IMS (impulse) and P1S (first peak)

	SNS				IMS				P1S			
	Median	25th	75th	IQR	Median	25th	75th	IQR	Median	25th	75th	IQR
TFM	1,22	1,20	1,29	0,09	1,32	1,20	1,55	0,36	0,91	0,90	1,06	0,16
TFC	1,11	1,05	1,15	0,09	1,16	1,00	1,24	0,24	0,98	0,80	1,04	0,24
TF									0,94	0,87	1,05	0,18
TT	1,03	1,00	1,06	0,06	1,02	0,96	1,13	0,17	1,07	0,98	1,24	0,26
CONTROLS	1,02	0,98	1,01	0,03	0,95	0,91	0,99	0,09	0,98	0,94	0,99	0,05

For each group, the median is reported together with the 25th, 75th and interquartile range (IQR). *TFM* transfemoral mechanical knee users, *TFC* transfemoral C-leg users, *TF* transfemoral, *TT* transtibial amputees

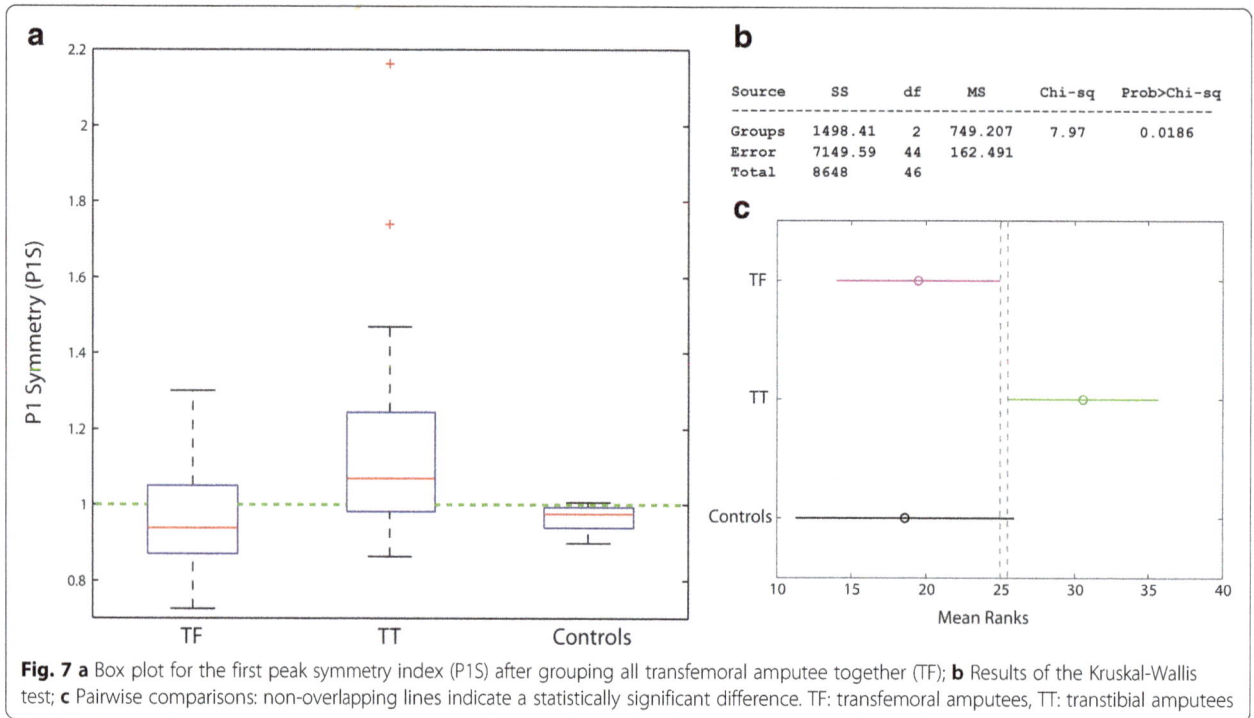

Fig. 7 a Box plot for the first peak symmetry index (P1S) after grouping all transfemoral amputee together (TF); **b** Results of the Kruskal-Wallis test; **c** Pairwise comparisons: non-overlapping lines indicate a statistically significant difference. TF: transfemoral amputees, TT: transtibial amputees

This is the first time that the SPS vs SNS regression is reported in the literature and that a quadratic relationship is described. The nonlinear fit is not surprising, because SPS is non-linearly related to the interplay of 1) the sounds and affected side stance durations and 2) the two double support durations. The quadratic fit stresses the importance of stance time symmetry, since it influences step asymmetry by a factor 2.

Question Q3

Question Q3 asked if the study of gait symmetry can be limited to just stance temporal symmetry, leaving out loading symmetry. Results support a negative answer.

When IMS vs SNS was examined considering the full set of subjects, a quadratic fit emerged: SNS explained as much as 79% of the variance in IMS. This is the first time this relationship is examined and reported. Since IMS is the integral of GRF over the stance phase, it is not surprising that IMS and SNS are related: a high stance time asymmetry is a leading factor for a high impulse asymmetry. However, GRF magnitude does not linearly increase with time, and has a shape which can differ between the sound and affected side. When all these elements become part of a ratio, it is not surprising that the relation between IMS and SNS can be non-linear.

This conclusion is valid for TFM and TFC at group level too, given the $R^2 > 0.64$. However, this is just partially true for TT, because R^2 decreases to 0.37 and

the RMSE is high (0.128): reporting SNS and not IMS can be misleading. This different evidence for TT can be ascribed to two factors only:

- The improvement in SNS asymmetry (1.03, IQR 0.06) compared to TFM (1.22, IQR 0.09) and TFC (1.11, IQR 0.09) (Table 3);
- A greater *asymmetry* in GRF magnitude between sides. This is supported by the evidences for P1S, as reported in Fig. 7. Further discussions are postponed to *Q6* below.

An adequate regression for P1S vs SNS was not found for none of the groups and ALL: the two indexes must measure different construct and therefore they must be separately reported.

Question Q4

Question Q4 asked if gait symmetry depends on the level of amputation. Results support a positive answer.

With reference to SNS, all amputee groups had statistically different median values. All TF spend more time on the sound side: TFM have the highest asymmetry (median asymmetry of 22%), which is twofold the TFC's (11%). As can be seen in Fig. 4, this is also true for 75% of TT, which means that ¼ of TT do spend more time on the *affected side*. This was never clearly reported in the literature. The TT asymmetry (3%) is 4 times less than TFC. Controls, in median, have a perfect symmetry, with a IQR of just 3%.

The SNS median for TFC (1.11) compares well with the median SNS that can be calculated from the results reported in [3] (1.09). Furthermore, our results can be compared with the study of Nolan et al. [2], that involved 4 transfemoral and 4 transtibial amputees using a single hinge knee and a SACH foot. Once appropriately converted to our indexes, Nolan's results are reported in Table 4. Results, can also be compared with Bateni et al. [41], which reported a mean stance asymmetry for TT of about 7% (calculated as the ratio of the mean between sides). Compared to these studies, our SNS values are lower. In particular, 63% of TT and 20% of TFC have a SNS lower than ±5%, which makes them unperceived by others as "impaired" walkers with regard to temporal symmetry [21]. This is not surprising given the different prosthetic components used and the fact that our patients followed a specialized rehabilitation training. Our SNS results for TT are also in very good agreement with results reported by Jarvis et al. [38] for young veterans (median 1.04, IQR = 0.03). For TFC, our SNS is higher (1.11 compared to 0.98) but the IQR is much smaller (0.09 compared to 0.20). This remarks that the training for transfemoral amputees is more challenging.

When looking at IMS, the TFM median was statistically different from TFC and TT: TFM asymmetry is *twice* that of TFC and *16 times* TT's. The comparison with Nolan et al. [2] is striking: our TFM had an impulse asymmetry which is half Nolan's; for TT it is 10 times less. This result points, again, in the direction of the benefits of energy-storage-and-return feet and more advanced knees. Improvement in loading asymmetry with energy-storage-and-return feet and feet with improved roll-over shape has been previously reported in [25, 27, 42], and match well with simulation studies [8].

Finally, P1S results show statistically significant differences between TF and TT (Fig. 7). About 59% of TF have a higher peak on the *prosthetic side*. Our results agree with Castro et al., which did not report an increased peak GRF on the sound side, but rather an increase in the GRF impulse. TT clearly show an asymmetric loading with higher values for the sound side (70% of patients), but 3 times less

than that reported by Nolan and co-workers. As previously reported, it is reasonable to ascribe this improvement to the use of energy-storage-and-return feet compared to SACH [27, 43].

Question Q5

Question Q5 asked if advanced prosthetic components improve temporal and loading symmetry, and if C-leg users have better results than mechanical knee users of the same mobility level. Results support a positive answer.

Results have been partially discussed while addressing Q1 and Q4 and can be summarized stating that TFC were statistically different from TFM for SNS and IMS. Results for IMS bring TFC to undistinguishable results to TT.

Also, the C-leg in combination with Variflex triggers a new GRF pattern that possibly ensures an increased comfort during walking (Question Q1). This requires further experimental confirmations.

Petersen et al. [44] have previously reported about SNS in C-leg users compared to TFM. However, that study was not able to prove a statistically significant improvement but just a trend, probably due to the small number of subjects included (5) with different amputation etiologies. Our results confirm that trend, with statistically significant differences. More generally, a considerable body of knowledge is available about the positive effects of the C-leg on amputees' mobility [31, 45–47], gait kinematic [32–40], kinetic [39] and step-length symmetry [32]. Our findings match well with this general trend toward improved symmetries.

As discussed in Q4, the comparison of the literature with our results for TT suggests a possible positive effect of energy-storage-and-return feet in comparison with SACH, for all the indexes of symmetry.

Question Q6

Question Q6 asked if it is always true that amputees overload the sound side both in terms of first peak and impulse of GRF, thus contributing to the development of osteoarthritis. Results support a negative answer.

As previously discussed about Q4, if we focus on IMS, 100% of TFM overload the *sound side*. This percentage decreases to 75% of TFC and 57% of TT. If we look at P1S, 41% TF load more the *sound side*. However, this percentage rises to 70% for TT. Based on these different percentages of TT and TF for IMS and P1S, it could be argued that two different mechanisms might be related to knee osteoarthritis for the two groups: peak overload for TT (measured by P1S), and extended duration of force action (impulse) for TF (measured by IMS). Given the higher prevalence of knee osteoarthritis in TF compared to TT [5, 10], it might be speculated that the second mechanism is more detrimental than the first.

Table 4 Results from Nolan et al. [2], converted to the indexes of symmetry used in this study. SNS (stance), IMS (impulse) and P1S (first peak)

	SNS	IMS	P1S
TFM	1,27	1,69	1,22
TT	1,05	1,36	1,25
CONTROLS	1,03	1,08	1,08

Having named *N* the indexes in [2], the new values follow from this equation: $New = (2 + N)/(2-N)$

TFM transfemoral mechanical knee users, *TT* transtibial amputees

Conclusions

In the Introduction, we posed three methodological and three clinical questions regarding the gait temporal and loading symmetry of lower-limb amputees. Based on the results collected on traumatic, K3-K4, transfemoral (mechanical knees and C-leg users) and transtibial patients successfully fit and trained in using their prosthesis, we can answer as follows.

The three *methodological* questions wanted to establish a minimum set of symmetry indexes to study and if there are limitations in their calculations. *First*, the first peak of the vertical ground reaction force at loading response cannot be clearly identified in all amputees, and the calculation of its index of symmetry was limited to patients with the typical M-Shaped pattern of the ground reaction force. *Second*, the analysis of temporal symmetry can be limited to stance, leaving out step symmetry. *Third*, stance, impulse and first peak symmetries should be separately reported.

The three *clinical* questions wanted to establish if "typical" levels of temporal and loading symmetry exist and change with the level of amputation and prosthetic components. *First*, the symmetries of stance, impulse and first peak are all influenced by the level of amputation. In particular, the time spent on the sound side decreases significantly from transfemoral mechanical knee users, to C-leg users, to transtibial patients. The impulse on the sound side decreases significantly from mechanical knee users to C-leg and transtibial patients. Transtibial patients have a higher first peak at loading response on their sound side, while most transfemoral patients do not. *Second*, advanced prosthetic component seem to positively influence the temporal and loading symmetry. In particular, the C-leg in combination with the Vari-flex foot improves stance, impulse symmetry and for about 60% of patients smooths the first peak at loading response. About 20% of C-leg users have a stance asymmetry which is below the level of perceived impaired gait, compared to 0% of mechanical knee users. For transtibial patients, comparisons of our results with the literature point toward an improvement of all indexes of symmetry, possibly due to the use of energy-storage-and-return feet instead of SACH feet. *Third*, it is not always true that amputees overload the sound side. Percentagewise, transfemoral amputees tend to overload the sound side with increased impulse, while TT with increased peak GRF. This might be suggestive of two separate mechanisms for the onset of knee osteoarthritis.

We think that our results can be exploited in the clinical routine. *First*, clinicians can use our results to set reasonable targets for rehabilitation. Specifically, they can compare the level of symmetry of a new patient with the ranges provided, and put the patient's performance and advancements during rehabilitation in perspective. Moreover, technical and healthcare professionals might use our findings to compare the effect of different prosthetic components and potentially the effect of different rehabilitation programs. *Second*, it is often required by payers (e.g. insurances, public healthcare services, or patients), to justify the use of advanced prosthetic components. We think that our results support the use of C-leg and energy-storage-and-return feet on K3-K4 traumatic patients: thanks to the improvement in temporal and loading symmetry compared to mechanical knees and SACH foot, these components can potentially have a positive effect on the asymmetry-related comorbidities analyzed in the Introduction and decrease social stigma. Further research is required to extend these results to other groups of patients, such as K2 and non-traumatic amputees. *Finally*, our results might suggest possible strategies to mitigate knee osteoarthritis of the sound side. Pending further research, transfemoral amputees might take advantage of prosthetic components with an improved knee-foot coordination to specifically tackle stance time asymmetry. Transtibial patients might benefit from improved socket construction that does not limit knee extension, and prosthetic feet with improved push-off, roll-over shape and range of motion to reduce the first peak at loading response.

Funding
This research was conducted with internal institutional funds of INAIL. The publication cost of this article was funded by the American Orthotic & Prosthetic Association (AOPA).

Authors' contributions
AGC, MR and GV designed the experiment. MR and AGC collected and processed the data. All Authors contributed to data analysis and manuscript preparation. All authors read and approved the final manuscript.

Competing interests
The authors declare that they have no competing interests.

References
1. Winter DA, Sienko SE. Biomechanics of below-knee amputee gait. J Biomech. 1988;21(5):361-7.
2. Nolan L, Wit A, Dudziñski K, Lees A, Lake M, Wychowañski M. Adjustments in gait symmetry with walking speed in trans-femoral and trans-tibial amputees. Gait Posture. 2003;17(2):142-51.
3. Schmid M, Beltrami G, Zambarbieri D, Verni G. Centre of pressure displacements in trans-femoral amputees during gait. Gait Posture. 2005; 21(3):255-62.
4. Hof AL, van Bockel RM, Schoppen T, Postema K. Control of lateral balance in walking. Experimental findings in normal subjects and above-knee amputees. Gait Posture. 2007;25(2):250-8.
5. Gailey R, Allen K, Castles J, Kucharik J, Roeder M. Review of secondary physical conditions associated with lower-limb amputation and long-term prosthesis use. J Rehabil Res Dev. 2008;45(1):15-29.

6. Castro MP, Soares D, Mendes E, Machado L. Plantar pressures and ground reaction forces during walking of individuals with unilateral transfemoral amputation. PM&R. 2014;6(8):698–707.

7. Wezenberg D, Cutti AG, Bruno A, Houdijk H. Differentiation between solid-ankle cushioned heel and energy storage and return prosthetic foot based on step-to-step transition cost. J Rehabil Res Dev. 2014;51(10):1579–90.

8. Adamczyk PG, Kuo AD. Mechanisms of gait asymmetry due to push-off deficiency in unilateral amputees. IEEE Trans Neural Syst Rehabil Eng. 2015; 23(5):776–85.

9. Highsmith MJ, Andrews CR, Millman C, Fuller A, Kahle JT, Klenow TD, Lewis KL, Bradley RC, Orriola JJ. Gait training interventions for lower extremity amputees: a systematic literature review. Technol Innov. 2016;18(2–3):99–113.

10. Morgenroth DC, Gellhorn AC, Suri P. Osteoarthritis in the disabled population: a mechanical perspective. PM&R. 2012;4(5 Suppl):S20–7.

11. Vanicek N, Strike S, McNaughton L, Polman R. Gait patterns in transtibial amputee fallers vs. non-fallers: biomechanical differences during level walking. Gait Posture. 2009;29(3):415–20.

12. Norvell DC, Czerniecki JM, Reiber GE, Maynard C, Pecoraro JA, Weiss NS. The prevalence of knee pain and symptomatic knee osteoarthritis among veteran traumatic amputees and nonamputees. Arch Phys Med Rehabil. 2005;86:487–93.

13. Struyf PA, van Heugten CM, Hitters MW, Smeets RJ. The prevalence of osteoarthritis of the intact hip and knee among traumatic leg amputees. Arch Phys Med Rehabil. 2009;90:440–6.

14. Lemaire ED, Fisher FR. Osteoarthritis and elderly amputee gait. Arch Phys Med Rehabil. 1994;75(10):1094–9.

15. Burke MJ, Roman V, Wright V. Bone and joint changes in lower limb amputees. Ann Rheum Dis. 1978;37(3):252–4.

16. Rush PJ, Wong JS, Kirsh J, Devlin M. Osteopenia in patients with above knee amputation. Arch Phys Med Rehabil. 1994;75(1):112–5.

17. Shojaei I, Hendershot BD, Wolf EJ, Bazrgari B. Persons with unilateral transfemoral amputation experience larger spinal loads during level-ground walking compared to able-bodied individuals. Clin Biomech (Bristol, Avon). 2016;32:157–63. https://doi.org/10.1016/j.clinbiomech.2015.11.018.

18. Yoder AJ, Petrella AJ, Silverman AK. Trunk-pelvis motion, joint loads, and muscle forces during walking with a transtibial amputation. Gait Posture. 2015;41(3):757–62.

19. Russell Esposito E, Wilken JM. The relationship between pelvis-trunk coordination and low back pain in individuals with transfemoral amputations. Gait Posture. 2014;40(4):640–6.

20. Rabuffetti M, Recalcati M, Ferrarin M. Trans-femoral amputee gait: socket-pelvis constraints and compensation strategies. Prosthetics Orthot Int. 2005; 29(2):183–92.

21. Handžić I, Reed KB. Perception of gait patterns that deviate from normal and symmetric biped locomotion. Front Psychol. 2015;6:199.

22. Marinakis GN. Interlimb symmetry of traumatic unilateral transtibial amputees wearing two different prosthetic feet in the early rehabilitation stage. J Rehabil Res Dev. 2004;41(4):581–90.

23. Esquenazi A. Gait analysis in lower-limb amputation and prosthetic rehabilitation. Phys Med Rehabil Clin N Am. 2014;25(1):153–67.

24. Hof AL. The 'extrapolated center of mass' concept suggests a simple control of balance in walking. Hum Mov Sci. 2008;27(1):112–25.

25. Powers MC, Torburn L, Perry J, Ayyappa E. Influence of prosthetic foot design on sound limb loading in adults with unilateral below-knee amputations. Arch Phys Med Rehabil. 1994;75(7):825–9.

26. Snyder RD, Powers CM, Fountain C, Perry J. The effect of five prosthetic feet on the gait and loading of the sound limb in dysvascular below-knee amputees. J Rehabil Res Dev. 1995;32:309–15.

27. Hansen AH, Meier MR, Sessoms PH, Childress DS. The effects of prosthetic foot roll-over shape arc length on the gait of trans-tibial prosthesis users. Prosthetics Orthot Int. 2006;30(3):286–99.

28. Gard SA. Use of quantitative gait analysis for the evaluation of prosthetic walking performance. J Prosthet Orthot. 2006;18(6):P93–P104.

29. Perry J, Burnfield J. Gait analysis: normal and pathological function: Thorofare: SALCK Inc.; 2010.

30. Evans JD. Straightforward statistics for the behavioral sciences. Pacific Grove: Brooks/Cole Publishing; 1996.

31. Cutti AG, Lettieri E, Del Maestro M, Radaelli G, Luchetti M, Verni G, Masella C. Stratified cost-utility analysis of C-leg versus mechanical knees: findings from an Italian sample of transfemoral amputees. Prosthetics Orthot Int. 2017;41(3):227–36.

32. Segal AD, Orendurff MS, Klute GK, McDowell ML, Pecoraro JA, Shofer J, Czerniecki JM. Kinematic and kinetic comparisons of transfemoral amputee gait using C-leg and Mauch SNS prosthetic knees. J Rehabil Res Dev. 2006; 43(7):857–70.

33. Putti AB, Arnold GP, Cochrane L, Abboud RJ. The Pedar in-shoe system: repeatability and normal pressure values. Gait Posture. 2007;25(3):401–5.

34. Hurkmans HL, Bussmann JB, Benda E, Verhaar JA, Stam HJ. Accuracy and repeatability of the Pedar Mobile system in long-term vertical force measurements. Gait Posture. 2006;23(1):118–25.

35. Dekel S, Weissman SL. Joint changes after overuse and peak overloading of rabbit knees in vivo. Acta Orthop Scand. 1978;49(6):519–28.

36. Guilak F. Biomechanical factors in osteoarthritis. Best Pract Res Clin Rheumatol. 2011;25(6):815–23.

37. Buckwalter JA, Anderson DD, Brown TD, Tochigi Y, Martin JA. The roles of mechanical stresses in the pathogenesis of osteoarthritis: implications for treatment of joint injuries. Cartilage. 2013;4(4):286–94.

38. Jarvis HL, Bennett AN, Twiste M, Phillip RD, Etherington J, Baker R. Temporal spatial and metabolic measures of walking in highly functional individuals with lower limb amputations. Arch Phys Med Rehabil. 2016;98(7):1389–99.

39. Kaufman KR, Frittoli S, Frigo CA. Gait asymmetry of transfemoral amputees using mechanical and microprocessor-controlled prosthetic knees. Clin Biomech (Bristol, Avon). 2012;27(5):460–5.

40. Kaufman KR, Levine JA, Brey RH, Iverson BK, McCrady SK, Padgett DJ, Joyner MJ. Gait and balance of transfemoral amputees using passive mechanical and microprocessor-controlled prosthetic knees. Gait Posture. 2007;26(4):489–93.

41. Bateni H, Olney SJ. Kinematic and kinetic variations of below-knee amputee gait. J Prosthet Orthot. 2004;14(1):2–10.

42. Underwood HA, Tokuno CD, Eng JJ. A comparison of two prosthetic feet on the multi-joint and multi-plane kinetic gait compensations in individuals with a unilateral trans-tibial amputation. Clin Biomech (Bristol, Avon). 2004;19:609–16.

43. Lehmann JF, Price R, Boswell-Bessette S, Dralle A, Questad K, deLateur BJ. Comprehensive analysis of energy storing prosthetic feet: flex foot and Seattle foot versus standard SACH foot. Arch Phys Med Rehabil. 1993;74(11):1225–31.

44. Petersen AO, Comins J, Alkjær T. Assessment of gait symmetry in transfemoral amputees using C-leg compared with 3R60 prosthetic knees. J Prosthet Orthot. 2010;22(2):106–12.

45. Hahn A, Lang M. Effects of mobility grade, age, and etiology on functional benefit and safety of subjects evaluated in more than 1200 C-leg trial fittings in Germany. J Prosthet Orthot. 2015;27(3):86–94.

46. Hafner BJ, Willingham LL, Buell NC, Allyn KJ, Smith DG. Evaluation of function, performance, and preference as transfemoral amputees transition from mechanical to microprocessor control of the prosthetic knee. Arch Phys Med Rehabil. 2007;88(2):207–17. Erratum in: Arch Phys Med Rehabil. 2007 Apr;88(4):544

47. Highsmith MJ, Kahle JT, Bongiorni DR, Sutton BS, Groer S, Kaufman KR. Safety, energy efficiency, and cost efficacy of the C-leg for transfemoral amputees: a review of the literature. Prosthetics Orthot Int. 2010;34(4):362–77.

20

The impact of ankle–foot orthoses on toe clearance strategy in hemiparetic gait

Kannit Pongpipatpaiboon[1], Masahiko Mukaino[1*] , Fumihiro Matsuda[2], Kei Ohtsuka[2], Hiroki Tanikawa[2], Junya Yamada[3], Kazuhiro Tsuchiyama[2] and Eiichi Saitoh[1]

Abstract

Background: Ankle–foot orthoses (AFOs) are frequently used to improve gait stability, toe clearance, and gait efficiency in individuals with hemiparesis. During the swing phase, AFOs enhance lower limb advancement by facilitating the improvement of toe clearance and the reduction of compensatory movements. Clinical monitoring via kinematic analysis would further clarify the changes in biomechanical factors that lead to the beneficial effects of AFOs. The purpose of this study was to investigate the actual impact of AFOs on toe clearance, and determine the best strategy to achieve toe clearance (including compensatory movements) during the swing phase.

Methods: This study included 24 patients with hemiparesis due to stroke. The gait performance of these patients with and without AFOs was compared using three-dimensional treadmill gait analysis. A kinematic analysis of the paretic limb was performed to quantify the contribution of the extent of lower limb shortening and compensatory movements (such as hip elevation and circumduction) to toe clearance. The impact of each movement related to toe clearance was assessed by analyzing the change in the vertical direction.

Results: Using AFOs significantly increased toe clearance ($p = 0.038$). The quantified limb shortening and pelvic obliquity significantly differed between gaits performed with versus without AFOs. Among the movement indices related to toe clearance, limb shortening was increased by the use of AFOs ($p < 0.0001$), while hip elevation due to pelvic obliquity (representing compensatory strategies) was diminished by the use of AFOs ($p = 0.003$). The toe clearance strategy was not significantly affected by the stage of the hemiparetic condition (acute versus chronic) or the type of AFO (thermoplastic AFOs versus adjustable posterior strut AFOs).

Conclusions: Simplified three-dimensional gait analysis was successfully used to quantify and visualize the impact of AFOs on the toe clearance strategy of hemiparetic patients. AFO use increased the extent of toe clearance and limb shortening during the swing phase, while reducing compensatory movements. This approach to visualization of the gait strategy possibly contributes to clinical decision-making in the real clinical settings.

Keywords: Orthosis, Hemiplegia, Gait, Rehabilitation, Compensation, Swing phase

* Correspondence: mmukaino@fujita-hu.ac.jp
[1]Department of Rehabilitation Medicine I, School of Medicine, Fujita Health University, 1-98 Dengakugakubo, Kutsukake, Toyoake, Aichi 470-1192, Japan
Full list of author information is available at the end of the article

Background

Impaired paretic limb advancement is a clearly observable manifestation of gait pathology in individuals with hemiparesis due to stroke [1–3]. Previous studies have reported specific gait changes following hemiparesis, such as decreased knee flexion, hip flexion, and ankle dorsiflexion during the swing phase, which can negatively influence the achievement of toe clearance [1–6]. Reduction in toe clearance of the affected limb leads to tripping while walking, which is a major cause of falls [7, 8]. In healthy individuals, toe clearance is mainly achieved by limb shortening, which is affected by hip flexion, knee flexion, and ankle dorsiflexion. On the other hand, to obtain sufficient toe clearance during the swing phase, individuals with hemiparesis often require compensatory strategies that modify the kinematic pattern, including hip hiking and circumduction, which are common gait deviations [3, 9]. These changes during the swing phase have a reciprocal relationship. When the limb shortening is reduced due to paresis, the compensatory movements will be increased to contribute to toe clearance; hence, they are in a trade-off relationship [10].

Ankle–foot orthoses (AFOs) are frequently prescribed to improve walking ability in hemiparetic patients, as they provide passive or dynamic support of ankle movement. AFOs provide support not only during the stance phase of gait by encouraging lateral stability or improving early stance knee moments, but also in the swing phase to maintain ankle dorsiflexion and facilitate toe clearance [11–17]. The effect of AFOs on the swing phase is additionally reflected in the compensatory movements. Cruz et al. [18] demonstrated that the compensatory pelvic obliquity observed in response to impaired ankle dorsiflexion in hemiplegic patients was minimized when the patients wore an AFO. Improved joint motions and decreased compensatory movement when using AFOs could potentially contribute to an efficient gait and promote walking activity in hemiparetic patients.

Clarification of the mechanical effect of AFOs on these gait parameters, and quantifications of compensatory movements would be helpful for clinical decision-making in rehabilitation clinics. For example, understanding the influence of rehabilitative training and the use of AFOs on gait indices (i.e., ankle angle, knee angle, hip elevation, or toe clearance) would help to determine the best rehabilitative strategy and to identify the need for AFO use in individual patients.

The aim of this study was to clarify the mechanical effect of AFOs and to quantify the impact of AFO use on hemiparetic gait pattern during the swing phase, as this information would be helpful for clinical decision-making in rehabilitation clinics. For example, understanding the

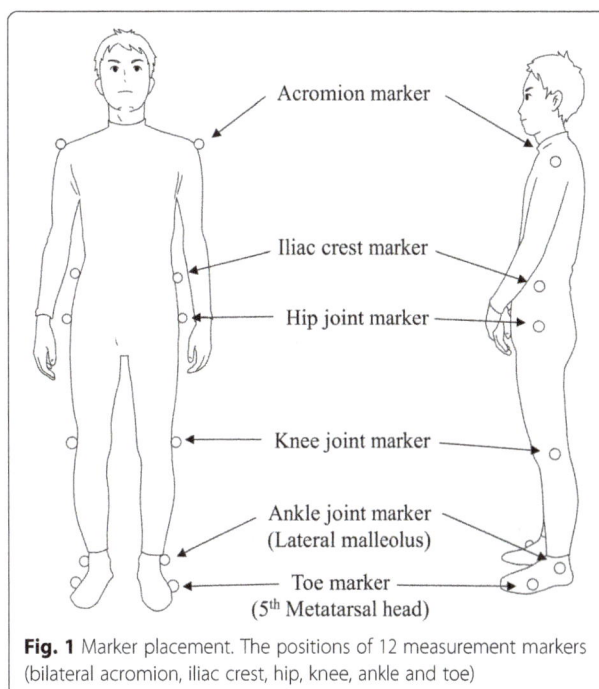

Fig. 1 Marker placement. The positions of 12 measurement markers (bilateral acromion, iliac crest, hip, knee, ankle and toe)

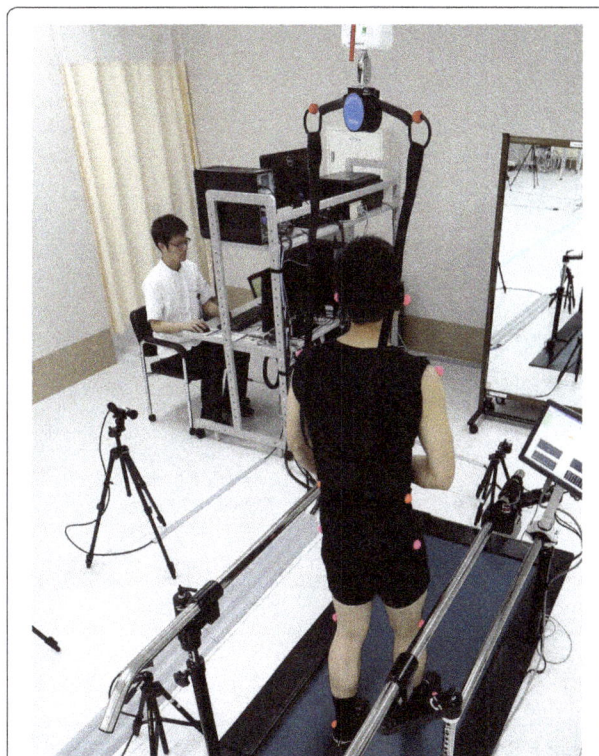

Fig. 2 Measurement using the simplified gait analysis system. The patients walk on the treadmill for the measurement. Safety suspension and a handrail are provided to prevent falls during the measurement

influence of rehabilitative training and the AFO and its types on gait indices (i.e., ankle angle, knee angle, hip elevation, or toe clearance) would help to determine the best rehabilitative strategy and to investigate the need for AFO use in individual patients. Based on a prior study showing the relationship between limb shortening and compensatory movements [10], we hypothesized that the AFOs would positively affect functional limb shortening in a way that would consequently impact on toe clearance and compensatory maneuvers, particularly represented by hip elevation. Previous studies have shown the effects of AFOs and a relationship between limb shortening and compensatory movements. In the normal gait pattern, functional limb shortening (representing lower limb joint movement) is a main strategy for toe clearance. However, patients with hemiparesis have impaired lower limb function, and thus require compensatory strategies (e.g., hip hiking, circumduction of the paretic limb) to promote swing phase propulsion [19, 20]. Additionally, the extent of toe clearance is mainly determined by the extent of functional limb shortening and hip elevation as compensatory movements, which are in a trade-off relationship [10]. AFO usage reduces the gait pattern deviation and increases the walking ability, thereby reducing energy costs [21, 22]. In this study, we hypothesized that the AFOs

would positively affect functional limb shortening in a way that would consequently impact on toe clearance and compensatory maneuvers, particularly represented by hip elevation. To determine the actual impact of limb shortening and compensatory movements on toe clearance, the vertical component of the movements that comprised toe clearance was calculated using three-dimensional kinematic motion analysis. The changes in joint angles were also investigated.

Methods
Participants
Twenty-four patients with post-stroke hemiparesis in either the subacute (time after onset; TAO ≤ 90 days) or chronic (TAO > 90 days) stages who received rehabilitation training at the Fujita Health University Rehabilitation Complex Center were recruited for this study. The study participants were 18 males and 6 females aged 47 ± 19 years (mean ± SD). Eleven patients had right hemiplegia, and 13 had left hemiplegia. The duration of hemiparesis ranged from 1 to 81 months. Nine participants were in the subacute stage, and the remaining 15 participants were in the chronic stage. The participants were evaluated on a range of neurological motor impairments with the

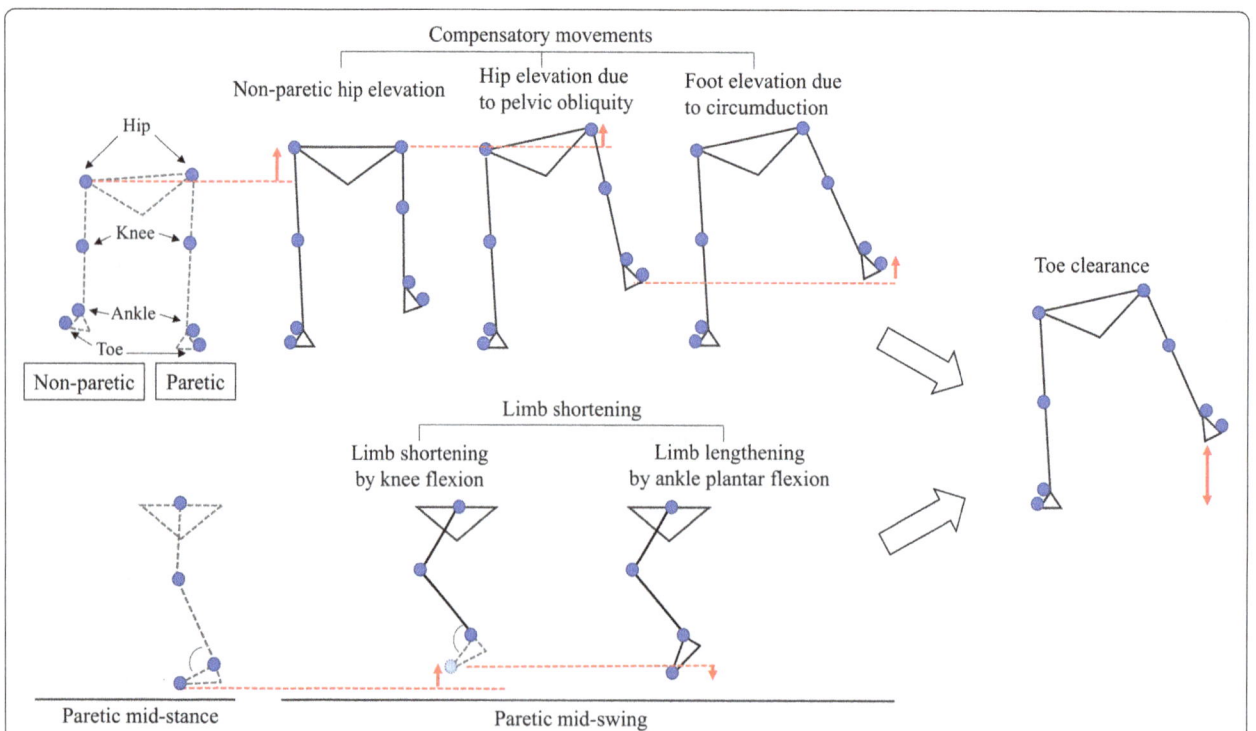

Fig. 3 Schematic diagram of analysis of the components of toe clearance. The two components of limb shortening (limb shortening by knee flexion and limb lengthening by ankle plantar flexion) and the three components of compensatory movements (non-paretic hip elevation, hip elevation due to pelvic obliquity, and foot elevation due to circumduction) are visualized. All indices were calculated from the difference in the vertical position of the markers between the paretic mid-stance and the paretic mid-swing

stroke impairment assessment set (SIAS). In evaluating the lower extremity, three items including hip flexion, knee extension, and foot tap were tested, and each item was rated from 0 (severely impaired) to 5 (normal) for expressing motor function of lower extremities (maximum score 15) [23]. All participants used their personal AFOs in daily life and had the ability to walk independently on a treadmill without orthoses, handrails, or any assistive devices. The types of AFOs were classified into two groups: thermoplastic AFOs (tAFOs) or adjustable posterior strut AFOs (APS-AFOs). The APS-AFO is an articulated AFO that is used for gait rehabilitation in hemiparetic patients [24–26]. The APS-AFO allows easy adjustment of the ankle-hinge joint, as the length and thickness of the strut can be changed to suit the patient (Additional file 1: Figure S1). Half of the participants (12 patients) used tAFOs during the walking trial, and the other half used APS-AFOs. Patients were excluded if they marked cardio-respiratory or metabolic disease, history of previous neuromuscular diseases or orthopedic conditions that may limit walking ability, or impaired cognitive or communicative ability to follow instructions. This study was approved by the Medical Ethics Committee board of Fujita Health University. All patients provided written informed consent prior to participation.

Procedure

Kinematic data was acquired via three-dimensional treadmill gait analysis performed using a simplified gait analysis system (KinemaTracer˚; Kissei Comtec Co., Ltd., Matsumoto, Japan). The KinemaTracer® system is composed of a computer for recording and data analysis, and four charge-coupled device cameras with 60 Hz frame rates installed around both sides of the treadmill. The measurement error for this system was determined using a modified protocol based on the evaluation protocol of measurement error developed by The Clinical Gait Analysis Forum of Japan [27]. The averaged absolute error for each axis ranged from 0.5 to 2.4 mm, which is comparable to existing systems [27, 28] (Additional file 2: Supplemental methods and Additional file 3: Figure S2).

A total of 12 markers (30 mm in diameter) were placed bilaterally on the acromion processes, iliac crests (on a vertical line passing through the hips), hip joints (at points one-third from the greater trochanter on the line between the greater trochanter and the anterior superior iliac spine), knee joints (on the midline of the anteroposterior diameter of the lateral epicondyle of the femur), lateral malleoli, and the fifth metatarsal heads (Fig. 1). Although the first toe is more commonly used to put the toe marker, the fifth metatarsal heads are selected in this study, for the following reasons: the marker tracking with this system would be more stable with the markers placed on the 5th metatarsal head than on the 1st metatarsal head. The foot marker at the

5th metatarsal head also will better reflect the real floor-to-floor clearance (toe clearance) in patients with equinovarus, which is frequently seen in hemiparetic patients. The feasibility of this method in real clinical settings has been verified in previous studies [29, 30]. All participants practiced walking on the treadmill until they became accustomed to it. A rest interval of 5 to 10 min was provided prior to test initiation. Each patient was then asked to walk at a comfortable self-selected speed with and without their AFO. To reduce the variability in kinematic adaptations, we applied the same process for all the patients to select the speed: 1) The ground gait speed without AFO was measured during a 10 m walk. 2) The treadmill speed was set at 70% of that ground gait speed. 3) If the patients did not feel comfortable, the speed was gradually increased until the patients felt comfortable at the maximum of the ground gait speed.

The order of these two conditions (with or without an AFO) was selected randomly. The appropriate footwear was prescribed to match the AFO for each patient during trials performed with and without AFOs. There was a 5-min rest

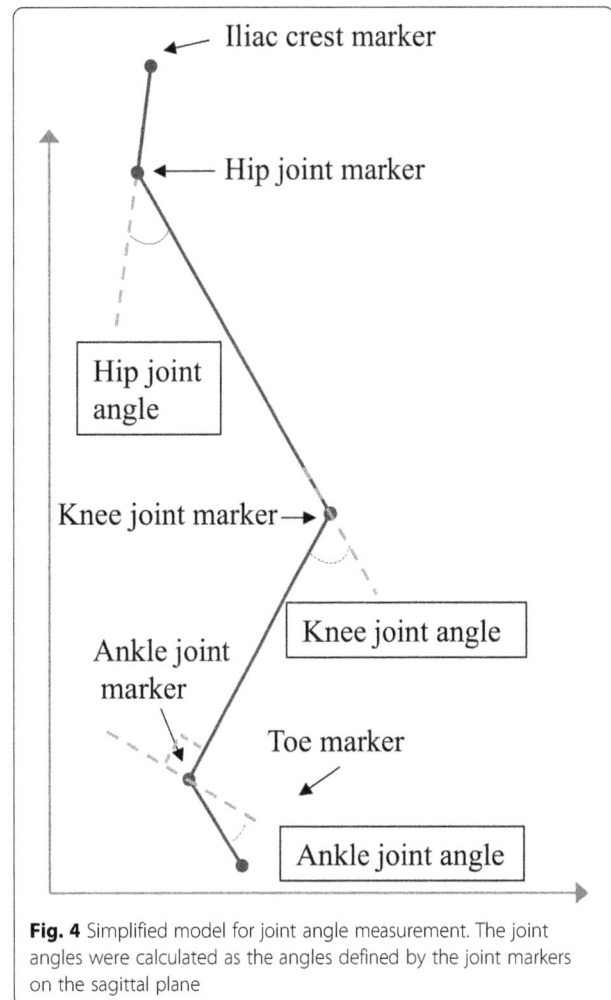

Fig. 4 Simplified model for joint angle measurement. The joint angles were calculated as the angles defined by the joint markers on the sagittal plane

period between trials. Additional assistive devices or handrails were not allowed during the walking trial. The duration of the gait measuring time was 20 s, and data capture was started when patients achieved a steady state walking speed in each trial. The average number of gait cycles was 16.7 ± 1.8 without the AFO and 16.3 ± 1.9 with the AFO. A single measurement session took about 20 min to complete, making this a feasible procedure for use in a real clinic. During each measurement, a technician managed the measurements and treadmill controls and a physical therapist stood by to supervise the patient and to prevent falls. Safety suspension and handrail was also prepared (Fig. 2). Additional procedures for checking marker tracking errors, when necessary, required 10 to 20 min for each patient.

Outcome measures and statistics

The present study calculated the following as indices of lower-limb function and compensatory movements of the paretic limb during the swing phase: toe elevation from the walking surface, the vertical component of functional limb shortening in terms of hip-toe distance, hip elevation due to pelvic obliquity, non-paretic hip elevation, and foot elevation due to foot lateral shift (circumduction). The mid-swing values were calculated at the time point at which the swing toe of the paretic side crossed beneath the hip marker on the sagittal plane. At this time, the vertical component of the lateral foot shift by circumduction could be calculated independently of the limb movement on the sagittal axis, without considering the effect of the

inclination of the hip-toe line on the sagittal plane. The mid-stance values were calculated at the time point at which the stance toe of the paretic side crossed the vertical line drawn from the hip marker on the sagittal plane. All the indicators of dynamic movement were calculated with respect to the vertical direction (Fig. 3). All values were calculated using an automated process.

Indices for limb shortening

Limb shortening was divided into two components: limb shortening due to knee/hip joint movement and limb shortening or lengthening due to ankle joint movement. The limb shortening due to knee joint movement was derived by calculating virtual limb shortening assuming the ankle joint angles to be fixed. The limb shortening or lengthening was derived by calculating the difference between the actual total limb shortening and the limb shortening due to knee joint movements.

Indices for compensatory movements

Hip elevation due to pelvic obliquity, non-paretic hip elevation, and foot elevation due to foot lateral shift (circumduction) can be understood as movements compensating for toe clearance, because these movements are not observed in normal gait patterns [10].

Hip elevation due to obliquity on the paretic side was calculated from the vertical movement of the hip marker on the paretic side, which was taken to represent hip hiking. Non-paretic hip elevation, which is seen in hemiplegic patients with severe lower-limb dysfunction [31],

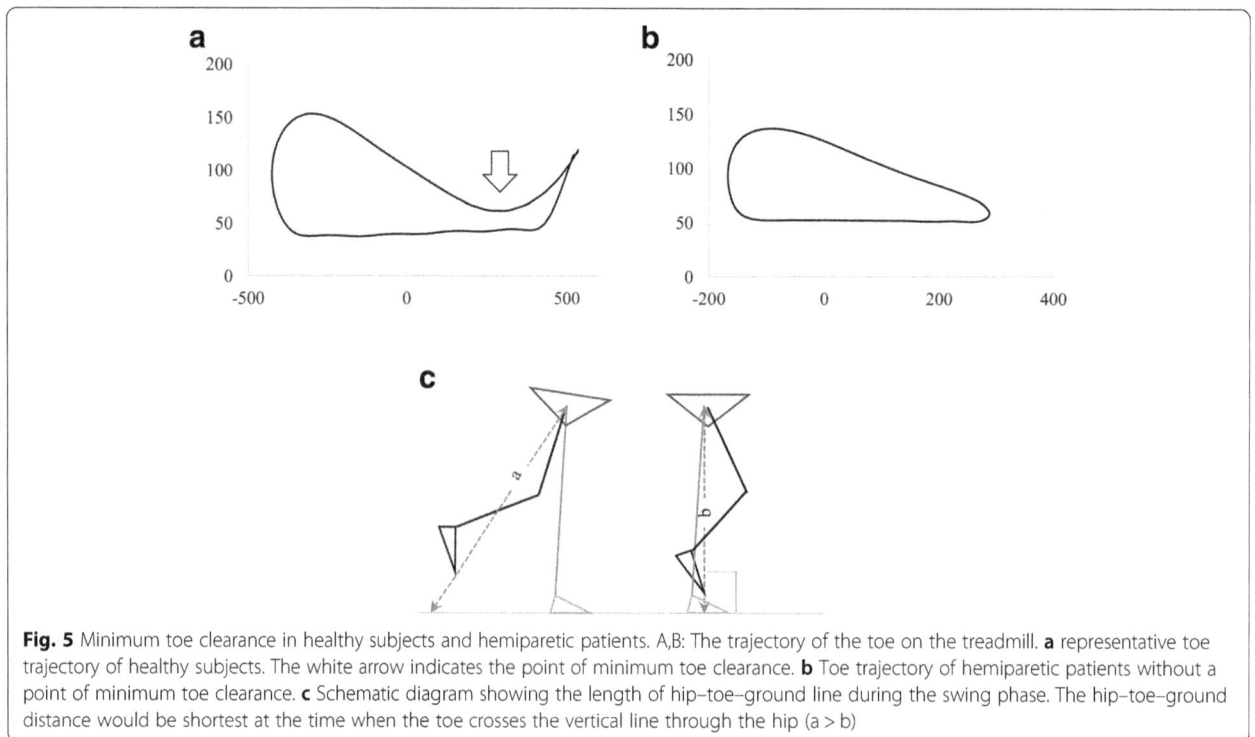

Fig. 5 Minimum toe clearance in healthy subjects and hemiparetic patients. A,B: The trajectory of the toe on the treadmill. **a** representative toe trajectory of healthy subjects. The white arrow indicates the point of minimum toe clearance. **b** Toe trajectory of hemiparetic patients without a point of minimum toe clearance. **c** Schematic diagram showing the length of hip–toe–ground line during the swing phase. The hip–toe–ground distance would be shortest at the time when the toe crosses the vertical line through the hip (a > b)

was calculated as the difference in vertical position of the non-paretic hip marker between the mid-stance and the mid-swing of the paretic limb. The foot elevation due to foot lateral shift was calculated from the vertical value due to the displacement of the lateral malleolus.

Index of toe clearance

The elevation in the vertical axis of the fifth metatarsal heads from the walking surface was measured as an indicator of toe clearance.

Calculation of joint angles

The joint angles of the hip, knee, and ankle were represented by the trunk-thigh angle, thigh-crus angle, and crus-foot angle, respectively, which were defined by the marker positions in the sagittal plane, as follows: the hip joint angles were defined as the angles between the iliac crest marker, hip marker, and knee marker; the knee joint angles were determined from the angles between the hip marker, knee marker, and ankle marker; and the ankle

joint angles were calculated from the angles between the knee marker, ankle marker, and toe marker (Fig. 4).

Unlike prior studies that commonly used minimum toe clearance (MTC) as a representation of toe clearance ability during mid-swing [32, 33], the present study evaluated toe clearance at the time when the toe crosses the vertical line from the hip marker. The vertical trajectory of the toe, which follows a downward-pointing curve during mid-swing in healthy individuals, was absent in some of our post-stroke patients, and instead showed an upward-pointing curve during swing phase trajectory which precluded calculation of the MTC (Fig. 5a,b). For this reason, we identified toe clearance at the time when the toe passed directly underneath the hip marker, when the hip–floor distance through the toe (dotted line) would be the shortest without hip elevation (Fig. 5c). This timing is also ideal for calculating the impact of limb shortening and compensatory movement because the hip and the toe markers are both in the same frontal plane at this time. Therefore, the impact of the circumduction on toe movement in the

Table 1 Patient characteristics and self-selected speed used at walking trial with and without AFO

ID	Age (years)	Gender	Diagnosis	Affected side	SIAS-LE /15	TAO (days)	Self-selected speed on treadmill (km/hr)	Type of AFO
1	58	M	Hemorrhage	L	5	2313	1.0	APS-AFO
2	41	M	Hemorrhage	L	12	32	1.7	tAFO
3	58	M	Hemorrhage	R	10	57	1.7	tAFO
4	80	M	Hemorrhage	R	9	104	1.8	APS-AFO
5	60	M	Infarction	R	8	765	1.9	APS-AFO
6	21	F	Hemorrhage	R	8	2439	2.0	tAFO
7	43	F	Hemorrhage	L	8	38	2.2	APS-AFO
8	18	M	Hemorrhage	L	8	81	2.3	APS-AFO
9	15	F	Hemorrhage	R	11	1809	2.3	tAFO
10	58	M	Hemorrhage	R	9	413	2.4	tAFO
11	74	M	Hemorrhage	L	11	876	2.4	APS-AFO
12	52	F	Hemorrhage	R	11	543	2.5	tAFO
13	55	M	Hemorrhage	L	10	1579	2.5	tAFO
14	38	F	Hemorrhage	L	8	2260	2.5	tAFO
15	79	F	Infarction	L	10	84	2.6	tAFO
16	53	M	Infarction	L	9	322	2.6	tAFO
17	64	M	Hemorrhage	L	11	1768	2.6	APS-AFO
18	14	M	Infarction	L	10	233	2.7	APS-AFO
19	53	M	Hemorrhage	R	12	47	2.8	APS-AFO
20	47	M	Infarction	R	10	80	2.8	APS-AFO
21	47	M	Hemorrhage	L	8	341	2.8	tAFO
22	43	M	Infarction	R	12	73	3.3	tAFO
23	26	M	Hemorrhage	L	12	81	4.0	APS-AFO
24	33	M	Hemorrhage	R	10	200	4.2	APS-AFO

AFO Ankle–foot orthosis, *APS-AFO* Adjustable posterior strut AFO, *F* Female, *M* Male, *No* Number, *TAO* Time after onset, *tAFO* Thermoplastic AFO

vertical axis could be easily calculated independently from the impact of other toe clearance-related limb movements.

Subgroup analyses were performed to compare the effect of AFOs between subacute and chronic stroke patients, and between tAFOs and APS-AFOs.

Statistical analyses were performed using SPSS version 19.0 (SPSS, Chicago, IL) and JMP 12 (SAS Institute Inc. Cary, NC, USA). Descriptive statistics were used to describe patients' demographic characteristics. To enable further analysis of parameters, the mean and standard deviation (SD) were presented. The changes in gait parameters were evaluated using the paired t-test. The Student's t-test (unpaired t-test) was used to compare the effect of AFOs on the alterations of joint displacement between two subgroups: stroke patients in the subacute vs the chronic stage, and patients with a tAFO vs an APS-AFO. The goodness of fit was computed using the Shapiro-Wilk test, and showed normal distribution of data. Values of $P < 0.05$ were considered to indicate statistically significant differences.

Results

Patient characteristics and comfortable self-selected speeds used at walking trial both with and without AFO in each participant are presented in Table 1.

Representative trajectories of toe clearance, shortening of hip-toe distance, and paretic hip elevation due to pelvic obliquity are presented in Fig. 6.

The gait indices (mid-swing–mid-stance) are summarized in Fig. 7. The toe clearance was significantly increased by the use of an AFO (Fig. 7a: 33.9 ± 19.6 vs. 37.6 ± 16.9, $p = 0.038$). The toe clearance could be divided into two parts: the limb shortening and compensatory movements. The compensatory movements were significantly decreased by the use of the AFO (Fig. 7b; 33.0 ± 19.4 vs. 28.1 ± 17.2: $p = 0.001$), whereas the limb shortening was increased (Fig. 7c; 2.2 ± 25.6 vs. 10.3 ± 23.7: $p < 0.001$). Among the three components of compensatory movements (pelvic obliquity on paretic side, non-paretic hip elevation, and foot elevation due to circumduction), a significant difference was noted with and without the AFO for the pelvic obliquity on the paretic side (19.8 ± 18.9 vs. 16.4 ± 19.7, $p = 0.003$), and a weak tendency was noted for a reduction in the non-paretic hip elevation by the AFO (12.6 ± 17.4 vs. 11.2 ± 18.6, $p = 0.234$). No difference was observed in the foot elevation due to circumduction (Fig. 7b'). The limb lengthening by ankle movement was significantly decreased by the use of AFO (-13.6 ± 7.4 vs. -7.6 ± 5.4, $p < 0.0001$), contributing to limb shortening. No significant change was observed in limb

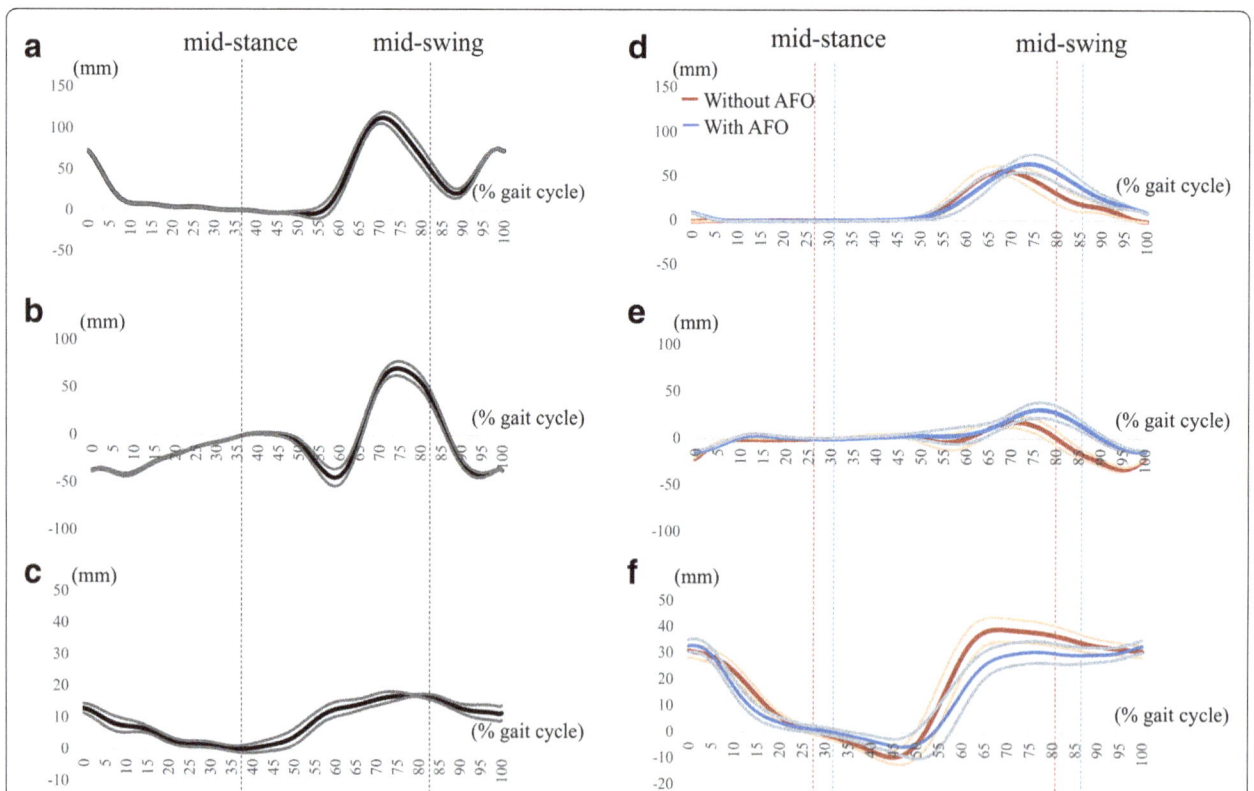

Fig. 6 Representative trajectories of gait indices: The representative trajectories (mean ± SD) of 1) Toe clearance (**a, d**), 2) Shortening of hip-toe distance (**b, e**) and 3) Paretic hip elevation due to pelvic obliquity (**c, f**) in a healthy subject (**a-c**) and a hemiparetic patient with (Blue line) and without (Red line) AFO(**d-f**)

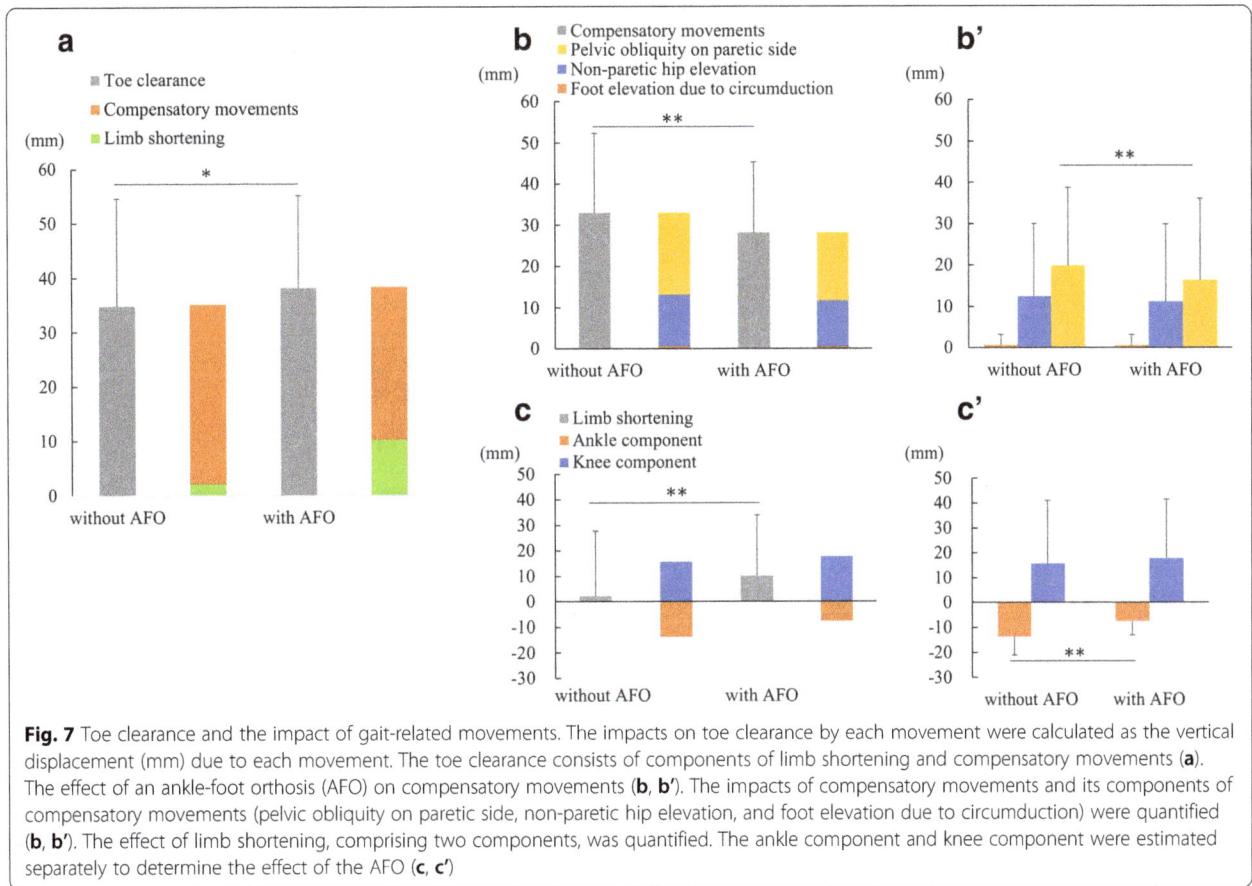

Fig. 7 Toe clearance and the impact of gait-related movements. The impacts on toe clearance by each movement were calculated as the vertical displacement (mm) due to each movement. The toe clearance consists of components of limb shortening and compensatory movements (**a**). The effect of an ankle-foot orthosis (AFO) on compensatory movements (**b**, **b'**). The impacts of compensatory movements and its components of compensatory movements (pelvic obliquity on paretic side, non-paretic hip elevation, and foot elevation due to circumduction) were quantified (**b**, **b'**). The effect of limb shortening, comprising two components, was quantified. The ankle component and knee component were estimated separately to determine the effect of the AFO (**c**, **c'**)

shortening due to knee movement (15.8 ± 25.3 vs. 17.9 ± 23.6, $p = 0.183$; Fig. 7c').

The joint angle changes on the paretic limb in walking trials performed with and without AFOs was shown in Fig. 8. There were significant quantitative differences between trials performed with AFOs and those performed without AFOs in the decreases in hip flexion (13.6 ± 6.9 (with) vs 14.5 ± 7.3 (without), $p = 0.019$), knee flexion (25.7 ± 14.3 (with) vs 29.1 ± 15.9 (without), $p = 0.001$), and ankle plantar flexion (6.1 ± 5.4 (with) vs 10.4 ± 5.4 (without), $p = 0.007$) during the swing phase.

The subgroup analyses regarding the effect of AFOs on kinematic components revealed no significant differences in any of the measured indices in subacute vs chronic stroke patients, or in tAFOs vs APS-AFOs.

Discussion

The present study confirmed the positive influence of AFOs on functional limb shortening, with resulting improvements in toe clearance and compensatory movement. The average toe elevation in hemiparetic gait was enhanced by the use of AFOs, irrespective of the stage of hemiparesis and/or the type of AFO used. Using an AFO resulted in an increase in ankle dorsiflexion during the swing phase and a subsequent decrease in compensatory

movements, which was consistent with previous studies [17, 18, 34]. Furthermore, the present findings manifested the simple relationship between the changes in limb shortening and compensatory movements to achieve toe clearance, by breaking down each movement into the actual impact on toe clearance. As shown in this study, the toe clearance was increased by the use of AFOs (33.9 vs. 37.6, $P = 0.038$), due to the increase in vertical gain by limb shortening (2.2 vs. 10.3, $p < 0.001$). The compensatory movements account for the rest. This type of visualization could be useful for monitoring the beneficial effects of AFOs.

Improved joint motions and decreased compensatory movement when using AFOs could potentially contribute to efficient gait and promote walking activity in hemiparetic patients.

The degree of limb shortening is mainly determined by the degree of knee flexion, especially in the healthy subjects or patients with mild paresis [10]. Conversely, AFOs achieve limb shortening due to the mechanical property that limits ankle plantarflexion, which could be referred to as another compensatory approach to improve limb shortening. The present and previous findings indicate that toe clearance in hemiparetic patients with the use of AFOs could be achieved by the following mechanism. First, decreased knee flexion in hemiparetic

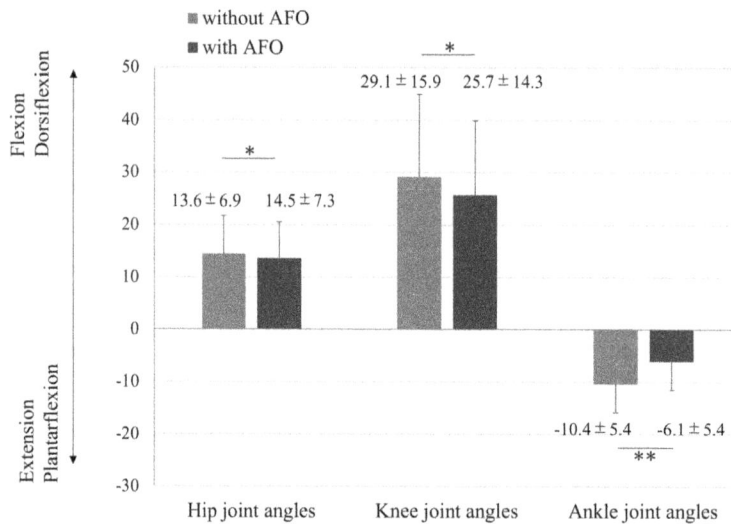

Fig. 8 Joint angle changes on the paretic limb in walking trials performed with and without ankle-foot orthoses (AFOs). The joint angle changes from mid-stance to mid-swing on a paretic limb. Error bar: SD *:< 0.05, **:< 0.01. *P* values were obtained by a paired t-test

gait may be compensated for by the AFO's effect on decreasing ankle plantar flexion and subsequently maintaining the optimal hip-toe distance. Second, hip hiking (as a compensatory gait pattern) is consequently minimized because of acquired optimal limb shortening, as shown in the present study. The interrelationship of relevant gait indices are hypothesized as shown in Fig. 9.

Decreased knee flexion may be considered a negative effect of AFOs on the hemiparetic gait. The possible explanations for this include the following: First, ankle plantar flexion that has been decreased by AFO decreases limb lengthening, so the patient might not need to flex the knee as much to shorten the limb, because the same toe clearance can be achieved with less effort.

In fact, in the present study, the use of AFO decreased limb lengthening due to ankle plantar flexion (Fig. 7c). In addition, the weight of the orthosis might influence knee flexion by making it more difficult for the paretic limb to flex the knee against gravity. Another possibility is the discrepancy between the knee-flexion angle and the effect of the knee flexion, which is seen when the knee-flexion angle is very small. In this case, slight knee flexion does not merit the toe clearance. For example, if the hip-knee-toe markers were aligned on the vertical line (Fig. 10a) and the ankle angle was fixed, the knee flexion could lengthen the hip-toe distance (Fig. 10b). In this situation, a discrepancy would arise between the knee-flexion angle and the limb shortening; a small knee

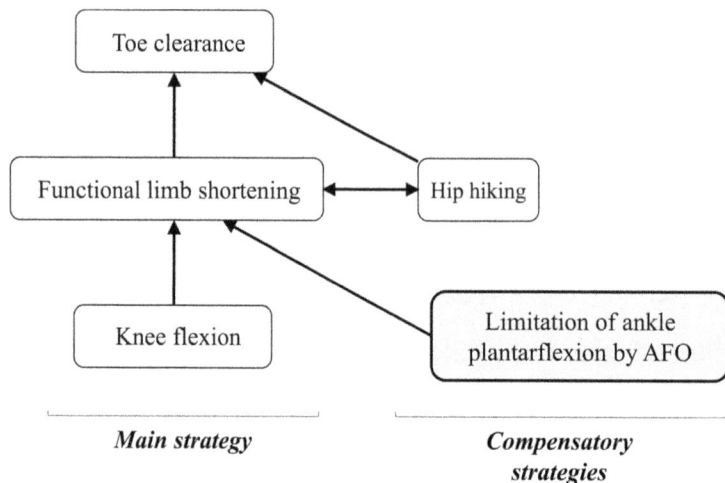

Fig. 9 The possible discrepancy between the knee flexion angle and its impact on limb shortening. The positional relationships between the hip, knee, ankle and toe markers at the mid-swing(**a**,**b**). Reduced knee flexion angle (θ1 > θ2) could lead to increased limb shortening (L1 > L2), in cases where the ankle angles are fixed

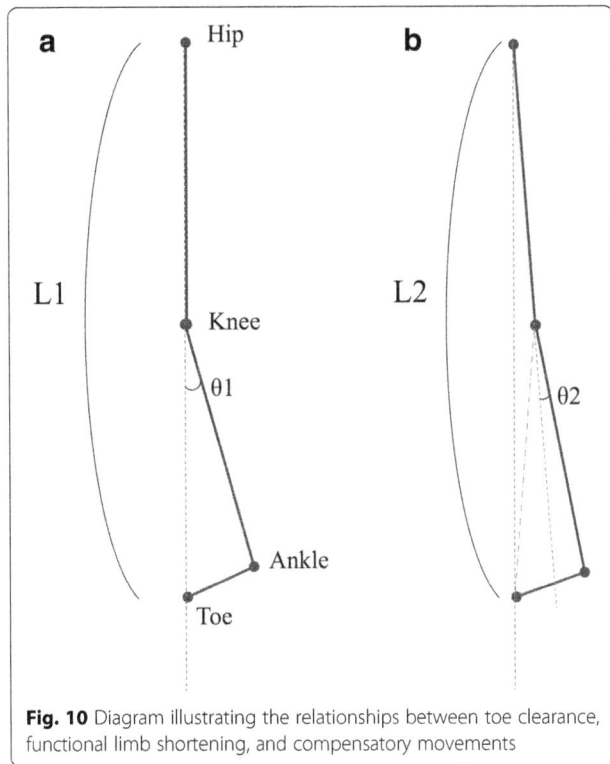

Fig. 10 Diagram illustrating the relationships between toe clearance, functional limb shortening, and compensatory movements

flexion may not have a beneficial effect on limb shortening. The present study identified a conflict between the effect of AFO on reducing knee flexion and the relative increase in limb shortening due to knee movement (Figs. 7c and 8), which might have been influenced by this paradoxical relationship between joint angle and limb shortening.

In addition, the effect of AFO use on knee angles itself could have influenced by the different characteristics of the participant groups. A previous study showed an increase in knee flexion by AFO use in hemiplegic patients; Gatti et al. reported a positive effect of AFO use on knee flexion angle (26.316 without AFO vs. 30.785 with AFO) in the patient group with paresis scores of 4–5 on the Scandinavian Stroke Scale, which is milder paresis than in the present study [35].The effect of AFO use on knee movements should be further investigated, including whether the reduction in knee flexion has a negative impact on the recovery of knee movement.

The use of an AFO had a weak tendency to reduce the elevation of the non-paretic limb. Non-paretic hip elevation may occur in the following situations. First, it can occur if there is unusual elevation of the pelvis at the mid-swing of the paretic limb. This can be achieved either by ankle plantar flexion or by over-extension of the knee at the mid-stance of the non-paretic limb. However, the data did not evidence either of these causes.

Second, this can occur when the vertical position of the pelvis is lowered at the mid-stance of the paretic limb and elevated during the swing phase of the paretic limb. The lowered vertical position of the pelvis can occur due to the knee flexion of the paretic limb or the drop of the non-paretic side of the pelvis (Trendelenburg's sign). In this case, the non-paretic hip drop showed significant correlation with the extent of the non-paretic hip elevation, while paretic knee flexion did not, indicating that the lowered pelvic position caused by the drop of the non-paretic side of the pelvis during the stance phase of the paretic limb was the main reason for the non-paretic hip elevation during the swing phase of the paretic limb. There was a weak, non-significant tendency of this drop of the pelvis to be decreased by the use of AFO (Additional file 4: Figure S3). The AFO effect on this non-paretic limb elevation must be confirmed in studies that have larger samples.

The present study clarified the real clinical picture of AFO-affected gait patterns, contributing a deepened understanding of the systematically balanced relationship between the enhancement of paretic limb clearance and the ability to reduce compensatory movement during the swing phase. Recognition and quantification of the interrelationships among the changes in joint kinematics, joint displacement, functional limb shortening, and the actual impacts on toe clearance would contribute to the comprehensive understanding of the effects of intervention and help clinicians to develop strategies to guide patients toward improving the advancement of the paretic limb during the swing phase. For example, when toe clearance is insufficient due to paresis, clinicians could consider facilitating improvements in the ability to effect limb shortening; otherwise, they could prepare AFOs for that purpose. If the effects are insufficient, compensatory movements could be encouraged. Conversely, once the clinician can confirm that the patient has gained sufficient toe clearance, the focus of the intervention could be redirected to the reduction of compensatory movements. With the use of gait analysis systems, we can quantify the actual impact and monitor the effect of each intervention and set goals for the patient. This will require further quantitative investigations in future studies for development, but this structured quantification may enable tailor-made rehabilitation training for individual patients. In addition to facilitating toe clearance in the swing phase, AFOs assist in other aspects of gait such as gait stability during the stance phase. Further analysis of the effect of AFOs should be encouraged to further the comprehensive understanding of the holistic effect of AFO use.

This study had a number of limitations. First, all included patients were able to independently ambulate on the treadmill without gait aids or orthoses. The findings may not be representative of those with severe hemiparesis. Further analysis of patients with more impaired gait abilty would facilitate further understanding of the effect of AFOs. Second, there was a relatively small sample population with heterogeneity. However, subgroup analyses found that the type of AFO and stage of hemiparesis did not significantly affect the kinematic parameters. Third, there was a small number of markers compared with commonly-used marker sets such as plug-in gait and Helen Hayes [36, 37], and the joint angles were indirectly estimated from the positions of the joint markers in the sagittal plane. We consider that this would not be critical enough to negate the present results, as the validity of measuring abnormal gait patterns, including the degree of joint angle movements, using this simple marker set has been shown previously [29, 38–40]. However, the limitations of this simplified method should be further confirmed in future studies.

Conclusion

The present study quantified the impact of AFOs on toe clearance strategy in hemiparetic patients, and investigated the interrelationships between movement parameters. The results offer an insight into the effects of AFOs on the overall biomechanism of hemiparetic gait during the swing phase. Furthermore, these attempts to quantify and visualize the gait strategy could contribute to the clinical judgment and decision-making regarding rehabilitation strategy, which will help achieve better outcomes in rehabilitation practice.

Additional files

Additional file 1: Figure S1. Adjustable posterior strut ankle–foot orthosis (APS-AFO). (TIFF 22671 kb)

Additional file 2: Supplemental methods and results. The details of additional experiment for clarifying measurement error. (DOCX 16 kb)

Additional file 3: Figure S2. Experimental setting for clarifying measurement error. A: A 1-m-long aluminum bar with four markers on it. B-D: The participant held the aluminium bar in three ways while walking; parallel to his torso, parallel to the sagittal and horizontal planes, or parallel to the coronal and horizontal planes. (PNG 1540 kb)

Additional file 4: Figure S3. Correlation among non-paretic hip elevation (at mid-swing), paretic knee flexion, and non-paretic hip drop at paretic mid-stance. A. Correlation between the non-paretic hip elevation at the paretic mid-swing and the paretic knee flexion at the paretic mid-stance. The correlation coefficient was 0.10 ($p = 0.80$). B. Correlation between the non-paretic hip elevation at the paretic mid-swing and the non-paretic hip drop at the paretic mid-stance. The correlation coefficient was − 0.60 ($p < 0.01$). C. Comparison of the non-paretic hip drop at the paretic mid-stance with and without AFO ($p = 0.23$). (PNG 1140 kb)

Funding
This work was supported by the Fujita Health University fund (grant number 2015100341).

Authors' contributions
MM, ES, and KO supervised the study. MM, KP, and FM conceptualized and designed the study. FM and KT recruited the participants, ran the experiments, collected the data, and performed the software analysis. MM and KP interpreted results from the data. KP computed the statistical analysis, drafted the original manuscript and finalized the manuscript. All authors have read and approved the final version of the manuscript.

Competing interests
The authors declare that they have no competing interests.

Author details
[1]Department of Rehabilitation Medicine I, School of Medicine, Fujita Health University, 1-98 Dengakugakubo, Kutsukake, Toyoake, Aichi 470-1192, Japan. [2]Faculty of Rehabilitation, School of Health Sciences, Fujita Health University, Toyoake, Aichi, Japan. [3]Department of Rehabilitation, Fujita Health University Hospital, Toyoake, Aichi, Japan.

References
1. Perry J. Gait analysis: normal and pathological function. 1st ed. Thorofare: Slack, Inc.; 1992.
2. Balaban B, Tok F. Gait disturbances in patients with stroke. PM&R. 2014;6: 635–42.
3. Chen G, Patten C, Kothari DH, Zajac FE. Gait differences between individuals with post-stroke hemiparesis and non-disabled controls at matched speeds. Gait Posture. 2005;22:51–6.
4. De Quervain IA, Simon SR, Leurgans S, Pease WS, McAllister D. Gait pattern in the early recovery period after stroke. J Bone Joint Surg Am. 1996;78: 1506–14.
5. Sulzer JS, Gordon KE, Dhaher YY, Peshkin MA, Patton JL. Preswing knee flexion assistance is coupled with hip abduction in people with stiff-knee gait after stroke. Stroke. 2010;41:1709–14. https://doi.org/10.1161/STROKEAHA.110.586917.
6. Campanini I, Merlo A, Damiano B. A method to differentiate the causes of stiff-knee gait in stroke patients. Gait Posture. 2013;38:165–9. https://doi.org/10.1016/j.gaitpost.2013.05.003.
7. Begg RK, Tirosh O, Said CM, Sparrow WA, Steinberg N, Levinger P, Galea MP. Gait training with real-time augmented toe-ground clearance information decreases tripping risk in older adults and a person with chronic stroke. Front Hum Neurosci. 2014;8:1–6.
8. Cohen L, Miller T, Sheppard MA, Gordon E, Gantz T, Atnafou R. Bridging the gap: bringing together intentional and unintentional injury prevention efforts to improve health and well being. J Saf Res. 2003;34:473–83.
9. Kerrigan DC, Frates EP, Rogan S, Riley PO. Hip hiking and circumduction: quantitative definitions. Am J Phys Med Rehabil. 2000;79:247–52.
10. Matsuda F, Mukaino M, Ohtsuka K, Tanikawa H, Tsuchiyama K, Teranishi T, Kanada Y, Kagaya H, Saitoh E. Biomechanical factors behind toe clearance during the swing phase in hemiparetic patients. Top Stroke Rehabil. 2017; 24:177–82.
11. Tyson SF, Sadeghi-Demneh E, Nester CJ. A systematic review and meta-analysis of the effect of an ankle-foot orthosis on gait biomechanics after stroke. Clin Rehabil. 2013;27:879–91.
12. Leung J, Moseley AM. Impact of ankle-foot orthoses on gait and leg muscle activity in adults with hemiplegia. Physiotherapy. 2003;89:39–55.
13. Tyson SF, Kent RM. Effects of an ankle-foot orthosis on balance and walking after stroke: a systematic review and pooled meta-analysis. Arch Phys Med Rehabil. 2013;94:1377–85.
14. Gök H, Küçükdeveci A, Altinkaynak H, Yavuzer G, Ergin S. Effects of ankle-foot orthoses on hemiparetic gait. Clin Rehabil. 2003;17:137–9.
15. Yokoyama O, Sashika H, Hagiwara A, Yamamoto S, Yasui T. Kinematic effects on gait of a newly designed ankle-foot orthosis with oil damper resistance: a case series of 2 patients with hemiplegia. Arch Phys Med Rehabil. 2005;86:162–6.
16. Fatone S, Gard SA, Malas BS. Effect of ankle-foot orthosis alignment and foot-plate length on the gait of adults with poststroke hemiplegia. Arch Phys Med Rehabil. 2009;90:810–8.

17. Park JH, Chun MH, Ahn JS, Yu JY, Kang SH. Comparison of gait analysis between anterior and posterior ankle foot orthosis in hemiplegic patients. Am J Phys Med Rehabil. 2009;88:630–4.

18. Cruz TH, Dhaher YY. Impact of ankle-foot-orthosis on frontal plane behaviors post-stroke. Gait Posture. 2009;30:312–6.

19. Burpee JL, Lewek MD. Biomechanical gait characteristics of naturally occurring unsuccessful foot clearance during swing in individuals with chronic stroke. Clin Biomech. 2015;30:1102–7.

20. Olney SJ, Richards CL. Hemiparetic gait following stroke. Part I: Charac Gait Posture. 1996;4:136–48.

21. Thijssen DH, Paulus R, van Uden CJ, Kooloos JG, Hopman MT. Decreased energy cost and improved gait pattern using a new orthosis in persons with long-term stroke. Arch Phys Med Rehabil. 2007;88:181–6.

22. Franceschini M, Massucci M, Ferrari L, Agosti M, Paroli C. Effects of an ankle-foot orthosis on spatiotemporal parameters and energy cost of hemiparetic gait. Clin Rehabil. 2003;17:368–72.

23. Chino N, Sonoda S, Domen K, Saitoh E, Kimura A. Stroke impairment assessment set: a new evaluation instrument for stroke patients. Jpn J Rehabil Med. 1994;31:119–25.

24. Mizuno M, Saitoh E, Iwata E, Okada M, Teranishi T, Itoh M, Hayashi M, Oda Y. The development of a new posterior strut AFO with an adjustable joint: its concept and a consideration of basic function. Bull Jap Soc Prosthet Orthot. 2005;21:225–33.

25. Tanino G, Tomita Y, Mizuno S, Maeda H, Miyasaka H, Orand A, Takeda K, Sonoda S. Development of an ankle torque measurement device for measuring ankle torque during walking. J Phys Ther Sci. 2015;27:1477–80. https://doi.org/10.1589/jpts.27.1477.

26. Maeshima S, Okazaki H, Okamoto S, Mizuno S, Asano N, Maeda H, Masaki M, Matsuo H, Tsunoda T, Sonoda S. A comparison of knee-ankle-foot orthoses with either metal struts or an adjustable posterior strut in hemiplegic stroke patients. J Stroke Cerebrovasc Dis. 2015;24:1312–6. https://doi.org/10.1016/j.jstrokecerebrovasdis.2015.02.003.

27. Ehara Y, Fujimoto H, Miyazaki S, Mochimaru M, Tanaka S, Yamamoto S. Comparison of the performance of 3D camera systems II. Gait Posture. 1997; 5(3):251–5.

28. Carse B, Meadows B, Bowers R, Rowe P. Affordable clinical gait analysis: an assessment of the marker tracking accuracy of a new low-cost optical 3D motion analysis system. Physiotherapy. 2013;99(4):347–51.

29. Mukaino M, Ohtsuka K, Tsuchiyama K, Matsuda F, Inagaki K, Yamada J, Saitoh E. Feasibility of a simplified, clinically oriented, three-dimensional gait analysis system for the gait evaluation of stroke patients. Prog Rehabil Med. 2016;1:1.

30. Ohtsuka K, Saitoh E, Kagaya H, Itoh N, Tanabe S, Matsuda F, Tanikawa H, Yamada J, Aoki T, Kanada Y. Application of Lissajous overview picture in treadmill gait analysis. Jpn J Compr Rehabili Sci. 2015;6:33–42.

31. Matsuda F, Mukaino M, Ohtsuka K, Tanikawa H, Tsuchiyama K, Teranishi T, Kanada Y, Kagaya H, Saitoh E. Analysis of strategies used by hemiplegic stroke patients to achieve toe clearance. Jpn J Compr Rehabil Sci. 2016;7:111–8.

32. Begg R, Best R, Dell'Oro L, Taylor S. Minimum foot clearance during walking: strategies for the minimisation of trip-related falls. Gait Posture. 2007;25:191–8.

33. Mills PM, Barrett RS, Morrison S. Toe clearance variability during walking in young and elderly men. Gait Posture. 2008;28:101–7.

34. Bleyenheuft C, Caty G, Lejeune T, Detrembleur C. Assessment of the chignon dynamic ankle-foot orthosis using instrumented gait analysis in hemiparetic adults. Ann Readapt Med Phys. 2008;51:154–60.

35. Gatti MA, Freixes O, Fernández SA, Rivas ME, Crespo M, Waldman SV, Olmos LE. Effects of ankle foot orthosis in stiff knee gait in adults with hemiplegia. J Biomech. 2012;45:2658–61.

36. Kadaba MP, Ramakrishnan HK, Wootten ME. Measurement of lower extremity kinematics during level walking. J Orthop Res. 1990;8:383–92.

37. Davis RB III, Õunpuu S, Tyburski D, Gage JR. A gait analysis data collection and reduction technique. Hum Mov Sci. 1991;10:575–87.

38. Itoh N, Kagaya H, Saitoh E, Ohtsuka K, Yamada J, Tanikawa H, Tanabe S, Itoh N, Aoki T, Kanada Y. Quantitative assessment of circumduction, hip hiking, and forefoot contact gait using Lissajous figures. Jpn J Compr Rehabil Sci. 2012;3:78–84.

39. Tanikawa H, Ohtsuka K, Mukaino M, Inagaki K, Matsuda F, Teranishi T, Kanada Y, Kagaya H, Saitoh E. Quantitative assessment of retropulsion of the hip, excessive hip external rotation, and excessive lateral shift of the trunk over the unaffected side in hemiplegia using three-dimensional treadmill

gait analysis. Top Stroke Rehabil. 2016;23:311–7.

40. Hishikawa N, Tanikawa H, Ohtsuka K, Mukaino M, Inagaki K, Matsuda F, Teranishi T, Kanada Y, Kagaya H, Saitoh E. Quantitative assessment of knee extensor thrust, flexed-knee gait, insufficient knee flexion during the swing phase, and medial whip in hemiplegia using three-dimensional treadmill gait analysis. Top Stroke Rehabil; 2018. (in press)

Permissions

All chapters in this book were first published in JNER, by BioMed Central; hereby published with permission under the Creative Commons Attribution License or equivalent. Every chapter published in this book has been scrutinized by our experts. Their significance has been extensively debated. The topics covered herein carry significant findings which will fuel the growth of the discipline. They may even be implemented as practical applications or may be referred to as a beginning point for another development.

The contributors of this book come from diverse backgrounds, making this book a truly international effort. This book will bring forth new frontiers with its revolutionizing research information and detailed analysis of the nascent developments around the world.

We would like to thank all the contributing authors for lending their expertise to make the book truly unique. They have played a crucial role in the development of this book. Without their invaluable contributions this book wouldn't have been possible. They have made vital efforts to compile up to date information on the varied aspects of this subject to make this book a valuable addition to the collection of many professionals and students.

This book was conceptualized with the vision of imparting up-to-date information and advanced data in this field. To ensure the same, a matchless editorial board was set up. Every individual on the board went through rigorous rounds of assessment to prove their worth. After which they invested a large part of their time researching and compiling the most relevant data for our readers.

The editorial board has been involved in producing this book since its inception. They have spent rigorous hours researching and exploring the diverse topics which have resulted in the successful publishing of this book. They have passed on their knowledge of decades through this book. To expedite this challenging task, the publisher supported the team at every step. A small team of assistant editors was also appointed to further simplify the editing procedure and attain best results for the readers.

Apart from the editorial board, the designing team has also invested a significant amount of their time in understanding the subject and creating the most relevant covers. They scrutinized every image to scout for the most suitable representation of the subject and create an appropriate cover for the book.

The publishing team has been an ardent support to the editorial, designing and production team. Their endless efforts to recruit the best for this project, has resulted in the accomplishment of this book. They are a veteran in the field of academics and their pool of knowledge is as vast as their experience in printing. Their expertise and guidance has proved useful at every step. Their uncompromising quality standards have made this book an exceptional effort. Their encouragement from time to time has been an inspiration for everyone.

The publisher and the editorial board hope that this book will prove to be a valuable piece of knowledge for researchers, students, practitioners and scholars across the globe.

List of Contributors

Jeffrey R. Koller and C. David Remy
Department of Mechanical Engineering, University of Michigan, 2350 Hayward, 48109 Ann Arbor, MI, USA

Daniel P. Ferris
J. Crayton Pruitt Family Department of Biomedical Engineering, University of Florida, 1275 Center Drive, 32611 Gainesville, FL, USA
Department of Mechanical Engineering, University of Florida, 1275 Center Drive, 32611 Gainesville, FL, USA

Han Houdijk and Laura Hak
Department of Human Movement Sciences, Faculty of Behavioral and Movement Sciences, Vrije Universiteit Amsterdam, Van der Boechorststraat 9, 1081 BT Amsterdam, The Netherlands

Han Houdijk
Department of Research and Development, Heliomare Rehabilitation, Wijk aan Zee, the Netherlands

Daphne Wezenberg
Department of Health and Technology | Human Kinetic Technology, The Hague University of Applied Sciences, The Hague, The Netherlands

Andrea Giovanni Cutti
Production Directorate, Applied Research, INAIL Prosthesis Center, Vigorso di Budrio, Bologna, Italy

Christine Chen, Mark Hanson and Richard Hillestad
RAND Corporation, 1776 Main Street, Santa Monica, CA 90401, USA

Ritika Chaturvedi
RAND Corporation, 1200 South Hayes Street, Arlington, VA 22202-5050, USA

Soeren Mattke and Harry H. Liu
RAND Corporation, 20 Park Plaza, Suite 920, Boston, MA 02116, USA

Allen Dobson, Kennan Murray, Nikolay Manolov and Joan E. DaVanzo
Dobson DaVanzo and Associates, LLC, 450 Maple Avenue East, Suite 303, Vienna, VA 22180, USA

Ahmed W. Shehata, Erik J. Scheme and Jonathon W. Sensinger
Institute of Biomedical Engineering, University of New Brunswick, Fredericton, NB E3B 5A3, Canada
Department of Electrical and Computer Engineering, University of New Brunswick, Fredericton, NB E3B 5A3, Canada

Ahmed W. Shehata
Division of Physical Medicine and Rehabilitation, Department of Medicine, University of Alberta, Edmonton, AB T6G 2E1, Canada

Leonard F. Engels, Marco Controzzi and Christian Cipriani
Scuola Superiore Sant'Anna, The BioRobotics Institute, V.le R. Piaggio 34, 56025 Pontedera, PI, Italy

Andrea M. Kuczynski, Adam Kirton, Jennifer A. Semrau and Sean P. Dukelow
University of Calgary, Calgary, AB T2N 2T9, Canada

Andrea M. Kuczynski and Adam Kirton
Section of Neurology, Department of Pediatrics, Alberta Children's Hospital Research Institute, Calgary, AB, Canada

Adam Kirton, Jennifer A. Semrau and Sean P. Dukelow
Department of Clinical Neurosciences, Foothills Medical Centre, Hotchkiss Brain Institute, 1403 – 29th St. NW, Calgary, AB, Canada

Yushin Kim
Major in Sport, Health and Rehabilitation, Department of Health Administration and Healthcare, Cheongju University, Cheongju 28503, Republic of Korea

Yushin Kim, Hang-Jun Cho and Hyung-Soon Park
Department of Mechanical Engineering, Korea Advanced Institute of Science and Technology (KAIST), Daejeon 34141, Republic of Korea

Marko Markovic, Meike A. Schweisfurth, Dario Farina and Strahinja Dosen
Applied Rehabilitation Technology Lab (ART-Lab), Department of Trauma Surgery, Orthopedics and Plastic Surgery, University Medical Center Göttingen, Georg-August-University, 37075 Göttingen, Germany

Meike A. Schweisfurth
Faculty of Life Sciences, Hochschule für Angewandte Wissenschaften Hamburg, Ulmenliet 20, 21033 Hamburg, Germany

Leonard F. Engels
Biorobotics Institute, Scuola Superiore Sant'Anna, Viale R. Piaggio, 34, 56025 Pontedera, PI, Italy

Dario Farina
Neurorehabilitation Engineering Department of Bioengineering Imperial College London, London SW7 2AZ, UK

Strahinja Dosen
Faculty of Medicine, Department of Health Science and Technology, Center for Sensory-Motor Interaction, Aalborg University, DE-9220 Aalborg, Denmark

Thomas Matheve and Annick Timmermans
Rehabilitation Research Center - Biomed, Faculty of Medicine and Life Sciences, Hasselt University, Hasselt, Belgium.

Simon Brumagne
Department of Rehabilitation Sciences, KU Leuven–University of Leuven, Leuven, Belgium

Christophe Demoulin
Department of Sport and Rehabilitation Sciences, University of Liege, Liege, Belgium

Nicolas Schweighofer
Biokinesiology and Physical Therapy, University of Southern California, Los Angeles, USA

Chunji Wang
Neuroscience graduate Program, University of Southern California, Los Angeles, USA

Denis Mottet
STAPS, Université de Montpellier, Euromov, Montpellier, France

Isabelle Laffont and Karima Bakthi
Montpellier University Hospital, Euromov, IFRH, Montpellier University, Montpellier, France

David J. Reinkensmeyer
Departments of Mechanical and Aerospace Engineering, Anatomy and Neurobiology, University of California, Irvine, USA

Olivier Rémy-Néris
Université de Bretagne Occidentale, Centre hospitalier universitaire, LaTIM-INSERM UMR1101, Brest, France

Kristen M Trianda ilou, Alexander J Barry, Kelly N Thielbar and Nikolay Stoykov
Shirley Ryan Ability Lab, Arms + Hands Lab, Chicago, IL, USA

Daria Tsoupikova
School of Design, University of Illinois at Chicago (UIC), Chicago, IL, USA

Derek G Kamper
UNC/NC State Joint Department of Biomedical Engineering, University of North Carolina at Chapel Hill, Chapel Hill, NC, USA
Closed-Loop Engineering for Advanced Rehabilitation Research Core, University of North Carolina at Chapel Hill, Chapel Hill, NC, USA

Bruno Bonnechère, Inès Haack and Serge Van Sint Jan
Laboratory of Anatomy, Biomechanics and Organogenesis (LABO) [CP 619], Université Libre de Bruxelles, Lennik Street 808, 1070 Brussels, Belgium

Bruno Bonnechère, Bart Jansen and Lubos Omelina
Department of Electronics and Informatics – ETRO, Vrije Universiteit Brussel, Brussels, Belgium
imec, Leuven, Belgium

Véronique Feipel
Laboratory of Functional Anatomy (LAF), Université Libre de Bruxelles, Brussels, Belgium

Massimo Pandolfo
Department of Neurology, Erasme Hospital, Brussels, Belgium

Kostas Georgiadis and Nikos Laskaris
AIIA lab, Informatics Department, AUTH, Thessaloniki, Greece

Kostas Georgiadis, Spiros Nikolopoulos and Ioannis Kompatsiaris
Information Technologies Institute (ITI), Centre for Research and Technology Hellas, Thessaloniki-Thermi, Greece

Nikos Laskaris
Neuro Informatics.GRoup, AUTH, Thessaloniki, Greece

Christian Werner, Jürgen M. Bauer and Klaus Hauer
Department of Geriatric Research, Agaplesion Bethanien Hospital Heidelberg, Geriatric Center at the Heidelberg University, Heidelberg, Germany

Christian Werner and Jürgen M. Bauer
Center for Geriatric Medicine, Heidelberg University, Heidelberg, Germany

Rebekka Rosner
Department of Radiological Diagnostics, Theresien Hospital Mannheim, Mannheim, Germany

Stefanie Wiloth
Institute of Gerontology, Heidelberg University, Heidelberg, Germany

Nele Christin Lemke
Network of Aging Research (NAR), Heidelberg University, Heidelberg, Germany

Michael H. Li and Babak Taati
Toronto Rehabilitation Institute, University Health Network, 550 University Ave, Toronto, ON M5G 2A2, Canada
Institute of Biomaterials and Biomedical Engineering, University of Toronto, 164 College St, Room 407, Toronto, ON M5S 3G9, Canada

Tiago A. Mestre and Susan H. Fox
Edmond J. Safra Program in Parkinson's Disease, Toronto Western Hospital, University Health Network, 399 Bathurst St, Toronto, ON M5T 2S8, Canada

Tiago A. Mestre
The Ottawa Hospital Research Institute, 1053 Carling Ave, Ottawa, ON K1Y 4E9, Canada
Division of Neurology, Department of Medicine, 1053 Carling Ave, Ottawa, ON K1Y 4E9, Canada

Tiago A. Mestre and Susan H. Fox
Division of Neurology, University of Toronto, Suite RFE 3-805, 200 Elizabeth St, Toronto, ON M5G 2C4, Canada

Babak Taati
Department of Computer Science, University of Toronto, 10 King's College Road, Room 3302, Toronto, ON M5S 3G4, Canada

Christopher M. Frost, Daniel C. Ursu, Andrej Nedic, Cheryl A. Hassett, Jana D. Moon, Patrick J. Buchanan, Theodore A. Kung, Stephen W. P. Kemp, Paul S. Cederna and Melanie G. Urbanchek
University of Michigan Department of Surgery, Section of Plastic Surgery, 570 MSRB II Level A, 1150 W. Medical Center Drive, Ann Arbor, MI 48109-5456, USA

Daniel C. Ursu and R. Brent Gillespie
University of Michigan Department of Mechanical Engineering, Ann Arbor, MI, USA

Shane M. Flattery
Vassar College, Poughkeepsie, NY, USA

Stephen W. P. Kemp and Paul S. Cederna
Department of Biomedical Engineering, University of Michigan, Ann Arbor, MI, USA

Mike D. Rinderknecht, Olivier Lambercy and Roger Gassert
Rehabilitation Engineering Laboratory, Department of Health Sciences and Technology, ETH Zurich, Zurich, Switzerland

Vanessa Raible, Imke Büsching, Aida Sehle and Joachim Liepert
Department of Neurorehabilitation, Kliniken Schmieder, Allensbach, Germany

Imke Büsching, Aida Sehle and Joachim Liepert
Lurija Institut, Konstanz, Germany

Marco Germanotta, Arianna Cruciani, Cristiano Pecchioli, Simona Loreti, Albino Spedicato, Matteo Meotti, Rita Mosca, Gabriele Speranza, Giorgia Giannarelli, Luca Padua and Irene Aprile
IRCCS Fondazione Don Carlo Gnocchi, Piazzale Morandi 6, 20121 Milan, Italy

Simona Loreti
Physical Medicine and Rehabilitation Unit, Sant'Andrea Hospital, "Sapienza" University of Rome, Via di Grottarossa, 1035, 00189 Rome, Italy

Francesca Cecchi
IRCCS Fondazione Don Carlo Gnocchi, Via di Scandicci, 269, 50143 Florence, Italy

Luca Padua
Department of Geriatrics, Neurosciences and Orthopaedics, Università Cattolica del Sacro Cuore, Largo Francesco Vito 1, 00168 Rome, Italy

Andrea Giovanni Cutti, Gennaro Verni, Gian Luca Migliore, Amedeo Amoresano and Michele Raggi
INAIL Prosthetic Center, Via Rabuina 14, 40054 Vigorso di Budrio, BO, Italy

Kannit Pongpipatpaiboon, Masahiko Mukaino and Eiichi Saitoh
Department of Rehabilitation Medicine I, School of Medicine, Fujita Health University, 1-98 Dengakugakubo, Kutsukake, Toyoake, Aichi 470-1192, Japan

Fumihiro Matsuda, Kei Ohtsuka, Hiroki Tanikawa and Kazuhiro Tsuchiyama
Faculty of Rehabilitation, School of Health Sciences, Fujita Health University, Toyoake, Aichi, Japan

Junya Yamada
Department of Rehabilitation, Fujita Health University Hospital, Toyoake, Aichi, Japan

Index

www.ingramcontent.com/pod-product-compliance
Lightning Source LLC
Chambersburg PA
CBHW061304190326
41458CB00011B/3762